BASIC AND CLINICAL SCIENCE COURSE

Pediatric Ophthalmology and Strabismus

Section 6

2010–2011

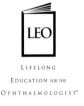

LEO

LIFELONG
EDUCATION FOR THE
OPHTHALMOLOGIST®

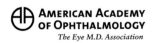

AMERICAN ACADEMY
OF OPHTHALMOLOGY
The Eye M.D. Association

The Basic and Clinical Science Course is one component of the Lifelong Education for the Ophthalmologist (LEO) framework, which assists members in planning their continuing medical education. LEO includes an array of clinical education products that members may select to form individualized, self-directed learning plans for updating their clinical knowledge. Active members or fellows who use LEO components may accumulate sufficient CME credits to earn the LEO Award. Contact the Academy's Clinical Education Division for further information on LEO.

The American Academy of Ophthalmology is accredited by the Accreditation Council for Continuing Medical Education to provide continuing medical education for physicians.

The American Academy of Ophthalmology designates this educational activity for a maximum of 15 *AMA PRA Category 1 Credits*™. Physicians should only claim credit commensurate with the extent of their participation in the activity.

The Academy provides this material for educational purposes only. It is not intended to represent the only or best method or procedure in every case, nor to replace a physician's own judgment or give specific advice for case management. Including all indications, contraindications, side effects, and alternative agents for each drug or treatment is beyond the scope of this material. All information and recommendations should be verified, prior to use, with current information included in the manufacturers' package inserts or other independent sources, and considered in light of the patient's condition and history. Reference to certain drugs, instruments, and other products in this course is made for illustrative purposes only and is not intended to constitute an endorsement of such. Some material may include information on applications that are not considered community standard, that reflect indications not included in approved FDA labeling, or that are approved for use only in restricted research settings. **The FDA has stated that it is the responsibility of the physician to determine the FDA status of each drug or device he or she wishes to use, and to use them with appropriate, informed patient consent in compliance with applicable law.** The Academy specifically disclaims any and all liability for injury or other damages of any kind, from negligence or otherwise, for any and all claims that may arise from the use of any recommendations or other information contained herein.

Basic and Clinical Science Course

Gregory L. Skuta, MD, Oklahoma City, Oklahoma, *Senior Secretary for Clinical Education*

Louis B. Cantor, MD, Indianapolis, Indiana, *Secretary for Ophthalmic Knowledge*

Jayne S. Weiss, MD, Detroit, Michigan, *BCSC Course Chair*

Section 6

Faculty Responsible for This Edition

Edward L. Raab, MD, JD, *Chair,* New York, New York
Aazy A. Aaby, MD, Portland, Oregon
Jeffrey N. Bloom, MD, Cleveland, Ohio
Jane C. Edmond, MD, Houston, Texas
Gregg T. Lueder, MD, St Louis, Missouri
Scott E. Olitsky, MD, Kansas City, Missouri
Paul H. Phillips, MD, Little Rock, Arkansas
Robert E. Wiggins, MD, Asheville, North Carolina
  Practicing Ophthalmologists Advisory Committee for Education
Kanwal K. Nischal, MBBS, *Consultant,* London, United Kingdom

The authors state the following financial relationships:

Dr Bloom: WMR Biomedical, consultant, equity ownership/stock options

Dr Edmond: Inspire, consultant, lecturer/honoraria recipient

Dr Nischal: Massie Research Laboratories, lecturer/honoraria recipient; Merck, lecturer/honoraria recipient

Dr Wiggins: Ophthalmic Mutual Insurance Company, consultant

The other authors state that they have no significant financial interest or other relationship with the manufacturer of any commercial product discussed in the chapters that they contributed to this course or with the manufacturer of any competing commercial product.

Recent Past Faculty

Arlene V. Drack, MD
Amy K. Hutchinson, MD
David A. Plager, MD
John W. Simon, MD

In addition, the Academy gratefully acknowledges the contributions of numerous past faculty and advisory committee members who have played an important role in the development of previous editions of the Basic and Clinical Science Course.

American Academy of Ophthalmology Staff

Richard A. Zorab, *Vice President, Ophthalmic Knowledge*

Hal Straus, *Director, Publications Department*

Carol L. Dondrea, *Publications Manager*

Christine Arturo, *Acquisitions Manager*

D. Jean Ray, *Production Manager*

Stephanie Tanaka, *Medical Editor*

Steven Huebner, *Administrative Coordinator*

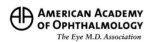

AMERICAN ACADEMY
OF OPHTHALMOLOGY
The Eye M.D. Association

655 Beach Street
Box 7424
San Francisco, CA 94120-7424

Contents

General Introduction xix

Objectives 1

**Introduction—Rapport With Children: Tips for a
Productive Examination** 3
Preparation 3
The Examination 3
Eyedrops 5
Use of Topical Anesthesia for Foreign-Body Removal 5

PART I   Strabismus .7

1 Strabismus Terminology 9
Prefixes and Suffixes 9
   Prefixes 9
   Suffixes 10
Strabismus Classification Terms 10
   Fusional Status 10
   Variation of the Deviation With Gaze Position or Fixating Eye 10
   Fixation 11
   Age of Onset 11
   Type of Deviation 11
   Abbreviated Designations for Types of Strabismus 11
Important Axes of the Eye 11

2 Anatomy of the Extraocular Muscles
   and Their Fascia 13
Origin, Course, Insertion, Innervation, and Action of the
   Extraocular Muscles 13
   Horizontal Rectus Muscles 13
   Vertical Rectus Muscles 14
   Oblique Muscles 14
   Levator Palpebrae Superioris Muscle 15
   Insertion Relationships of the Rectus Muscles 16
Blood Supply of the Extraocular Muscles 16
   Arterial System 16
   Venous System 18
Structure of the Extraocular Muscles 18

Orbital and Fascial Relationships 19
    Adipose Tissue 19
    Muscle Cone 19
    Muscle Capsule 19
    The Tenon Capsule 20
    Pulley System 21
Anatomical Considerations During Surgery 24

3   Motor Physiology **27**
Basic Principles and Terms 27
    Axes of Fick, Center of Rotation, and Listing's Plane 27
    Positions of Gaze 27
    Extraocular Muscle Action 28
Eye Movements 32
    Motor Units 32
    Monocular Eye Movements 33
    Binocular Eye Movements 34
    Supranuclear Control Systems for Eye Movement 37

4   Sensory Physiology and Pathology **39**
Physiology of Normal Binocular Vision 39
    Retinal Correspondence 39
    Fusion 41
Selected Aspects of the Neurophysiology of Vision 42
    Retinogeniculocortical Pathway 42
    Visual Development 44
    Effects of Abnormal Visual Experience on the
        Retinogeniculocortical Pathway 46
Abnormalities of Binocular Vision 49
    Confusion 49
    Diplopia 49
Sensory Adaptations in Strabismus 50
    Suppression 50
    Anomalous Retinal Correspondence 52
    Subjective Testing for Sensory Adaptations 53
    Monofixation Syndrome 59

5   Amblyopia **61**
Classification 62
    Strabismic Amblyopia 62
    Anisometropic Amblyopia 63
    Ametropic Amblyopia 64
    Stimulus Deprivation Amblyopia 64
Diagnosis 64
Treatment 65
    Cataract Removal 65
    Refractive Correction 66

Occlusion and Optical Degradation 66
Complications of Therapy 67

**6 Diagnostic Techniques for Strabismus
and Amblyopia** **71**
History and Characteristics of the Presenting Complaint 71
Assessment of Visual Acuity 71
Distance Visual Acuity 71
Near Visual Acuity 74
Assessment of Ocular Alignment 74
Cover Tests 74
Light Reflex Tests 76
Dissimilar Image Tests 78
Dissimilar Target Tests 79
Positions of Gaze 80
Assessment of Eye Movements 81
Ocular Rotations 81
Convergence 81
Fusional Vergence 82
Special Tests 83
Motor Tests 83
3-Step Test 83
Prism Adaptation Test 86
Tests of Binocular Sensory Cooperation 86
Worth 4-Dot Testing 87
Stereoacuity Testing 87
Cycloplegic Refraction 87
Adverse Effects 88

7 Esodeviations **89**
Pseudoesotropia 89
Infantile (Congenital) Esotropia 89
Pathogenesis 91
Management 91
Nystagmus and Esotropia 92
Accommodative Esotropia 93
Refractive Accommodative Esotropia 93
High Accommodative Convergence/Accommodative Esotropia 94
Partially Accommodative Esotropia 95
Nonaccommodative Acquired Esotropia 95
Basic (Acquired) Esotropia 95
Acute Esotropia 96
Cyclic Esotropia 96
Sensory Deprivation Esodeviation 96
Divergence Insufficiency 97
Spasm of the Near Synkinetic Reflex 97
Surgical (Consecutive) Esodeviation 97

Incomitant Esotropia 98
   Sixth Cranial Nerve (Abducens) Paralysis. 98
   Other Forms of Incomitant Esotropia 98

8 Exodeviations **99**
Pseudoexotropia 99
Exophoria 99
Intermittent Exotropia. 99
   Clinical Characteristics 99
   Evaluation 100
   Classification 101
   Treatment 101
Constant Exotropia 103
   Infantile Exotropia 104
   Sensory Exotropia. 104
   Consecutive Exotropia 105
Exotropic Duane Syndrome 105
Neuromuscular Abnormalities 105
Dissociated Horizontal Deviation 105
Convergence Insufficiency 106
Convergence Paralysis. 106

9 A- and V-Pattern Horizontal Strabismus **107**
Clinical Features and Identification 107
Management. 110
   Summary of Treatment Plans 112

10 Vertical Deviations **113**
Inferior Oblique Muscle Overaction 113
   Clinical Features 114
   Management 114
Superior Oblique Muscle Overaction 115
   Clinical Features 115
   Management 116
Oblique Muscle Pseudo-Overaction 116
Dissociated Vertical Deviation 116
   Clinical Features 116
   Management 117
Superior Oblique Muscle Paralysis (Palsy or Paresis). 118
   Clinical Features 118
   Management 120
Inferior Oblique Muscle Paralysis 121
   Clinical Features 122
   Management 122
Monocular Elevation Deficiency (Double Elevator Palsy). 123
   Clinical Features 123
   Management 124

Orbital Floor Fractures 124
    Clinical Features 125
    Management 126

11 Special Forms of Strabismus **127**
Duane Syndrome 127
    Clinical Features 128
    Management 129
Brown Syndrome 130
    Clinical Features 130
    Management 131
Third Cranial Nerve Paralysis 132
    Clinical Features 132
    Management 132
Sixth Cranial Nerve Paralysis 134
    Clinical Features 134
    Management 134
Thyroid Eye Disease 135
    Clinical Features 135
    Management 135
Chronic Progressive External Ophthalmoplegia 137
    Clinical Features 137
    Management 137
Myasthenia Gravis 137
    Clinical Features 137
    Management 138
Congenital Fibrosis Syndrome 138
    Clinical Features 139
    Management 140
Möbius Syndrome 140
    Clinical Features 140
    Management 141
Esotropia Associated With High Myopia 141
Internuclear Ophthalmoplegia 141
    Clinical Features 141
    Management 141
Ocular Motor Apraxia 141
    Clinical Features 142
Superior Oblique Myokymia 142
    Clinical Features 142
    Management 142
Other Settings for Strabismus 143

12 Surgery of the Extraocular Muscles **145**
Indications for Surgery 145
Planning Considerations 145
    Visual Acuity 145
    Incomitance 146

Cyclovertical Strabismus 146
Prior Surgery 147
Surgical Techniques for the Muscles and Tendons 147
Weakening Procedures 147
Strengthening Procedures 147
Adjustable Sutures 148
Pull-Over (Stay) Sutures 149
Transposition Procedures 149
Posterior Fixation 149
Guidelines for Strabismus Surgery 149
Esodeviation and Exodeviation 150
Oblique Muscle Weakening Procedures 151
Oblique Muscle Tightening (Strengthening) Procedures 152
Vertical Rectus Muscle Surgery for Hypotropia and Hypertropia 152
Other Rectus Muscle Surgery 153
Approaches to the Extraocular Muscles 154
Fornix Incision 154
Limbal or Peritomy Incision 154
Complications of Strabismus Surgery 154
Unsatisfactory Alignment 155
Refractive Changes 155
Diplopia 155
Perforation of the Sclera 155
Postoperative Infections 156
Foreign-Body Granuloma and Allergic Reaction 156
Conjunctival Inclusion Cyst 157
Conjunctival Scarring 157
Adherence Syndrome 158
Dellen 158
Anterior Segment Ischemia 158
Change in Eyelid Position 159
Lost and Slipped Muscles 159
Anesthesia for Extraocular Muscle Surgery 160
Methods 160
Postoperative Nausea and Vomiting 161
Oculocardiac Reflex 161
Malignant Hyperthermia 161

**13 Chemodenervation Treatment of Strabismus
and Blepharospasm Using Botulinum Toxin** **163**
Pharmacology and Mechanism of Action 163
Indications, Techniques, and Results 163
Complications 164

PART II Pediatric Ophthalmology 165

14 Growth and Development of the Eye 167
Normal Growth and Development 167
    Dimensions of the Eye .167
    Refractive State 169
    Orbit and Ocular Adnexa 169
    Iris, Pupil, and Anterior Chamber 169
    Intraocular Pressure .170
    Extraocular Muscle Anatomy and Physiology 170
    Retina 170
    Visual Acuity and Stereoacuity 170
Abnormal Growth and Development 171

15 Orbital Dysmorphology and Eyelid Disorders 173
Terminology and Associations of Abnormal Interocular Distance 173
    Hypotelorism 173
    Hypertelorism 173
    Exorbitism 173
    Telecanthus 174
    Dystopia Canthorum .175
Eyelid Disorders 175
    Cryptophthalmos 175
    Congenital Coloboma of the Eyelid 175
    Ankyloblepharon 176
    Congenital Ectropion 176
    Congenital Entropion 176
    Epiblepharon 176
    Congenital Tarsal Kink 176
    Distichiasis 177
    Trichotillomania 177
    Euryblepharon 177
    Epicanthus 177
    Palpebral Fissure Slants 178
    Blepharophimosis Syndrome 178
    Ptosis 178
    Marcus Gunn Jaw-Winking 180

16 Infectious and Allergic Ocular Diseases 181
Intrauterine and Perinatal Infections of the Eye 181
    Toxoplasmosis 181
    Rubella 183
    Cytomegalic Inclusion Disease 184
    Herpes Simplex Infection 185
    Syphilis 185
    Lymphocytic Choriomeningitis 186

Ophthalmia Neonatorum 186
    Etiology 187
    Most Important Agents 187
    Prophylaxis for Ophthalmia Neonatorum. 188
Conjunctivitis 188
    Bacterial Conjunctivitis 189
    Viral Conjunctivitis 190
    Blepharitis 193
Orbital and Adnexal Infections 194
    Preseptal Cellulitis 194
    Orbital Cellulitis 195
Ocular Allergy 197
    Seasonal Allergic Conjunctivitis. 198
    Vernal Keratoconjunctivitis. 198
    Atopic Keratoconjunctivitis. 200
Stevens-Johnson Syndrome 200
Kawasaki Disease 201

17 The Lacrimal Drainage System **203**
Developmental Anomalies 203
    Atresia or Stenosis of the Lacrimal Puncta or Canaliculi 203
    Supernumerary Puncta 204
    Congenital Lacrimal Fistula 204
Dacryocele. 204
    Clinical Features 204
    Management 205
Nasolacrimal Duct Obstruction. 205
    Clinical Features 205
    Nonsurgical Management 206
    Surgical Management 206

18 Diseases of the Cornea and Anterior Segment. **211**
Congenital Corneal Anomalies 211
    Abnormalities of Corneal Size and Shape 211
    Peripheral Developmental Abnormalities: Anterior
        Segment Dysgenesis. 212
    Central Corneal Developmental Abnormalities 214
Infantile Corneal Opacities. 216
    Sclerocornea 216
    Tears, Breaks, or Ruptures of Descemet's Membrane 217
    Mucopolysaccharidosis and Mucolipidosis 217
    Congenital Hereditary Endothelial Dystrophy. 217
    Dermoids 218
    Congenital or Infantile Glaucoma 218
    Congenital Hereditary Stromal Dystrophy 219
    Corneal Ulcers 219
    Amniocentesis 219
    Treatment of Corneal Opacities 219

Systemic Diseases With Corneal Manifestations in Childhood 220
    Cystinosis 220
    Hepatolenticular Degeneration 220
    Congenital Syphilis 221
    Familial Dysautonomia 221

19 Iris Abnormalities. **223**
Dyscoria. 223
Aniridia 223
Coloboma of the Iris 224
Iris Nodules 225
    Lisch Nodules 225
    Juvenile Xanthogranuloma 226
    Iris Mamillations 226
Primary Iris Cysts. 226
    Cysts of Iris Pigment Epithelium 226
    Central (Pupillary) Cysts 227
    Cysts of Iris Stroma 227
Secondary Iris Cysts. 227
Brushfield Spots 227
Pediatric Iris Heterochromia 227
Persistent Pupillary Membranes 228
Abnormalities in the Size, Shape, or Location of the Pupil 228
    Congenital Miosis. 228
    Congenital Mydriasis 229
    Anisocoria 229
    Corectopia 230
    Polycoria and Pseudopolycoria 230
Congenital Iris Ectropion 231
Iris Transillumination 231
Posterior Synechiae 231

20 Pediatric Glaucomas **233**
Genetics. 233
Primary Congenital Glaucoma 233
    Pathophysiology 234
    Clinical Manifestations and Diagnosis 234
    Natural History 238
Secondary Pediatric Glaucomas. 238
    Secondary to Ocular Anomalies. 238
    Secondary to Systemic Disease 238
    Secondary Mechanical Glaucomas. 239
    Other Secondary Glaucomas 239
    Aphakic Glaucoma 239
Treatment 240
    Surgical Therapy 240
    Medical Therapy 242
Prognosis and Follow-Up 243

21 Childhood Cataracts and Other Pediatric Lens Disorders **245**
   Pediatric Cataracts 245
      Systemic Implications 245
      Onset 245
      Inheritance 246
      Laterality 246
      Morphology 246
      Persistent Fetal Vasculature 250
      Evaluation 250
      History 251
      Visual Function 252
      Ocular Examination 252
      Workup 253
   Surgery 254
      Management of the Anterior Capsule 255
      Lensectomy Without Intraocular Lens Implantation 255
      Lensectomy With Intraocular Lens Implantation 257
      Intraocular Lens Implantation 258
      Postoperative Care 259
      Visual Outcome After Cataract Extraction 260
   Structural or Positional Lens Abnormalities 260
      Congenital Aphakia 260
      Spherophakia 260
      Coloboma 260
   Dislocated Lenses in Children 261
      Simple Ectopia Lentis 262
      Ectopia Lentis et Pupillae 262
      Marfan Syndrome 263
      Homocystinuria 263
      Weill-Marchesani Syndrome 264
      Sulfite Oxidase Deficiency 264
      Treatment 264

22 Uveitis in the Pediatric Age Group **267**
   Classification 267
   Anterior Uveitis 267
      Juvenile Idiopathic Arthritis 267
      Tubulointerstitial Nephritis and Uveitis Syndrome 271
      Orbital Pseudotumor 272
      Other Causes of Anterior Uveitis 272
   Intermediate Uveitis 272
   Posterior Uveitis 272
      Toxoplasmosis 272
      Toxocariasis 273
   Panuveitis 274
      Sarcoidosis 274
      Familial Juvenile Systemic Granulomatosis 274

Vogt-Koyanagi-Harada Syndrome 275
Other Causes of Posterior Uveitis and Panuveitis 275
Masquerade Syndromes 275
Diagnosis of Pediatric Uveitis. 275
Treatment of Pediatric Uveitis 275
Medical Management 276
Surgical Treatment of Uveitis Complications 278

23 Vitreous and Retinal Diseases and Disorders **279**
Early-Onset Retinal Disease 279
Persistent Fetal Vasculature. 279
Retinopathy of Prematurity. 280
Coats Disease. 287
Hereditary Retinal Disease. 288
Leber Congenital Amaurosis 289
Achromatopsia 291
Congenital Stationary Night Blindness 291
Foveal Hypoplasia. 292
Aicardi Syndrome. 292
Hereditary Macular Dystrophies 292
Stargardt Disease 292
Best Disease 293
Hereditary Vitreoretinopathies 294
Juvenile Retinoschisis 294
Stickler Syndrome. 295
Familial Exudative Vitreoretinopathy 296
Norrie Disease 296
Goldmann-Favre Vitreoretinal Dystrophy 296
Systemic Diseases and Disorders With Retinal Manifestations. 296
Diabetes Mellitus 296
Leukemia 297
Albinism. 298
Familial Oculorenal Syndromes 302
Neurometabolic Disorders 302
Gangliosidoses 303
HIV/AIDS 304

24 Optic Disc Abnormalities **305**
Developmental Anomalies 305
Morning Glory Disc Anomaly 305
Coloboma of the Optic Nerve. 306
Myelinated (Medullated) Retinal Nerve Fibers 306
Tilted Disc Syndrome 307
Bergmeister Papilla 307
Megalopapilla. 307
Optic Nerve Hypoplasia 308
Optic Nerve Aplasia 309

Optic Nerve Pits or Holes 310
Peripapillary Staphyloma. 310
Optic Atrophy 310
Dominant Optic Atrophy. 310
Behr Optic Atrophy 311
Leber Hereditary Optic Neuropathy 311
Optic Neuritis 311
Papilledema 312
Idiopathic Intracranial Hypertension (Pseudotumor Cerebri) 312
Pseudopapilledema 313
Drusen 314

25 Childhood Nystagmus **317**
Nomenclature 317
Evaluation 318
History 318
Ocular Examination 318
Childhood Nystagmus Types 320
Congenital Nystagmus (Infantile Nystagmus Syndrome) 321
Acquired Nystagmus 324
Differential Diagnosis 326
Treatment 326
Prisms. 326
Nystagmus Surgery 328
Low Vision Rehabilitation 330

26 Ocular and Periocular Tumors in Childhood **331**
Orbital Tumors. 331
Differential Diagnosis 331
Primary Malignant Neoplasms 334
Metastatic Tumors. 336
Benign Tumors 338
Ectopic Tissue Masses 343
Childhood Orbital Inflammations 346
Eyelid and Epibulbar Lesions 347
Papillomas 348
Conjunctival Epithelial Inclusion Cysts. 348
Epibulbar Limbal Dermoid Tumors 348
Lipodermoid 348
Conjunctival Nevi. 349
Congenital Nevocellular Nevi of the Skin 349
Ocular Melanocytosis 350
Inflammatory Conditions 350
Intraocular Tumors 351
Iris and Ciliary Body Lesions 351
Choroidal and Retinal Pigment Epithelial Lesions 352

    Leukemia 354
    Retinoblastoma 354

27 Phakomatoses **363**
  Neurofibromatosis 363
    Neurofibromatosis Type 1 365
    Neurofibromatosis Type 2 371
  Tuberous Sclerosis 371
  von Hippel–Lindau Disease 374
  Sturge-Weber Syndrome 375
    Ocular Involvement 377
    Management 377
  Ataxia-Telangiectasia 378
  Incontinentia Pigmenti 379
  Wyburn-Mason Syndrome 381

28 Craniofacial Malformations **383**
  Craniosynostosis 383
    Etiology of Craniosynostosis 386
  Craniosynostosis Syndromes 387
    Crouzon Syndrome 387
    Apert Syndrome 388
    Saethre-Chotzen Syndrome 388
  Ocular Complications 388
    Proptosis 388
    Corneal Exposure 388
    Globe Luxation 389
    Vision Loss 390
    Strabismus 390
    Optic Nerve Abnormalities 391
    Ocular Adnexa Abnormalities 391
  Management 392
  Nonsynostotic Craniofacial Conditions 392
    Branchial Arch Syndromes 392
    Pierre Robin Sequence 394
    Fetal Alcohol Syndrome 394

29 Ocular Findings in Inborn Errors of Metabolism **397**
  Treatment 399

30 Ocular Trauma in Childhood **403**
  Child Abuse 404
    Shaking Injury 404
  Superficial Injury 407
  Penetrating Injury 408
  Blunt Injury 409
    Hyphema 409
    Orbital Fractures 411

31 Decreased Vision in Infants and Children **413**
Normal Visual Development 413
Approach to the Infant With Decreased Vision 414
   Pregeniculate Visual Loss. 414
   Retrogeniculate Visual Loss, or Cortical Visual Impairment 415
   Delayed Visual Maturation 416
Low Vision Rehabilitation 416

Basic Texts. 419
Related Academy Materials 421
Credit Reporting Form 425
Study Questions 429
Answers 438
Index 443

General Introduction

The Basic and Clinical Science Course (BCSC) is designed to meet the needs of residents and practitioners for a comprehensive yet concise curriculum of the field of ophthalmology. The BCSC has developed from its original brief outline format, which relied heavily on outside readings, to a more convenient and educationally useful self-contained text. The Academy updates and revises the course annually, with the goals of integrating the basic science and clinical practice of ophthalmology and of keeping ophthalmologists current with new developments in the various subspecialties.

The BCSC incorporates the effort and expertise of more than 80 ophthalmologists, organized into 13 Section faculties, working with Academy editorial staff. In addition, the course continues to benefit from many lasting contributions made by the faculties of previous editions. Members of the Academy's Practicing Ophthalmologists Advisory Committee for Education serve on each faculty and, as a group, review every volume before and after major revisions.

Organization of the Course

The Basic and Clinical Science Course comprises 13 volumes, incorporating fundamental ophthalmic knowledge, subspecialty areas, and special topics:

1 Update on General Medicine
2 Fundamentals and Principles of Ophthalmology
3 Clinical Optics
4 Ophthalmic Pathology and Intraocular Tumors
5 Neuro-Ophthalmology
6 Pediatric Ophthalmology and Strabismus
7 Orbit, Eyelids, and Lacrimal System
8 External Disease and Cornea
9 Intraocular Inflammation and Uveitis
10 Glaucoma
11 Lens and Cataract
12 Retina and Vitreous
13 Refractive Surgery

In addition, a comprehensive Master Index allows the reader to easily locate subjects throughout the entire series.

References

Readers who wish to explore specific topics in greater detail may consult the references cited within each chapter and listed in the Basic Texts section at the back of the book.

These references are intended to be selective rather than exhaustive, chosen by the BCSC faculty as being important, current, and readily available to residents and practitioners.

Related Academy educational materials are also listed in the appropriate sections. They include books, online and audiovisual materials, self-assessment programs, clinical modules, and interactive programs.

Study Questions and CME Credit

Each volume of the BCSC is designed as an independent study activity for ophthalmology residents and practitioners. The learning objectives for this volume are given on page 1. The text, illustrations, and references provide the information necessary to achieve the objectives; the study questions allow readers to test their understanding of the material and their mastery of the objectives. Physicians who wish to claim CME credit for this educational activity may do so by mail, by fax, or online. The necessary forms and instructions are given at the end of the book.

Conclusion

The Basic and Clinical Science Course has expanded greatly over the years, with the addition of much new text and numerous illustrations. Recent editions have sought to place a greater emphasis on clinical applicability while maintaining a solid foundation in basic science. As with any educational program, it reflects the experience of its authors. As its faculties change and as medicine progresses, new viewpoints are always emerging on controversial subjects and techniques. Not all alternate approaches can be included in this series; as with any educational endeavor, the learner should seek additional sources, including such carefully balanced opinions as the Academy's Preferred Practice Patterns.

The BCSC faculty and staff are continuously striving to improve the educational usefulness of the course; you, the reader, can contribute to this ongoing process. If you have any suggestions or questions about the series, please do not hesitate to contact the faculty or the editors.

The authors, editors, and reviewers hope that your study of the BCSC will be of lasting value and that each Section will serve as a practical resource for quality patient care.

Objectives

Upon completion of BCSC Section 6, *Pediatric Ophthalmology and Strabismus*, the reader should be able to

- describe evaluation techniques for young children that provide the maximum gain of information with the least trauma and frustration

- outline the anatomy and physiology of the extraocular muscles and their fascia

- explain the classification, diagnosis, and treatment options for amblyopia

- describe the commonly used diagnostic and measurement tests for strabismus

- classify the various esodeviations and exodeviations, and describe the management of each type

- identify vertical strabismus and special forms of strabismus, and formulate a treatment plan for each type

- list the possible complications of strabismus surgery, and describe guidelines to minimize them

- differentiate among various causes of congenital and acquired ocular infections in children, and formulate a logical plan for the diagnosis and management of each type

- list the most common diseases and malformations of the cornea, lacrimal drainage system, anterior segment, and iris seen in children

- describe the diagnostic findings and treatment options for childhood glaucoma

- identify common types of childhood cataracts and other lens disorders

- outline a diagnostic and management plan for childhood cataracts

- identify appropriate diagnostic tests for pediatric uveitis
- differentiate among various optic disc, vitreoretinal, and metabolic diseases and disorders found in children
- describe the features of the various forms of nystagmus and understand their significance
- list the characteristics of ocular tumors and phakomatoses seen in children
- describe the characteristic findings of accidental and nonaccidental childhood trauma
- design an approach to the diagnosis of decreased vision in children, and be familiar with the resources available to these patients

Rapport With Children: Tips for a Productive Examination

Children are not merely small adults, and most common ophthalmologic problems in children are different from the most common problems in adults. The varying developmental levels of children require different approaches to the ophthalmic examination. Proper preparation and attitude can make the ophthalmic examination of pediatric patients both enjoyable and rewarding.

Preparation

If at all possible, have a small room or corner of the waiting area designated for children. Both the parents and the adult patients will be relieved by this separation. A small table and chairs, some books, and some toys are sufficient.

A dedicated long pediatric examination lane with different types of distance fixation targets is optimal. Following the *one toy, one look* rule, have several small toys readily available for near fixation (Fig I-1). Light-colored plastic finger puppets become silent accommodative near targets that can also provide a corneal light reflex if placed over a muscle light or penlight.

Some children fear the white coat. You may choose to enter the room without yours.

The Examination

Examination of the pediatric patient begins with observing children at ease in the play area, as they navigate their way to the lane, and in their parent's arms as you enter the room. This may be the best look you get before children cry and bury their face in the parent's shoulder. Observe the parents and siblings. Some ophthalmic conditions tend to run in families.

Seat yourself at the child's eye level and introduce yourself to the child and the parent. Establish and maintain eye contact with the child. Be relaxed, open, honest, and playfully engaging during the examination. Gaining the child's confidence makes for a faster and better examination, easier follow-up visits, and greater parental support. Some children are more comfortable sitting in a parent's lap.

Initiate verbal contact by asking children easy questions with simple answers. For example, children enjoy being regarded as "big" and correcting adults when they are wrong.

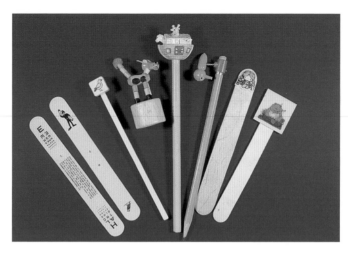

Figure I-1 Small toys, pictures, and reduced letter and E charts are used as near fixation targets. *(Reproduced with permission from Haldi BA, Mets MB. Nonsurgical treatment of strabismus. Focal Points: Clinical Modules for Ophthalmologists. San Francisco: American Academy of Ophthalmology; 1997, module 4. Photograph courtesy of Betty Anne Haldi, CO.)*

Tell them they look "so grown up"; grossly overestimate their age or grade level and then ask, "Is that right?" A simple joke can relax both child and parent.

To initiate physical contact with children, you can ask them to "give me five" or admire an article of their clothing, such as their shoes. Pushing the "magic button" on the nose of a child as you surreptitiously activate video presentations or mechanical animals with your foot pedal allows you to work close to the child's face while he or she is distracted.

Go where the action is—you may have only a few moments of cooperation, so check what you most need to see at the beginning of the examination. If fusion is in doubt, check it first before disrupting it with other tests, including those for vision. While checking vision, make children feel successful by initially giving them objects they can readily discern; then say, "That's too easy—let's try this one."

Copies of whatever optotypes are appropriate for children (Allen cards, picture chart, tumbling E) can be given to the parent for at-home rehearsal to help differentiate not seeing the test object from not understanding the test.

Develop a different vocabulary for working with children, such as "I want to show you something special" instead of "I want to examine you." Use "magic sunglasses" for the Polaroid stereo glasses, "special flashlight" for the retinoscope, "funny hat" for the indirect ophthalmoscope, and "magnifying glass" for the indirect lens. Confrontation visual fields can be performed as a counting-fingers game or Simon Says. Talk children into a slit-lamp examination by saying that they can "drive the motorcycle" by having them grab the handles of the slit lamp. Use your imagination to "play" with children as you rapidly proceed with the examination. Children will be more cooperative if you are sharing an experience instead of doing something to them.

Save the most threatening or most unpleasant part of the examination for the end. The least expensive test you can order is a return office visit. Children who become totally uncooperative can return later to finish the examination.

For the follow-up examination of a child who was fussy during the first visit, ask the parent to bring the child in hungry and then feed him or her during the examination.

When dealing with a vision-threatening or life-threatening problem, you must persist with the examination and even use sedation or anesthesia when necessary.

Eyedrops

The answers to the most common pediatric ophthalmic problems seen in the office will usually be found in the cycloplegic examination. Almost all children are apprehensive about eyedrops. However, they do not have to *like* the drops; the important thing is to instill them. There are many approaches to giving eyedrops. If possible, someone other than the examining physician should administer the drops. Some practitioners use a cycloplegic spray, some use a topical anesthetic drop first, and some simply use the cycloplegic drop. The drops can be described as being "like a splash of swimming pool water" that will "feel funny for about 30 seconds." Do not give children a long time to think about it. Dark irides are more difficult to dilate. In some cases, the parent can put the cycloplegic drops in at home, or the practitioner can perform an atropine refraction. (See Table 17-2 in BCSC Section 2, *Fundamentals and Principles of Ophthalmology,* for a complete listing of mydriatics and cycloplegics. See also Chapter 6 in this book.)

Use of Topical Anesthesia for Foreign-Body Removal

Procedures that provoke anxiety or are painful are best performed if children know that it is possible to numb the area. For example, the following process to remove foreign bodies can comfort the child:

1. Explain to the child that the eyes can be made numb.
2. Show the child the drop to be used while telling him or her that the drop is cold but most children say it is also comfortable. You can call it a "magic drop." Put a drop on the back of the child's hand first, before putting the drop in the eye. Tell the patient he or she might have felt that first drop in the eye but probably won't notice a second drop so much because the eye is already numb.
3. Demonstrate with a second drop that the eye has become numb. Show the child that a soft cotton-tipped applicator with drops on it can touch the eye without hurting or even being felt.
4. Introduce instruments for foreign-body removal in the same way.

Day SH, Sami DA. History, examination, and further investigation. In: Taylor D, Hoyt CS, eds. *Pediatric Ophthalmology and Strabismus.* 3rd ed. Cambridge, MA: Saunders; 2005:66–77.

McKeown CA. The pediatric eye examination. In: Albert DM, Jakobiec FA, eds. *Principles and Practice of Ophthalmology.* 2nd ed. Philadelphia: Saunders; 2000.

Pediatric Ophthalmology Panel. *Pediatric Eye Evaluations.* Preferred Practice Patterns. San Francisco: American Academy of Ophthalmology; 2002.

PART I

Strabismus

CHAPTER 1

Strabismus Terminology

The term *strabismus* is derived from the Greek word *strabismos,* "to squint, to look obliquely or askance." Strabismus means ocular misalignment, whether caused by abnormalities in binocular vision or by anomalies of neuromuscular control of ocular motility. Many terms are employed in discussions of strabismus, and unless these terms are used correctly and uniformly, confusion and misunderstanding can occur.

Orthophoria is the ideal condition of ocular alignment under binocular conditions. In reality, orthophoria is seldom encountered; a small heterophoria (see below) can be documented in most persons. Some ophthalmologists therefore prefer *orthotropia* to mean correct direction or position of the eyes. Both terms are commonly used to describe eyes without strabismus. *Heterophoria* is an ocular deviation kept latent by the fusional mechanism (latent strabismus). *Heterotropia* is a deviation that is manifest and not kept under control by the fusional mechanism *(manifest strabismus).*

It is important to identify the deviating eye, especially when seeking to call attention to the "offending" eye as causing the deviation. This usage is particularly helpful when dealing with vertical deviations, restrictive or paretic strabismus, or amblyopia in a preverbal child.

Prefixes and Suffixes

A detailed nomenclature has evolved to describe types of ocular deviations. This vocabulary uses many prefixes and suffixes based on the relative positions of the visual axes of both eyes to account for the multiple strabismic patterns encountered.

Prefixes

Eso- The eye is rotated so that the cornea is deviated nasally and the fovea is rotated temporally. Because the visual axes converge at a point closer than the fixation target, this is also known as *convergent strabismus.*

Exo- The eye is rotated so that the cornea is deviated temporally and the fovea is rotated nasally. Because the visual axes are still diverging at the fixation target, this is also known as *divergent strabismus.*

Hyper-   The eye is rotated so that the cornea is deviated superiorly and the fovea is rotated inferiorly. This is also known as *vertical strabismus.*

Hypo-   The eye is rotated so that the cornea is deviated inferiorly and the fovea is rotated superiorly. This is also known as *vertical strabismus.*

Incyclo-   The eye is rotated so that the superior pole of the vertical meridian is torted nasally and the inferior pole of the vertical meridian is torted temporally. This is also known as *intorsional strabismus.*

Excyclo-   The eye is rotated so that the superior pole of the vertical meridian is torted temporally and the inferior pole of the vertical meridian is torted nasally. This is also known as *extorsional strabismus.*

Suffixes

-phoria   A latent deviation (eg, esophoria, exophoria, right hyperphoria) that is controlled by the fusional mechanism so that the eyes remain aligned under normal binocular vision

-tropia   A manifest deviation (eg, esotropia, exotropia, right hypertropia, excyclotropia) that exceeds the control of the fusional mechanism so that the eyes are not aligned under binocular conditions

Strabismus Classification Terms

No classification is perfect or all-inclusive, and several methods of classifying eye alignment and motility disorders are used. Following are terms used in these classifications.

Fusional Status

Phoria   A latent deviation in which fusional control is always present

Intermittent tropia   A deviation in which fusional control is present part of the time

Tropia   A manifest deviation in which fusional control is not present

Variation of the Deviation With Gaze Position or Fixating Eye

Comitant (concomitant)   The size of the deviation does not vary by more than a few prism diopters with direction of gaze or with the eye used for fixating.

Incomitant (noncomitant)   The deviation varies in size with the direction of gaze or with the eye used for fixating. Most incomitant strabismus is paralytic or restrictive.

Fixation

Alternating   Spontaneous alternation of fixation from one eye to the other

Monocular   Definite preference for fixation with one eye

Age of Onset

Congenital   A deviation documented before age 6 months, presumably related to a defect present at birth; the term *infantile* might be more appropriate.

Acquired   A deviation with later onset, after a period of apparently normal visual development

Type of Deviation

Horizontal   Esodeviation or exodeviation

Vertical   Hyperdeviation or hypodeviation

Torsional   Incyclodeviation or excyclodeviation

Combined   Horizontal, vertical, torsional, or any combination thereof

Abbreviated Designations for Types of Strabismus

The addition of a prime (′) to any of the following indicates near fixation (eg, E′ indicates esophoria at near).

E, X, RH, LH   Esophoria, exophoria, right hyperphoria, left hyperphoria at distance fixation, respectively

ET, XT, RHT, LHT   Constant esotropia, exotropia, right hypertropia, left hypertropia at distance fixation, respectively

E(T), X(T), RH(T), LH(T)   Intermittent esotropia, exotropia, right hypertropia, left hypertropia at distance fixation, respectively

RHoT, LHoT   Right hypotropia, left hypotropia at distance fixation, respectively

0, EX = 0   Orthophoria (orthoptropia)

Important Axes of the Eye

There is occasionally confusion in the ophthalmic literature regarding terms used to describe the axes of the eye. Following are some important definitions (see also BCSC Section 3, *Clinical Optics*).

Optical axis   A line that best approximates the line passing through the optical centers of the cornea, lens, and fovea. Because the lens is usually decentered with respect to the cornea and the visual axis, no single line can precisely pass through each of these points. However, because the amount of decentration is small, the best approximation of this line is taken to be the optical axis.

Pupillary axis   The imaginary line perpendicular to the corneal surface and passing through the midpoint of the entrance pupil

Visual axis   The imaginary line connecting the fixation point and the fovea

CHAPTER 2

Anatomy of the Extraocular Muscles and Their Fascia

Origin, Course, Insertion, Innervation, and Action of the Extraocular Muscles

There are 7 extraocular muscles: the 4 rectus muscles, the 2 oblique muscles, and the levator palpebrae superioris muscle. Cranial nerve (CN) VI (abducens) innervates the lateral rectus muscle; CN IV (trochlear), the superior oblique muscle; and CN III (oculomotor), the levator palpebrae, superior rectus, medial rectus, inferior rectus, and inferior oblique muscles. CN III has an upper and a lower division: the upper division supplies the levator palpebrae and superior rectus muscles; the lower division supplies the medial rectus, inferior rectus, and inferior oblique muscles. The parasympathetic innervation of the sphincter pupillae and ciliary muscle travels with the branch of the lower division of CN III that supplies the inferior oblique muscle. BCSC Section 5, *Neuro-Ophthalmology,* discusses the ocular motor nerves in more detail, and Section 2, *Fundamentals and Principles of Ophthalmology,* extensively illustrates the anatomical structures mentioned in this chapter.

When the eye is directed straight ahead and the head is also straight, the eye is said to be in *primary position*. The *primary action* of a muscle is its major effect on the position of the eye when the muscle contracts while the eye is in primary position. The secondary and tertiary actions of a muscle are the additional effects on the position of the eye in primary position (see also Chapter 3 and Table 3-1). The globe usually can be moved about 50° in each direction from primary position. Under normal viewing circumstances, however, the eyes move only about 15°–20° from primary position before head movement occurs.

Horizontal Rectus Muscles

The horizontal rectus muscles are the medial and lateral rectus muscles. Both arise from the annulus of Zinn. The *medial rectus muscle* courses along the medial orbital wall. The proximity of the medial rectus muscle to the medial orbital wall means the medial rectus can be injured during ethmoid sinus surgery. The *lateral rectus muscle* courses along the lateral orbital wall. In primary position, the medial rectus is an adductor, and the lateral rectus is an abductor. The medial rectus muscle is the only rectus muscle that does not have an oblique muscle running tangential to it. This makes surgery on the medial rectus less complicated, but means that there is neither a point of reference if the surgeon becomes disoriented nor a point of attachment if the muscle is lost.

Vertical Rectus Muscles

The vertical rectus muscles are the superior and inferior rectus muscles. The *superior rectus muscle* originates from the annulus of Zinn and courses anteriorly, upward over the eyeball, and laterally, forming an angle of 23° with the visual axis of the eye in primary position (Fig 2-1; see also Chapter 3, Fig 3-4). In primary position, this muscle's primary action is elevation, secondary action is intorsion (incycloduction), and tertiary action is adduction.

The *inferior rectus muscle* also arises from the annulus of Zinn, and it then courses anteriorly, downward, and laterally along the floor of the orbit, forming an angle of 23° with the visual axis of the eye in primary position (see Chapter 3, Fig 3-5). In primary position, the inferior rectus muscle's primary action is depression, secondary action is extorsion (excycloduction), and tertiary action is adduction.

Oblique Muscles

The *superior oblique muscle* originates from the orbital apex above the annulus of Zinn and passes anteriorly and upward along the superomedial wall of the orbit. The muscle becomes tendinous before passing through the trochlea, a cartilaginous saddle attached to the frontal bone in the superior nasal orbit. A bursa-like cleft separates the trochlea from the loose fibrovascular sheath surrounding the tendon. The discrete fibers of the tendon telescope as they move through the trochlea, the central fibers moving farther than the

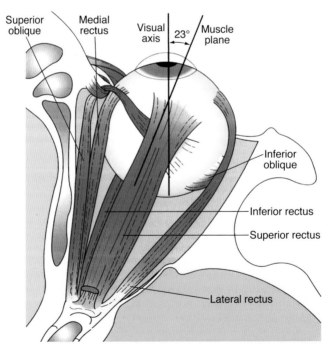

Figure 2-1 The extrinsic muscles of the right eyeball in primary position, seen from above. *(Modified with permission from Yanoff M, Duker J, eds. Ophthalmology. 2nd ed. London: Mosby; 2004:549.)*

peripheral ones (Fig 2-2). The function of the trochlea is to redirect the tendon inferiorly, posteriorly, and laterally, forming an angle of 51° with the visual axis of the eye in primary position (see Chapter 3, Fig 3-6). The tendon penetrates the Tenon capsule 2 mm nasally and 5 mm posteriorly to the nasal insertion of the superior rectus muscle. Passing under the superior rectus muscle, the tendon inserts in the posterosuperior quadrant of the eyeball, almost or entirely laterally to the midvertical plane or center of rotation. In primary position, the primary action of the superior oblique muscle is intorsion (incycloduction), secondary action is depression, and tertiary action is abduction.

The *inferior oblique muscle* originates from the periosteum of the maxillary bone, just posterior to the orbital rim and lateral to the orifice of the lacrimal fossa. It passes laterally, superiorly, and posteriorly, going inferior to the inferior rectus muscle and inserting under the lateral rectus muscle in the posterolateral portion of the globe, in the area of the macula. The inferior oblique muscle forms an angle of 51° with the visual axis of the eye in primary position (see Chapter 3, Fig 3-7). In primary position, the muscle's primary action is extorsion (excycloduction), secondary action is elevation, and tertiary action is abduction.

Helveston EM. The influence of superior oblique anatomy on function and treatment. The 1998 Bielschowsky Lecture. *Binocul Vis Strabismus Q.* 1999;14(1):16–26.

Levator Palpebrae Superioris Muscle

The levator palpebrae superioris muscle arises at the apex of the orbit from the lesser wing of the sphenoid bone just superior to the annulus of Zinn. The origin of this muscle blends with the superior rectus muscle inferiorly and with the superior oblique muscle medially. The levator palpebrae superioris passes anteriorly, lying just above the superior rectus muscle; the fascial sheaths of these 2 muscles are connected. The levator palpebrae

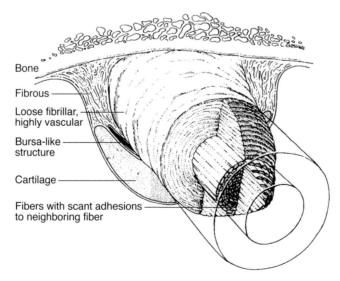

Bone
Fibrous
Loose fibrillar, highly vascular
Bursa-like structure
Cartilage
Fibers with scant adhesions to neighboring fiber

Figure 2-2 Components of the trochlea. *(Reproduced with permission from Helveston EM, Merriam WW, Ellis FD, et al. The trochlea: a study of the anatomy and physiology. Ophthalmology. 1982;89:124–133.)*

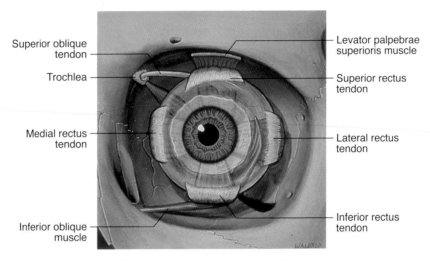

Figure 2-3 Extraocular muscles, frontal composite view, left eye. *(Reproduced with permission from Dutton JJ. Atlas of Clinical and Surgical Orbital Anatomy. Philadelphia: Saunders; 1994:23.)*

superioris muscle becomes an aponeurosis in the region of the superior fornix. This muscle has both a cutaneous and a tarsal insertion. BCSC Section 7, *Orbit, Eyelids, and Lacrimal System,* discusses this muscle in detail.

Figure 2-3 shows the extraocular muscles and their relationship to one another; Table 2-1 summarizes their characteristics.

Insertion Relationships of the Rectus Muscles

Starting at the medial rectus and proceeding to inferior rectus, lateral rectus, and superior rectus muscles, the rectus muscle tendons insert progressively farther from the limbus. A continuous curve drawn through these insertions yields a spiral, known as the *spiral of Tillaux* (Fig 2-4). The temporal side of the vertical rectus muscle insertion is farther from the limbus (ie, more posterior) than is the nasal side.

Blood Supply of the Extraocular Muscles

Arterial System

The muscular branches of the ophthalmic artery provide the most important blood supply for the extraocular muscles. The *lateral muscular branch* supplies the lateral rectus, superior rectus, superior oblique, and levator palpebrae superioris muscles; the *medial muscular branch,* the larger of the 2, supplies the inferior rectus, medial rectus, and inferior oblique muscles.

The lateral rectus muscle is partially supplied by the *lacrimal artery;* the *infraorbital artery* partially supplies the inferior oblique and inferior rectus muscles. The muscular branches give rise to the *anterior ciliary arteries* accompanying the rectus muscles; each rectus muscle has 1 to 3 anterior ciliary arteries. These pass to the episclera of the globe

Table 2-1 Extraocular Muscles

Muscle	Approx. Length of Active Muscle (mm)	Origin	Anatomical Insertion	Direction of Pull*	Tendon Length (mm)	Arc of Contact (mm)	Action From Primary Position	Innervation
Medial rectus (MR)	40	Annulus of Zinn	5.5 mm from medial limbus	90°	4.5	7	Adduction	Lower CN III
Lateral rectus (LR)	40	Annulus of Zinn	6.9 mm from lateral limbus	90°	7	12	Abduction	CN VI
Superior rectus (SR)	40	Annulus of Zinn	7.7 mm from superior limbus	23°	6	6.5	Elevation Intorsion Adduction	Upper CN III
Inferior rectus (IR)	40	Annulus of Zinn	6.5 mm from inferior limbus	23°	7	6.5	Depression Extorsion Adduction	Lower CN III
Superior oblique (SO)	32	Orbital apex above annulus of Zinn (functional origin at the trochlea)	Posterior to equator in superotemporal quadrant	51°	26	7–8	Intorsion Depression Abduction	CN IV
Inferior oblique (IO)	37	Behind inferior orbital rim lateral to lacrimal fossa	Macular area	51°	1	15	Extorsion Elevation Abduction	Lower CN III
Levator palpebrae superioris (LPS)	40	Orbital apex above annulus of Zinn	Septa of pretarsal orbicularis and anterior surface of tarsus	—	14–20	—	Eyelid elevation	Upper CN III

*Relative to visual axis in primary position. See also Chapter 3, Figs 3-3 through 3-7, in this volume.

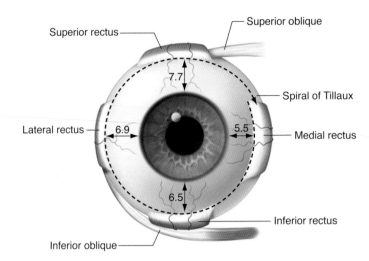

Figure 2-4 Spiral of Tillaux, right eye. *Note:* The distances, given in millimeters, are averages only and may vary greatly in individuals. *(Illustration by Christine Gralapp.)*

and then supply blood to the anterior segment. The superior and inferior rectus muscles carry the bulk of the blood supply.

Venous System

The venous system parallels the arterial system, emptying into the *superior* and *inferior orbital veins.* Generally, 4 *vortex veins* are located posterior to the equator; these are usually found near the nasal and temporal margins of the superior rectus and inferior rectus muscles.

Structure of the Extraocular Muscles

The important functional characteristics of muscle fibers are contraction speed and fatigue resistance. The eye muscles participate in motor acts that are among the fastest (saccadic eye movements) in the body and in those that are among the most sustained (gaze fixation and vergence movements). Like skeletal muscle, extraocular muscle is voluntary striated muscle. However, developmentally, biochemically, structurally, and functionally, it is different from typical skeletal muscle. The extraocular muscles are innervated at a ratio of nerve fiber to muscle fiber up to 10 times that of skeletal muscle. This difference may allow for more accurate eye movements controlled by an array of systems ranging from the primitive vestibulo-ocular reflex to highly evolved vergence movements.

The extraocular muscles exhibit a distinct 2-layer organization: an outer *orbital layer,* which acts only on connective tissue pulleys (see the section Pulley System), and an inner *global layer,* whose tendon inserts on the sclera to move the globe. The muscle fibers comprising the orbital and global layers can be either singly or multiply innervated.

Singly innervated fibers are fast-twitch generating and resistant to fatigue. Eighty percent of the fibers comprising the orbital layer muscle are singly innervated. Ninety percent of the fibers making up the global layer muscle are singly innervated, and they can be subdivided into 3 groups (red, intermediate, and white), based on mitochondrial content, with the red fibers being the most fatigue resistant and the white fibers, the least. The orbital singly innervated fibers are considered the major contributor to sustained extraocular muscle force in primary and deviated positions, and, of all muscle fiber types, this type is the most affected by denervation from damage to the motor nerves or from damage to the end plates, occurring after botulinum toxin injection.

The function of the multiply innervated fibers of the orbital and global layers is not clear. These fibers are not seen in the levator palpebrae superioris, and it is thought that they are involved in the finer control of fixation and in the smooth and finely graded eye movements, particularly vergence control.

These novel properties of eye muscles lead to differential responses to pharmaceuticals such as botulinum toxin, channel blockers, or local anesthetics, as well as disease processes such as myasthenia gravis and muscular dystrophy.

Lennerstrand G. Strabismus and eye muscle function. *Acta Ophthalmol Scand.* 2007;85(7): 711–723.

Orbital and Fascial Relationships

Within the orbit, a complex musculofibroelastic structure suspends the globe, supports the extraocular muscles, and compartmentalizes the fat pads (Fig 2-5). In the past, the distinctness of these layers has been overstated. The extent and complexity of the interconnectedness of the orbital tissues has recently come to light and is still being investigated. Clinically, the consequences of tissue entrapment in blowout fractures and post–retrobulbar hemorrhage fibrosis of delicate fibrous septa illustrate the intense fibrous connections throughout the orbit.

Adipose Tissue

The eye is supported and cushioned in the orbit by a large amount of fatty tissue. External to the muscle cone, fatty tissue comes forward with the rectus muscles, stopping about 10 mm from the limbus. Fatty tissue is also present inside the muscle cone, kept away from the sclera by the Tenon capsule (see Fig 2-5).

Muscle Cone

The muscle cone lies posterior to the equator. It consists of the extraocular muscles, the extraocular muscle sheaths, and the intermuscular membrane. The muscle cone extends posteriorly to the annulus of Zinn at the orbital apex.

Muscle Capsule

Each rectus muscle has a surrounding fascial capsule that extends with the muscle from its origin to its insertion. These capsules are thin posteriorly, but near the equator they thicken as they pass through the sleeve of the Tenon capsule, continuing anteriorly with

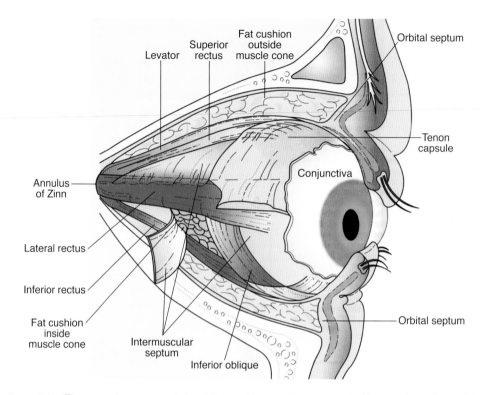

Figure 2-5 The muscle cone contains 1 fat cushion and is surrounded by another; these 2 fat cushions are separated by the rectus muscles and intermuscular septa. *(Reproduced with permission from Yanoff M, Duker J, eds.* Ophthalmology. *2nd ed. London: Mosby; 2004:553.)*

the muscles to their insertions. Anterior to the equator between the undersurface of the muscle and the sclera there is almost no fascia, only connective tissue footplates that connect the muscle to the globe. The smooth avascular surface of the muscle capsule allows the muscles to slide smoothly over the globe.

The Tenon Capsule

The Tenon capsule *(fascia bulbi)* is the principal orbital fascia and forms the envelope within which the eyeball moves (Fig 2-6A). The Tenon capsule fuses posteriorly with the optic nerve sheath and fuses anteriorly with the intermuscular septum at a position 3 mm from the limbus (Fig 2-6B). The posterior portion of the Tenon capsule is thin and flexible, allowing for free movement of the optic nerve, ciliary nerves, and ciliary vessels as the globe rotates, while separating the orbital fat inside the muscle cone from the sclera. At and just posterior to the equator, the Tenon capsule is thick and tough, suspending the globe like a trampoline by means of connections to the periorbital tissues. The global layer of the 4 rectus muscles penetrates this thick musculofibroelastic tissue approximately 10 mm posterior to their insertions. The oblique muscles penetrate the Tenon capsule anterior to the equator. The Tenon capsule continues forward over these 6 extraocular muscles and separates them from the orbital fat and structures lying outside the muscle cone.

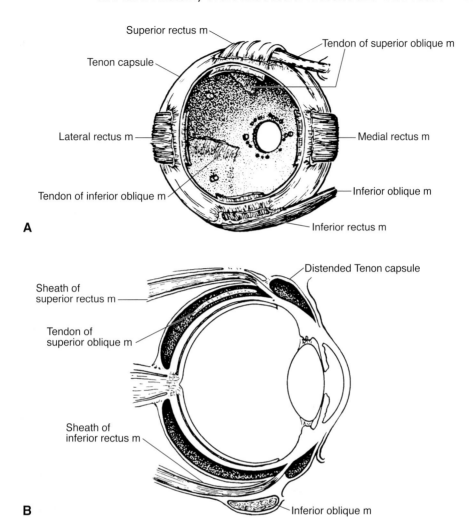

Figure 2-6   A, Anterior and posterior orifices of the Tenon capsule shown after enucleation of the globe. **B,** The Tenon space shown by injection with India ink. *(Modified with permission from von Noorden GK, Campos EC. Binocular Vision and Ocular Motility: Theory and Management of Strabismus. 6th ed. St Louis: Mosby; 2002:45.)*

Pulley System

The 4 rectus muscles are surrounded by distinct fibroelastic pulleys. Though not as distinct as the trochlea of the superior oblique, these pulleys maintain the position of the extraocular muscles relative to the orbit. They consist of collagen, elastin, and smooth muscle, which allows them to contract and relax. As the orbital muscle layer contracts, this pulley must be pulled back so that the distance between the location of the pulley and the insertion of the muscle on the globe remains approximately constant. Just as the trochlea acts as the functional origin of the superior oblique muscle, these pulleys act mechanically as the rectus muscle origins. The pulleys consist of discrete rings of dense collagen, which encircle the extraocular muscles, transitioning into less substantial but broader collagen sleeves both posteriorly and anteriorly. These sleeves stabilize the muscle path, preventing sideslipping or movement perpendicular to the muscle axis (Fig 2-7). Anteriorly, the sleeves thin to form slings between the rectus muscles (the *intermuscular septum*), which fuse with the conjunctiva 3 mm posterior to the limbus. The posterior section of the intermuscular septum separates the intraconal fat pads from the extraconal fat pads. Numerous extensions from all of the extraocular muscle sheaths attach to the orbit and help support the globe.

The inferior oblique muscle originates anteriorly from the inferonasal orbital rim adjacent to the anterior lacrimal crest, continuing laterally to enter its connective tissue pulley inferior to the inferior rectus at a site where the inferior oblique penetrates the Tenon capsule. The inferior oblique pulley and inferior rectus pulley are coupled to form the Lockwood ligament (Fig 2-8). The orbital layer of the inferior oblique muscle inserts partly on the conjoined inferior oblique/inferior rectus pulleys, partly on the inferior oblique sheath temporally, and partly on the inferior aspect of the lateral rectus pulley, forming a connective tissue "hammock" across the inferior orbit. The smooth muscle retractors of the lower eyelid (the Müller inferior tarsal muscle) and connective tissues extending to the inferior tarsal plate are also coupled to the conjoined inferior rectus/inferior oblique

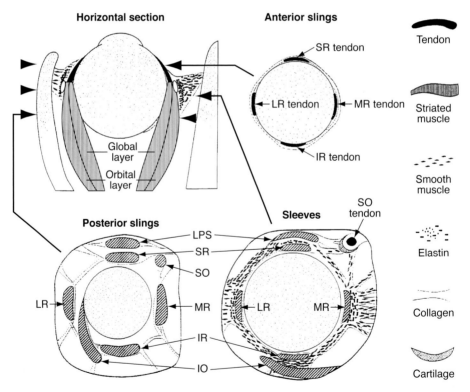

Figure 2-7 Structure of orbital connective tissues. IO, inferior oblique; IR, inferior rectus; LPS, levator palpebrae superioris; LR, lateral rectus; MR, medial rectus; SO, superior oblique; SR, superior rectus. The 3 coronal views are represented at the levels indicated by arrows in horizontal section. *(Modified with permission from Demer JL, Miller JM, Poukens V. Surgical implications of the rectus extraocular muscle pulleys.* J Pediatr Ophthalmol Strabismus. *1996;33(4):208–218.)*

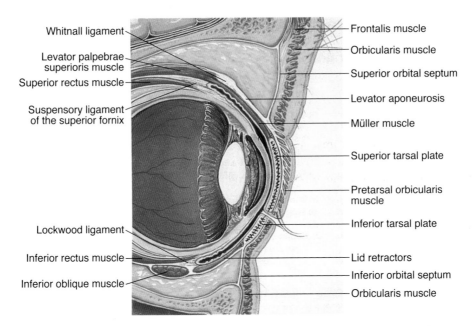

Whitnall ligament

Levator palpebrae superioris muscle

Superior rectus muscle

Suspensory ligament of the superior fornix

Lockwood ligament

Inferior rectus muscle

Inferior oblique muscle

Frontalis muscle

Orbicularis muscle

Superior orbital septum

Levator aponeurosis

Müller muscle

Superior tarsal plate

Pretarsal orbicularis muscle

Inferior tarsal plate

Lid retractors

Inferior orbital septum

Orbicularis muscle

Figure 2-8 Attachments of the upper and lower eyelids to the vertical rectus muscles. *(Reproduced with permission from Buckley EG, Freedman S, Shields MB, eds. Atlas of Ophthalmic Surgery, Vol III: Strabismus and Glaucoma. St Louis: Mosby-Year Book; 1995:15.)*

pulleys, coordinating lower eyelid positioning with vertical eye positioning during vertical gaze shift. In addition, a dense neurofibrovascular bundle containing the oblique motor nerve also attaches to the conjoined inferior oblique and inferior rectus pulley complex. It has been proposed that the neurofibrovascular bundle's connection to the orbital apex allows this bundle to function as an ancillary inferior oblique origin, tethering it inferiorly.

The *active pulley hypothesis* proposes that the pulley positions are shifted by the contraction of the orbital layer against the elasticity of the pulley suspension. Pathology of the pulley system is associated with patterns of strabismus. Since pulleys are located only a short distance from the globe center, small shifts in pulley location confer large shifts in extraocular muscle pulling direction. *Heterotopy (malpositioning)* of the rectus pulleys is a cause of incomitant strabismus and can mimic oblique muscle dysfunction by misdirecting the forces of the rectus muscle. Bony abnormalities can alter the extraocular muscle pulling direction by malpositioning the pulleys. Extorsion of the pulley array is associated with a V pattern; intorsion of the pulley array, with an A pattern. Strabismus is prevalent in craniosynostosis, particularly large A and V patterns, and it responds poorly to oblique extraocular muscle surgery. In the "heavy eye syndrome," high axial myopia is associated with esotropia and hypotropia, as the lateral rectus pulley shifts inferiorly toward the inferior rectus and the globe shifts superotemporally out of the rectus muscle array. Normal pulleys shift only slightly in the coronal plane, even during large ductions. Large gaze-related shifts due to instability in 1 or more pulleys are associated with incomitant strabismus. Inferior shifts of the lateral rectus pulley in adduction can produce a restrictive hypotropia closely resembling Brown syndrome, or they can produce an X-pattern exotropia.

Another recognized pathologic state of the pulley system is *pulley hindrance,* in which normal posterior shift with extraocular muscle contraction is mechanically impeded. Intentionally created hindrance can be therapeutic, however. The fadenoperation, or posterior fixation of an extraocular muscle through the underlying sclera, was designed to reduce an extraocular muscle's effect in its field of action by reducing the extraocular muscle's arc of contact and its rotational lever arm. Magnetic resonance imaging suggests that the actual effect of the fadenoperation is to hinder the posterior shift of the contracting extraocular muscle pulley, mechanically restricting extraocular muscle action.

Demer JL. Mechanics of the orbita. *Dev Ophthalmol.* 2007;40:132–157.

Anatomical Considerations During Surgery

The nerves to the rectus muscles and the superior oblique muscle enter the muscles approximately one-third of the distance from the origin to the insertion (or trochlea, in the case of the superior oblique muscle). Damaging these nerves during anterior surgery is difficult but not impossible. An instrument thrust more than 26 mm posterior to the rectus muscle's insertion may cause injury to the nerve.

Cranial nerve IV is outside the muscle cone and would not be affected by a retrobulbar block.

The nerve supplying the inferior oblique muscle enters the lateral portion of the muscle, where it crosses the inferior rectus muscle; the nerve can be damaged by surgery in this area. Because the parasympathetic innervation to the sphincter pupillae and ciliary muscle accompanies the nerve to the inferior oblique muscle, surgery in this area may also result in pupillary abnormalities. These nerves and the inferior oblique can be injured by an inferotemporal retrobulbar block. Any extraocular muscle could be reached by a retrobulbar needle and injured by injection of local anesthetic.

Maintaining the integrity of the muscle capsules decreases bleeding during surgery and provides a smooth muscle surface with less risk of adhesion formation. If only the muscle capsule is sutured to the globe, the muscle can retract backward, causing a "slipped muscle."

The intermuscular septum connections, especially between rectus muscles and oblique muscles, can help locate a lost muscle during surgery. Extensive intermuscular septum dissections are not necessary for rectus recession surgery. During resection surgery, the intermuscular septum connections should be severed to prevent, for example, the inferior oblique muscle from being advanced with the lateral rectus muscle.

The inferior rectus muscle is distinctly bound to the lower eyelid by the fascial extension from its sheath. *Recession,* or weakening, of the inferior rectus muscle tends to widen the palpebral fissure with an associated lower lid retraction; *resection,* or strengthening, of the inferior rectus muscle tends to narrow the fissure by elevating the lower eyelid. Therefore, any alteration of the inferior rectus muscle may be associated with palpebral fissure change (see Fig 2-8).

The superior rectus muscle is loosely bound to the levator palpebrae superioris muscle. The eyelid may be pulled downward following resection of the superior rectus muscle, thus narrowing the palpebral fissure, and pulled upward with a recession, widening the fissure. In hypotropia, a pseudoptosis may be present because the upper eyelid tends to follow the superior rectus (see Fig 2-8).

The blood supply to the extraocular muscles provides almost all of the temporal half of the anterior segment circulation and the majority of the nasal half of the anterior segment circulation, which also receives some blood from the long posterior ciliary artery. Therefore, simultaneous surgery on 3 rectus muscles may induce anterior segment ischemia, particularly in older patients.

Whenever muscle surgery is performed, special care must be taken to avoid penetration of the Tenon capsule 10 mm or more posterior to the limbus. If the integrity of the Tenon capsule is violated posterior to this point, fatty tissue may prolapse through the capsule and form a restrictive adhesion to sclera, muscle, intermuscular membrane, or conjunctiva, limiting ocular motility.

When surgery is performed near the vortex veins, accidental severing of a vein is possible. The procedures that present the greatest risk for damaging a vortex vein are inferior rectus and superior rectus muscle recession or resection, inferior oblique muscle weakening procedures, and exposure of the superior oblique muscle tendon. Hemostasis can be achieved with cautery or with an absorbable hemostatic sponge.

The sclera is thinnest just posterior to the 4 rectus muscle insertions. This area is the site for most muscle surgery, especially for recession procedures. Therefore, scleral perforation is always a risk during eye muscle surgery. The surgeon can minimize this risk by

- using spatulated needles with swedged sutures
- working with a clean, dry, and blood-free surgical field
- using loupe magnification or the operating microscope

Chapter 12 discusses these procedures and complications in greater detail.

Bron AJ, Tripathi RC, Tripathi BJ, eds. *Wolff's Anatomy of the Eye and Orbit.* 8th ed. London: Chapman & Hall; 1997.

Buckley EG, Freedman S, Shields MB, eds. *Atlas of Ophthalmic Surgery, Vol III: Strabismus and Glaucoma.* St Louis: Mosby-Year Book; 1995.

CHAPTER 3

Motor Physiology

Basic Principles and Terms

Axes of Fick, Center of Rotation, and Listing's Plane

A movement of the eye around a theoretical center of rotation is described with specific terminology. Two helpful concepts are the axes of Fick and Listing's plane (Fig 3-1). The *axes of Fick* are designated as *x, y,* and *z*. The *x-axis* is a transverse axis passing through the center of the eye at the equator; vertical rotations of the eye occur about this axis. The *y-axis* is a sagittal axis passing through the pupil; involuntary torsional rotations occur about this axis. The *z-axis* is a vertical axis; horizontal rotations occur about this axis. *Listing's equatorial plane* contains the center of rotation and includes the x and z axes. The y-axis is perpendicular to Listing's plane.

Positions of Gaze

- Primary position is the position of the eyes when fixating straight ahead.
- Secondary positions are straight up, straight down, right gaze, left gaze.

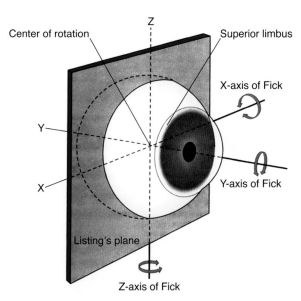

Figure 3-1   Axes of Fick, center of rotation, Listing's plane. *(Reproduced with permission from Yanoff M, Duker J, eds.* Ophthalmology. *2nd ed. London: Mosby; 2004:557.)*

27

- Tertiary positions are the 4 oblique positions of gaze: up and right, up and left, down and right, down and left.
- Cardinal positions are up and right, up and left, right, left, down and right, down and left (Fig 3-2).

See Chapter 6 for additional discussion of positions of gaze.

Extraocular Muscle Action

The 4 rectus muscles have traditionally been thought of as fixed straight strings running directly from the orbital apex to the muscle insertions. The oblique muscles, historically, were thought to simply attach obliquely to the globe. In light of ongoing discoveries that lend support to the active pulley hypothesis (see Chapter 2), some of the older concepts and descriptions of extraocular muscles and their actions are currently undergoing revision. In the following sections, however, we use the traditional concepts and terminology to help the novice acquire the vocabulary needed to form a basic understanding of this subject.

Arc of contact

The point of effective, or physiologic, insertion is the tangential point where the muscle first contacts the globe. The action of the eye muscle may be considered a vector of force that acts at this tangential point to rotate the eye. The length of muscle actually in contact with the globe constitutes the arc of contact. The traditional concepts of arc of contact and muscle plane, based on straight-line 2-dimensional models of orbital anatomy, do not take into account the recently discovered effective muscle pulleys and their effect on linearity of muscle paths.

Primary, secondary, and tertiary action

With the eye in primary position, the horizontal rectus muscles are purely horizontal movers around the z-axis (the vertical axis), and they have a primary action only. The vertical rectus muscles have a direction of pull that is mostly vertical as their primary action, but the angle of pull from origin to insertion is inclined 23° to the visual axis, giving rise

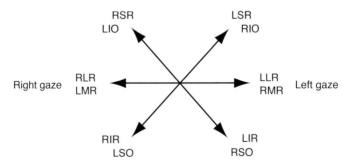

Figure 3-2 Cardinal positions and yoke muscles. RSR, right superior rectus; LIO, left inferior oblique; LSR, left superior rectus; RIO, right inferior oblique; RLR, right lateral rectus; LMR, left medial rectus; LLR, left lateral rectus; RMR, right medial rectus; RIR, right inferior rectus; LSO, left superior oblique; LIR, left inferior rectus; RSO, right superior oblique.

also to torsion, which is defined as any rotation of the vertical corneal meridians. *Intorsion* (also called *incycloduction*) is the secondary action for the superior rectus; *extorsion* (also called *excycloduction*) is the secondary action for the inferior rectus; and *adduction* is the tertiary action for both muscles. Because the oblique muscles are inclined 51° to the visual axis, torsion is their primary action. Vertical rotation is their secondary and horizontal rotation their tertiary action (Table 3-1).

Field of action

The term *field of action* has been used in 2 ways to describe entirely separate and distinct concepts:

- to indicate the direction of rotation of the eye from primary position if the muscle was the only one to contract
- to refer to the gaze position (one of the cardinal positions) in which the effect of the muscle is most readily observed

For the lateral rectus muscle, the direction of rotation and the gaze position are both abduction; for the medial rectus, they are both adduction. However, the direction of rotation and the gaze position are not the same for all muscles. For example, the inferior oblique muscle, acting alone, is an abductor and elevator, pulling the eye up and out—but its elevation action is best observed in adduction. Similarly, the superior oblique muscle, acting alone, is an abductor and depressor, pulling the eye down and out—but its depression action is best observed in adduction.

The clinical significance of fields of action is that a deviation (strabismus) that increases with gaze in some directions may result from the weakness of the muscle normally pulling the eye in that direction. For example, an acute left sixth nerve palsy in an adult can be diagnosed by asking the patient with diplopia 3 questions:

1. Is the diplopia horizontal or vertical? *Patient's answer:* Horizontal [eliminating all but the medial and lateral recti].
2. Is the diplopia worse at distance or at near? *Patient's answer:* Distance [implicating the lateral recti, which act more at distance viewing than in convergence].
3. Is the diplopia worse on looking to the left or to the right? *Patient's answer:* Looking to the left [the field of action of the left lateral rectus].

Table 3-1 Action of the Extraocular Muscles from Primary Position

Muscle*	Primary	Secondary	Tertiary
Medial rectus	Adduction	—	—
Lateral rectus	Abduction	—	—
Inferior rectus	Depression	Extorsion	Adduction
Superior rectus	Elevation	Intorsion	Adduction
Inferior oblique	Extorsion	Elevation	Abduction
Superior oblique	Intorsion	Depression	Abduction

*The superior muscles are intortors; the inferior muscles, extortors. The vertical rectus muscles are adductors; the oblique muscles, abductors.

Changing muscle action with different gaze positions

The gaze position determines the effect of extraocular muscle contractions on the rotation of the eye. The different positions are primary gaze and the 6 cardinal positions (see Fig 3-2). In each of these 6 cardinal positions, each of the 6 extraocular muscles has different effects on the eye rotation based on the relationship between the *visual axis* of the eye and the orientation of the muscle plane to the visual axis. Each cardinal position minimizes the angle between the visual axis and the muscle plane of the muscle being tested, thus maximizing the horizontal effect of the medial or lateral rectus or the vertical effect of the superior rectus, inferior rectus, superior oblique, or inferior oblique. By having the patient move the eyes to the 6 cardinal positions, the clinician can isolate and evaluate the ability of each of the 6 extraocular muscles to move the eye. See also Binocular Eye Movements later in the chapter.

With the eye in primary position, the horizontal rectus muscles share a common horizontal plane that contains the visual axis (Fig 3-3). The relative strength of the horizontal rectus muscles can be assessed by observing the horizontal excursion of the eye as it moves medially from primary position to test the medial rectus and laterally to test the lateral rectus.

The muscle actions of the vertical rectus muscles and the oblique muscles are more complex because, in primary position, the muscle axes are not parallel with the visual axis (see Figs 3-4 through 3-7).

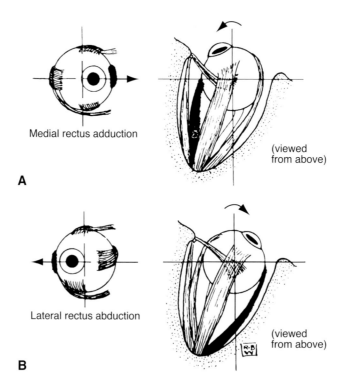

Medial rectus adduction

(viewed from above)

A

Lateral rectus abduction

(viewed from above)

B

Figure 3-3   The right horizontal rectus muscles. **A,** Right medial rectus muscle. **B,** Right lateral rectus muscle. *(Reproduced with permission from von Noorden GK. Atlas of Strabismus. 4th ed. St Louis: Mosby; 1983:3.)*

In primary position, the superior and inferior rectus muscle planes form an angle of 23° with the visual axis (y-axis) and insert slightly anterior to the z-axis (Figs 3-4, 3-5). Therefore, from primary position, the contraction of the superior rectus has 3 effects: primary elevation around the x-axis, secondary intorsion around the y-axis, and adduction around the z-axis. The relative strength of the superior rectus muscle can be most readily observed by aligning the visual axis parallel to the muscle plane axis—that is, when the eye is rotated 23° in abduction. In this position, the superior rectus becomes a pure elevator and its elevating action is maximal. To minimize the elevation action of the superior rectus, the visual axis should be perpendicular to the muscle axis at a position of 67° of adduction. In this position, the superior rectus would become a pure intorter. Because the globe cannot be adducted this far, there is still a superior rectus elevating action in maximal adduction.

The action of the inferior rectus muscle is similar to that of the superior rectus. Because the inferior rectus is attached to the globe inferiorly, its action from primary position is primarily depression, secondarily extorsion, and tertiarily adduction (see Fig 3-5). Its action as a depressor is maximally demonstrated in 23° of abduction and minimized in adduction.

The 2 oblique muscle planes course in a direction from the anteromedial aspect of the globe to the posterolateral, forming an angle of approximately 51° with the visual axis (Figs 3-6, 3-7). Because of the large angle formed in primary position, the primary action of the superior oblique is intorsion, with a secondary depression and tertiary

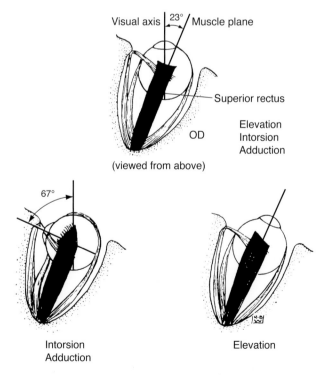

Figure 3-4 The right superior rectus muscle, viewed from above. *(Modified with permission from von Noorden GK. Atlas of Strabismus. 4th ed. St Louis: Mosby; 1983:3.)*

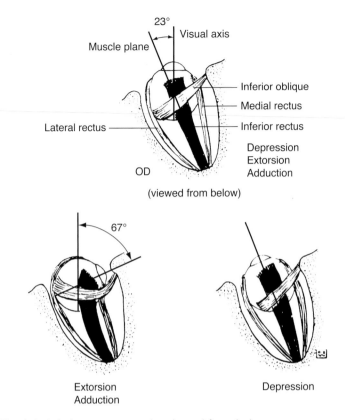

Figure 3-5 The right inferior rectus muscle, viewed from below. *(Modified with permission from von Noorden GK. Atlas of Strabismus. 4th ed. St Louis: Mosby; 1983:5.)*

abduction. As the muscle plane is aligned with the visual axis in extreme adduction, the superior oblique muscle action can be seen as a depressor. With abduction of the eye, the visual axis becomes perpendicular to the muscle plane, and the muscle action is one of intorsion.

The action of the inferior oblique is similar to that of the superior oblique (see Fig 3-7). In primary position, the primary action is extorsion, with secondary elevation and tertiary abduction. The inferior oblique's action as an elevator is best seen in adduction and, as an extorter, in abduction.

Eye Movements

Motor Units

An individual motor nerve fiber and its several muscle fibers constitute a motor unit. *Electromyography* records motor unit electrical activity. An electromyogram is useful in investigating normal and abnormal innervation and can be helpful in documenting paralysis, recovery from paralysis, and abnormalities of innervation in myasthenia gravis and muscle atrophy. However, this test is not helpful in ordinary comitant strabismus.

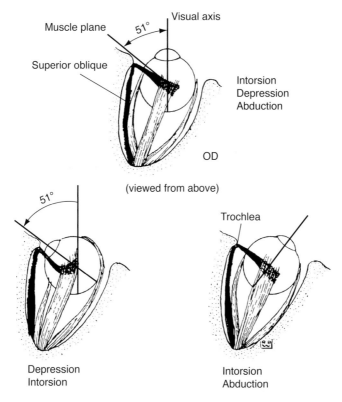

Figure 3-6 The right superior oblique muscle, viewed from above. *(Modified with permission from von Noorden GK. Atlas of Strabismus. 4th ed. St Louis: Mosby; 1983:7.)*

Recruitment during fixation or following movement

As the eye moves farther into abduction, more and more lateral rectus motor units are activated and brought into play by the brain to help pull the eye. This process is called *recruitment.* In addition, as the eye fixates farther into abduction, the frequency of activity of each motor unit increases until it reaches a peak (for some motor units, several hundred contractions per second).

Monocular Eye Movements

Ductions

Ductions are monocular rotations of the eye. *Adduction* is movement of the eye nasally; *abduction* is movement of the eye temporally. *Elevation (supraduction* or *sursumduction)* is an upward rotation of the eye; *depression (infraduction* or *deorsumduction)* is a downward rotation of the eye. *Intorsion (incycloduction)* is defined as a nasal rotation of the superior portion of the vertical corneal meridian. *Extorsion (excycloduction)* is a temporal rotation of the superior portion of the vertical corneal meridian.

The following terms relating to the muscles used in monocular eye movements are also important:

- *agonist:* the primary muscle moving the eye in a given direction

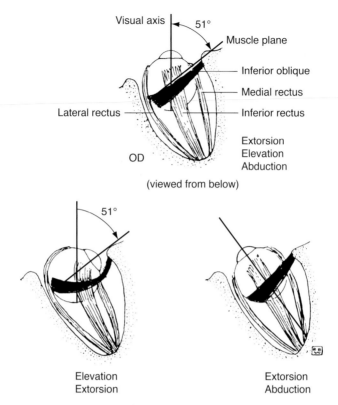

Visual axis — 51° — Muscle plane

Inferior oblique

Medial rectus

Lateral rectus — Inferior rectus

Extorsion
Elevation
Abduction

OD

(viewed from below)

51°

Elevation
Extorsion

Extorsion
Abduction

Figure 3-7 The right inferior oblique muscle, viewed from below. *(Modified with permission from von Noorden GK. Atlas of Strabismus. 4th ed. St Louis: Mosby; 1983:9.)*

- *synergist:* the muscle in the same eye as the agonist that acts with the agonist to produce a given movement (eg, the inferior oblique muscle is a synergist with the agonist superior rectus muscle for elevation of the eye)
- *antagonist:* the muscle in the same eye as the agonist that acts in the direction opposite to that of the agonist; the medial rectus and lateral rectus muscles are antagonists

Sherrington's law of reciprocal innervation states that increased innervation and contraction of a given extraocular muscle are accompanied by a reciprocal decrease in innervation and contraction of its antagonist. For example, as the right eye abducts, the right lateral rectus muscle receives increased innervation while the right medial rectus receives decreased innervation.

Binocular Eye Movements

When binocular eye movements are conjugate and the eyes move in the same direction, such movements are called *versions.* When the eye movements are disconjugate and the eyes move in opposite directions, such movements are known as *vergences* (eg, convergence and divergence).

Versions

Right gaze *(dextroversion)* is movement of both eyes to the patient's right. Left gaze *(levoversion)* is movement of both eyes to the patient's left. *Elevation,* or *upgaze (sursumversion),* is an upward rotation of both eyes; *depression,* or *downgaze (deorsumversion),* is a downward rotation of both eyes. In *dextrocycloversion,* both eyes rotate so that the superior portion of the vertical corneal meridian moves to the patient's right. Similarly, *levocycloversion* is movement of both eyes so that the superior portion of the vertical corneal meridian rotates to the patient's left.

The term *yoke muscles* is used to describe 2 muscles (1 in each eye) that are the prime movers of their respective eyes in a given position of gaze. For example, when the eyes move or attempt to move into right gaze, the right lateral rectus muscle and the left medial rectus muscle are simultaneously innervated and contracted. These muscles are said to be "yoked" together.

Each extraocular muscle in 1 eye has a yoke muscle in the other eye. Because the effect of a muscle is usually best seen in a given direction of gaze, the concept of yoke muscles is used to evaluate the contribution of each extraocular muscle to eye movement. See Figure 3-2, which shows the 6 cardinal positions of gaze and the yoke muscles whose primary actions are in that field of gaze.

Hering's law of motor correspondence states that equal and simultaneous innervation flows to yoke muscles concerned with the desired direction of gaze. The most useful application of this law is in evaluating binocular eye movements and, in particular, the yoke muscles involved.

Hering's law has important clinical implications, especially when the practitioner is dealing with a paralytic or restrictive strabismus. Because the amount of innervation to both eyes is always determined by the fixating eye, the angle of deviation varies according to which eye is fixating. When the normal eye is fixating, the amount of misalignment is called the *primary deviation.* When the paretic or restrictive eye is fixating, the amount of misalignment is called the *secondary deviation.* The secondary deviation is larger than the primary deviation because of the increased innervation necessary to move the paretic or restrictive eye to the position of fixation.

Hering's law is also necessary to explain the following example. If a patient has a right superior oblique muscle paresis and uses the right eye to fixate an object that is located up and to the patient's left, the innervation of the right inferior oblique muscle required to move the eye into this gaze position is reduced because the right inferior oblique does not have to overcome the normal antagonistic effect of the right superior oblique muscle. Therefore, according to Hering's law, less innervation is also received by the right inferior oblique muscle's yoke muscle, the left superior rectus muscle. This decreased innervation could lead to the incorrect impression that the left superior rectus muscle is paretic (Fig 3-8).

Vergences

Convergence is movement of both eyes nasally relative to a given starting position; *divergence* is movement of both eyes temporally relative to a given starting position. *Incyclovergence* is a rotation of both eyes so that the superior portion of each vertical corneal meridian rotates nasally; *excyclovergence* is a rotation of both eyes so that the superior pole of each vertical

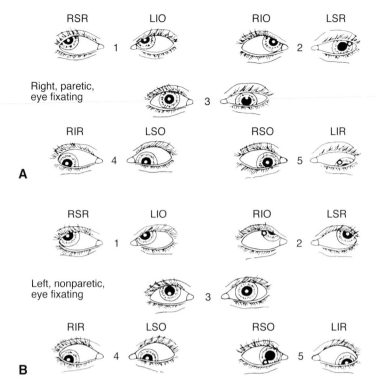

Figure 3-8 Paresis of right superior oblique muscle. **A,** With right paretic eye fixating, little or no vertical difference appears between the 2 eyes in the right (uninvolved) field of gaze (*1* and *4*). In primary position *(3)*, a left hypotropia may be present because the right elevators require less innervation and thus the left elevators will receive less than normal innervation. When gaze is up and left *(2)*, the RIO needs less than normal innervation to elevate the right eye because its antagonist, the RSO, is paretic. Consequently, its yoke, the LSR, will be apparently underacting, and pseudoptosis with pseudoparesis of the LSR will be present. When gaze is toward the field of action of the paretic muscle *(5)*, maximal innervation is required to move the right eye down during adduction, and thus the LIR will be overacting. **B,** With left sound eye fixating, no vertical difference appears in the right field of gaze (*1* and *4*). In primary position *(3)*, the right eye is elevated because of unbalanced elevators. When gaze is up and left *(2)*, the RIO shows marked overaction because its antagonist is paretic and there is contracture of the unopposed muscle. The action of the LSR is normal. When gaze is down and left *(5)*, normal innervation required by the fixating normal eye does not suffice to fully move the paretic eye. (See also Chapter 6, Fig 6-8.) *(Reproduced with permission from von Noorden GK. Atlas of Strabismus. 4th ed. St Louis: Mosby; 1983:24–25.)*

corneal meridian rotates temporally. *Vertical vergence* movement, though less frequently encountered, can also occur: 1 eye moves upward and the other downward. (See also Chapter 4.) Other important terms and concepts related to vergences include the following:

Tonic convergence The constant innervational tone to the extraocular muscles when a person is awake and alert. Because of the anatomical shape of the bony orbits and the position of the rectus muscle origins, the alignment of the eyes under complete muscle paralysis is divergent. Therefore, convergence tone is necessary in the awake state to maintain straight eyes even in the absence of strabismus.

Accommodative convergence of the visual axes   Part of the synkinetic near reflex. A fairly consistent increment of accommodative convergence (AC) occurs for each diopter of accommodation (A), giving the *accommodative convergence/accommodation (AC/A) ratio.*

Abnormalities of this ratio are common, and they are an important cause of strabismus. With an abnormally high AC/A ratio, the excess convergence tends to produce esotropia during accommodation on near targets. An abnormally low AC/A ratio tends to make the eyes exotropic when the person looks at near targets. For techniques of measuring this ratio, see the discussion of the AC/A ratio under Convergence in Chapter 6.

Voluntary convergence   A conscious application of the near synkinesis.

Proximal (instrument) convergence   An induced convergence movement caused by a psychological awareness of near; this movement is particularly apparent when a person looks through an instrument such as a binocular microscope.

Fusional convergence   A movement to converge and position the eyes so that similar retinal images project on corresponding retinal areas. Fusional convergence is accomplished without changing the refractive state of the eyes and is prompted by bitemporal retinal image disparity. See also Chapter 4.

Fusional divergence   The only clinically significant form of divergence. It is an optomotor reflex to diverge and align the eyes so that similar retinal images project on corresponding retinal areas. Fusional divergence is accomplished without changing the refractive state of the eyes and is prompted by binasal retinal image disparity. See also Chapter 4.

Supranuclear Control Systems for Eye Movement

There are several supranuclear eye movement systems. The *saccadic system* generates all fast (up to 400°–500°/sec) eye movements, such as eye movements of refixation. This system functions to place the image of an object of interest on the fovea or to move the eyes from one object to another. Saccadic movements require a sudden strong pulse of force from the extraocular muscles to move the eye rapidly against the viscosity produced by the fatty tissue and the fascia in which the globe lies. The study of saccadic velocity is of practical value in determining paresis of muscles and abnormal innervation.

The *smooth pursuit system* generates all following, or pursuit, eye movements. Pursuit latency is shorter than for saccades, but the maximum peak velocity of these slow pursuit movements is limited to 30°–60°/sec. The *vergence system* controls disconjugate eye movement, as in convergence or divergence. Supranuclear control of vergence eye movements is not yet fully understood. The *nonoptic reflex systems* integrate eye movements and body movements. The most clinically important of these systems is the *labyrinthine reflex system,* which involves the semicircular canals of the inner ears. Other, less important, systems involve the utricle and saccule of the inner ears. The cervical, or neck, receptors also provide input for this nonoptic reflex control.

These systems are discussed in depth in BCSC Section 5, *Neuro-Ophthalmology.*

von Noorden GK, Campos EC. *Binocular Vision and Ocular Motility: Theory and Management of Strabismus.* 6th ed. St Louis: Mosby; 2002:55.

CHAPTER 4

Sensory Physiology and Pathology

Physiology of Normal Binocular Vision

If an area of the retina is stimulated by any means—externally by light or internally by mechanical pressure or electrical processes—the resulting sensation is always one of light, and the light is subjectively localized as coming from a specific visual direction in space. This directional value of the retinal elements is an intrinsic physiologic property of the retina and the brain. Thus, the stimulation of any retinal area results in a visual sensation from a subjective visual direction relative to the visual direction of the fovea. The imaginary line connecting the fixation point and the fovea is termed the *visual axis,* and normally, with central fixation, it is subjectively localized straight ahead. BCSC Section 12, *Retina and Vitreous,* illustrates and discusses in depth the anatomy and physiology of the retina.

Retinal Correspondence

If retinal areas in the 2 eyes share a common subjective visual direction—that is, if their simultaneous stimulation results in the subjective sensation that the stimulating target or targets come from the same direction in space—these retinal areas or points are said to be *corresponding.* If the simultaneous stimulation of retinal areas in the 2 eyes results in the sensation of 2 separate visual directions for a target, or diplopia, these retinal areas or points are said to be *noncorresponding,* or *disparate.* If corresponding retinal areas in the 2 eyes bear identical relationships to the fovea in each eye (eg, both corresponding areas are located equidistantly to the right or left of and above or below the fovea), *normal retinal correspondence (NRC)* exists. Dissimilar relationships in the 2 eyes, between corresponding retinal areas and their respective foveas, indicate *anomalous retinal correspondence (ARC).* (ARC is discussed at length later in the chapter.) Correspondence, normal or anomalous, is necessary for single binocular vision.

If the 2 eyes have NRC and each fovea fixates the identical point, this point is seen singly. Points to both sides of this fixation point likewise fall on corresponding retinal areas and also are seen singly, as long as these points lie on a horizontal construct known as the *Vieth-Müller circle.* This circle passes through the optical center of each eye and the point of fixation. When attempts are made to duplicate the Vieth-Müller circle experimentally, the locus of all points seen singly falls not on the circle but on a curved surface called the *empirical horopter* (Fig 4-1). The horopter not only exists in 2 dimensions but is actually a 3-dimensional space. Each fixation point determines a specific horopter. By definition,

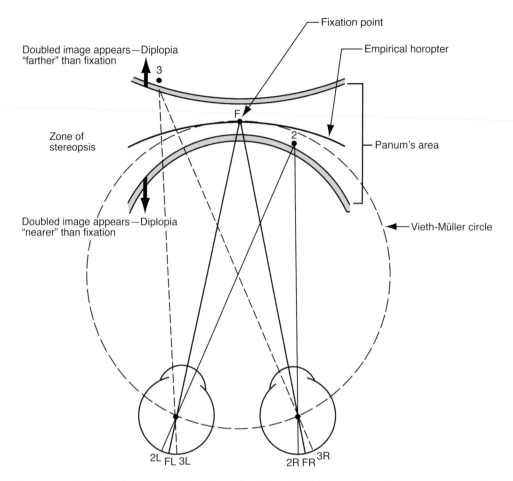

Figure 4-1 Empirical horopter. *F*, Fixation point; *FL* and *FR*, left and right foveas, respectively. Point 2, falling within Panum's area, is seen singly and stereoscopically. Point 3 falls outside Panum's area and is therefore seen double.

all points lying on the horopter curve stimulate corresponding retinal elements and thus are seen singly. All points not lying on the horopter fall on disparate retinal elements and would therefore be expected to create double vision. However, double vision does not occur physiologically within a limited area surrounding the horopter curve because the visual system fuses the 2 disparate retinal images, resulting in single binocular vision with stereopsis. The slightly different images caused by the 3-dimensional object stimulate stereoscopic perception.

Figure 4-1 shows objects in this space that fall mathematically on disparate retinal areas but are physiologically seen singly. This space is called *Panum's area of single binocular vision*. Objects outside Panum's area fall on widely disparate retinal areas and are seen as coming from 2 different visual directions, causing physiologic diplopia.

A 3-dimensional object is partly in front of and partly behind the empirical horopter and thus stimulates disparate retinal points and is seen stereoscopically. As long as the

3-dimensional object falls entirely within Panum's area, it is seen singly. Objects that fall outside Panum's area are seen double because the images are too disparate to be fused cortically into a single image. Stereopsis is a response to horizontally disparate retinal stimulation.

Fusion

Fusion is the cortical unification of visual objects into a single percept that is made possible by the simultaneous stimulation of corresponding retinal areas. For retinal images to be fused, they must be similar in size and shape. Because of their small receptive fields (see Chapter 1 in BCSC Section 12, *Retina and Vitreous*), the areas near the fovea (central fusion) allow very little overlap before diplopia is elicited. More overlap due to larger receptive fields is tolerated toward the periphery (peripheral fusion). Fusion has been artificially divided into sensory fusion, motor fusion, and stereopsis.

Sensory fusion

Sensory fusion is based on the innate orderly topographic relationship between the retinas and the visual cortex, whereby corresponding retinal points project to the same cortical locus, and corresponding adjacent retinal points have adjacent cortical representations.

Motor fusion

Motor fusion is a vergence movement that causes similar retinal images to fall and be maintained on corresponding retinal areas even though natural (eg, heterophorias) or artificial causes tend to induce disparities. For example, if progressive base-out prism is introduced before both eyes while a target is viewed, the retinal images move temporally over both retinas if the eyes remain in fixed position. However, fusional convergence movements maintain similar retinal images on corresponding retinal areas, and the eyes are observed to converge. This response is called *fusional convergence*. Motor fusion may be thought of as a diplopia avoidance mechanism and is the exclusive function of the extrafoveal retinal periphery. Fusional vergence amplitudes can be measured with rotary prisms, by major haploscopes, and by other devices. Representative normal values are given in Table 4-1. Fusional vergences are also discussed in Chapter 6.

Stereopsis

Stereopsis should not be thought of as a form of simple fusion. As discussed, stereopsis occurs when retinal disparity is too great to permit the simple superimposition or fusion of the 2 visual directions but is not great enough to elicit diplopia. Stereopsis, therefore, is a

Table 4-1 **Average Normal Fusional Amplitudes in Prism Diopters (Δ)**			
Testing Distance	Convergence Fusional Amplitudes	Divergence Fusional Amplitudes	Vertical Fusional Amplitudes
6 m	14	6	2.5
25 cm	38	16	2.6

bridge between simple sensory and motor fusion and diplopia. Stereopsis allows a subjective ordering of visual objects in depth, or 3 dimensions. It is the highest form of binocular cooperation, and it adds a new quality to vision.

Stereopsis and depth perception should not be considered synonymous. Monocular clues contribute to depth perception. These monocular clues include object overlap, relative object size, highlights and shadows, motion parallax, and perspective. Stereopsis is a *binocular* sensation of relative depth caused by horizontal retinal image disparity. Nasal disparity between 2 similar retinal images is interpreted by the brain as farther away from the fixation point, temporal disparity as nearer. At distances farther than 20 ft, we rely almost entirely on monocular clues for depth perception.

Selected Aspects of the Neurophysiology of Vision

The decussation of the optic nerves at the chiasm is essential for the development of binocular vision and stereopsis. With decussation, visual information from corresponding retinal areas in each eye runs via adjacent parallel separate circuits through the lateral geniculate body and optic tracts to the visual cortex, where the information from both eyes is finally commingled and modified by various inputs coming together.

Substantial research has recently focused on the neurophysiology of vision. We will focus on the retinal ganglion cell layer; the *lateral geniculate body (LGB)*, which is classically represented as 6 purely monocular laminae (4 dorsal parvocellular and 2 ventral magnocellular laminae with koniocellular laminae separating them [see the section Retinogeniculocortical Pathway]); and the primary visual cortex, also called the *striate cortex, V1,* or *Brodmann area 17*. This retinogeniculocortical pathway provides the neural substrate for visual perception (Fig 4-2).

The LGB is the principal thalamic visual nucleus linking the retina and the striate cortex. Of the approximately 1 million ganglion cells in the retina, approximately 90% of these terminate in the LGB. The LGB contains about 1.8 million neurons, yielding a ratio of ganglion cells to geniculate neurons of approximately 1:2. After a relatively direct transfer through the LGB, the signal activates a unit in the striate cortex containing approximately 1000 processing elements. According to the classic view, the striate cortex performs the basic analysis of geniculate input and then transmits its essence to higher peristriate cortical areas for further interpretation. These areas have been called *Brodmann areas 18* and *19*, or *V2, V3, V3a, V4,* and *V5*.

Retinogeniculocortical Pathway

The *magnocellular (M) system* and the *parvocellular (P) system* are the main neural systems in the retinogeniculocortical pathway (see Fig 4-2). Less is known about the *koniocellular (K) system*. The M system originates with the *parasol retinal ganglion cells*. These cells have large somas with large dendritic fields and large axons; they are rare in the foveal area and increase in number toward the near periphery. They synapse with the magnocellular neurons in the LGB. The M geniculate axons terminate in the striate cortex (V1) layer 4Cα. The neurons in this system have a fast response time, but these responses decay rapidly

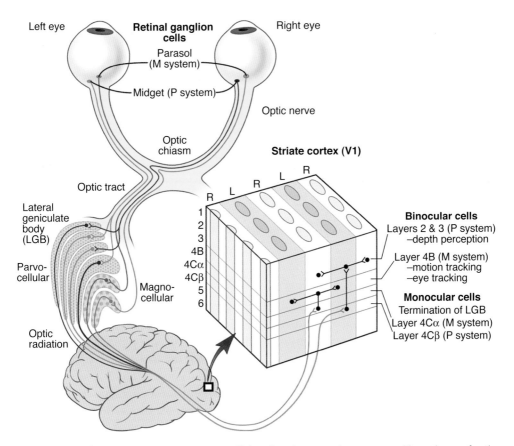

Figure 4-2 The magnocellular and parvocellular visual processing system. Note the perfectly parallel monocular separation of corresponding retinal areas that exists from the optic tract through the lateral geniculate body and optic radiation. The first binocular cells appear in layers 2, 3, and 4B of the ocular dominance columns in the striate cortex (V1). *(Redrawn with permission from Lawton A. The afferent visual system cortical representation of vision. In: Yanoff M, Duker J, eds. Ophthalmology. 2nd ed. London: Mosby; 2004:1299; and with permission from Horton J. The central visual pathways. In: Hart WM, ed. Adler's Physiology of the Eye: Clinical Applications. 9th ed. St Louis: Mosby; 1992:751. Illustration by Christine Gralapp.)*

when the stimulus is maintained, making the M system especially sensitive to moving stimuli but not to stationary images. The M system is also relatively insensitive to color. In macaque monkeys and probably also in humans, approximately 10% of the retinal input to the LGB comes from M cells.

The P system originates in the *midget retinal ganglion cells,* which have small somas and small dendritic fields; these cells are of relatively high density in the fovea and decrease in number as retinal eccentricity increases. The P retinal ganglion cells synapse with the parvocellular LGB cells. The P geniculate axons terminate in layer 4Cβ of V1. The P system gives a slow tonic response to visual stimulation, carries high-resolution information about object borders and color contrast, and is important for shape perception and the ability to see standing objects in detail. Approximately 80% of retinal input is from P ganglion cells.

The K system originates in the small, bistratified retinal ganglion cells, which have large dendritic fields. These cells synapse with the koniocellular LGB cells. The geniculate axons terminate in layers 3 and 1 of V1. This system is involved with aspects of color vision, especially blue color.

The fibers of the optic tract terminate in the LGB. Geniculate laminae 1 (parvo), 4 (parvo), and 6 (magno) receive axons from the contralateral nasal retina; laminae 2 (parvo), 3 (parvo), and 5 (magno) receive axons from the ipsilateral temporal retina. This monocular separation of corresponding retinal areas continues through the lateral geniculate laminae into the striate cortex (V1), where the geniculate axon terminals from the right and left eyes are segregated into a system of alternating parallel stripes called *ocular dominance columns* (see Fig 4-2). From there, the paired right and left monocular cells finally converge on the first binocular cells in layers 2, 3, 4Cα, and 4Cβ of V1. Binocular vision and binocular motor fusion are made possible by horizontal connections that enable information from these 2 monocular columns to be shared.

Visual Development

In the human retina, most of the ganglion cells are generated between the 8th and 15th weeks of gestation, reaching a plateau of 2.2–2.5 million by week 18. After week 30, the ganglion cell population falls dramatically during a period of rapid cell death that lasts 6–8 weeks. Thereafter, cell death continues at a low rate into the first few postnatal months. The retinal ganglion cell population is reduced to a final count of about 1 to 1.5 million. The loss of about 1 million optic axons may serve to refine the topography and specificity of the retinogeniculate projection by eliminating inappropriate connections.

The neurons of the human LGB are probably formed between the 8th and 11th weeks of gestation. By week 10, the first retinal ganglion cells invade the developing LGB. Segregation of the M, P, and K system retinal ganglion cells occurs on a timetable that parallels the lamination in the LGB. Retinal afferents prune back their axon terminals so that the synaptic connections are preserved only within the appropriate geniculate laminae, which emerge between weeks 22 and 25. It is thought that ganglion cells die if their axons do not successfully synapse with the appropriate targets in the brain. The LGB laminae become so precisely oriented that a properly positioned straight needle passing through all 6 layers would skewer only cells from corresponding retinal areas from each eye.

The cells that will become the striate cortex are probably formed between the 10th and 25th weeks of gestation. Initially, the geniculate afferents representing each eye overlap extensively in layer 4C (Fig 4-3). The maturation of the ocular dominance columns requires thousands of left and right eye geniculate afferents to gradually disentangle their overlapping axon terminals. This segregation transpires during the last few weeks of pregnancy and is almost complete at birth.

The continued development of visual function after birth is accompanied by major anatomical changes occurring simultaneously at all levels of the central visual pathways. The fovea is still covered by multiple cell layers and is sparsely packed with cones, which may account for the estimated visual acuity of 20/400 at birth. During the first years of life, the photoreceptors redistribute within the retina, and peak foveal cone density increases fivefold to achieve the configuration found in the adult retina, with an improvement in

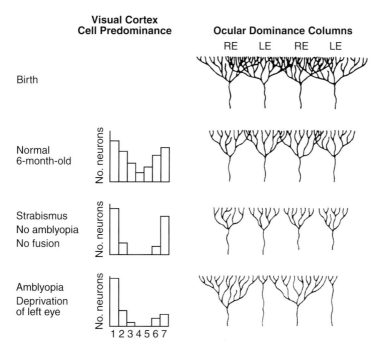

Figure 4-3 Anatomical and physiologic maturation of ocular dominance columns of the primary visual cortex in normal and deprived monkeys. *Birth:* Broad overlap of afferents from the lateral geniculate nucleus, hence little dominance by right *(RE)* vs left *(LE). Normal 6-month-old:* Regression of overlapping afferents from both eyes with distinct areas of monocular dominance. The bar graph shows the classic U-shaped distribution obtained by single-cell recordings from the visual cortex. About half the cells are driven predominantly by the right eye and the other half by the left eye. A small number are driven equally by the 2 eyes. *1* = driven only by right eye; *7* = driven only by left eye; *2–6* = driven binocularly. *Strabismus:* Effect of artificial eye misalignment in the neonatal period on ocular dominance. The monkey alternated fixation (no amblyopia) and lacked fusion. Lack of binocularity is evident as exaggerated segregation into dominance columns. The bar graph shows the results of single-cell recordings obtained from this animal after age 1 year. Almost all neurons are driven exclusively by the right or left eye, with little binocular activity. *Amblyopia:* Effect of suturing the left eyelid shut shortly after birth. Dominance columns of the normal right eye are much wider than those of the deprivationally amblyopic left eye. The bar graph shows markedly skewed ocular dominance and little binocular activity. *(Modified with permission from Tychsen L. Binocular vision. In: Hart WM, ed. Adler's Physiology of the Eye: Clinical Application. 9th ed. St Louis: Mosby; 1992:810.)*

visual acuity to the 20/20 level. In newborns, the white matter of the visual pathways is not fully myelinated. For the first 2 years after birth, myelin sheaths enlarge rapidly and then continue at a slower rate through the first decade of life. At birth, the neurons of the LGB are only 60% of their average size. Their volume gradually increases until age 2 years. Striate cortex refinement of synaptic connections continues for many years after birth. The density of synapses declines by 40% over several years to attain final adult levels at about age 10 years.

Physiologic activity in the fetus is vital to the development of normal anatomical connections in the visual system. In utero, mammalian retinal ganglion cells discharge spontaneous action potentials in the absence of any visual stimulation. Abolishing these action potentials with tetrodotoxin prevents the normal prenatal segregation of the retinogeniculate axons into appropriate geniculate laminae and blocks the formation of ocular dominance columns in the striate cortex. Thus, although the functional architecture of the visual system is ordained by genetics, the specificity and refinement are molded by physiologic vision-independent activity occurring in the fetus, as well as by postnatal vision-dependent experience.

Effects of Abnormal Visual Experience on the Retinogeniculocortical Pathway

Abnormal visual experience can powerfully affect retinogeniculocortical development. Abnormal development produced by visual deprivation, anisometropia, or strabismus appears to result in changes in the primary visual cortex, which ceases to be a faithful relay of visual signals. The developing visual system uses patterns of activity to refine neural connections and is extremely sensitive to unequal binocular competition and competitive inhibition.

If a newborn monkey is reared in the dark or with both eyes sutured closed, cells in the striate cortex eventually lose sharp orientation tuning and normal binocular responses. Some of the cells become unresponsive to visual stimulation and activate erratically and spontaneously. The remaining units give sluggish and unpredictable responses, with minimal potential for recovery. Cells in the striate cortex do not recover their normal responses.

Following the postnatal critical period, the visual system becomes impervious to the effects of sensory deprivation. If an adult monkey is visually deprived by the suturing of both eyelids, the cells in the striate cortex remain unaffected.

Single eyelid suturing in baby macaque monkeys usually produces axial myopia but no other significant changes in the eye. There is minor shrinkage of both the M and P cells of the lateral geniculate laminae receiving input from that deprived eye, but these cells respond briskly to visual stimulation, implying that a defect in the LGB is not likely to account for amblyopia. In the striate cortex, monocular visual deprivation causes the ocular dominance columns of the closed eye to appear radically narrowed (Fig 4-4; also see Fig 4-3). The explanation is that the 2 eyes compete for synaptic contacts in the cortex. As a result, the deprived eye loses many of the connections already formed at birth with postsynaptic cortical targets. This leads to excessive pruning of the terminal arbors of geniculate cells driven by the deprived eye. In turn, the ocular dominance columns of the deprived eye begin to shrink, which leads to a reduction in the cell size of the LGB cells required to sustain a reduced arbor of axon terminals in layer 4C. The open eye profits by the sprouting of terminal arbors beyond their usual boundaries to occupy territory relinquished by the deprived eye. However, the benefit derived by invading the cortical territory of the deprived eye is unclear because visual acuity does not improve beyond normal. Positron emission testing (PET) has shown a reduction in the cortical blood flow and glucose metabolism during stimulation of the amblyopic eye compared with the normal eye, suggesting the visual cortex as the primary site of amblyopia. This monocular deprivation also devastates binocularity in that few cells can be driven by both eyes.

There is a critical period in which visual development of the macaque monkey eye is vulnerable to the effects of eyelid suturing. This critical period corresponds to that in

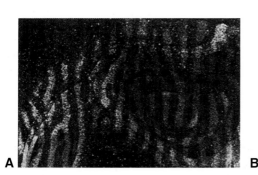 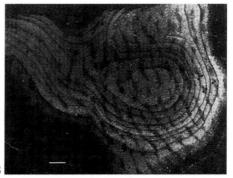

Figure 4-4 Change of ocular dominance columns in macaque monkey visual cortex after monocular deprivation. Radioactive proline was injected into the normal eye and transported to the visual cortex to reveal the projections of that eye. In these sections, cut parallel to the cortical surface, white areas show labeled terminals in layer 4. **A,** Normal monkey. The stripes representing the injected eye (bright) and noninjected eye (dark) have roughly equal spacing. **B,** Monocularly deprived monkey that had 1 eye sutured closed from birth for 18 months. The bright stripes (representing label in layer 4 from the open, injected eye) are widened; the dark ones (closed eye) are greatly narrowed, showing the devastating physical effect of deprivation amblyopia. (Scale bar = 1 mm). *(Reproduced with permission from Kaufman PL, Alm A. Adler's Physiology of the Eye. 10th ed. St Louis: Mosby; 2003:699. Originally from Hubel DH, Wiesel TN, LeVay S. Plasticity of ocular dominance columns in monkey striate cortex. Philos Trans R Soc Lond B Biol Sci. 1977;278(961):377–409.)*

which the wiring of the striate cortex is still vulnerable to the effects of visual deprivation. During the critical period, the deleterious effects of eyelid closure are correctable by reversal of the eyelid suture—that is, opening the sutured eye and closing the fellow eye. After this reversal, the ocular dominance columns of the initially closed eye appear practically normal, indicating that anatomical recovery of the initially shrunken columns was induced by opening the right eye and penalizing the left eye. However, when the right eye is sewn closed beyond the critical period and then is reopened and the fellow eye closed, the deprived eye columns do not reexpand.

Eyelid suturing in the baby macaque monkey is a good model for visual-deprivation amblyopia. In children, this condition can be caused by any dense opacity of the ocular media or occlusion by the eyelid. Visual deprivation can cause a rapid and profound amblyopia.

Amblyopia in children also has other causes. Optical defocus resulting from anisometropia causes the cortical neurons driven by the defocused eye to be less sensitive (particularly to higher spatial frequencies because they are most affected by blur) and to send out a weaker signal. This results in a binocular neural imbalance, causing reduced binocular activity, little if any narrowing of the ocular dominance columns, and cell shrinkage in the parvocellular laminae. Only the function of the P system is abnormal in anisometropic amblyopia. Deficits in binocular processing are also more pronounced when tested with stimuli of high spatial frequency.

The critical period for anisometropic amblyopia begins when the unilateral optical blur exceeds the lessening bilateral neural blur, which improves as the visual system develops sensitivity to high spatial frequency. This critical period may have a later onset than strabismic amblyopia and may require a prolonged period of unilateral blur. Meridional (astigmatic) amblyopia does not develop during the first year of life and may not develop until age 3.

Strabismus can be artificially created in monkeys by the sectioning of an extraocular muscle. Some monkeys develop alternating fixation after this procedure; they maintain normal acuity in each eye. Examination of the striate cortex reveals cells with normal receptive fields and an equal number of cells responsive to stimulation of either eye. However, the cortex is bereft of binocular cells (Fig 4-5; also see Fig 4-3). After 1 extraocular muscle is cut, some monkeys do not alternately fixate but constantly fixate with the same eye, and the deviating eye develops amblyopia. An important factor in the development of strabismic amblyopia is interocular suppression due to image uncorrelation. Strabismus causes abnormal input to the striate cortex by preventing the synchronous firing provided by simultaneous correlated images from the 2 foveas. Another factor is the optical defocus of the deviated eye. The dominant eye is focused on the object of regard while the deviated eye is pointed in a different direction; for the deviated eye, an object may be too near or too far to be in focus. Either mechanism can cause asynchrony or inhibition of 1 set of signals in the striate cortex layer 4C. In strabismic amblyopia, layer 4C, especially the parvocellular recipient layer, appears less active and binocular activity is reduced, but there is little change in the width of the ocular dominance columns.

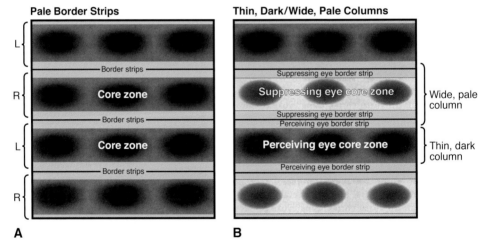

Figure 4-5   Schematic diagram of ocular dominance columns in macaque monkey cortex showing the effects of experimental strabismus (with and without monocular suppression) on metabolic activity. **A,** Strabismus without fixation preference: pale left- and right-eye binocular border strips showing decreased metabolic activity from disruption of ocular alignment but no monocular suppression, as revealed by strong metabolic activity in the monocular core zones serving each eye. **B,** Strabismus with left-eye fixation preference: weak metabolic activity in suppressed central core of the right eye as well as the binocular border strips of both eyes. *(Reproduced with permission from Kaufman PL, Alm A. Adler's Physiology of the Eye. 10th ed. St Louis: Mosby; 2003:703. Originally from Horton JC, Hocking DR, Adams DL. Metabolic mapping of suppression scotomas in striate cortex of macaques with experimental strabismus. J Neurosci. 1999;19:7111–7129.)*

The critical period for developing strabismic amblyopia appears to begin at approximately 4 months of age, during the time of ocular dominance segregation and sensitivity to binocular correlation.

Abnormal sensory input alone is sufficient to alter the normal anatomy of the visual cortex. Other areas of the cerebral cortex may also depend on sensory stimulation to form the proper anatomical circuits necessary for normal adult visual function. This notion underscores the importance of providing children with an adequate and healthful sensory environment.

Booth R, Fulton A. Amblyopia. In: Albert D, Jakobiec F, eds. *Principles and Practice of Ophthalmology.* 2nd ed. Philadelphia: Saunders; 2000:4340–4354.

Bron A, Tripathi RC, Tripathi BJ, eds. *Wolff's Anatomy of the Eye and Orbit.* 8th ed. London: Chapman & Hall; 1997:551–594.

Matsubara J. Central visual pathways. In: Kaufman P, Alm A, eds. *Adler's Physiology of the Eye: Clinical Application.* 10th ed. St Louis: Mosby; 2003:641–709.

Shan Y, Moster ML, Roemer RA, et al. Abnormal function of the parvocellular visual system in anisometropic amblyopia. *J Pediatr Ophthalmol Strabismus.* 2000;37(2):73–78.

Abnormalities of Binocular Vision

When a manifest deviation of the eyes occurs, the corresponding retinal elements of the eyes are no longer directed at the same object. This places the patient at risk for 2 different visual phenomena: visual confusion and diplopia.

Confusion

Visual confusion is the simultaneous perception of 2 different objects projected onto corresponding retinal areas. The 2 foveal areas are physiologically incapable of simultaneous perception of dissimilar objects. The closest foveal equivalent is retinal rivalry, wherein the 2 perceived images rapidly alternate (Fig 4-6). Confusion may be a phenomenon of nonfoveal retinal areas only. Clinically significant visual confusion is rare.

Diplopia

Double vision, or diplopia, usually results from an acquired misalignment of the visual axes that causes an image to fall simultaneously on the fovea of 1 eye and on a nonfoveal point in the other eye. The object that falls on these noncorresponding points must be outside Panum's area to be seen double. The same object is seen as having 2 different locations in subjective space, and the foveal image is always clearer than the nonfoveal image of the nonfixating eye. The symptom of diplopia depends on the age at onset, duration, and subjective awareness. The younger the child, the greater the ability to suppress, or inhibit, the nonfoveal image.

Central fusional disruption (horror fusionis) is an intractable diplopia that features the avoidance of bifoveal stimulation, an absence of suppression, and a loss of fusional amplitudes. The angle of strabismus may be small or may vary. Horror fusionis can occur in a

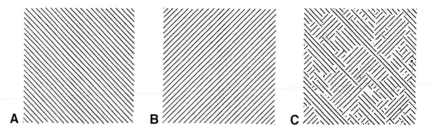

Figure 4-6 Rivalry pattern. **A,** Pattern seen by the left eye. **B,** Pattern seen by the right eye. **C,** Binocular vision. *(Reproduced with permission from von Noorden GK, Campos EC.* Binocular Vision and Ocular Motility: Theory and Management of Strabismus. *6th ed. St Louis: Mosby; 2002:12.)*

number of clinical settings: after disruption of fusion for a prolonged period; after head trauma; and, rarely, in long-standing strabismus. Management can be challenging.

> Lee MC. Acquired central fusional disruption with spontaneous recovery. *Strabismus.* 1998; 6(4):175–179.

Sensory Adaptations in Strabismus

To avoid confusion and diplopia, the visual system can use the mechanisms of suppression and ARC (Fig 4-7). It is important to realize that pathologic suppression and ARC develop only in the immature visual system.

Suppression

Suppression is the alteration of visual sensation that occurs when the images from 1 eye are inhibited or prevented from reaching consciousness during binocular visual activity. Pathologic suppression results from strabismic misalignment of the visual axes. Such suppression can be seen as an adaptation of a visually immature brain to avoid diplopia. Physiologic suppression is the mechanism that prevents physiologic diplopia (diplopia elicited by objects outside Panum's area) from reaching consciousness.

The following classification of suppression may be useful for the clinician:

- *Central versus peripheral. Central suppression* is the term used to describe the mechanism that keeps the foveal image of the deviating eye from reaching consciousness, thereby preventing confusion. *Peripheral suppression* is the mechanism that eliminates diplopia by preventing awareness of the image that falls on the peripheral retina in the deviating eye, the image that resembles the image falling on the fovea of the fixating eye. This form of suppression is clearly pathologic, developing as a cortical adaptation only within an immature visual system. Adults may be unable to develop peripheral suppression and therefore may be unable to eliminate the peripheral second image of the object viewed by the fixating eye (the object of regard) without closing or occluding the deviating eye.
- *Nonalternating versus alternating.* If suppression is unidirectional or always causes the image from the dominant eye to predominate over the image from the deviating

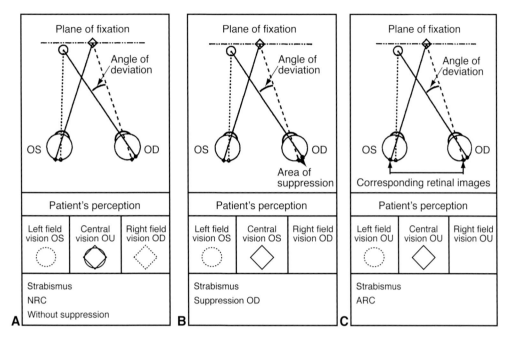

Figure 4-7 Retinal correspondence and suppression in strabismus. **A,** A strabismic patient with normal retinal correspondence (NRC) and without suppression would have diplopia and visual confusion, a common visual direction for 2 separate objects (represented by the superimposition of the images of the fixated diamond and the circle, which is imaged on the fovea of the deviating eye). **B,** The elimination of diplopia and confusion by suppression of the retinal image of the deviating right eye. **C,** The elimination of diplopia and confusion by anomalous retinal correspondence (ARC), an adaptation of visual directions of the deviated right eye. *(Adapted with permission from Kaufman PL, Alm A. Adler's Physiology of the Eye. 10th ed. St Louis: Mosby; 2003:490.)*

eye, the suppression is nonalternating. This type of mechanism may lead to the establishment of strabismic amblyopia. If the process is bidirectional or switches over time between the images of the 2 eyes, the suppression is described as *alternating*.

- *Facultative versus obligatory.* Suppression may be considered *facultative* if present only when the eyes are in the deviated state and absent in all other states. Patients with intermittent exotropia, for instance, often experience suppression when the eyes are divergent but may enjoy high-grade stereopsis when the eyes are straight. In contrast, *obligatory* suppression is present at all times, whether the eyes are deviated or aligned. The suppression scotoma in the deviating eye may be either *relative* (in the sense of permitting some visual sensation) or *absolute* (permitting no perception of light).

Tests of suppression

If a patient with strabismus and NRC does not have diplopia, suppression is present provided the sensory pathways are intact. In less clear-cut situations, several simple tests are available for clinical diagnosis of suppression. (See Subjective Testing for Sensory Adaptations, later in this chapter.)

Management of suppression

Therapy for suppression often involves the treatment of the strabismus itself:

- proper refractive correction
- occlusion or pharmacologic penalization, to permit equal and alternate use of each eye and to overcome any amblyopia that may be present
- alignment of the visual axes, to permit simultaneous stimulation of corresponding retinal elements by the same object

Orthoptic exercises may be attempted to overcome the tendency of the image from one eye to suppress the image from the other eye when both eyes are open. These exercises are designed to make the patient aware of diplopia first, then attempt to fuse the images—both on an instrument and in free space. The role of orthoptics in the therapy of suppression is controversial.

Anomalous Retinal Correspondence

Anomalous retinal correspondence (ARC) can be described as a condition wherein the fovea of the fixating eye has acquired an anomalous common visual direction with a peripheral retinal element in the deviated eye; that is, the 2 foveas have different visual directions. ARC is an adaptation that restores some sense of binocular cooperation. Anomalous binocular vision is a functional state superior to that prevailing in the presence of total suppression. In the development of ARC, the normal sensory development is replaced only gradually and not always completely. The more long-standing the deviation, the more deeply rooted the ARC may become. The period during which ARC may develop probably extends through the first decade of life.

Paradoxical diplopia can occur when ARC persists after surgery. When esotropic patients whose eyes have been set straight or nearly straight report, postoperatively, a crossed diplopic localization of foveal or parafoveal stimuli, they are experiencing paradoxical diplopia (Fig 4-8). Clinically, paradoxical diplopia is a fleeting postoperative phenomenon, seldom lasting longer than a few days to weeks. However, in rare cases, this condition has persisted for much longer.

Testing for ARC

Testing in patients with ARC is performed to determine how patients use their eyes in normal life and to seek out any vestiges of normal correspondence. As discussed earlier, ARC is a sensory adaptation to abnormal ocular alignment. Because the depth of the sensory rearrangement can vary widely, an individual can test positive for both NRC and ARC. Tests that closely simulate everyday use of the eyes are more likely to give evidence of ARC. The more dissociative the test, the more likely the test will produce an NRC response unless the ARC is deeply rooted. Some of the more common tests, in order of most dissociating to least dissociating, are the afterimage test, Worth 4-dot test, red-glass test (dissociation increases with the density of the red filter), amblyoscope, and Bagolini striated glasses. If the patient gives an anomalous localization response in the more dissociative tests, then the depth of ARC is greater. (See the section Subjective Testing for Sensory Adaptations.)

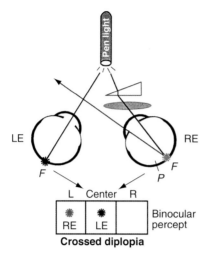

Figure 4-8 Paradoxical diplopia. Diagram of esotropia and ARC, wherein the deviation is being neutralized with a base-out prism. A red glass and base-out prism are placed over the right eye. The prism neutralizes the deviation by moving the retinal image of the pen-light temporally, off the pseudofovea *(P)* to the true fovea *(F)*. Because the pseudofovea is the center of orientation, the image is perceived to fall on the temporal retina and is projected to the opposite field, thus resulting in crossed diplopia. *(Reproduced with permission from Wright KW, Spiegel PH.* Pediatric Ophthalmology and Strabismus. *St Louis: Mosby; 1999:219.)*

The tests for ARC can basically be divided into 2 groups: those that stimulate the fovea of 1 eye and an extrafoveal area of the other eye, and those that stimulate the foveal area in each eye. Note that ARC is a binocular phenomenon, tested for and documented in both eyes simultaneously. Eccentric fixation is a monocular phenomenon found on testing 1 eye alone; it is not necessarily related to ARC. In eccentric fixation, patients do not fixate with the fovea when the fellow eye is covered. On cover testing, the eye remains more or less deviated, depending on how far the nonfoveolar area of fixation is from the fovea. Because some tests for ARC depend on separate stimulation of each fovea, the presence of eccentric fixation can significantly affect the test results. (See also Chapter 5.)

Subjective Testing for Sensory Adaptations

All tests are tainted by the inability of the testing conditions to reproduce the patient's condition of casual seeing. The more dissociative the test, the less the test simulates everyday use of the eyes. These tests should always be performed in conjunction with a cover test to decide whether a fusion response is due to orthophoria or ARC.

Red-glass test

In a patient with strabismus, the red-glass (diplopia) test involves stimulation of both the fovea of the fixating eye and an extrafoveal area of the other eye. First, the patient's deviation is measured objectively. Then a red glass is placed before the nondeviating eye while the patient fixates on a white light. This test can be performed both at distance and at near. If the patient sees only 1 light (either red or white), suppression is present (Fig 4-9A). A 5Δ or 10Δ prism base-up in front of the deviated eye can be used to move the image out of the suppression scotoma, causing the patient to experience diplopia. With NRC, the white image will be localized correctly: the white image is seen below and to the right of the left image (Fig 4-9B). With ARC, the white image will be localized incorrectly: it is seen directly below the image (Fig 4-9C).

The following responses are possible with the red-glass test:

- The patient may see a red light and a white light. If the patient has esotropia, the images appear uncrossed (eg, the red light is to the left of the white light with the red glass over the left eye). This response is known as *homonymous*, or *uncrossed*, *diplopia*. This can easily be remembered because the esotropic patient sees the red light on the same side as the red glass (Fig 4-9D). If the patient has exotropia, the images appear crossed (eg, the red light is to the right of the white light with the red glass over the left eye). This response is known as *heteronymous*, or *crossed*, *diplopia* (Fig 4-9E). If the measured separation between the 2 images equals the previously determined deviation, the patient has NRC.

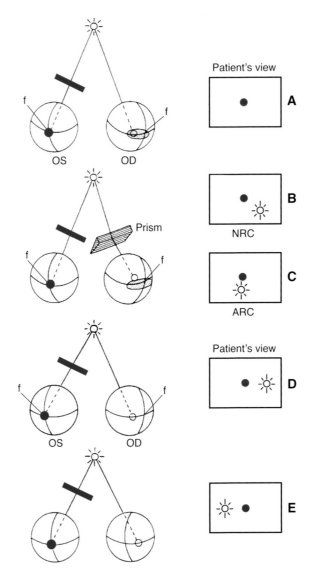

Figure 4-9 Red-glass test for suppression and ARC (see text for explanation; see also Fig 4-7). *(Modified with permission from von Noorden GK, Campos EC. Binocular Vision and Ocular Motility: Theory and Management of Strabismus. 6th ed. St Louis: Mosby; 2002:223.)*

- If the patient sees the 2 lights superimposed so that they appear pinkish despite a measurable esotropia or exotropia, an abnormal localization of retinal points is present. This condition is known as *harmonious anomalous retinal correspondence*.
- If the patient sees 2 lights (with uncrossed diplopia in esotropia and with crossed diplopia in exotropia), but the separation between the 2 images is found to be less than the previously determined deviation, the patient has *unharmonious anomalous retinal correspondence*. Some investigators consider unharmonious ARC to be an artifact of the testing situation.

Worth 4-dot test

In the Worth 4-dot test, a red glass is worn in front of 1 eye and a green glass in front of the other (Fig 4-10). The eye behind the red glass can see red light but not green light because the red glass blocks this wavelength. Similarly, the eye behind the green glass can see green light but not red light. A polarized Worth 4-dot test is available; it is administered and interpreted much like the traditional test except that polarized glasses are worn rather than red and green ones. As with the red-glass test, the Worth 4-dot test can produce a diplopic response in nonsuppression heterotropic NRC and either a diplopic or a fusion response in ARC, depending on the depth of the ARC adaptation. As mentioned earlier, this test must be performed in conjunction with cover testing.

When testing a patient for *monofixation syndrome* (see the section Monofixation Syndrome later in this chapter), the Worth 4-dot test can be used to demonstrate both the presence of peripheral fusion and the absence of bifixation. The standard Worth 4-dot flashlight projects onto a central retinal area of 1° or less when viewed at 10 ft, well within the 1°–4° scotoma characteristic of monofixation syndrome. Therefore, patients with monofixation syndrome will report 2 or 3 lights when viewing at 10 ft, depending on their ocular fixation preference. As the Worth 4-dot flashlight is brought closer to the patient, the dots begin to project onto peripheral retina outside the central monofixation scotoma until a fusion response (4 lights) is obtained. This usually occurs between 2 and 3 ft.

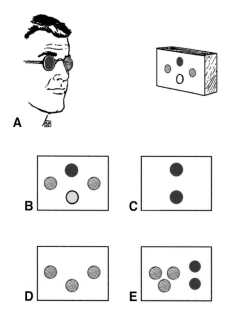

Figure 4-10 The Worth 4-dot test. **A,** Looking through a pair of red and green goggles, the patient views a box with 4 lights (1 red, 2 green, 1 white) at 6 m and at 33 cm (with the 4 lights mounted on a flashlight). The possible responses are given in B to E. **B,** Patient sees all 4 lights: peripheral fusion with orthophoria or strabismus with ARC. Depending on ocular dominance, the light in the 6 o'clock position is seen as white or pink. **C,** Patient sees 2 red lights: suppression in OS. **D,** Patient sees 3 green lights: suppression in OD. **E,** Patient sees 5 lights. The red lights may appear to the right, as in this figure (uncrossed diplopia with esotropia), or to the left of the green lights (crossed diplopia with exotropia). *(Reproduced with permission from von Noorden GK, Campos EC. Binocular Vision and Ocular Motility: Theory and Management of Strabismus. 6th ed. St Louis: Mosby; 2002:221.)*

Bagolini glasses

Bagolini striated glasses are glasses of no dioptric power that have many narrow stria-
tions running parallel in one meridian. These glasses cause the fixation light to appear as
an elongated streak, like micro-Maddox cylinders. The glasses are usually placed at 135°
in front of the right eye and at 45° in front of the left eye. The advantages of the Bagolini
glasses are that they afford the most lifelike testing conditions and permit the examiner
to perform cover testing during the examination. Figure 4-11 summarizes some of the

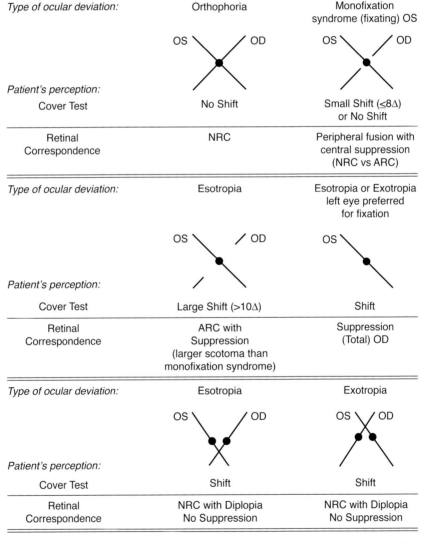

Figure 4-11 Bagolini striated glass test for retinal correspondence and suppression. For these
figures, the Bagolini lens is oriented at 135° in front of the right eye and at 45° in front of the
left eye. The perception of the oblique lines seen by each eye under binocular conditions is
shown. Examples of the types of strabismus in which these responses are commonly found
are given.

possible subjective results of this test. Note that in monofixation syndrome, the central scotoma is perceived as a gap in one of the lines surrounding the fixation light.

4Δ base-out prism test

The 4Δ base-out prism test is a diagnostic maneuver performed primarily to document the presence of a small facultative scotoma in a patient with monofixation syndrome and no manifest small deviation (see the section Monofixation Syndrome later in this chapter). In this test, a 4Δ base-out prism is quickly placed before 1 eye and then the other during binocular viewing, and motor responses are observed (Fig 4-12). Patients with bifixation usually show a version (bilateral) movement away from the eye covered by the prism followed by a unilateral fusional convergence movement of the eye not behind the prism. A similar response occurs regardless of which eye the prism is placed over. Often, no movement is seen in patients with monofixation syndrome when the prism is placed before the nonfixating eye. A refixation version movement is seen when the prism is placed before the fixating eye, but the expected fusional convergence does not occur.

The 4Δ base-out prism test is the least reliable method used to document the presence of a macular scotoma. An occasional patient with bifixation recognizes diplopia when

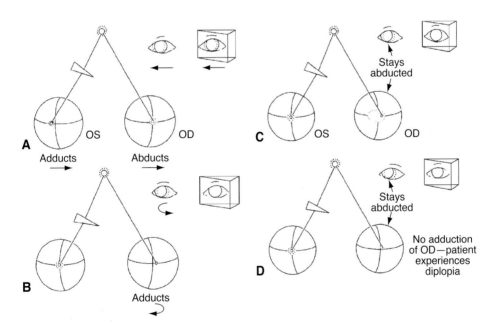

Figure 4-12 The 4Δ base-out prism test. **A,** When a prism is placed over the left eye, dextroversion occurs during refixation of that eye, indicating absence of foveal suppression in the left eye. If a suppression scotoma is present in the left eye, there will be no movement of either eye when placing the prism before the left eye. **B,** A subsequent slow fusional adduction movement of the right eye is observed, indicating absence of foveal suppression in the right eye. **C,** In a second patient, the right eye stays abducted, and the absence of an adduction movement **(B)** indicates foveal suppression in the right eye. **D,** Another cause of absence of the adduction movement is weak fusion, and such patients experience diplopia until refusion occurs spontaneously. *(Reproduced with permission from von Noorden GK, Campos EC. Binocular Vision and Ocular Motility: Theory and Management of Strabismus. 6th ed. St Louis: Mosby; 2002:220.)*

the prism is placed before an eye but makes no convergence movement to correct for it. Patients with monofixation syndrome may switch fixation each time the prism is inserted and show no movement, regardless of which eye is tested.

Afterimage test

The test can be performed by covering a camera flash with black paper and then exposing only a narrow slit, the center of which is covered with black tape to serve as a fixation point, as well as to protect the fovea from exposure. This test involves the stimulation, or labeling, of the macula of each eye with a different linear afterimage, 1 horizontal and 1 vertical. Because suppression scotomata extend along the horizontal retinal meridian and may obscure most of a horizontal afterimage, the vertical afterimage is placed on the deviating eye and the horizontal afterimage on the fixating eye simply by having each eye fixate the linear light filament separately.

The central zone of the linear light is occluded to allow the fovea to fixate and remain unlabeled. The patient is then asked to draw the relative positions of the perceived afterimages. Possible perceptions are shown in Figure 4-13.

Amblyoscope testing

Although its use has declined in recent years, the major amblyoscope (Fig 4-14) in various forms (eg, Clement Clarke synoptophore, American Optical troposcope), was for decades a mainstay in the field of strabismus. The amblyoscope can be used in the measurement of horizontal, vertical, and torsional deviations; in the diagnosis of suppression and retinal correspondence; and in the determination of fusional amplitudes and the

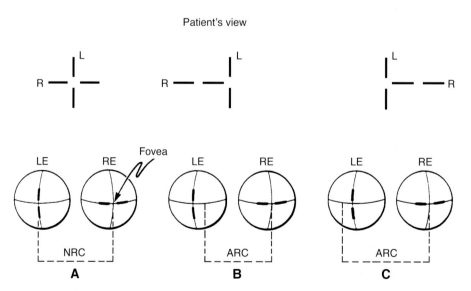

Figure 4-13   Afterimage test. **A,** Normal localization (cross) in normal correspondence (NRC). **B,** Anomalous crossed localization (ARC) in a case of esotropia. **C,** Anomalous uncrossed localization in a case of exotropia. *(Reproduced with permission from von Noorden GK, Campos EC. Binocular Vision and Ocular Motility: Theory and Management of Strabismus. 6th ed. St Louis: Mosby; 2002:227.)*

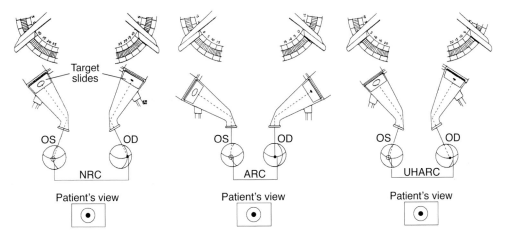

Figure 4-14 Testing with a major amblyoscope for retinal correspondence in a patient with 20 diopters of esotropia. *(Reproduced with permission from von Noorden GK, Campos EC. Binocular Vision and Ocular Motility: Theory and Management of Strabismus. 6th ed. St Louis: Mosby; 2002:229.)*

degree of stereopsis, with testing usually performed by an orthoptist. The major amblyoscope can also be used in exercises designed to overcome suppression and expand fusional amplitudes. A description of this instrument and its uses can be found in the following reference.

von Noorden GK, Campos EC. *Binocular Vision and Ocular Motility: Theory and Management of Strabismus.* 6th ed. St Louis: Mosby; 2002.

Monofixation Syndrome

The term *monofixation syndrome* is used to describe a particular presentation of a sensory state in strabismus. The essential feature of this syndrome is the presence of peripheral fusion with the absence of bimacular fusion due to a physiologic macular scotoma.

A patient with monofixation syndrome may have no manifest deviation but usually has a small heterotropia (less than 8Δ), most commonly esotropia. Stereoacuity is present but reduced. Amblyopia is a common finding. The original description of this entity states that retinal correspondence is normal regardless of whether there is a manifest deviation; this has been questioned by other authors.

Monofixation may be a primary condition. It is a favorable outcome of infantile strabismus surgery. This syndrome can also result from anisometropia or macular lesions. It can be the cause of unilaterally reduced vision when no obvious strabismus is present. If amblyopia is clinically significant, occlusion therapy is indicated.

Diagnosis

To make the diagnosis of monofixation syndrome, the clinician must demonstrate the absence of bimacular fusion by documenting a macular scotoma in the nonfixating eye under binocular conditions; and the presence of peripheral binocular vision (peripheral fusion). Several binocular perimetric techniques have been described to plot the monofixation scotoma. However, they are rarely used clinically.

Vectographic projections of Snellen letters can be used clinically to document the facultative scotoma of the monofixation syndrome. Snellen letters are viewed through polarized analyzers or goggles equipped with liquid crystal shutters in such a way that some letters are seen with only the right eye, some with only the left eye, and some with both eyes. Patients with monofixation syndrome delete letters that are imaged only in the nonfixating eye.

Testing stereoacuity is an important part of the monofixation syndrome evaluation. Any amount of gross stereopsis confirms the presence of peripheral fusion. Most patients with monofixation syndrome demonstrate 200–3000 sec of arc stereopsis. However, because some patients with this syndrome have no demonstrable stereopsis, other tests for peripheral fusion, such as the Worth 4-dot test and Bagolini glasses, must be used in conjunction with stereoacuity measurement. Fine stereopsis (better than 67 sec of arc) is present only in patients with bifixation.

Parks MM. The monofixation syndrome. *Trans Am Ophthalmol Soc.* 1969;67:609–657. (This classic thesis outlines early studies of small-angle deviations and central versus peripheral binocular vision. The development of the various terms used to describe these conditions is also covered in detail.)

von Noorden GK, Campos EC. *Binocular Vision and Ocular Motility: Theory and Management of Strabismus.* 6th ed. St Louis: Mosby; 2002:340–345.

CHAPTER 5

Amblyopia

Amblyopia is a unilateral or, less commonly, bilateral reduction of best-corrected visual acuity that cannot be attributed directly to the effect of any structural abnormality of the eye or the posterior visual pathways. Amblyopia is caused by abnormal visual experience early in life resulting from one of the following:

- strabismus
- anisometropia or high bilateral refractive errors (isometropia)
- stimulus deprivation

Amblyopia is responsible for more unilaterally reduced vision of childhood onset than all other causes combined, with a prevalence of 2%–4% in the North American population. This fact is particularly distressing because, in principle, most amblyopic vision loss is preventable or reversible with timely detection and appropriate intervention. Children with amblyopia or at risk for amblyopia should be identified at a young age, when the prognosis for successful treatment is best. Screening plays an important role in detecting amblyopia and other vision problems at an early age and can be performed in the primary care practitioner's office, allowing the primary care physician to help coordinate the care of these patients, or in community-based vision screening programs. Repeated screening is important for continuing to check for the development of vision problems and is also helpful in detecting false-positive results. A consensus about the best method and the appropriate age to screen has not yet emerged.

Amblyopia is primarily a defect of central vision; the peripheral visual field is usually normal. Experimental studies on animals and clinical studies of infants and young children support the concept of critical periods for sensitivity in developing amblyopia. These critical periods correspond to the period when the child's developing visual system is sensitive to abnormal input caused by stimulus deprivation, strabismus, or significant refractive errors. In general, the critical period for stimulus deprivation amblyopia occurs earlier than that for ocular misalignment or anisometropia. Furthermore, the time necessary for amblyopia to occur during the critical period is shorter for stimulus deprivation than for strabismus or anisometropia.

Although the neurophysiologic mechanisms that underlie amblyopia are far from clear, the study of experimental modification of visual experience in animals and laboratory testing of humans with amblyopia have provided some insights. Animal models have revealed that a variety of profound disturbances of visual system neuron function may result from abnormal early visual experience. Cells of the primary visual cortex can completely lose their innate ability to respond to stimulation of 1 or both eyes, and cells that remain responsive may show significant functional deficiencies. Abnormalities also occur in neurons in the lateral geniculate body. Evidence concerning involvement at the retinal level remains inconclusive; if present, changes in the retina make at most a minor contribution to the overall visual defect.

Several findings from both animals and humans, such as increased spatial summation and lateral inhibition when light detection thresholds are measured using different-sized spots, suggest that the receptive fields of neurons in the amblyopic visual system are abnormally large. This disturbance may account for the *crowding phenomenon* (also known as *contour interaction*), whereby Snellen letters or equivalent symbols of a given size become more difficult to recognize if they are closely surrounded by similar forms, such as a full line or field of letters.

Daw NW. Critical periods and amblyopia. *Arch Ophthalmol.* 1998;116(4):502–505.

Simons K. Preschool vision screening: rationale, methodology, and outcome. *Surv Ophthalmol.* 1996;41(1):3–30.

von Noorden GK. Amblyopia: a multidisciplinary approach. Proctor lecture. *Invest Ophthalmol Vis Sci.* 1985;26(12):1704–1716.

Classification

Amblyopia has traditionally been subdivided in terms of the major disorders that may be responsible for its occurrence.

Strabismic Amblyopia

The most common form of amblyopia develops in the consistently deviating eye of a child with strabismus. Constant, nonalternating heterotropias (typically esodeviations) are most likely to cause significant amblyopia. Strabismic amblyopia is thought to result from competitive or inhibitory interaction between neurons carrying the nonfusible inputs from the 2 eyes, which leads to domination of cortical vision centers by the fixating eye and chronically reduced responsiveness to input by the nonfixating eye. Amblyopia itself does not as a rule prevent diplopia. Older patients with long-standing deviations might develop double vision after strabismus surgery despite the presence of substantially reduced visual acuity from amblyopia.

Several features of typical strabismic amblyopia are uncommon in other forms of amblyopia. In strabismic amblyopia, grating acuity, the ability to detect patterns composed of uniformly spaced stripes, is often reduced considerably less than Snellen acuity. Apparently, the affected eye sees forms in a twisted or distorted manner that interferes more with letter recognition than with the simpler task of determining whether a grating pattern is present. This discrepancy must be considered when the results of tests based on grating detection, such as Teller card preferential looking (a method of estimating acuity in infants and toddlers), are interpreted (Fig 5-1).

When visual acuity is checked with the use of a neutral-density filter, the acuity of an eye with amblyopia tends to decline less sharply than that of a normal eye. This phenomenon is called the *neutral-density filter effect.*

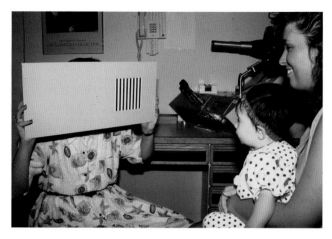

Figure 5-1 Teller acuity card being used to measure the visual acuity in a preverbal child. *(Courtesy of John W. Simon, MD.)*

Eccentric fixation refers to the consistent use of a nonfoveal region of the retina for monocular viewing by an amblyopic eye. Minor degrees of eccentric fixation, detectable only with special tests such as visuscopy, are seen in many patients with strabismic amblyopia and relatively mild acuity loss. A visuscope projects a target with an open center surrounded by 2 concentric circles onto the retina, and the patient is asked to fixate on the target. If the target is not directed at the fovea, the degree of eccentric fixation can be measured using the concentric circles as a guide. Many ophthalmoscopes are equipped with a visuscope. Clinically evident eccentric fixation, detectable by observing the noncentral position of the corneal reflection from the amblyopic eye while it fixates a light with the dominant eye covered, generally implies visual acuity of 20/200 or worse. See Chapter 6 for a discussion of clinical testing. Use of the nonfoveal retina for fixation cannot, in general, be regarded as the primary cause of reduced acuity in affected eyes. The mechanism of this interesting phenomenon, long a source of speculation, remains unknown.

Anisometropic Amblyopia

Second in frequency to strabismic amblyopia, anisometropic amblyopia develops when unequal refractive errors in the 2 eyes causes the image on 1 retina to be chronically defocused. This condition is thought to result partly from the direct effect of image blur on visual acuity development in the involved eye and partly from interocular competition or inhibition similar (but not necessarily identical) to that responsible for strabismic amblyopia. Relatively mild degrees of hyperopic or astigmatic anisometropia (1–2 D) can induce mild amblyopia. Mild myopic anisometropia (less than –3 D) usually does not cause amblyopia, but unilateral high myopia (–6 D or greater) often results in severe amblyopic vision loss. Unless strabismus is present, the eyes of a child with anisometropic amblyopia look normal to the family and primary care physician, typically causing a delay in detection and treatment.

Ametropic Amblyopia

Ametropic amblyopia, a bilateral reduction in acuity that is usually relatively mild, results from large, approximately equal, uncorrected refractive errors in both eyes of a young child. Its mechanism involves the effect of blurred retinal images alone. Hyperopia exceeding about 5 D and myopia in excess of 6 D carry a risk of inducing bilateral amblyopia. Uncorrected bilateral astigmatism in early childhood may result in loss of resolving ability limited to the chronically blurred meridians *(meridional amblyopia)*. The degree of cylindrical ametropia necessary to produce meridional amblyopia is not known, but most ophthalmologists recommend correction of greater than 2 D of cylinder.

Stimulus Deprivation Amblyopia

Deprivation amblyopia may occur when the visual axis is obstructed. The most common cause is a congenital or early acquired cataract, but corneal opacities and vitreous hemorrhage may also be implicated. Deprivation amblyopia is the least common but most damaging and difficult to treat of the various forms of amblyopia. Amblyopic vision loss resulting from a unilateral occlusion of the visual axis tends to be worse than that produced by bilateral deprivation of similar degree because interocular effects add to the direct developmental impact of severe image degradation. Even in bilateral cases, however, acuity can be 20/200 or worse.

In children younger than 6 years, dense congenital cataracts that occupy the central 3 mm or more of the lens must be considered capable of causing severe amblyopia. Similar lens opacities acquired after age 6 years are generally less harmful. Small polar cataracts, around which retinoscopy can be readily performed, and lamellar cataracts, through which a reasonably good view of the fundus can be obtained, may cause mild to moderate amblyopia or may have no effect on visual development. *Occlusion amblyopia* is a form of deprivation amblyopia that may be seen after therapeutic patching.

Diagnosis

Amblyopia is diagnosed when a patient is found to have a condition known to increase the risk of amblyopia and when reduced visual acuity cannot be explained entirely on the basis of physical abnormalities of the eye. Characteristics of vision alone cannot be used to reliably differentiate amblyopia from other forms of vision loss. The crowding phenomenon, for example, is typical of amblyopia but is not pathognomonic or uniformly demonstrable. Afferent pupillary defects rarely occur in amblyopia, and then, only in severe cases. Amblyopia sometimes coexists with vision loss directly caused by an uncorrectable structural abnormality of the eye such as optic nerve hypoplasia or coloboma. When the clinician encounters doubtful or borderline cases of this type ("organic amblyopia") in a young child, it is appropriate to undertake a trial of occlusion therapy. Improvement in vision confirms that amblyopia was indeed present.

Multiple assessments using a variety of tests or performed on different occasions are sometimes required to make a final judgment concerning the presence and severity of amblyopia. General techniques for visual acuity assessment in children are discussed in

Chapter 6, but the clinician trying to determine the degree of amblyopic vision loss in a young patient should keep certain special considerations in mind. The fixation pattern, which indicates the strength of preference for 1 eye or the other under binocular viewing conditions, is a test for estimating the relative level of vision in the 2 eyes for preverbal children with strabismus. This test is quite sensitive for detecting amblyopia, but results can be falsely positive, showing a strong preference when vision is equal or nearly equal in the 2 eyes, particularly with small-angle strabismus.

A variety of optotypes can be used to directly measure acuity in children 3–6 years old. When possible, it is best to use linear symbols to measure visual acuity. Often, however, only isolated symbols can be used, which may lead to underestimated amblyopic vision loss due to the crowding phenomenon. Crowding bars help alleviate this problem (Fig 5-2). In addition, the young child's brief attention span frequently results in measurements that fall short of the true limits of acuity; these results can mimic bilateral amblyopia or obscure or falsely suggest a significant interocular difference.

Treatment

Treatment of amblyopia involves the following steps:

1. Eliminate (if needed) any obstacle to vision, such as a cataract.
2. Correct any significant refractive error.
3. Force use of the poorer eye by limiting use of the better eye.

Cataract Removal

Cataracts capable of producing amblyopia require surgery without unnecessary delay. In young children, amblyopia may develop as quickly as 1 week per age of life. Removal of visually significant congenital lens opacities during the first 4–6 weeks of life is necessary for optimal recovery of vision. In symmetric bilateral cases, the interval between operations on the first and second eyes should be no more than 1–2 weeks. Acutely developing severe traumatic cataracts in children younger than 6 years should be removed within a few weeks of injury, if possible. Significant cataracts with uncertain time of onset also deserve prompt and aggressive treatment during childhood if recent development is at least a possibility (eg, in the case of an opacity that appears to have originated from a posterior

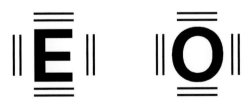

Figure 5-2 Crowding bars, or contour interaction bars, allow the examiner to test crowding phenomenon with isolated optotypes. Bars surrounding the optotype mimic the full row of optotypes to the amblyopic child. *(Reproduced with permission from Coats DK, Jenkins RH. Vision assessment of the pediatric patient. Refinements.* San Francisco: American Academy of Ophthalmology; 1997,1:1.)

lenticonus deformity). Chapter 21 of this volume and BCSC Section 11, *Lens and Cataract,* discuss the special considerations of cataract surgery in children.

Refractive Correction

In general, optical prescription for amblyopic eyes should be based on the refractive error as determined with cycloplegia. Because an amblyopic eye's ability to control accommodation tends to be impaired, this eye cannot be relied on to compensate for uncorrected hyperopia as would a normal child's eye. Sometimes, however, symmetric decreases in plus lens power may be required to foster acceptance of spectacle wear by a child. Refractive correction for aphakia following cataract surgery in childhood must be provided promptly to avoid compounding the visual deprivation effect of the lens opacity with that of a severe optical deficit. Both anisometropic and ametropic amblyopia may improve or resolve with refractive correction alone over several months. Given this, many ophthalmologists wait to initiate patching or penalization (discussed in the following section) in order to see whether the vision improves with spectacle correction alone. The role of refractive surgery in those patients who fail conventional treatment with spectacles and/or contact lenses is under investigation.

Cotter SA; Pediatric Eye Disease Investigator Group. Treatment of anisometropic amblyopia in children with refractive correction. *Ophthalmology.* 2006;113(6):895–903.

Paysse EA. Photorefractive keratectomy for anisometropic amblyopia in children. *Trans Am Ophthalmol Soc.* 2004;102:341–371.

Occlusion and Optical Degradation

Full-time occlusion of the sound eye is defined as occlusion during all waking hours. This treatment is usually performed using commercially available adhesive patches. Spectacle-mounted occluders or special opaque contact lenses can be used as an alternative to full-time patching if skin irritation or inadequate adhesion is a significant problem, provided that close supervision ensures that the spectacles remain in place consistently. (Switching to a different brand of patch or preparing the skin with tincture of benzoin or ostomy adhesive before application can eliminate most skin-related problems.) Rarely, strabismus may result during full-time patching; it is not known whether strabismus would have occurred with other forms of amblyopia treatment. Therefore, the child whose eyes are consistently or intermittently straight may benefit by being given some opportunity to see binocularly. Modest reductions in patching are employed by many ophthalmologists (removing the patch for an hour or two a day) to reduce the likelihood of occlusion amblyopia or of inducing strabismus.

Part-time occlusion, defined as occlusion for 1–6 hours per day, has been shown to achieve the same results as the prescription of full-time occlusion. The relative duration of patch-on and patch-off intervals should reflect the degree of amblyopia; for moderate to severe deficits, at least 6 hours per day is preferred.

Compliance with occlusion therapy for amblyopia declines with increasing age. The effectiveness of more acceptable part-time patching regimens in older children is being actively investigated. Furthermore, studies in older children with amblyopia have shown that treatment can still be beneficial beyond the first decade of life. This is especially true in children who have not previously undergone treatment.

Other methods of amblyopia treatment involve optical degradation of the better eye's image to the point that it becomes inferior to the amblyopic eye's, an approach often called *penalization.* Use of the amblyopic eye is thus promoted within the context of binocular seeing. Studies have demonstrated that pharmacologic penalization can be used to successfully treat moderate levels of amblyopia. The improvement in vision has been shown to be similar to that obtained with the prescription of patching. A cycloplegic agent (usually atropine 1% drops or homatropine 5% drops) is administered to the better-seeing eye so that it is unable to accommodate. As a result, the better eye experiences blur with near viewing and, if uncorrected hyperopia is present, with distance viewing. This form of treatment has been demonstrated to be as effective as patching for mild to moderate amblyopia (visual acuity of 20/100 or better in the amblyopic eye). Depending on the depth of amblyopia and the response to prior treatment, the hyperopic correction of the dominant eye can be reduced to enhance the effect. Regular follow-up of patients whose amblyopia is being treated with cycloplegia is important to avoid reverse amblyopia in the previously preferred eye.

Pharmacologic penalization offers the particular advantage of being difficult to thwart even if the child objects. Alternative methods of treatment based on the same principle involve prescribing excessive plus-power lenses (fogging) or diffusing filters. These methods avoid potential pharmacologic side effects and may be capable of inducing greater blur. If the child is wearing glasses, application of translucent tape or a Bangerter foil (a neutral-density filter) to the spectacle lens can be tried. Proper utilization (no peeking!) of spectacle-borne devices must be closely monitored.

Another benefit of pharmacologic penalization and other nonoccluding methods in patients with straight eyes is that the eyes can work together, a great practical advantage in children with latent nystagmus.

Pediatric Eye Disease Investigator Group. A randomized trial of atropine vs. patching for treatment of moderate amblyopia in children. *Arch Ophthalmol.* 2002;120(3):268–278.

Scheiman MM, Hertle RW, Beck RW, et al. Randomized trial of treatment of amblyopia in children aged 7 to 17 years. *Arch Ophthalmol.* 2005:123(4):437–447.

Complications of Therapy

Any form of amblyopia therapy introduces the possibility of overtreatment leading to amblyopia in the originally better eye. Full-time occlusion carries the greatest risk of this complication and requires close monitoring, especially in the younger child. The first follow-up visit after initiation of treatment should occur within 1 week for an infant and after an interval corresponding to 1 week per year of age for the older child (eg, 4 weeks for a 4-year-old). Subsequent visits can be scheduled at longer intervals based on early response. Part-time occlusion and optical degradation methods allow for less frequent observation, but regular follow-up is still critical. The parents of a strabismic child should be instructed to watch for a switch in fixation preference and to report its occurrence promptly. Iatrogenic amblyopia can usually be treated successfully with judicious patching of the better-seeing eye or by alternating occlusion. Sometimes, simply stopping treatment altogether for a few weeks leads to equalization of vision.

The desired endpoint of therapy for unilateral amblyopia is free alternation of fixation (although 1 eye may still be used somewhat more frequently than the other), linear Snellen acuity that differs by no more than 1 line between the 2 eyes, or both. The time required for completion of treatment depends on the following:

- degree of amblyopia
- choice of therapeutic approach
- compliance with the prescribed regimen
- age of the patient

More severe amblyopia, less complete obstruction of the dominant eye's vision, and older age are all associated with a need for more prolonged treatment. Full-time occlusion during infancy may reverse substantial strabismic amblyopia in 1 week or less. In contrast, an older child who wears a patch only after school and on weekends may require a year or more of treatment to overcome a moderate deficit.

Compliance issues

Lack of compliance with the therapeutic regimen is a common problem that can prolong the period of treatment or lead to outright failure. If difficulties derive from a particular treatment method, a suitable alternative should be sought. Families who appear to lack sufficient motivation should be counseled concerning the importance of the project and the need for firmness in carrying it out. They can be reassured that once an appropriate routine is established and maintained for a short time, the daily effort required is likely to diminish, especially if the amblyopia improves.

The problems associated with an unusually resistant child vary according to age. In infancy, restraining the child through physical methods such as arm splints or mittens or merely making the patch more adhesive with tincture of benzoin may be useful. For children older than 3 years, creating goals and offering rewards tends to work well, as does linking patching to play activities (eg, decorating the patch each day or patching while the child plays a video game). Authoritative words directed specifically toward the child by the doctor may also help. The toddler period (1–3 years) is particularly challenging.

Unresponsiveness

In some cases, even conscientious application of an appropriate therapeutic program fails to improve vision at all or beyond a certain level. Complete or partial unresponsiveness to treatment occasionally affects younger children but most often occurs in patients older than 5 years. The decision of whether to initiate or continue treatment in a prognostically unfavorable situation should take into account the wishes of the patient and family. Primary therapy should generally be terminated if there is a lack of demonstrable progress over 3–6 months with good compliance.

Before it is concluded that intractable amblyopia is present, refraction should be rechecked, the pupils carefully reevaluated, and the macula and optic nerve critically inspected for subtle evidence of hypoplasia or other malformation that might have been previously overlooked. Neuroimaging might be considered in cases that inexplicably fail to respond to treatment. Amblyopia associated with unilateral high myopia and extensive myelination of retinal nerve fibers is a specific syndrome in which treatment failure is particularly common.

Recurrence

When amblyopia treatment is discontinued after fully or partially successful completion, approximately 25% of patients show some degree of recurrence, which can usually be reversed with renewed therapeutic effort. Institution of a maintenance regimen such as patching for 1–3 hours per day, optical penalization with spectacles, or pharmacologic penalization with atropine 1 or 2 days per week can prevent backsliding. If the need for maintenance treatment is established, treatment must be continued until stability of visual acuity is demonstrated with no treatment other than regular spectacles. This may require periodic monitoring until age 8–10 years. As long as vision remains stable, intervals of up to 6 months between follow-up visits are acceptable. The improvement in visual acuity that is obtained in most children treated between 7 and 12 years of age is sustained following cessation of treatment.

CHAPTER 6

Diagnostic Techniques for Strabismus and Amblyopia

History and Characteristics of the Presenting Complaint

When the patient is a child, it is especially important to obtain information regarding the mother's pregnancy, paying close attention to maternal health, gestational age at the time of birth, birth weight, and neonatal history. The physician should also ask about the child's developmental milestones.

It is desirable to document the age of onset of a deviation or symptom. Old photographs may be useful for this purpose. In addition, the physician should seek to answer the following questions about the deviation or symptom:

- Did its onset coincide with trauma or illness?
- Is the deviation constant or intermittent?
- Is it present for distance or near vision or both?
- Is it unilateral or alternating?
- Is it present only when the patient is inattentive or fatigued?
- Does the child close 1 eye?
- Is the deviation associated with double vision?

Earlier treatment should be reviewed, such as amblyopia therapy, spectacle correction, use of miotics, orthoptic therapy, or prior eye muscle surgery. While obtaining the history, the physician should observe the patient continually, noting such behaviors as head posturing, head movement, attentiveness, and motor control.

Past and present medications should be recorded, along with drug sensitivities and allergic responses. Any history of thyroid or neurologic problems should be particularly emphasized. It is also important to document anesthetic methods used for previous surgeries and any related problems, and a detailed family history of strabismus or other eye disorders.

Assessment of Visual Acuity

Distance Visual Acuity

Several tests are available for distance visual acuity determination. The system used to measure vision should be properly calibrated for the test distance to be utilized. Table 6-1 lists the expected acuity for various tests at different ages.

Table 6-1 Normal Visual Acuity Using Various Tests in Children

Age (Years)	Vision Test	Normal
0–2	Visually evoked potential (VEP)	20/30 (age 1)
0–2	Preferential looking	20/30 (age 2)
0–2	Fixation behavior	CSM (see text)
2–5	Allen pictures	20/40–20/20
2–5	HOTV	20/40–20/20
2–5	E-game	20/40–20/20
5+	Snellen	20/30–20/20

By convention, visual acuity is determined first for the right eye and then for the left. A patch or occluder is used in front of the left eye as the acuity of the right eye is checked, then vice versa. An adhesive patch is the most effective occluder. The line with the smallest figures in which the majority of letters can be read accurately is recorded; if the patient misses a few of the figures on a line, a notation is made. If the patient does not have corrective lenses, a pinhole may be used to estimate the best visual acuity potential.

Patients with poor vision may need to walk to the chart until they can see the 20/400 line. In such cases, visual acuity is recorded as the distance in feet (numerator) over the size of the letter (denominator); for example, if the patient is able to read the big E at 5 ft, the acuity would be recorded as 5/400. Because the selection of large figures is limited, it is advisable to confirm measurements slightly closer to the chart using figures that can be changed.

Visual acuity assessment of children is often difficult, and the clinician must resort to various means of evaluation. In preverbal or nonverbal children, acuity can be evaluated by the *CSM method. C* refers to the location of the corneal light reflex as the patient fixates the examiner's light under monocular conditions (opposite eye covered). Normally, the reflected light from the cornea is near the *center* of the cornea, and it should be positioned symmetrically in both eyes. If the fixation target is viewed eccentrically, fixation is termed *uncentral (UC). S* refers to the *steadiness* of fixation on the examiner's light as it is held motionless and as it is slowly moved about. The S evaluation is also done under monocular conditions. *M* refers to the ability of the strabismic patient to *maintain* alignment first with 1 eye, then with the other, as the opposite eye is uncovered. Maintenance of fixation is evaluated under binocular conditions. Inability to maintain fixation with either eye with the opposite eye uncovered is presumptive evidence of a difference in acuity between the 2 eyes. Thus, preverbal or nonverbal patients with strong fixation preference in 1 eye should be suspected of having amblyopia in the other eye. An eye that has eccentric fixation and nystagmoid movements when attempting fixation would have its visual acuity designated *uncentral, unsteady,* and *unmaintained (UC, US, UM).*

In a child with straight eyes, it is impossible to tell whether he or she will maintain fixation with either eye unless the *induced tropia test* is used. This test is performed by placing a base-vertical prism of 10–15 prism diopters (Δ) over 1 eye to induce a vertical deviation. An alternative method involves holding a prism with base in to induce esotropia. The patient is then tested for the ability to maintain fixation with either eye under binocular, albeit dissociated, viewing conditions. It is also important to determine whether each eye can maintain fixation through smooth pursuit or a blink; strong fixation preference for 1 eye indicates amblyopia in the nonpreferred eye.

Occasionally, avoidance movements can be demonstrated when the good eye is occluded. The patient may attempt to maneuver around the occluder when the good eye is occluded but not when the poorly seeing eye is covered. A child with poor vision in the right eye, for example, might be noted to "fix and follow" (F and F) more poorly using that eye and to object to occlusion of the left eye.

The visual acuity of preschool-aged and older children can be tested using the illiterate E test (the *E-game*), letters, numbers, or symbols, all generically referred to as *optotypes*. Children being tested with the E-game are asked to point their hand or fingers in the direction of the E. This test can be difficult to use because of developmental status and confusion of right versus left even among children with good acuity. Visual acuity testing with Snellen letters or numbers requires the child to name each letter or number, whereas visual acuity testing with the HOTV test or with LEA symbols can be done by matching, a cognitively easier task. Whenever possible, a line of optotypes or single optotypes surrounded by *contour interaction bars* ("crowding bars") should be used to prevent the overestimation of visual acuity of an amblyopic eye that often occurs with isolated optotypes (see Chapter 5, Fig 5-2). Isolated optotypes should be used only if the child cannot be tested with any other class of optotype; Allen pictures do not provide any contour interaction, and their overall size and the width of their underlying components fail to conform to accepted parameters of optotype design.

In addition to recording the results, the clinician should identify the type of test used in order to facilitate comparisons with measurements taken at other times. Most pediatric ophthalmologists consider Snellen acuity most reliable, followed by HOTV, LEA symbols, the illiterate E test, Allen pictures, and fixation behavior. The most reliable test that the child can perform should be used. Preferential looking techniques using Teller acuity cards can be a useful adjunctive test for comparing visual acuity between fellow eyes in infants and preverbal children. The Cardiff Acuity Test, which uses vanishing optotypes and preferential looking techniques, is popular in Europe.

LogMAR testing is becoming more popular. LogMAR is expressed as the logarithm of the minimum angle of resolution and converts the geometric sequence of a traditional test chart to a linear scale. The use of LogMAR allows more effective analysis of visual acuity scores and more precise comparisons of results. This system is often utilized in research protocols.

Patients with latent nystagmus may show better visual acuity with both eyes together than with 1 eye occluded. To assess distance monocular visual acuity in this situation, it is helpful to fog the eye not being tested with a lens that is +5 D greater than the refractive error in that eye.

Wright KW, Walonker F, Edelman P. 10-Diopter fixation test for amblyopia. *Arch Ophthalmol.* 1981;99(7):1242–1246.

Near Visual Acuity

Uncorrected and corrected near visual acuity are determined, again using age-appropriate symbols. Because of inaccuracy related to viewing distance, near visual acuities should never be compared with distance acuities in children. A measurement of near visual acuity in children with reduced vision is important in helping determine how they function at school.

Assessment of Ocular Alignment

Ocular alignment tests can be grouped into 4 basic types: cover tests, corneal light reflex tests, dissimilar image tests, and dissimilar target tests.

Cover Tests

Eye movement capability, image formation and perception, foveal fixation in each eye, attention, and cooperation are all necessities for cover testing. If a patient is unable to maintain constant fixation on an accommodative target, the results of cover testing may not be valid, and this battery of tests therefore should not be used.

There are 3 types of cover tests: the cover-uncover test, the alternate cover test, and the simultaneous prism and cover test. All can be performed with fixation at distance or near.

The monocular *cover-uncover test* is the most important test for detecting the presence of manifest strabismus and for differentiating a heterophoria from a heterotropia (Fig 6-1). As 1 eye is covered, the examiner watches carefully for any movement in the opposite, *noncovered* eye; such movement indicates the presence of a heterotropia. With movement of the noncovered eye assumed to be absent, movement of the *covered* eye in one direction just after the cover is applied and a movement in the opposite direction (a fusional movement) as the cover is removed indicate a heterophoria that becomes manifest only when binocularity is interrupted. If the patient has a heterophoria, the eyes will be straight before and after the cover-uncover test; the deviation that appears during the test is a result of interruption of binocular vision. A patient with a heterotropia, however, starts out with a deviated eye and ends up (after the test) with either the same or the opposite eye deviated (if the opposite eye is the deviated one, the condition is termed *alternating heterotropia*). Some patients may have straight eyes and start out with a heterophoria prior to the cover-uncover test; however, after prolonged testing—and therefore prolonged interruption of binocular vision—dissociation into a manifest heterotropia can occur.

The *alternate cover test (prism and cover test)* measures the total deviation, regardless of whether it is latent or manifest (Fig 6-2). This test does not specify how much of each type of deviation is present (ie, it does not separate the heterophoria from the heterotropia). This test should be done at both distance and near fixation. Once dissociation is achieved, the amount of deviation is measured using prisms to eliminate the eye movement as the cover is alternately switched from eye to eye. It may be necessary to use both horizontally and vertically placed prisms. The amount of prism power required is the measure of deviation. Two horizontal or 2 vertical prisms should not be superimposed on each other because this can induce significant measurement errors. Their values cannot

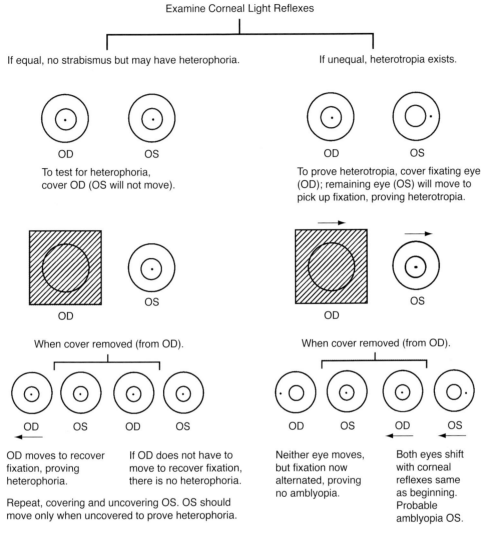

Figure 6-1 The monocular cover-uncover test.

be directly added. A more accurate method for measuring large deviations is to place prisms in front of each eye, although it should be noted that these are not perfectly additive either. However, it is acceptable to superimpose a horizontal prism on a vertical prism before the same eye if necessary.

Whereas the alternate cover test measures the total deviation (heterophoria and heterotropia), the *simultaneous prism and cover test* is helpful in determining the actual heterotropia when both eyes are uncovered (heterotropia alone). The test is performed by covering the fixating eye at the same time the prism is placed in front of the deviating eye. The test is repeated using increasing prism powers until the deviated eye no longer shifts. This test has special application in monofixation syndrome, which may include a small-angle heterotropia. Patients with this condition may reduce the amount of deviation measured in the alternate cover test by exerting at least partial control over a coexisting

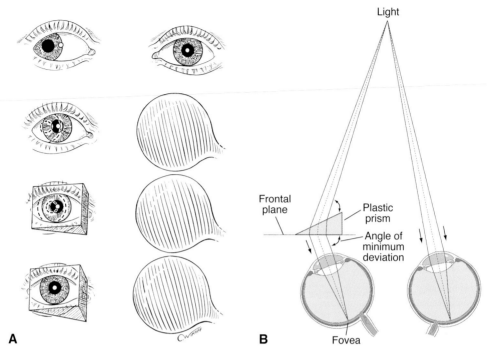

Figure 6-2 The alternate cover test. **A,** Top row: A right exotropia. Second row: The cover test shows movement of the right eye to fixate when the left eye is covered. Third row: A small prism introduced before the right eye begins to neutralize the deviation. Bottom row: The correct prism has been introduced, and no more movement is seen when the cover is alternated between eyes. **B,** The diagram shows how the prism eliminates movement on cover testing by aligning rays of light from the fixation target with the fovea in the exotropic right eye. The size of the prism gives a measurement of the exotropia. *(Reproduced with permission from Simon JW, Calhoun JH. A Child's Eyes: A Guide to Pediatric Primary Care. Gainesville, FL: Triad Publishing; 1997:72.)*

heterophoria through peripheral fusion when both eyes are open. In this instance, the simultaneous prism and cover test measures the amount of heterotropia in a deviation that has a superimposed heterophoria. This test may be useful in assessing the deviation under real-life conditions with both eyes viewing.

Thompson JT, Guyton DL. Ophthalmic prisms. Measurement errors and how to minimize them. *Ophthalmology*. 1983;90(3):204–210.

Light Reflex Tests

Corneal light reflex tests are useful in assessing ocular alignment in patients who cannot cooperate sufficiently to allow cover testing or who have poor fixation. The main tests of this type are the Hirschberg, modified Krimsky, Brückner, and major amblyoscope methods.

The *Hirschberg method* is based on the premise that 1 mm of decentration of the corneal light reflection corresponds to approximately 7°, or 15Δ, of ocular deviation of the visual axis. Therefore, a light reflex at the pupillary margin is about 2 mm from the pupillary center (with a 4-mm pupil), which corresponds to 15°, or approximately 30Δ, of deviation. A reflex in the mid-iris region is about 4 mm from the pupillary center, which is roughly 30°, or 60Δ, of deviation; similarly, a reflex at the limbus is about 45°, or 90Δ, of deviation (Fig 6-3).

The *Krimsky method* uses reflections produced on both corneas by a penlight and is ideally used at near fixation. The original method involved placing prisms in front of the deviating eye. More common modifications today involve holding prisms before the fixating eye or split between the 2 eyes. By adjusting the prisms to center the corneal reflection in the deviated eye, it is possible to approximate and quantitate the near deviation (Fig 6-4). The Hirschberg and Krimsky methods can be inaccurate even when used by experienced strabismologists. Therefore, their use is often limited to patients who are uncooperative or have vision that is too poor to allow for a measurement with other techniques.

The angle kappa can affect light reflex measurements. *Angle kappa* is the angle between the visual axis and the anatomical pupillary axis of the eye. If the fovea is temporal to the pupillary axis (as is usually the case), the corneal light reflection will be slightly nasal to the center of the cornea. This is termed *positive angle kappa* and simulates exodeviation. If the position of the fovea is nasal to the pupillary axis, the corneal light reflection will be slightly temporal to the center of the cornea. This is termed *negative angle kappa* and simulates esodeviation (Fig 6-5). An angle kappa will not affect any of the cover tests.

In the *Brückner* test, the direct ophthalmoscope is used to obtain a red reflex simultaneously in both eyes. If strabismus is present, the deviated eye will have a lighter and brighter reflex than the fixating eye. Note that this test detects, but does not measure, the deviation. This test also identifies opacities in the visual axis and moderate to severe anisometropia. The Brückner test is primarily used by primary care practitioners to screen for strabismus and anisometropia.

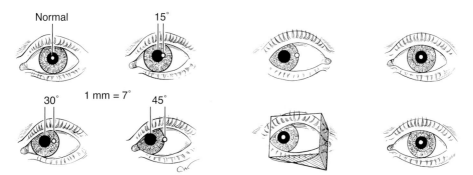

Figure 6-3 Hirschberg test. The extent to which the corneal light reflex is displaced from the center of the pupil provides an approximation of the angular size of the deviation (in this example, a left esotropia). *(Reproduced with permission from Simon JW, Calhoun JH. A Child's Eyes: A Guide to Pediatric Primary Care. Gainesville, FL: Triad Publishing; 1997:72.)*

Figure 6-4 Original Krimsky test. The right exotropia is measured by the size of the prism required to center the pupillary reflexes, as shown at bottom. *(Reproduced with permission from Simon JW, Calhoun JH. A Child's Eyes: A Guide to Pediatric Primary Care. Gainesville, FL: Triad Publishing; 1997:72.)*

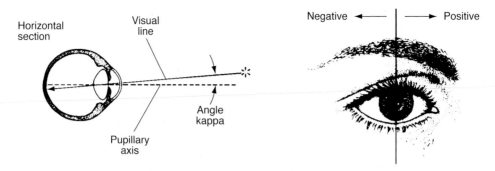

Figure 6-5 Angle kappa. A positive angle (light reflex medial to the vertical line) simulates exotropia, whereas a negative angle (light reflex lateral to the vertical line) simulates esotropia. *(Reprinted from Parks MM.* Ocular Motility and Strabismus. *Hagerstown, MD: Harper & Row; 1975.)*

The *major amblyoscope method* uses separate target illumination, which can be moved to center the corneal light reflection. The amount of deviation is then read directly from the scale of the amblyoscope (see Chapter 4).

Choi RY, Kushner BJ. The accuracy of experienced strabismologists using the Hirschberg and Krimsky tests. *Ophthalmology.* 1998;105(7):1301–1306.

Dissimilar Image Tests

Dissimilar image tests are 1-target tests in which the image of the target is made artificially dissimilar in both eyes. Because one image falls on the fovea of one eye and on a nonfoveal region of the other eye in strabismic patients, esotropic patients perceive the images homonymously, and exotropic patients perceive them as crossed. All vertical deviations result in vertically crossed diplopia. The 3 most commonly used of these tests are the Maddox rod test, the double Maddox rod test, and the red glass test.

The *Maddox rod test* uses a specially constructed device consisting of a series of parallel cylinders that converts a point source of light into a line image. The optical properties of the cylinders cause the streak of light to be situated 90° to the orientation of the parallel cylinders. Because fusion is precluded by the Maddox rod, heterophorias and heterotropias cannot be differentiated. The Maddox rod can be used to test for horizontal and vertical deviations, and, when used in conjunction with another Maddox rod, for cyclodeviations.

To test for horizontal deviations, the Maddox rod is placed in front of one eye (for this example, the right eye) with the cylinders in the horizontal direction. The patient fixates a point source of light and then sees a vertical line with the right eye and a white light with the left eye. If the light superimposes the line, orthophoria is present. In this example, if the light is on the left side of the line, an esodeviation is present; and if the light is on the right side of the line, an exodeviation is present. A similar procedure with the cylinders aligned vertically is used to test for vertical deviations. To measure the amount of deviation, the examiner holds prisms of different powers until the line superimposes the point source. The Maddox rod test is not a satisfactory test for horizontal deviations, however, because accommodative convergence cannot be controlled.

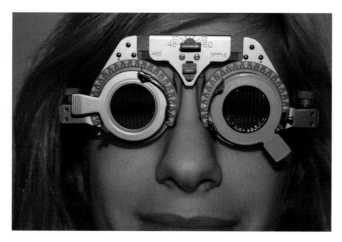

Figure 6-6 Double Maddox rod. Cylinders are aligned vertically to produce 2 horizontal lines. *(Courtesy of Scott Olitsky, MD.)*

The *double Maddox rod test* is used to determine cyclodeviations. A Maddox rod is placed in a trial frame or phoropter and positioned in front of each eye, with the rods aligned vertically so that the patient sees horizontal line images (Fig 6-6). The patient or examiner rotates the axes of the rods until the lines are perceived to be parallel. To facilitate the patient's recognition of the 2 lines, it is often helpful to dissociate the lines by placing a small prism base-up or base-down in front of 1 eye. The degrees of deviation and the direction (incyclo or excyclo) can be determined by the angle of rotation that causes the line images to appear horizontal and parallel. Traditionally, a red Maddox rod was placed before the right eye and a white Maddox rod before the left, but evidence suggests the different colors can cause fixation artifacts that do not occur if the same color is used bilaterally.

In the *red glass test,* a red glass is placed in front of the right eye. This test is used for the same purpose as the Maddox rod test but is not applicable to cyclodeviations. As in the Maddox rod test, prisms are used to eliminate the horizontal or vertical diplopia, and the amount of deviation is recorded.

Dissimilar Target Tests

Dissimilar target tests are based on the patient's response to the dissimilar images created by each eye viewing a different target; the deviation is measured first with 1 eye fixating and then with the other. In these tests, in contrast to dissimilar image tests, diplopia is created by having the patient observe 2 different targets simultaneously, with each target seen by 1 eye only. Esotropic patients will have crossed diplopia, and exotropic patients homonymous diplopia. Confusion in interpreting the results will occur if this distinction is not recognized by the examiner. There are several dissimilar target tests, but the 3 most frequently encountered are the Lancaster red-green projection test, the Hess screen test, and the major amblyoscope test. Though used less commonly in clinical practice than cover and light reflex tests, they may be useful in the evaluation of patients with complex strabismus.

The *Lancaster red-green test* uses red-green goggles that can be reversed, a red-slit projector, a green-slit projector, and a screen ruled into squares. The patient's head is held steady; by convention, the test is begun with the red filter in front of the right eye. The examiner projects a red slit onto the screen, and the patient is asked to place the green slit so that it appears to coincide with the red slit. The relative positions of the 2 streaks are then recorded. The test is repeated for the diagnostic positions of gaze (these positions are discussed in the next section), and the goggles are then reversed so that the deviation with the fellow eye fixating can be recorded. The Lancaster red-green test is used primarily for patients with diplopia caused by incomitant strabismus and requires that the patient have normal retinal correspondence (see Chapter 4). The *Hess screen test* uses a principle similar to that used in the Lancaster red-green test.

The *major amblyoscope test* uses dissimilar targets that the patient is asked to superimpose. If the patient has normal retinal correspondence, the horizontal, vertical, and torsional deviations can be read directly from the calibrated scale of the amblyoscope (see Chapter 4, Fig 4-14).

Positions of Gaze

The *primary position of gaze* is the position of the eyes when fixating straight ahead on an object at infinity. For practical purposes, infinity is considered to be 20 ft (6 m), and for this position the head should be straight.

Cardinal positions are those 6 positions of gaze in which the prime mover is 1 muscle of each eye, together called *yoke muscles* (see Chapter 3, Fig 3-2). *Midline positions* are straight up and straight down from primary position. These latter 2 gaze positions help determine the elevating and depressing capabilities of the eye, but they do not isolate any 1 muscle because 2 elevator and 2 depressor muscles affect midline gaze positions.

The phrase *diagnostic positions of gaze* has been applied to the composite of these 9 gaze positions: the 6 cardinal positions, straight up and down, and primary position. For patients with vertical strabismus, the diagnostic positions of gaze include forced head tilt to the right and left (see the section 3-Step Test, later in the chapter). Several schemes have been devised to record the results of ocular alignment and motility in the various diagnostic positions of gaze (Fig 6-7).

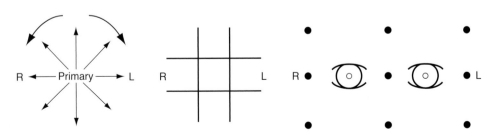

Figure 6-7 Three examples of methods for recording the results of ocular alignment testing.

Assessment of Eye Movements

Ocular Rotations

Generally, when eye movements are assessed, versions are tested first. The examiner should pay particular attention to the movements of both eyes into the 9 diagnostic positions of gaze. Limitations of movement into these positions and asymmetry of excursion of the 2 eyes should be noted. Spinning the child, or provoking the doll's head phenomenon, may be helpful in eliciting the vestibular-stimulated eye movements. If versions are not full, duction movements should be tested for each eye separately. BCSC Section 5, *Neuro-Ophthalmology,* also discusses testing of the ocular motility system.

Convergence

Alignment at near is usually measured at 13 in (33 cm) directly in front of the patient in the horizontal plane. Comparison of the alignment in the primary position at both distance and near fixation helps assess the accommodative convergence (synkinetic near) reflex. The *near point of convergence* is determined by placing a fixation object at 40 cm in the midsagittal plane of the patient's head. As the subject fixates on the object, it is moved toward the subject until 1 eye loses fixation and turns out. The point at which this action occurs is the near point of convergence. The eye that is able to maintain fixation is considered to be the dominant eye. The normal near point of convergence is 8–10 cm or less. This determination does not distinguish between fusional and accommodative convergence, and any heterophoria that is present should be taken into account and corrected for algebraically.

Accommodative convergence/accommodation ratio

The *accommodative convergence/accommodation (AC/A) ratio* is defined as the amount of convergence measured in prism diopters per unit (diopter) change in accommodation. There are 2 methods of clinical measurement (see also BCSC Section 3, *Clinical Optics*): the gradient method and the heterophoria method.

1. The *gradient method* arrives at the AC/A ratio by dividing the change in deviation in prism diopters by the change in lens power. An accommodative target must be used, and the working distance (typically at 1/3 m or 6 m) is held constant. Plus or minus lenses (eg, +1, +2, +3, −1, −2, −3) are used to vary the accommodative requirement. This method measures the *stimulus AC/A ratio,* which is not necessarily identical to the *response AC/A ratio.* The latter can be determined only with the use of an optometer that records the change in accommodation actually produced.
2. The *heterophoria method* employs the distance–near relationship, measuring the distance and near deviations. A similar alignment is normally present for distance and near fixation. If the patient is more exotropic or less esotropic at near, too little convergence, or a low AC/A ratio, is present; if the patient is more esotropic or less

exotropic at near, a high AC/A ratio is present. In accommodative esotropia, an increase of esotropia of 10Δ or more from distance to near fixation is considered to represent a high AC/A ratio.

An abnormally high AC/A ratio can be managed optically, pharmacologically, or surgically. For example, plus lens spectacles for hyperopia reduce accommodation and therefore reduce accommodative convergence. This principle is the mainstay of the medical management of esotropia. Bifocals reduce or eliminate the need to accommodate for near fixation. This optical management may be used for excess convergence at near—that is, an esodeviation greater at near. Underplussed or overminused spectacles create the need for greater-than-normal accommodation. This excess accommodation creates more accommodative convergence and is occasionally used to reduce an exodeviation.

Long-acting cholinesterase inhibitors (eg, echothiophate iodide) can be used to decrease accommodative convergence. These drugs act directly on the ciliary body, facilitating transmission at the myoneural junction. They reduce the central demand for accommodative innervation and thus reduce the amount of convergence induced by accommodation.

Fusional Vergence

Vergences move the 2 eyes in opposite directions. Fusional vergences are motor responses used to eliminate horizontal, vertical, or torsional image disparity. They can be grouped by the following functions:

- *Fusional convergence* eliminates bitemporal retinal disparity and controls an exophoria.
- *Fusional divergence* eliminates binasal retinal disparity and controls an esophoria.
- *Vertical fusional vergence* controls a hyperphoria or hypophoria.
- *Torsional fusional vergence* controls incyclophoria or excyclophoria.

Fusional vergences can be measured by using a haploscopic device (major amblyoscope), a rotary prism, or a bar prism, and gradually increasing the prism power until diplopia occurs. Accommodation must be controlled during fusional vergence testing. Fusional vergences can be changed by the following:

- *Compensatory mechanisms:* As a tendency to deviate evolves, the patient gradually develops a larger-than-normal fusional vergence for that deviation. Very large fusional vergences are common in compensated, long-standing vertical deviations and in exodeviations.
- *Change in visual acuity:* Improved acuity improves the fusional vergence mechanism. The treatment of reduced vision may change a symptomatic intermittent deviation to an asymptomatic heterophoria.
- *State of awareness:* Fatigue, illness, or drug and alcohol ingestion may decrease the fusional vergence mechanism, converting a heterophoria to a heterotropia.
- *Orthoptics:* The magnitude of the fusional vergence mechanism (mainly fusional convergence) may be increased by exercises. This treatment works best for near fusional convergence, particularly for the relief of the symptoms of convergence insufficiency.

- *Optical stimulation of fusional vergence:* (1) In controlled accommodative esotropia, reducing the strength of the hyperopia or bifocal correction induces an esophoria that stimulates fusional divergence. (2) The power of prisms used to control diplopia may be gradually reduced to stimulate a compensatory fusional vergence.

Special Tests

Motor Tests

Special motor tests include forced ductions, active force generation, and saccadic velocity. See also BCSC Section 5, *Neuro-Ophthalmology.*

- *Forced ductions* are performed by using forceps to move the eye into various positions, thus determining resistance to passive movement. This test is usually performed at the time of surgery but can sometimes be performed preoperatively with topical anesthesia in cooperative patients.
- *Active force generation* assesses the relative strength of a muscle. The patient is asked to move the eye in a given direction while the observer grasps the eye with an instrument. If the muscle tested is paretic, the examiner feels less than normal tension.
- *Saccadic velocity* can be recorded using a special instrument that graphically records the speed and direction of eye movement. This test is useful to differentiate paralysis from restriction. A paralyzed muscle generates a reduced saccadic velocity throughout the movement of the involved eye, whereas a restricted muscle produces an initially normal velocity that rapidly decelerates when the eye reaches the limit of its movement.

The field of single binocular vision may be tested on either a Goldmann perimeter or a tangent screen. These tests are useful for following the recovery of a paretic muscle or for measuring the outcome of surgery to alleviate diplopia. A small white test object is followed by both eyes in the various cardinal positions throughout the visual field. When the patient indicates that the test object is seen double, the point is plotted. The examiner then repeats the same procedure until he or she has plotted the entire visual field, noting the area in which the patient reported single vision and the area of double vision. The field of binocular fixation normally measures about 45°–50° from the fixation point except where it is blocked by the nose (Fig 6-8).

3-Step Test

Cyclovertical muscle paralyses, especially those involving the superior oblique muscles, are often responsible for hyperdeviations. The 3-step test is an algorithm that can be used to help identify the paretic cyclovertically acting muscle. As helpful as this test is, however, it is not always diagnostic and can be misleading, especially in patients in whom more than 1 muscle is paralyzed, in patients who have undergone strabismus surgery, in the presence of a skew deviation, and in the presence of restrictions or dissociated vertical deviation (see Chapter 10).

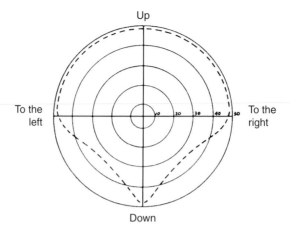

Figure 6-8 The normal field of single binocular vision.

The examiner must be familiar with the anatomy and motor physiology of the extraocular muscles in order to understand the test. There are 8 cyclovertically acting muscles: 4 work as depressors (2 in each eye), and 4 work as elevators (2 in each eye). The 2 *depressors* of each eye are the *inferior rectus (IR)* and *superior oblique (SO) muscles;* the 2 *elevators* of each eye are the *superior rectus (SR)* and the *inferior oblique (IO) muscles.* The 3-step test is performed as described in the following sections (Fig 6-9).

Step 1

If the case is one of paralysis, determine which eye is hypertropic by using the cover-uncover test (see Fig 6-1 and the discussion earlier in this chapter). Step 1 narrows the number of possible underacting muscles from 8 to 4. In the example shown in Figure 6-9, the right eye has been found to be hypertropic. This means that the paralysis will be found in either the depressors of the right eye (RIR, RSO) or the elevators of the left eye (LIO, LSR). Draw an oval around these 2 muscle groups (Fig 6-9A).

Step 2

Determine whether the vertical deviation is greater in right gaze or in left gaze. In the example, the deviation is larger in left gaze. This implicates 1 of the 4 vertically acting muscles used in left gaze. Draw an oval around the 4 vertically acting muscles that are used in left gaze (Fig 6-9B). At the end of step 2, the 2 remaining possible muscles (1 in each eye) are both intortors or extortors and both superior or inferior muscles (1 rectus and 1 oblique). Note that in Figure 6-9B, the increased left-gaze deviation eliminates 2 inferior muscles and implicates 2 superior muscles.

Step 3

Known as the *Bielschowsky head-tilt test,* the final step involves tilting the head to the right and then to the left during distance fixation. Head tilt to the right stimulates intorsion of the right eye (RSR, RSO) and extorsion of the left eye (LIR, LIO). Head tilt to the left stimulates extorsion of the right eye (RIR, RIO) and intorsion of the left eye (LSR, LSO).

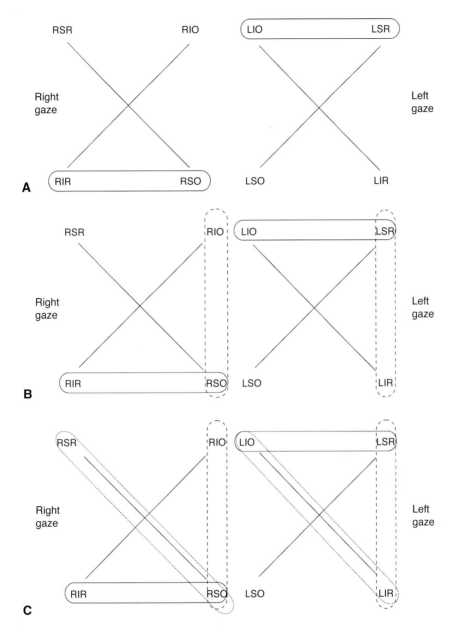

Figure 6-9 The 3-step test. **A,** Step 1: A right hypertropia suggests weakness in 1 of the 2 depressors of the right eye (RIR or RSO) or in 1 of the 2 elevators of the left eye (LIO or LSR). **B,** Step 2: Worsening of the right hypertropia on left gaze implicates either the RSO or the LSR. Note that, at the end of step 2, 1 depressor and 1 elevator of opposite eyes will be the possible weak muscle. **C,** Step 3: The right head tilt causes intorsion (incycloduction) of the right eye. Because this rotation depends on activation of both the RSO (a depressor) and the RSR (an elevator), weakness of the RSO will cause the right hypertropia to increase.

Normally, the 2 intortors and the 2 extortors of each eye have *opposite* vertical actions that cancel each other. If 1 intortor or 1 extortor is weak, it cannot act vertically, and the vertical action of the other ipsilateral torting muscle becomes manifest.

Figure 6-9C illustrates the results if step 2 had demonstrated that the deviation was greater in left gaze and the right superior oblique was the paretic muscle. In this case, when the head is tilted to the right, in order to maintain fixation, the right eye must intort and the left eye must extort. Because the right superior oblique is weak, the vertical action of the right superior rectus is unopposed. Contraction of this muscle in an attempt to incycloduct the eye results in an upward movement of the right eye, thus increasing the vertical deviation.

Because the oblique muscles are minor elevators and depressors, the difference in vertical alignment of the eyes will be smaller during head-tilt testing when there is a paresis of the vertical rectus muscles as compared to the oblique muscles.

Parks MM. Isolated cyclovertical muscle palsy. *AMA Arch Ophthalmol.* 1958;60(6):1027–1035.

Prism Adaptation Test

In prism adaptation, the patient is fitted with prisms of sufficient magnitude to permit alignment of the visual axes. In many cases, this step provokes a restoration of sensory binocular cooperation in a form of fusion and even stereopsis. This technique simulates orthotropia and possibly offers some predictive value of whether fusion may be restored when the patient undergoes surgical alignment.

In some patients, however (especially those with acquired esotropia), placement of such prisms increases the deviation. In such cases, anomalous retinal correspondence based on the objective angle may drive the eyes to maintain this adaptive alignment even with prismatic correction. After wearing such prisms, the patient returns with a greater angle of deviation. Prism adaptation is used by some ophthalmologists in patients with acquired esotropia. The patient is reexamined every 1–2 weeks and given larger prism correction, if needed, until the deviation no longer increases. Surgery is then performed on the new, larger, prism-adapted angle. The Prism Adaptation Study demonstrated a smaller undercorrection rate when surgery was based on this deviation compared to standard surgery.

Repka MX, Connett JE, Scott WE. The one-year surgical outcome after prism adaptation for the management of acquired esotropia. *Ophthalmology.* 1996;103(6):922–928.

Tests of Binocular Sensory Cooperation

Assessment of the vergence system indicates the extent to which the 2 eyes can be directed at the same object. Sensory binocularity involves the use of both eyes together to form 1 perception. In general, normal sensory binocularity depends on normal fusional vergence. Ideally, testing should therefore be performed before binocularity is disrupted by occlusion of either eye. Two classes of tests are commonly used to assess sensory binocularity: Worth 4-dot testing (and its equivalents) and stereoacuity testing.

Worth 4-Dot Testing

The mechanics of Worth 4-dot testing are described in Chapter 4. Only patients who are using both eyes together can appreciate all 4 lights being projected (see Chapter 4, Fig 4-10). If the right eye is suppressed, as often occurs if that eye is deviated, the patient will report seeing 3 green lights because the white light appears green. If the left eye is suppressed, the patient will report seeing 2 red lights because the white light appears red. If alternate eyes are suppressed, the patient may see 2 red and 3 green lights alternating. Patients with diplopia may report seeing 5 lights simultaneously.

Stereoacuity Testing

Worth 4-dot testing is best at detecting suppression, but stereoacuity testing assesses the use of the 2 eyes for stereopsis. Stereopsis occurs when the 2 retinal images, slightly disparate because of the normally different views provided by the horizontal separation of the 2 eyes, are cortically integrated. There are 2 types of stereopsis tests: *contour* and *random dot*. *Contour stereopsis tests* involve actual horizontal separation of the targets presented to each eye (with polarized or red-green glasses) such that monocular clues to depth are present at lower stereoacuity levels. *Random-dot stereopsis tests* circumvent the problem of monocular clues by embedding the stereo figures in a background of random dots.

In the *Stereo Fly test* (a contour stereopsis test), a card with superimposed images of a fly is shown to the patient. Ability to detect the elevation of the fly's wings above the plane of the card indicates stereopsis. Because the separation of the superimposed images is 3000 seconds of arc, this test is one of gross stereopsis. In other figures on the card, there is less separation between the superimposed images. Thus, quantitation of finer stereoacuity may be possible in cooperative patients.

Several different types of random-dot stereopsis tests are clinically useful. The *Randot test,* in which polarized glasses are worn, can measure stereoacuity to 20 seconds of arc. The *Random-Dot E test* employs a preferential looking strategy to test stereopsis and is used in pediatric vision screening programs. Red-green glasses are used in the *TNO test* to provide separation of the images seen by each eye. The *Lang stereopsis tests* do not require glasses to produce a random-dot stereoscopic effect and therefore may be useful in young children who object to wearing glasses.

Stereopsis can also be measured at distance using the AO Project-O-Chart (American Optical, Buffalo, NY) with Vectograph slide or the Smart System II PC-Plus (M&S Technologies, Park Ridge, IL). Distance stereoacuity measurements, such as that used in the Frisby distance test, may be helpful in monitoring control of intermittent exotropia.

Cycloplegic Refraction

One of the most important tests in the evaluation of any patient with complaints pertinent to binocular vision and ocular motility is refraction with cycloplegic agents. *Cyclopentolate* (1.0%) is the preferred drug for routine use in children, especially when combined with phenylephrine, which has no cycloplegic effect itself. Use of 0.5% strength is suggested in

Table 6-2 Administration and Duration of Cycloplegics

Medication	Administration Schedule	Onset of Action	Duration of Cycloplegic Action
Tropicamide	1 drop q 5 min × 2; wait 30 min	20–40 min	4–6 hr
Cyclopentolate	1 drop q 5 min × 2; wait 30 min	30–60 min	6–24 hr
Scopolamine	1 drop q 5 min × 2; wait 1 hr	30–60 min	4–7 d
Homatropine	1 drop q 5 min × 2; wait 1 hr	30–60 min	1 d
Atropine*	1 drop tid × 3 days; then 1 drop morning of appointment	45–120 min	1–2 wk

*Some physicians think that atropine ointment is a safer vehicle for delivery of the drug, given once a day × 3 days.

infants, and the clinician should be aware that some adverse psychological effects have been observed in children receiving cyclopentolate. *Homatropine* (5.0%) and *scopolamine* (0.25%) are occasionally used instead of cyclopentolate, but neither is as rapid acting or as effective. *Tropicamide* (0.5% or 1.0%), which is used in conjunction with phenylephrine (2.5%) for routine dilation, is usually not strong enough for effective cycloplegia in children. Some ophthalmologists use a combination of cyclopentolate and tropicamide to achieve maximum dilation. Many ophthalmologists advocate *atropine* 1.0% drops or ointment, but this drug causes prolonged blurring and is more often associated with toxic or allergic side effects (see the following section). Nonetheless, 1% atropine drops are being used safely and with increasing frequency for the treatment of amblyopia (see Chapter 5).

Table 6-2 shows the schedule of administration and duration of action for commonly used cycloplegics. The duration of action varies greatly, and the pupillary effect occurs earlier and lasts longer than does the cycloplegic effect, so a dilated pupil does not necessarily indicate complete cycloplegia. For patients with accommodative esodeviations, frequent repeated cycloplegic examinations are essential when control is precarious, but not otherwise. Having the patient fixate at distance is helpful to prevent false readings caused by residual accommodative effort.

Adverse Effects

Adverse reactions to cycloplegic agents include allergic (or hypersensitivity) reaction with conjunctivitis, edematous eyelids, and dermatitis. These reactions are more frequent with atropine than with any of the other agents. Hypnotic effect can be seen with scopolamine and occasionally with cyclopentolate or homatropine.

Systemic intoxication from atropine manifests in fever, dry mouth, flushing of the face, rapid pulse, nausea, dizziness, delirium, and erythema. Treatment is discontinuation of the medicine, with supportive measures as necessary. If the reaction is severe, physostigmine may be given. Remember, 1 drop of 1.0% atropine is 0.5 mg atropine.

CHAPTER 7

Esodeviations

An *esodeviation* is a latent or manifest convergent misalignment of the visual axes. Esodeviations are the most common type of strabismus, accounting for more than 50% of ocular deviations in the pediatric population. Three commonly recognized forms of esodeviation are grouped according to variations in fusional capabilities:

- *Esophoria* is a latent esodeviation that is controlled by fusional mechanisms so that the eyes remain properly aligned under normal binocular viewing conditions.
- *Intermittent esotropia* is an esodeviation that is intermittently controlled by fusional mechanisms but becomes manifest under certain conditions, such as fatigue, illness, stress, or tests that interfere with the maintenance of normal fusional abilities (such as covering 1 eye).
- *Esotropia* is an esodeviation that is not controlled by fusional mechanisms, so the deviation is constantly manifest.

Esodeviations can result from innervational, anatomical, mechanical, refractive, and accommodative causes. Table 7-1 lists the major types of esodeviation.

Pseudoesotropia

Pseudoesotropia is characterized by the false appearance of esotropia when the visual axes are actually aligned accurately. The appearance may be caused by a flat, broad nasal bridge; prominent epicanthal folds; or a narrow interpupillary distance. The observer sees less sclera nasally than would be expected, which creates the impression that the eye is turned in toward the nose, especially when the child gazes to either side. Because no real deviation exists, both corneal light reflex testing and cover testing results are normal. True esotropia can develop in children with pseudoesotropia, as in any child, so parents and pediatricians should be cautioned that reassessment is required if the apparent deviation does not improve.

Infantile (Congenital) Esotropia

Few children who are eventually diagnosed with classic infantile esotropia are actually born with esotropia. Although the parents often describe the crossing as occurring at birth, the exact date is not precisely established in most cases, and they rarely remember seeing the

Table 7-1 Major Types of Esodeviation

Pseudoesotropia
Infantile (congenital) esotropia
Nystagmus and esotropia
  Ciancia syndrome
  Manifest latent nystagmus
  Nystagmus blockage syndrome
Accommodative esotropia
  Refractive (normal AC/A)
  Nonrefractive (high AC/A)
  Partially accommodative
Nonaccommodative acquired esotropia
  Basic
  Acute
  Cyclic
  Sensory deprivation
  Divergence insufficiency and divergence paralysis
  Spasm of the near synkinetic reflex
  Surgical (consecutive)
Incomitant esotropia
  Sixth cranial nerve (abducens) paralysis
  Medial rectus restriction
    Thyroid eye disease
    Medial orbital wall fracture
  High myopia with esotropia
  Duane syndrome and Möbius syndrome

deviation in the newborn nursery. Documented presence of esotropia by age 6 months has been accepted as a defining element of infantile esotropia by most ophthalmologists. This criterion has been used in clinical studies. Some ophthalmologists refer to this disorder as *congenital esotropia;* the term *infantile esotropia* will be used in this volume.

A family history of esotropia or strabismus is often present, but well-defined genetic patterns are unusual. Other than strabismus, children with infantile esotropia are usually normal. Esotropia, however, occurs in up to 30% of children with neurologic and developmental problems, including cerebral palsy and hydrocephalus.

Equal visual acuity associated with alternation of fixation from 1 eye to the other is common in children with infantile esotropia. Cross-fixation, in which a large-angle esotropia is associated with the use of the adducted eye for fixation of objects in the contralateral temporal field, is also frequent (Fig 7-1). Amblyopia usually is present when a constant in-turning of only 1 eye occurs.

The misalignment is often readily visible and the deviation is characteristically larger than 30 prism diopters (Δ). There may be an apparent abduction deficit because of cross-fixation; children with equal vision have no need to abduct either eye on side gaze. If amblyopia is present, only the better-seeing eye will fixate in all fields of gaze, making the amblyopic eye appear to have an abduction weakness. The child's ability to abduct each eye may be demonstrated with the doll's head maneuver or by observation with 1 eye patched; the clinician can also rotate the child. Inferior oblique muscle overaction

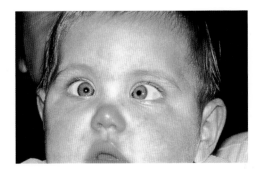

Figure 7-1 Infantile esotropia. *(Reproduced from Archer SM. Esotropia. Focal Points: Clinical Modules for Ophthalmologists. San Francisco: American Academy of Ophthalmology; 1994, module 12.)*

and dissociated vertical deviation may occur in more than 50% of patients with infantile esotropia but are not commonly recognized until age 1 year or older.

Asymmetry of monocular horizontal smooth pursuit is normal in infants up to age 6 months, with nasal-to-temporal smooth pursuit less well developed than temporal-to-nasal smooth pursuit. Patients with infantile esotropia have persistent monocular smooth pursuit asymmetry that does not resolve.

Pathogenesis

The cause of infantile esotropia remains unknown. The debate regarding its etiology has focused on the implications of 2 conflicting theories. Worth's "sensory" concept was that infantile esotropia resulted from a deficit in a supposed fusion center in the brain. According to this theory, the goal of restoring binocularity was considered hopeless, because there was no way to provide this absent neural function. Chavasse disagreed with Worth's theory and believed the primary problem was mechanical and potentially curable if the deviation could be eliminated in infancy. Several authors began to report favorable sensory results in some infants operated on between 6 months and 2 years of age. These encouraging results became the basis for the practice of early surgery for patients with infantile esotropia.

Management

Cycloplegic refraction characteristically reveals 1–2 D of hyperopia, which is the normal refractive error in young children. Significant astigmatism or myopia may be present and may require correction. Because accommodative esotropia can occur as early as age 4 months, significant refractive errors are corrected by prescribing the full cycloplegic retinoscopy findings. A small-angle esotropia that is variable or intermittent may be more likely to respond to hyperopic correction than a large-angle, constant esotropia.

Ocular alignment is rarely achieved without surgery in a child with early-onset esotropia. However, surgery should be undertaken only after correction of significant refractive errors and treatment of amblyopia. Failure to correct these problems may compromise stable surgical alignment of the eyes.

Most ophthalmologists agree that surgery should be undertaken early. The eyes should be aligned by age 24 months to optimize binocular cooperation. Surgery can be performed in healthy children between ages 4 and 6 months to maximize binocular function such as stereopsis. Patients with a constant and stable esotropia of at least 40Δ who present between ages 2 and 4 months are unlikely to improve spontaneously. Based on this observation, some surgeons suggest even earlier surgery in hopes of achieving a superior sensory outcome. Smaller angles may be observed, as they may improve spontaneously.

The child's psychological and motor development may improve and accelerate after the eyes are straightened. It is felt that bonding is improved between infant and parents after surgical straightening of the eyes. Improved techniques have minimized the risk of general anesthesia such that anesthetic concerns need not dictate the age at which surgery is performed in healthy infants.

Various surgical approaches have been suggested for infantile esotropia. The most common procedure is recession of both medial rectus muscles. Recession of a medial rectus muscle combined with resection of the ipsilateral lateral rectus muscle is an acceptable alternative. Two-muscle surgery spares horizontal rectus muscles for subsequent surgery should it be needed; this is a common occurrence in patients with infantile esotropia. Some surgeons operate on 3 or even 4 horizontal rectus muscles at the time of the initial surgery if the deviation is larger than 50Δ. Associated overaction of the inferior oblique muscles is often treated at the time of the initial surgery using inferior oblique muscle-weakening procedures. Chapter 12 discusses surgical procedures in greater detail.

Botulinum toxin injections into the medial rectus muscles have been used by some ophthalmologists in the treatment of infantile esotropia. Multiple injections may be required, and the long-term sensory and motor outcomes have not been shown to be superior to those from incisional surgery.

The goal of treatment in infantile esotropia is to reduce the deviation to orthotropia or as close to it as possible. Ideally, this results in normal sight in each eye and in the development of at least some degree of sensory fusion that will maintain motor alignment. However, many children will require multiple surgeries. Alignment within 8Δ of orthotropia frequently results in the development of the monofixation syndrome, characterized by peripheral fusion, central suppression, and favorable appearance, and is therefore considered a successful surgical result and the goal of treating children with infantile esotropia. This small-angle strabismus generally represents a stable, functional surgical outcome even though bifoveal fusion is not achieved.

Ing M, Costenbader FD, Parks MM, Albert DG. Early surgery for congenital esotropia. *Am J Ophthalmol*. 1966;61(6):1419–1427.

Pediatric Eye Disease Investigator Group. The clinical spectrum of early-onset esotropia: experience of the Congenital Esotropia Observational Study. *Am J Ophthalmol*. 2002;133(1): 102–108.

von Noorden GK. A reassessment of infantile esotropia. XLIV Edward Jackson Memorial Lecture. *Am J Ophthalmol*. 1988;105(1):1–10.

Nystagmus and Esotropia

Nystagmus occurs in up to one-third of patients with a history of early-onset esotropia. For a detailed discussion of nystagmus and esotropia, see Chapter 25 of this volume.

Accommodative Esotropia

Accommodative esotropia is defined as a convergent deviation of the eyes associated with activation of the accommodative reflex. All accommodative esodeviations are acquired, with the following characteristics:

- onset generally between 6 months and 7 years of age, averaging 2½ years of age (can be as early as age 4 months)
- usually intermittent at onset, becoming constant
- often hereditary
- sometimes precipitated by trauma or illness
- frequently associated with amblyopia
- diplopia may occur (especially in older children) but usually disappears as patient develops facultative suppression scotoma in the deviating eye

Types of accommodative esotropia are listed in Table 7-1 and discussed in the following sections.

Refractive Accommodative Esotropia

The mechanism of refractive accommodative esotropia involves 3 factors: (1) uncorrected hyperopia, (2) accommodative convergence, and (3) insufficient fusional divergence. The uncorrected hyperopia forces the patient to accommodate to sharpen the retinal image, thus inducing increased convergence. If the patient's fusional divergence mechanism is insufficient to compensate for the increased convergence tonus, esotropia results. The angle of esotropia is generally between 20Δ and 30Δ and approximately equal at distance and near fixation. The amount of hyperopia averages +4 D.

Treatment of refractive accommodative esotropia consists of correction of the full amount of hyperopia, as determined under cycloplegia. Any concomitant amblyopia should be treated as well. Significant delay in initiating treatment following the onset of esotropia increases the likelihood that a portion of the esodeviation will fail to respond to antiaccommodative therapy.

Parents must understand the importance of full-time wear of spectacle correction. The esodeviation, without glasses, may even increase initially after the correction is worn. Discussing this issue with parents at the time the prescription is first given is often more effective than offering the same explanation afterward. In addition, it is helpful to explain that the glasses help control the strabismus, not cure it. This will help eliminate potential frustration when the child's eyes continue to cross when he or she is not wearing glasses.

Surgical correction may be required when a patient with refractive accommodative esotropia fails to regain fusion with glasses or subsequently develops a nonaccommodative component to the deviation. However, the ophthalmologist must rule out latent uncorrected hyperopia before proceeding with surgery.

High Accommodative Convergence/Accommodative Esotropia

In patients with a *high accommodative convergence/accommodation (AC/A),* excess convergence tonus results from accommodation, and esotropia develops in the setting of insufficient fusional divergence. Because more accommodation is required at near fixation than at distance, the angle of esotropia is greater at near. It can be reduced by +3.00 D bifocal lenses. Measurement of the angle of esotropia with fixation targets that require appropriate accommodation is critical to making the diagnosis of this type of esotropia.

High AC/A esotropia may occur in patients with large degrees of hyperopia or in patients with normal levels of hyperopia, emmetropia, or even myopia. In these latter groups of patients, the disorder is also referred to as *nonrefractive accommodative esotropia.* The refractive error in these patients averages +2.25 D.

No consensus exists on the best management of high AC/A esotropia. Several options are available:

- *Bifocals.* The most commonly used treatment option for nonrefractive accommodative esotropia is bifocal spectacles. If bifocals are employed, they should initially be prescribed in the executive or 35-mm flat-top style with a power of +2.50 or +3.00 D. The top of the segment should cross the pupil, and the vertical height of the bifocal should not exceed that of the distance portion of the lens. Detailed instructions concerning the bifocal should be given to the optician. Progressive bifocal lenses have been used successfully, but conventional bifocals are preferred. If progressive bifocals are used, they should be fitted higher than adult lenses (about 4 mm) and with a power up to +3.00 or the power needed to achieve alignment at near fixation. An ideal response to bifocal glasses is restoration of normal binocular function (fusion and stereopsis) at both distance and near fixation. An acceptable response is fusion at distance with less than 10Δ of residual esotropia through the bifocal at near fixation.
- *Long-acting cholinesterase inhibitors.* Ophthalmologists who use long-acting cholinesterase inhibitors suggest starting with maximum strength (0.125% echothiophate iodide drops) in both eyes once daily for 6 weeks. If such treatment is effective, strength or frequency should be decreased to the minimum effective dose. Parents must be warned about the potentially serious adverse effects of these drugs, including deletion of pseudocholinesterase from the blood, which makes the patient highly susceptible to depolarizing muscle relaxants such as succinylcholine. Echothiophate iodide can also cause pupillary cysts to form; some ophthalmologists prescribe phenylephrine 2.5% drops twice daily concurrently to reduce the risk of cyst formation. Echothiophate has been difficult to obtain in the United States.
- *Surgery.* Some ophthalmologists advocate surgery for high AC/A esotropia. Surgery can normalize the AC/A ratio in these patients. It can be used in some patients to allow discontinuation of a bifocal and control of the esodeviation with single-vision glasses or contact lenses.
- *Observation.* Many patients will show a decrease in the near deviation with time and ultimately develop binocular vision at both distance and near fixation. Some ophthalmologists will observe the near deviation as long as the distance deviation allows for the development of fusion or if the patient is asymptomatic.

For the long-term management of both refractive and nonrefractive accommodative eso-tropia, it is important to remember that measured hyperopia usually increases until age 5–7 years. Therefore, if the esotropia with glasses increases, the cycloplegic refraction should be repeated and the full correction prescribed. After age 5–7 years, hyperopia may decrease, and the full cycloplegic refraction in place will thus blur vision and the prescription will need to be reduced.

If glasses or drugs correct all or nearly all of the esotropia and if some degree of sen-sory binocular cooperation or fusion is present, the clinician may begin to reduce the strength of the glasses or the drugs to create a small esophoria when the patient reaches age 5 or 6. This reduction may stimulate the fusional divergence mechanism to redevelop normal magnitude. An increase in the fusional divergence combined with the natural de-crease of both the hyperopia and the high AC/A ratio may enable the patient to maintain straight eyes without glasses or bifocals.

Partially Accommodative Esotropia

Patients with partially accommodative esodeviations show a reduction in the angle of esotropia with glasses but have a residual esotropia despite treatment of amblyopia and provision of full hyperopic therapy. Sometimes, partially accommodative esotropia re-sults from decompensation of a fully accommodative esotropia, but in other instances the child may have had an esotropia that subsequently developed an accommodative element. An interval of weeks to months between the onset of accommodative esotropia and the application of full cycloplegic refraction often results in some residual esotropia, even after the proper glasses are worn. Hence, prompt treatment of accommodative esotropia may offer substantial benefits. Patients with pure refractive accommodative esotropia who have been made orthotropic with glasses are less likely to develop a nonaccommodative component to their esodeviation than are patients with the type of accommodative esotro-pia with a high AC/A ratio.

Treatment of partially accommodative esotropia consists of amblyopia management and prescription of the full hyperopic correction. Strabismus surgery may be warranted for the nonaccommodative portion depending on the size of the deviation and the wishes of the patient and family. It is important that the patient and parents understand before surgery that its purpose is to produce straight eyes with glasses—not to allow the child to discontinue wearing glasses altogether.

Mulvihill A, MacCann A, Flitcroft I, O'Keefe M. Outcome in refractive accommodative esotro-pia. *Br J Ophthalmol.* 2000;84(7):746–749.

Trigler L. Managing accommodative esotropia patients and their parents. *Focal Points: Clinical Modules for Ophthalmologists.* San Francisco: American Academy of Ophthalmology; 2008, module 5.

Nonaccommodative Acquired Esotropia

Basic (Acquired) Esotropia

Esotropia that develops after age 6 months and that is not associated with an accommo-dative component is called *basic,* or *acquired, esotropia.* As with infantile esotropia, an accommodative factor is usually absent, the amount of hyperopia is not significant, and the near deviation is the same as the distance deviation. Although most children with this form of esotropia are otherwise healthy, central nervous system lesions must be considered. Therapy consists of amblyopia treatment and surgical correction as soon as possible after the onset of the deviation.

When planning surgery for patients with acquired esotropia, some ophthalmologists advocate prism adaptation (see Prism Adaptation Test in Chapter 6).

Acute Esotropia

Occasionally, an acquired esotropia is acute in onset. In such cases, the patient immediately becomes aware of the deviation and frequently has diplopia. A careful motility evaluation is important to rule out an accommodative or paretic component. Artificial disruption of binocular vision, such as may follow treatment of an ocular injury or patching for amblyopia, is one of the known causes of acute esotropia. Because the onset of comitant esotropia in an older child may indicate an underlying neurologic disorder, neurologic evaluation may be indicated. Most patients with acute onset of esotropia have a history of normal binocular vision, and therefore the prognosis for restoration of single binocular vision with prisms and surgery is good. Prisms may be used during a period of observation before surgery is performed.

Cyclic Esotropia

Cyclic esotropia is rare, with an estimated incidence of 1:3000–1:5000 strabismus cases. Onset typically occurs during the preschool years, although an infantile case and several adult cases have been reported. The esotropia is present intermittently, usually every other day (48-hour cycle). Variable cycles and 24-hour cycles have also been documented.

Fusion and binocular vision are usually absent or defective on the strabismic day, with marked improvement on the straight day. Diplopia on strabismic days is unusual and has been a prominent symptom only in patients of a relatively older age who are unable to develop suppression.

Cyclic esotropia is noted for its unpredictable response to various forms of therapy, with the exception of surgery, which is usually curative. Occlusion therapy may convert the cyclic deviation into a constant one.

Sensory Deprivation Esodeviation

Monocular vision loss from various causes, such as cataract, corneal scarring, optic atrophy, or prolonged blurred or distorted retinal images, may cause an esodeviation.

Obstacles preventing clear and focused retinal images and symmetric visual stimulation must be identified and remedied as soon as possible. Animal and clinical data indicate that restoration of normal, symmetric inputs must be accomplished at an early age if irreversible amblyopia is to be avoided. After all obstacles to balanced sensory inputs have been removed, any secondary amblyopia is treated, if possible. Surgery for residual esotropia may be indicated. The surgical management of these cases is similar to that of early-onset esotropia, except when good visual acuity cannot be restored as a result of irreversible amblyopia or organic defects. In such situations, strabismus surgery should generally be performed only on the abnormal eye.

Divergence Insufficiency

The characteristic finding of divergence insufficiency is an esodeviation, generally in adult patients, that is greater at distance than at near. The deviation does not change with vertical or horizontal gaze, and fusional divergence is reduced. Divergence paralysis may represent a more severe form of divergence insufficiency. Because true paralysis of divergence cannot generally be documented, the term *divergence insufficiency* is preferred. Divergence insufficiency can be divided into a primary isolated form and a secondary form associated with other neurologic abnormalities stemming from pontine tumors or severe head trauma. A thorough clinical evaluation can frequently distinguish between the 2 forms of divergence insufficiency. Primary isolated divergence insufficiency is frequently a benign condition that predominantly occurs in patients older than 50 years: symptoms may resolve within several months. Patients with secondary divergence insufficiency may obtain relief from symptoms with treatment of the underlying neurologic disorder (eg, corticosteroids for temporal arteritis, treatment of intracranial hypertension). Management of diplopia consists of base-out prisms and, sometimes, surgery.

Jacobson DM. Divergence insufficiency revisited: natural history of idiopathic cases and neurologic associations. *Arch Ophthalmol.* 2000;118(9):1237–1241.

Spasm of the Near Synkinetic Reflex

Spasm of the near reflex is a spectrum of abnormalities of the near response. Thus, patients can present with varying combinations of excessive convergence, excessive accommodation, and miosis. The etiology is generally thought to be functional, related to psychological factors, but, rarely, it can be associated with organic disease. Patients may present with acute, persistent esotropia alternating at other times with orthotropia. The characteristic movement is the substitution of a convergence movement for a gaze movement on horizontal versions. Monocular abduction is normal in spite of marked abduction limitation on versions. Pseudomyopia may occur. Treatment has consisted of cycloplegic agents such as atropine or homatropine, plus lenses for patients with significant hyperopia, and bifocals.

Surgical (Consecutive) Esodeviation

Esodeviation following surgery for exodeviation frequently improves spontaneously. Treatment includes base-out prisms, plus lenses or miotics (especially if the patient is hyperopic), alternate occlusion, and, finally, surgery. Unless the deviation is very large or symptomatic, surgery should be postponed for several months because of the possibility of spontaneous improvement.

A slipped or lost lateral rectus muscle produces varying amounts of esotropia, depending on the amount of slippage. A slipped muscle should be suspected in the case of consecutive esotropia with a large abduction deficit following surgery on a lateral rectus muscle. Surgical exploration and reattachment of the muscle to the globe is required.

Transposition procedures may be necessary when lost muscles cannot be found. For slipped muscles, advancement of the muscle on the globe is required. (See Chapter 12, Fig 12-9, and the accompanying text discussion.)

Incomitant Esotropia

The term *incomitant esotropia* is used when the esodeviation varies in size with different fields of gaze.

Sixth Cranial Nerve (Abducens) Paralysis

Paralysis of the lateral rectus muscle causes an incomitant esodeviation. Sixth cranial nerve paralysis occurring at birth has been reported but is uncommon. Most cases of suspected congenital sixth cranial nerve paralysis represent infantile esotropia with cross-fixation. Congenital sixth cranial nerve paralysis is thought to be caused by the increased intracranial pressure associated with the birth process and usually resolves spontaneously. Sixth cranial nerve paralysis occurs much more frequently in childhood than in infancy. Older patients may complain of double vision and often have a face turn toward the side of the paralytic sixth cranial nerve to avoid diplopia. Approximately one-third of these cases are associated with intracranial lesions and may have associated neurologic findings. Other cases may be related to infectious or immunologic processes that involve cranial nerve VI. Spontaneous benign lesions usually resolve over several months.

The vision in both eyes is usually equal unless strabismic amblyopia or associated structural defects are found. The esotropia increases in gaze toward the paralyzed lateral rectus muscle. Saccadic velocities show slowing of the affected lateral rectus muscle, and active force generation tests document the weakness of that muscle. Versions show limited or no abduction of the affected eye.

A careful history should be taken to define antecedent infections, head trauma, or other possible inciting factors for sixth cranial nerve weakness. Neurologic evaluation and computed tomography (CT) or magnetic resonance imaging (MRI) are indicated when neurologic signs or symptoms are present.

Patching may be required to maintain vision in the esotropic eye in children in the amblyopia age range, especially if the child has no face turn to maintain binocular fusion. Fresnel Press-On prisms are useful to correct the diplopia in primary position. Correction of a significant hyperopic refractive error may help prevent the development of an accommodative esotropia.

Additional features and treatments are discussed in Chapter 11. See also BCSC Section 5, *Neuro-Ophthalmology.*

Other Forms of Incomitant Esotropia

Medial rectus muscle restriction may result from thyroid eye disease, medial orbital wall fracture, or an excessively resected medial rectus muscle (see Chapter 12).

For discussions of *high myopia with esotropia, Duane syndrome,* and *Möbius syndrome,* see Chapter 11 and BCSC Section 5, *Neuro-Ophthalmology.*

Preferred Practice Patterns Committee, Pediatric Panel. *Esotropia and Exotropia.* San Francisco: American Academy of Ophthalmology; 2002.

CHAPTER 8

Exodeviations

An exodeviation is a divergent strabismus that can be latent (controlled by fusion) or manifest. Although the exact etiology of most exodeviations is unknown, proposed causes include anatomical and mechanical factors within the orbit as well as abnormalities of innervation such as excessive tonic divergence.

Pseudoexotropia

The term *pseudoexotropia* refers to an appearance of exodeviation when in fact the eyes are properly aligned. Pseudoexotropia may result from the following:

- wide interpupillary distance
- positive angle kappa without other ocular abnormalities (see the discussion of angle kappa in Chapter 6)
- positive angle kappa together with ocular abnormalities such as temporal dragging of the macula in retinopathy of prematurity

Exophoria

Exophoria is an exodeviation controlled by fusion under usual conditions of seeing. An exophoria is detected when binocular vision is interrupted, as during an alternate cover test. Exophoria may be asymptomatic if the angle of strabismus is small and fusional convergence amplitudes are adequate. Prolonged, detailed visual work may bring about asthenopia. Treatment is usually not necessary unless an exophoria progresses to an intermittent exotropia.

Intermittent Exotropia

With the possible exception of exophoria at near, the most common type of exodeviation is intermittent exotropia, which is latent at times and manifest at others.

Clinical Characteristics

The onset of intermittent exotropia usually occurs early, before age 5, but it may be detected for the first time even later in childhood. Because proper eye alignment with intermittent exotropia requires that compensatory fusional factors be active, the deviation often becomes manifest during times of visual inattention, fatigue, or stress. Parents of affected children often report that the exotropia occurs late in the day with fatigue or during illness, daydreaming, or drowsiness upon awakening. Exposure to bright light often causes a reflex closure of 1 eye.

During the early stages of the disorder, the deviation is usually larger for distance viewing than for near, and the exotropia is seen more frequently when the visual target is remote. Later, the near and distance exodeviations tend to be more equal in magnitude even if fusional control remains good. Intermittent exotropias can be associated with small hypertropias, A and V patterns, and oblique muscle dysfunction, all of which are discussed in Chapters 9 and 10.

In many patients, untreated intermittent exotropia progresses toward constant exotropia. During this progression, tropic episodes occur at lower levels of fatigue and last for longer periods. Children younger than 10 years may initially have diplopia but often develop the cortical adaptations of suppression and abnormal retinal correspondence (see Chapter 4) with time. However, normal retinal correspondence and good binocular function remain when the eyes are straight. Amblyopia is uncommon unless the intermittent exotropia progresses to constant or nearly constant exotropia at an early age or unless another amblyogenic factor, such as anisometropia, is present.

Evaluation

The clinical evaluation begins with a history of the age of onset of the strabismus and a determination as to whether the exotropia is becoming more frequent. The clinician records how often and under what circumstances the deviation is manifest. A qualitative measurement of the control of the exodeviation exhibited throughout the examination is an important component of the evaluation and can be categorized as

- *Good control:* Exotropia manifests only after cover testing, and the patient resumes fusion rapidly without blinking or refixating.
- *Fair control:* Exotropia manifests after fusion is disrupted by cover testing, and the patient resumes fusion only after blinking or refixating.
- *Poor control:* Exotropia manifests spontaneously and may remain manifest for an extended time.

The Newcastle Control Score is used by some ophthalmologists to quantitatively grade the control of patients with intermittent exotropia. It may also predict the future need for surgery in these patients.

Prism and alternate cover testing should be used to evaluate the exodeviation at fixation distances of 20 ft and 14 in. A far distance measurement at 100–200 ft (at the end of a long hallway or out a window) may more likely demonstrate a latent deviation or bring out an even larger one. The deviation at near fixation is often less than the deviation at distance fixation. This difference may be due to either a high accommodative convergence/accommodation (AC/A) ratio or tenacious proximal fusion. The high AC/A ratio is a compensatory mechanism to help maintain alignment at near fixation. *Tenacious proximal fusion* is a proximal vergence aftereffect that occurs in some patients with intermittent exotropia; this aftereffect is due to a slow-to-dissipate fusion mechanism that prevents intermittent exotropia from manifesting at near fixation with a brief cover test. For patients with significantly more exodeviation in the distance than at near, a near alternate cover test after 1 hour of monocular occlusion to eliminate the effects of tenacious proximal fusion may help distinguish between patients with a truly high AC/A ratio and those with a pseudo-high AC/A ratio. A patient with a pseudo-high AC/A ratio would have roughly equal distance and near measurements after occlusion; a patient with a truly high AC/A ratio would continue to have significantly less exodeviation at near. Testing with +3 D lenses at near or −2 D lenses at distance can confirm the abnormality of the AC/A ratio.

Haggerty H, Richardson S, Hrisos S, Strong NP, Clarke MP. The Newcastle Control Score: a new method of grading the severity of intermittent distance exotropia. *Br J Ophthalmol.* 2004;88(2):233–235.

Kushner BJ, Morton GV. Distance/near differences in intermittent exotropia. *Arch Ophthalmol.* 1998;116(4):478–486.

Mohney BG, Huffaker RK. Common forms of childhood exotropia. *Ophthalmology.* 2003; 110(11):2093–2096.

Classification

Intermittent exotropia has traditionally been classified into several groups, based on the difference between prism and alternate cover test measurements at distance and at near and the change in near measurement produced by unilateral occlusion or +3 D lenses:

- *Basic* type exotropia is present when the exodeviation is approximately the same at distance and near fixation.
- *Divergence excess* type consists of an exodeviation that is greater at distance fixation than at near and can be divided into *true divergence excess* and *simulated divergence excess,* as described previously (see the section Evaluation).
- *Convergence insufficiency* type is present when the exodeviation is greater at near than at distance. This type excludes isolated convergence insufficiency, which is discussed later in this chapter.

Sensory testing usually reveals excellent stereopsis with normal retinal correspondence when the exodeviation is latent and suppression with abnormal retinal correspondence when the exodeviation is manifest. However, if the deviation manifests rarely, diplopia may persist during those manifestations.

Treatment

Although many patients with intermittent exotropia will eventually require surgery, opinions vary widely regarding the timing of surgery and the use of nonsurgical methods to delay or possibly to prevent the need for surgical intervention. Some ophthalmologists prefer to delay surgery in young children in whom good preoperative visual acuity and stereopsis could be exchanged for a small-angle esotropia, amblyopia, and decreased stereopsis. However, other ophthalmologists worry that delaying surgery too long could allow the development of permanent suppression and loss of long-term stability following surgical correction.

Nonsurgical management

Corrective lenses are prescribed for significant myopic, astigmatic, and hyperopic refractive errors. Correction of even mild myopia may improve control of the exodeviation. Mild to moderate degrees of hyperopia are not routinely corrected in children with intermittent exotropia for fear of worsening the deviation. However, some patients with more than 4.0 D of hyperopia (or more than 1.5 D of hyperopic anisometropia) may actually gain better control of the exodeviation after optical correction. Children with severe hyperopia may be unable to sustain the necessary accommodation for a clear image, and the lack of accommodative effort produces a blurred retinal image and manifest exotropia. Optical correction may improve retinal image clarity and help control the exodeviation.

Some ophthalmologists use additional minus lens power, usually 2–4 D beyond refractive error correction, to stimulate accommodative convergence to help control the exodeviation. This therapy may cause asthenopia in school-aged children, but it can be effective as a temporizing measure to promote fusion and delay surgery during the visually immature years.

Part-time patching of the dominant (nondeviating) eye 4–6 hours per day, or alternate daily patching when no strong ocular preference is present, can be an effective treatment for small- to moderate-sized deviations, although the benefit produced is often temporary and these patients eventually require surgery. The exact mechanism by which patching improves control of intermittent exotropia is not known; presumably, patching disrupts suppression and constitutes a passive orthoptic treatment. On the other hand, patching completely prevents the exercise of fusion, which could accelerate progression.

Active orthoptic treatments, which consist of antisuppression therapy/diplopia awareness and fusional convergence training, can be used alone or in combination with patching, minus lenses, and surgery. For deviations of 20Δ or less, orthoptic treatment alone has been reported by some authors to have a long-term success rate comparable to that of surgery. Others have found no benefit and recommend surgery for any poorly controlled deviation.

Base-in prisms can be used to promote fusion in intermittent exotropia, but this treatment option is seldom chosen for long-term management because it can cause a reduction in fusional vergence amplitudes.

Surgical treatment

Surgery is customarily performed when progression toward constant exotropia is documented, as evidenced by the deviation being manifest more frequently, or when control is poor. No consensus exists regarding specific indications; however, the best sensory outcomes are probably achieved with motor alignment before age 7 or before 5 years of strabismus duration, or while the deviation is still intermittent. Many surgeons use manifestation of the deviation more than 50% of the time as criterion for surgery.

Symmetric recession of both lateral rectus muscles is the most common surgical procedure for intermittent exotropia. Recession of 1 lateral rectus muscle combined with resection of the ipsilateral medial rectus muscle is an acceptable alternative and may be pre-ferred for patients with basic type intermittent exotropia. Some strabismus surgeons per-form unilateral lateral rectus muscle recession for patients with smaller exodeviations.

Abroms AD, Mohney BG, Rush DP, Parks MM, Tong PY. Timely surgery in intermittent and constant exotropia for superior sensory outcome. *Am J Ophthalmol.* 2001;131(1):111–116.

Kushner BJ. Selective surgery for intermittent exotropia based on distance/near differences. *Arch Ophthalmol.* 1998;116(3):324–328.

Management of consecutive esotropia

An immediate overcorrection of up to 10Δ–15Δ is desirable after bilateral lateral rectus muscle recessions. Persistent esotropia (beyond 3–4 weeks), referred to as *consecutive eso-tropia,* may require treatment with base-out prisms (usually Fresnel Press-On prisms) or alternate patching to prevent amblyopia or relieve diplopia. Corrective lenses or miotics should be considered if hyperopia is significant. Bifocals can be used for a high AC/A ratio. Unless deficient ductions suggest a slipped or lost muscle, a delay of several months is recommended before reoperation because spontaneous improvement is common. If this does not occur, a medial rectus muscle recession in 1 or both eyes can be performed, provided abduction is normal in both eyes. Unilateral lateral rectus muscle recession/medial rectus muscle resection surgery can be followed by medial rectus muscle reces-sion/lateral rectus muscle resection surgery on the other eye. Botulinum toxin injection into 1 medial rectus muscle may be effective in the management of consecutive esotropia, particularly when fusion is present.

Raab EL, Parks MM. Recession of the lateral recti: early and late postoperative alignments. *Arch Ophthalmol.* 1969;82(2):203–208.

Management of residual exotropia

Mild to moderate residual exodeviation is often treated by observation alone if fusional control is good. However, manifest exotropia commonly returns in time. Therefore, some surgeons recommend base-in prism management for residual exotropia, with a gradual weaning of the prism dosage. Postoperative patching and orthoptic treatment can also be applied. In small doses, botulinum toxin injection has also been used to treat residual exotropia, but supportive data are limited. Indications for reoperation, usually on unoper-ated muscles, are the same as for initial surgery.

Constant Exotropia

Constant exotropia is encountered most often in older patients manifesting sensory exo-tropia or decompensated intermittent exotropia.

Surgical treatment for constant exotropia consists of appropriate bilateral recessions of the lateral rectus muscles or unilateral lateral rectus muscle recession combined with a medial rectus muscle resection. In some cases, patients with an enlarged field of periph-eral vision because of rapid alternation of fixation may notice a field constriction when the eyes are straight.

Infantile Exotropia

Infantile exotropia presents before age 6 months with a large-angle constant deviation (Fig 8-1). It has been reported to be uncommon in otherwise healthy infants, and many children with infantile exotropia have associated neurologic impairment or craniofacial disorders. Patients with constant infantile exotropia are operated on early in life in the same manner as are patients with infantile esotropia. Early surgery can lead to gross binocular vision, but perfect binocular function is rare. These patients also tend to develop dissociated vertical deviation and inferior oblique muscle overaction and should be observed closely for the development of these associated motility disturbances.

Hunter DG, Ellis FJ. Prevalence of systemic and ocular disease in infantile exotropia: comparison with infantile esotropia. *Ophthalmology.* 1999;106(10):1951–1956.

Sensory Exotropia

Any condition that severely reduces visual acuity in 1 eye can cause sensory exotropia. The causes include anisometropia, corneal or lens opacities, optic atrophy or hypoplasia, macular lesions, and amblyopia. It is not known why some persons become esotropic after unilateral vision loss and others become exotropic. Both sensory esotropia and sensory exotropia are common in children, but exotropia predominates in infants younger than 1 year, older children, and adults. If the disadvantaged eye can be visually rehabilitated, peripheral fusion may sometimes be reestablished after surgical realignment, provided the sensory exotropia has not been present for an extended period.

Loss of fusional abilities, known as *central fusional disruption,* or *horror fusionis,* can lead to constant and permanent diplopia when adult-onset sensory exotropia has been

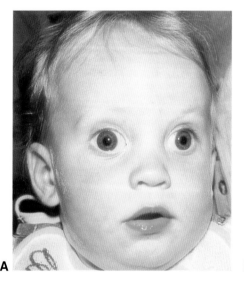
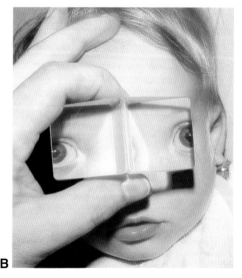

A   B

Figure 8-1 Infantile exotropia. **A,** This 10-month-old infant with infantile exotropia also shows developmental delay. **B,** Krimsky testing using 2 base-in prisms to measure the large exotropia. *(Reproduced with permission from Wilson ME.* Exotropia. *Focal Points: Clinical Modules for Ophthalmologists. San Francisco: American Academy of Ophthalmology; 1995, module 11.)*

present for several years prior to vision rehabilitation and realignment. In these patients, intractable diplopia may persist, even with well-aligned eyes.

Consecutive Exotropia

Consecutive exotropia is defined as exotropia that follows previous surgery for esotropia. Treatment of consecutive exotropia depends on many factors, including the size of the deviation, the type and amount of surgery that preceded its development, the presence of duction limitations, lateral incomitance, and the level of visual acuity in each eye. The planning of strabismus surgery is discussed in Chapter 12.

Exotropic Duane Syndrome

Duane syndrome can present with exotropia, usually accompanied by a face turn away from the affected eye. Adduction is most often markedly deficient; other signs include eyelid narrowing, globe retraction, and characteristic upshoots and downshoots. See Chapter 11 for further discussion of Duane syndrome.

Neuromuscular Abnormalities

A constant exotropia may result from third cranial nerve paralysis, internuclear ophthalmoplegia, or myasthenia gravis. These conditions are discussed in detail in Chapter 11 and in BCSC Section 5, *Neuro-Ophthalmology.*

Dissociated Horizontal Deviation

Dissociated strabismus may contain vertical, horizontal, and torsional components. When the dissociated abduction movement is predominant, it is called *dissociated horizontal deviation (DHD).* Though not a true exotropia, DHD can be confused with a constant or intermittent exotropia. Dissociated vertical deviation and latent nystagmus often coexist with DHD (Fig 8-2). Treatment usually consists of unilateral or occasionally bilateral lateral rectus recession in addition to any necessary oblique or vertical muscle surgery.

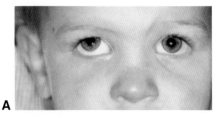 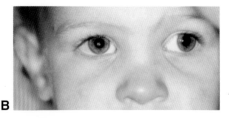

A   B

Figure 8-2 Dissociated strabismus complex. **A,** When the patient fixates with the left eye, a prominent dissociated vertical deviation is shown in the right eye. **B,** However, when the patient fixates with the right eye, a prominent dissociated horizontal deviation (DHD) is shown in the left eye. *(Reproduced with permission from Wilson ME. Exotropia.* Focal Points: Clinical Modules for Ophthalmologists. *San Francisco: American Academy of Ophthalmology; 1995, module 11.)*

Brodsky MC, Fray KJ. Dissociated horizontal deviation after surgery for infantile esotropia: clinical characteristics and proposed pathophysiologic mechanisms. *Arch Ophthalmol.* 2007; 125(12):1683–1692.

Wilson ME, Hutchinson AK, Saunders RA. Outcomes from surgical treatment for dissociated horizontal deviation. *J AAPOS.* 2000;4(2):94–101.

Convergence Insufficiency

Characteristics of convergence insufficiency include asthenopia, blurred near vision, and reading problems in the presence of poor near fusional convergence amplitudes and a remote near point of convergence. The patient, typically an older child or adult, may have an exophoria at near but, by definition, should not have an exotropia. Rarely, accommodative spasms may occur if accommodation and convergence are stimulated in an effort to overcome the convergence insufficiency. Convergence insufficiency, as discussed here, should not be confused with the convergence insufficiency type of intermittent exotropia discussed previously. Convergence insufficiency is seen more commonly in patients with Parkinson disease than in age-matched controls.

Treatment of convergence insufficiency usually involves orthoptic exercises. Base-out prisms can be used to stimulate fusional convergence during reading. Stereograms, "pencil push-ups," and other near point exercises are often used. If these exercises fail, base-in prism reading glasses may be needed. Medial rectus muscle resection, unilateral or bilateral, has been used in rare cases when nonsurgical treatments have been unsatisfactory, but this surgery carries a substantial risk of diplopia in distance viewing. Patients with combined convergence and accommodative insufficiency often benefit from plus lenses and base-in prisms for reading.

Convergence Paralysis

Convergence paralysis, a condition distinct from convergence insufficiency and usually secondary to an intracranial lesion, is characterized by normal adduction and accommodation with exotropia and diplopia on attempted near fixation only. Convergence paralysis differs from convergence insufficiency in its relatively acute onset and the patient's inability to overcome any base-out prism. Convergence paralysis usually results from a lesion in the corpora quadrigemina or the nucleus of cranial nerve III and may be associated with Parinaud syndrome (see BCSC Section 5, *Neuro-Ophthalmology*).

Treatment is limited to providing base-in prisms at near to alleviate the diplopia. Occasionally, accommodation also is weakened, particularly in a chronically ill patient, and plus lenses may also be required at near. These patients have little, if any, fusional vergence amplitudes, and it may not be possible to restore comfortable single binocular vision. Occlusion of 1 eye at near is indicated in such cases, and eye muscle surgery is contraindicated.

CHAPTER 9

A- and V-Pattern Horizontal Strabismus

Some patients have horizontal deviations that change in magnitude in upgaze and downgaze. An *A pattern* is present when a horizontal deviation shows a more convergent or less divergent alignment in upgaze than in downgaze. *V pattern* describes a horizontal deviation that is more convergent or less divergent in downgaze compared with upgaze. An A or V pattern is found in 15%–25% of horizontal strabismus cases. Other, less common variations of pattern horizontal strabismus include Y, λ, and X patterns.

Clinical Features and Identification

A and V patterns are determined by measurement of alignment while the patient fixates on an accommodative target at distance, with fusion prevented, in primary position and straight upgazes and downgazes. Proper refractive correction is necessary during measurement because an uncompensated accommodative component can introduce exaggerated convergence in downgaze.

An A pattern is considered clinically significant when the difference in measurement between upgaze and downgaze, each approximately 25° from the primary position, is at least 10 prism diopters (Δ); for a V pattern, the difference must be at least 15Δ.

Ophthalmologists have traditionally considered each of the following conditions to be a cause of A and V patterns, but these may merely be associations:

- *Bilateral oblique muscle dysfunction.* Inferior oblique muscle overaction is associated with V patterns (Figs 9-1, 9-2), and superior oblique muscle overaction with A patterns (Figs 9-3, 9-4), reflecting the ancillary abducting action in upgaze and downgaze, respectively, attributed to these muscles. Whether a true primary overaction of the oblique muscles exists, especially with respect to their vertical actions, is controversial (see Chapter 10).
- *Horizontal rectus muscle dysfunction.* One early school of thought attributed the patterns to varying effectiveness of the lateral rectus muscles in the upper half of the vertical gaze field, and of the medial rectus muscles in the lower half of this field. In this concept, for example, increases in lateral rectus or medial rectus muscle action produce a V pattern. Decreased action of these muscles produces an A pattern.

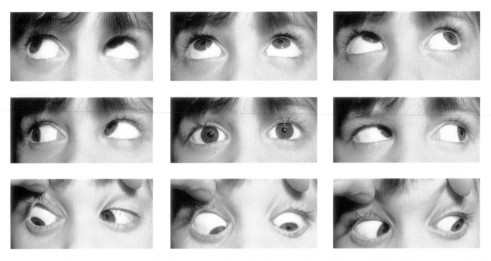

Figure 9-1 V-pattern esotropia. Note overelevation (overaction of the inferior oblique muscles) and limitation of depression (underaction of the superior oblique muscles) of each eye when in adduction.

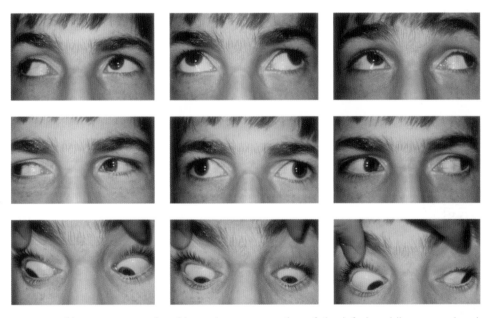

Figure 9-2 V-pattern exotropia with moderate overaction of the inferior oblique muscles. In this patient, there is no apparent underaction of either superior oblique muscle.

Although, empirically, horizontal rectus muscle surgery involving displacement of the reinsertions is somewhat effective as treatment of the underlying deviation (discussed later in this chapter), there is no convincing evidence that there are selective innervational influences on these muscles in vertical gazes.

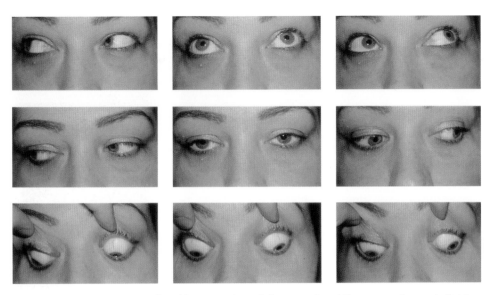

Figure 9-3 A-pattern exotropia with overaction of the superior oblique muscles and slight underaction of only the right inferior oblique muscle, with depression of the adducted right eye. Asymmetry of oblique muscle over- and underactions is common and often is ignored in the correction of A or V patterns when the discrepancy is small.

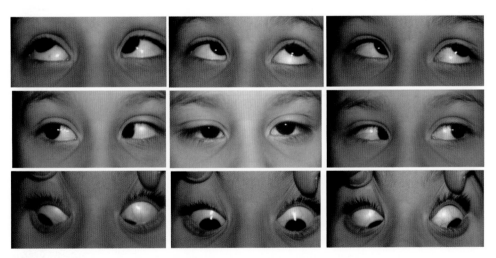

Figure 9-4 A-pattern esotropia with bilateral superior oblique muscle overaction and inferior oblique muscle underaction, left eye more so. *(Courtesy of Edward L. Raab, MD.)*

- *Vertical rectus muscle dysfunction.* Increases or decreases of the tertiary adducting action of these muscles can explain a less convergent or more divergent alignment in upgaze or downgaze and the corresponding pattern.

More recently, there has been extensive investigation of traditional concepts of extraocular muscle anatomy and function. Evidence of the existence of orbital pulleys that

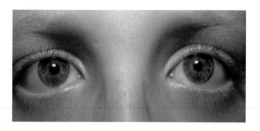

Figure 9-5 Downward slant of the palpebral fissures, often associated with a V-pattern horizontal deviation. *(Courtesy of Edward L. Raab, MD.)*

influence the paths of the rectus muscles has been extended to include the oblique muscles as well. Abnormalities (heterotopia) of the orbital pulley system have been postulated as the cause of simulated oblique muscle overactions and of altered rectus muscle pathways and functions, which can result in A or V patterns (see Chapter 2). These effects may also be linked to the observation that patients with upward- or downward-slanting palpebral fissures (Fig 9-5) also show A and V patterns because of an underlying variation in orbital configuration reflected in the orientation of the fissures. Patients with craniofacial anomalies (see Chapter 28) frequently have a V-pattern exotropia or esotropia with marked elevation of the adducting eye as an exaggeration of altered muscle pathways.

Demer JL. Mechanics of the orbita. *Dev Ophthalmol.* 2007;40:132–157.

Ron Y, Dagi LR. The etiology of V pattern strabismus in patients with craniosynostosis. *Int Ophthalmol Clin.* 2008;48(2):215–223.

Tan KP, Sargent MA, Poskitt KJ, Lyons CJ. Ocular overelevation in adduction in craniosynostosis: is it the result of excyclorotation of the extraocular muscles? *J AAPOS.* 2005;9(6): 550–557.

Management

Clinically significant patterns typically are treated surgically, in combination with correction of the underlying horizontal deviation (specific procedures are discussed in Chapter 12). The following are guidelines for planning surgical correction of A- and V-pattern deviations:

- The amount of horizontal rectus muscle surgery for the underlying horizontal deviation when the inferior oblique muscles are to be weakened should be the same as that for a deviation without an A or V pattern, because inferior oblique muscle weakening does not substantially change primary position alignment.
- Patients with large A or V patterns usually require weakening as part of the surgical plan. Weakening the inferior oblique muscles corrects up to 15Δ–20Δ of V pattern.
- Superior oblique muscle overaction is more likely to be observed in exotropia than in esotropia. Bilateral superior oblique tenotomies or lengthening procedures correct up to 35Δ–40Δ of A pattern (see also Chapter 12). There is a risk of induced torsional imbalance, especially in patients with fusional ability. Horizontal rectus muscle surgery with the appropriate displacement is an alternative treatment.

- The effect of bilateral superior oblique muscle weakening on primary position horizontal alignment remains somewhat controversial. Some surgeons think that this causes a change of 10Δ–15Δ toward convergence in primary position and suggest modifying horizontal surgery to compensate for this expected change. Because the appropriate amount of modification is difficult to determine, adjustable sutures on the horizontal rectus muscles can be helpful in a suitable patient.
- Displacing the horizontal rectus muscle insertions, usually one-half the width of the tendon, is indicated when oblique muscle dysfunction is absent or inconsistent with the pattern. The medial rectus muscles are always moved toward the "apex" of the pattern (ie, upward in A patterns and downward in V patterns). The lateral rectus muscles are moved toward the open end or "base" (ie, upward in V patterns and downward in A patterns). These rules apply whether the horizontal rectus muscles are weakened or tightened (Fig 9-6). Some surgeons have described a procedure in which, instead of displacing the reattached horizontal rectus muscles, one corner (upper or lower) of the insertion is placed farther from the limbus than the other (slanted insertion), giving an effect similar to that of displacement.
- When horizontal rectus muscle recession-resection surgery is the preferred choice because of other pertinent factors in the case (eg, prior surgery, unimprovable vision in 1 eye), displacement of the rectus muscle insertions should be in mutually opposite directions, according to the rules just stated. Unlike what occurs when both horizontal rectus muscles of an eye are moved in the same direction, this has little, if any, net vertical effect in the primary position. The same is thought to be true for torsion, although this has not been clearly shown.
- Vertical rectus procedures—for example, temporal displacement of the superior rectus muscles for A-pattern esotropia or temporal displacement of the inferior rectus muscles for V-pattern esotropia—are employed rarely, because the horizontal rectus muscle operations required for the underlying esotropia or exotropia can correct the pattern when appropriate displacements of the latter muscles are utilized.

Ohba M, Nakagawa T. Treatment for "A" and "V" exotropia by slanting muscle insertions. *Jpn J Ophthalmol.* 2000;44(4):433–438.

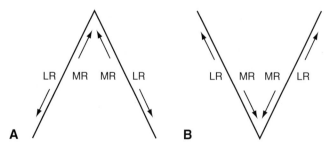

Figure 9-6   Direction of displacement of medial rectus (MR) and lateral rectus (LR) muscles in operations to treat A-pattern **(A)** and V-pattern deviations **(B)**. A useful mnemonic is MALE: *m*edial rectus muscle to the *a*pex, *l*ateral rectus muscle to the *e*mpty space. *(Reprinted from von Noorden GK, Campos EC.* Binocular Vision and Ocular Motility. *Theory and Management of Strabismus. 6th ed. St Louis: Mosby; 2002.)*

Summary of Treatment Plans

V-pattern esotropia and exotropia
- Appropriate horizontal rectus muscle procedure in usual amounts.
- Weakening of inferior oblique muscles if they are overacting.
- Horizontal rectus muscle insertion displacement if there is no inferior oblique muscle overaction.

A-pattern esotropia
- Appropriate horizontal rectus muscle procedure in usual amounts.
- Horizontal rectus muscle insertion displacement whether or not there is superior oblique muscle overaction (A pattern usually is small).

A-pattern exotropia
- Appropriate horizontal rectus muscle procedure in usual amounts or slightly less.
- Weakening of superior oblique muscles if large A pattern.
- Horizontal rectus muscle displacement if small A pattern, whether or not superior oblique muscles are overacting, especially in patients with fusional ability.

Additional discussion of A- and V-pattern horizontal deviations and an extensive bibliography can be found in the following references.

Biglan AW. Pattern strabismus. In: Rosenbaum AL, Santiago AP, eds. *Clinical Strabismus Management: Principles and Surgical Techniques.* Philadelphia: Saunders; 1999:202–215.

von Noorden GK, Campos EC. *Binocular Vision and Ocular Motility: Theory and Management of Strabismus.* 6th ed. St Louis: Mosby; 2002.

CHAPTER 10

Vertical Deviations

A vertical misalignment of the visual axes, or vertical deviation, may be comitant or incomitant (noncomitant). Either form can occur alone or be associated with a horizontal deviation, with the latter being the more typical setting for small comitant vertical deviations.

Most vertical deviations are incomitant. They are associated with so-called dysfunctional overactions or underactions of the superior and inferior oblique muscles, paralysis of 1 or more of these cyclovertical muscles, or restriction of vertical movement. Nearly every vertical paralytic deviation is incomitant at onset but may with time approach comitance unless there are associated restrictions, such as might occur with an orbital blowout fracture or thyroid eye disease.

A vertical deviation is described according to the direction of the deviating nonfixating eye. Accordingly, if the right eye is higher than the left and the left eye is fixating, the deviation is termed a *right hypertropia*. If the nonfixating right eye is lower than the fixating left eye, this is called a *right hypotropia*. If the ability to alternately fixate is present, the deviation is named for the usually hyperdeviating eye.

The following references give in-depth information on the entities discussed in this chapter, as well as on other topics in strabismus.

Rosenbaum AL, Santiago AP. *Clinical Strabismus Management: Principles and Surgical Techniques.* Philadelphia: Saunders; 1999.

von Noorden GK, Campos EC. *Binocular Vision and Ocular Motility: Theory and Management of Strabismus.* 6th ed. St Louis: Mosby; 2002.

Surgical treatment of these conditions is discussed in Chapter 12 of this volume.

Inferior Oblique Muscle Overaction

Overaction of the inferior oblique muscle is termed *primary* when it is not associated with superior oblique muscle paralysis. It is called *secondary* when it accompanies paresis or palsy of the inferior oblique muscle's antagonist superior oblique muscle or yoke superior rectus muscle. The eye is elevated in adduction, both horizontally and in upgaze (Fig 10-1).

One explanation of primary overaction involves vestibular influences governing postural tonus of the extraocular muscles. Some observers have questioned the concept of a true inferior oblique overaction, preferring to describe the movement merely

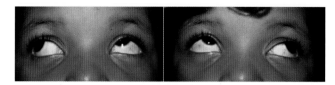

Figure 10-1 Bilateral inferior oblique overaction. Overelevation in adduction, seen best in the upper fields. *(Courtesy of Edward L. Raab, MD.)*

as *overelevation in adduction.* What appears to be an overaction may actually be due to abnormal function of a different extraocular muscle. Magnetic resonance imaging (MRI) studies have demonstrated connective tissue pulleys where the inferior oblique muscle's path crosses that of the inferior rectus muscle. This arrangement is said to lead to a dynamic interaction of these muscles during vertical rotation that could give the appearance of overaction (see Chapter 2). Nevertheless, in this chapter the traditional view of inferior oblique muscle overaction is retained. Chapter 9 discusses the traditional causative role of the oblique muscles in A- and V-pattern horizontal deviations.

Demer JL, Oh SY, Clark RA, Poukens V. Evidence for a pulley of the inferior oblique muscle. *Invest Ophthalmol Vis Sci.* 2003;44(9):3856–3865.

Kushner BJ. Multiple mechanisms of extraocular muscle "overaction." *Arch Ophthalmol.* 2006; 124(5):680–688.

Stager DR. Costenbader Lecture. Anatomy and surgery of the inferior oblique muscle: recent findings. *J AAPOS.* 2001;5(4):203–208.

Clinical Features

Primary inferior oblique muscle overaction has been reported to develop between ages 1 and 6 years in up to two-thirds of patients with infantile esotropia. The entity also occurs, less frequently, in association with acquired esotropia or exotropia and occasionally in patients with no other form of strabismus. A bilateral overaction can be asymmetric, because of either different times of onset or different degrees of severity.

With the eyes in lateral gaze to the opposite side, alternate cover testing shows that the higher eye refixates with a downward movement and that the lower eye does so with an upward movement. When inferior oblique overaction is bilateral, the higher and lower eyes reverse in the opposite lateral gaze. These features differentiate inferior oblique overaction from dissociated vertical deviation (DVD; see the discussion later in this chapter), in which neither eye refixates with an upward movement whether adducted, abducted, or in primary position. A V-pattern horizontal deviation and extorsion are common with overacting inferior oblique muscles.

Management

In all but the mildest cases, a weakening procedure on the inferior oblique muscle (recession, disinsertion, myectomy, or anterior transposition) is indicated, graded or not for the severity of the overaction according to the individual experience of the surgeon (see also Chapter 12). Variations in the structure or path of this muscle may affect the surgical result.

Some observers believe that a modest recession actually functions as an anterior transposition, an operation that has evolved in technique so that it is now useful for correcting marked overaction of the inferior oblique muscles and DVD, particularly when both are present simultaneously. Excyclotorsion can also be improved by this procedure. Actual results vary according to the new location of the anterior and posterior fibers of the reinserted inferior oblique muscle. A spread-out reinsertion, especially if closer to the limbus than is the inferior rectus muscle, can restrict elevation, especially when the eye is abducted (anti-elevation syndrome). Weakening of the inferior oblique muscles has an insignificant effect on primary position horizontal alignment. An associated horizontal deviation requiring surgical correction is treated at the same operative session.

Kushner BJ. Restriction of elevation in abduction after inferior oblique anteriorization. *J AAPOS.* 1997;1(1):55–62.

Santiago AP, Isenberg SJ, Apt L, Roh YB. The effect of anterior transposition of the inferior oblique muscle on ocular torsion. *J AAPOS.* 1997;1(4):191–196.

Superior Oblique Muscle Overaction

For clinical purposes, almost all cases of bilateral superior oblique muscle overaction can be considered primary, because paralysis of the inferior rectus and inferior oblique muscles is uncommon.

Clinical Features

A vertical deviation in primary position often occurs with unilateral or asymmetric bilateral overaction of the superior oblique muscles. The lower eye contains the unilaterally or more prominent bilaterally overacting superior oblique muscle. An associated horizontal deviation, most often exotropia, may be present. The overacting superior oblique muscle also results in hypotropia of the adducting eye in opposite lateral gaze, which is accentuated in the lower field (Fig 10-2). An alternative term for this finding is *overdepression in adduction*.

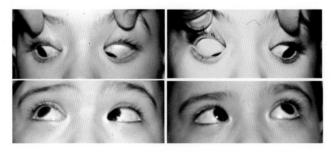

Figure 10-2 **Top row,** Bilateral superior oblique overaction. Overdepression in adduction, seen best in the lower fields. **Bottom row,** Associated bilateral inferior oblique underaction. *(Courtesy of Edward L. Raab, MD.)*

Management

In a patient with a clinically significant hypertropia or hypotropia or an A pattern, a superior oblique tendon weakening procedure (recession, tenotomy, tenectomy, or lengthening by insertion of a silicone expander or nonabsorbable suture or by Z-splitting) is appropriate (see also Chapter 12). However, many surgeons are reluctant to perform superior oblique muscle weakening in patients with binocular single vision, in whom the resulting, sometimes asymmetric torsional and/or vertical effects can cause diplopia. As with inferior oblique muscle overaction, the associated horizontal deviation is corrected at the same operative session. Some surgeons, anticipating a convergent effect, adjust their surgical amounts for horizontal rectus muscles when simultaneously weakening the superior oblique muscles.

Bardorf CM, Baker JD. The efficacy of superior oblique split Z-tendon lengthening for superior oblique overaction. *J AAPOS.* 2003;7(2):96–102.

Lee SY, Rosenbaum AL. Surgical results of patients with A-pattern horizontal strabismus. *J AAPOS.* 2003;7(4):251–255.

Oblique Muscle Pseudo-Overaction

There are occasions, such as in large-angle exotropia and thyroid eye disease, when clinical examination of ocular rotations indicates apparent overaction of both the superior and the inferior oblique muscles in the fields of their vertical action. This phenomenon can be explained as an attempt by the vertical rectus muscle of the opposite, abducting eye to overcome a relative restriction to elevation or depression (resulting from this muscle's confinement by the shape of the lateral portion of the bony orbit) through the exertion of extra innervation, which, by Hering's law, is distributed to the yoke oblique muscle as well. Unless it is severe, this condition does not require oblique muscle weakening as part of the surgical plan.

Dissociated Vertical Deviation

Dissociated vertical deviation (DVD) is an innervational disorder found in more than 50% of patients with infantile esotropia and in other forms of strabismus. One suggested explanation for DVD is that it may be the result of compensating mechanisms for latent nystagmus, with the oblique muscles having the principal role. Alternatively, recent work has suggested that deficient fusion allows the primitive dorsal light reflex, prominent in other species, to emerge.

Brodsky MC. Dissociated vertical divergence: a righting reflex gone wrong. *Arch Ophthalmol.* 1999;117(9):1216–1222.

Guyton DL. Ocular torsion reveals the mechanisms of cyclovertical strabismus: the Weisenfeld lecture. *Invest Ophthalmol Vis Sci.* 2008;49(3):847–857.

Clinical Features

DVD usually presents after age 2 years, whether or not the horizontal deviation it usually accompanies has been surgically corrected. Either eye slowly drifts upward and outward,

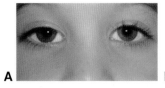 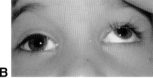 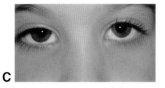

A   **B**   **C**

Figure 10-3 Dissociated vertical deviation, left eye. **A,** Straight eyes when binocular vision allowed. **B,** Large left hyperdeviation immediately after the eye is uncovered. **C,** Left eye drifts back down toward horizontal. The right eye behaves similarly (not shown).

with simultaneous extorsion, when occluded or during periods of visual inattention (Fig 10-3). Some patients attempt to compensate by tilting the head, for reasons that still have not been conclusively identified.

As the vertically deviated eye moves down (and intorts) to fixate when the previously fixating fellow eye is occluded, the latter makes no downward movement. Note that with true hypertropia, when the hypertropic eye refixates, the occluded fellow eye moves downward into a hypotropic position of equal magnitude. In contrast, eyes with DVD have no corresponding hypotropia of the fellow eye when the hypertropic eye refixates. The vertical movement usually predominates, but sometimes the principal dissociated movement is one of abduction *(dissociated horizontal deviation* or *DHD).*

The condition is usually bilateral though frequently asymmetric. It may occur spontaneously (manifest DVD) or only when 1 eye is occluded (latent DVD). In addition to DHD, latent nystagmus (see Chapter 25) and horizontal strabismus are often associated with DVD. These entities are manifestations of poor fusion.

Measurement of DVD is difficult and imprecise. One method uses base-down prism in front of the upwardly deviating eye while it is behind an occluder. The occluder is then switched to the fixating lower eye. The base-down prism power is adjusted until the deviating eye shows no downward movement to refixate. Results are similar when a red Maddox rod is used to generate a horizontal stripe viewed by the dissociated higher eye while the other eye fixates on a small light; vertical prism power is used to eliminate the separation of the light and the line. Each eye is tested separately in cases of bilateral DVD. The deviation can also simply be graded on a 1+ (least) to 4+ (most) scale.

Santiago AP, Rosenbaum AL. Dissociated vertical deviation and head tilts. *J AAPOS.* 1998; 2(1):5–11.

Management

Treatment for DVD is indicated if the deviation becomes manifest frequently. Changing fixation preference by penalization is effective mostly in unilateral or highly asymmetric bilateral DVD. Surgery on the vertical rectus muscles often improves the condition but rarely eliminates it. Distinguishing DVD from overaction of the inferior oblique muscles is important because the surgical approaches to these two conditions are different in most cases, although inferior oblique muscle anterior transposition is suitable for either entity.

Engman JH, Egbert JE, Summers CG, Young TL. Efficacy of inferior oblique anterior transposition placement grading for dissociated vertical deviation. *Ophthalmology.* 2001;108(11): 2045–2050.

Quinn AG, Kraft SP, Day C, Taylor RS, Levin AV. A prospective evaluation of anterior transposition of the inferior oblique muscle, with and without resection, in the treatment of dissociated vertical deviation. *J AAPOS.* 2000;4(6):348–353.

Superior Oblique Muscle Paralysis (Palsy or Paresis)

The most common single cyclovertical muscle paralysis encountered by the ophthalmologist is the fourth cranial (trochlear) nerve palsy, involving the superior oblique muscle. It can be congenital or acquired, the latter usually as a result of closed head trauma or, somewhat less commonly, central nervous system vascular problems, diabetes, and brain tumors. Direct trauma to the tendon or the trochlear area is an occasional cause of unilateral superior oblique muscle palsy.

The same clinical features can result from a congenitally lax, attenuated, or even absent superior oblique tendon; from an unusual course of the muscle; or from functional consequences of orbital pulleys, although strictly speaking, these are not paralytic entities. Superior oblique muscle underaction can also occur in several craniofacial abnormalities (see Chapter 28).

Kono R, Demer JL. Magnetic resonance imaging of the functional anatomy of the inferior oblique muscle in superior oblique palsy. *Ophthalmology.* 2003;110(6):1219–1229.

To differentiate congenital from acquired superior oblique muscle paralysis, the clinician will find it helpful to examine old family photographs to detect a compensatory head tilt present in childhood. Facial asymmetry from long-standing head tilting and large vertical fusional amplitudes also indicate chronicity. The distinction is important because recently diagnosed paralysis that cannot be attributed to known trauma suggests the possibility of a serious intracranial lesion and the need for neurologic investigation.

Neurologic aspects of superior oblique muscle paralysis are discussed in BCSC Section 5, *Neuro-Ophthalmology.*

Clinical Features

Either the normal or the affected eye can be preferred for fixation. Examination of versions usually reveals underaction of the involved superior oblique muscle and overaction of its antagonist inferior oblique muscle; however, the action of the superior oblique muscle can appear normal. If depression cannot be evaluated because of inability of the eye to adduct, for example in third cranial nerve paralysis, superior oblique function can be evaluated by observing whether there is intorsion of the eye, as judged by the movement of surface landmarks, when the patient looks downward from the primary position. The diagnosis of superior oblique muscle paralysis is further established by results of the 3-step determination (Fig 10-4) and double Maddox rod testing to measure torsional imbalance (see Chapter 6). However, 3-step test results can be confounded by DVD, entities involving restriction, and some cases of skew deviation. Intorsion of the higher eye—instead of the expected extorsion—determined by double Maddox rod testing and by ophthalmoscopy identifies skew deviation, especially when there are associated neurologic findings. Some

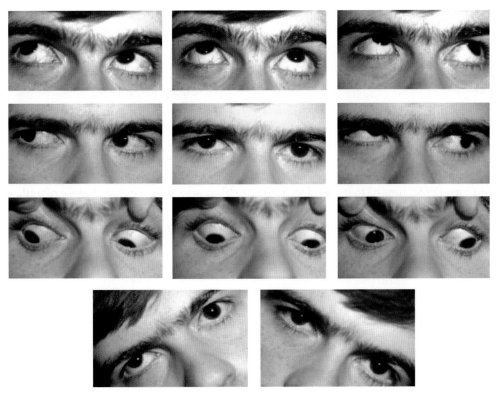

Figure 10-4 Right superior oblique palsy. There is a right hypertropia in primary position that increases on left gaze and with head tilted to the right. Note accompanying overaction of the right inferior oblique muscle. *(Courtesy of Edward L. Raab, MD.)*

ophthalmologists document serial changes in the deviation by means of the Hess screen or Lancaster red-green test, or plot the field of binocular single vision (see Chapter 6).

To differentiate bilateral from unilateral superior oblique muscle paresis or palsy, the following criteria are used:

- *Unilateral cases* usually show little if any V pattern (see Chapter 9) and less than 5° of excyclotorsion. The 3-step test yields positive results for the involved side only. Abnormal head positions are common, usually a tilt toward the shoulder opposite the side of the weakness. Amblyopia is common in congenital but not in acquired palsies.
- *Bilateral cases* usually show a V pattern. Excyclotorsion is at least 5° and is highly diagnostic when 10° or more. A complaint of apparent tilting of objects is common in acquired bilateral cases. The Bielschowsky head-tilt test yields positive results on tilt to each side—that is, right head tilt shows a right hypertropia and left head tilt a left hypertropia. Signs of bilaterality in cases initially thought to be unilateral include bilateral objective fundus excyclotorsion, esotropia in downgaze, and even the mildest degree of inferior oblique overaction (see earlier in the chapter) on the

presumed uninvolved side. Markedly asymmetric bilateral palsies that initially appear to be unilateral have prompted the term *masked bilateral.* This is especially to be anticipated when closed head trauma is the likely cause of the paralysis.

Management

Prisms that compensate the hyperdeviation in primary position may be used to overcome diplopia in small, symptomatic deviations that lack a prominent torsional component. Abnormal head position, significant vertical deviation, diplopia, and asthenopia are indications for surgery. Common operative strategies are discussed in the following sections.

Unilateral superior oblique muscle paralysis

The usual first approach to unilateral superior oblique muscle paralysis is weakening of the antagonist inferior oblique muscle alone when the hyperdeviation in primary position is no greater than 15Δ. The amount of deviation in primary position that is corrected by any weakening technique is proportional to the degree of overaction of the inferior oblique muscle. This procedure would be ineffective in skew deviation, as inferior oblique muscle weakening would aggravate the incyclotorsion of the higher eye.

If the primary position deviation is greater than 15Δ, or if there is an undercorrection after inferior oblique muscle weakening, one should add recession of the contralateral (yoke) inferior rectus muscle, which has the additional advantage of facilitating use of an adjustable suture, or tucking of the weak superior oblique muscle tendon if it is significantly lax. A variation of the forced duction test, described specifically for this purpose, helps identify a lax tendon.

Plager DA. Traction testing in superior oblique palsy. *J Pediatr Ophthalmol Strabismus.* 1990; 27(3):136–140.

As a basic guideline, each millimeter of recession of a vertical rectus muscle results in approximately 3Δ of vertical correction in the primary position. Determining the quantity of tuck for a superior oblique tendon is less exact, but the objective is to tuck the tendon until forced ductions on both sides are comparable. Excessive tucking risks the possibility of Brown syndrome (see Chapter 11).

The surgical plan should include recession of the ipsilateral superior rectus muscle if a forced duction test shows limited depression on the side of the hypertropia. This finding is expected in long-standing superior oblique palsy, because of ipsilateral superior rectus muscle contracture, in which case there is deficient depression across the lower field and the amount of deviation in right lateral gaze is closer to that in left lateral gaze, a so-called *spread of comitance.* On version testing, Hering's law may cause this to appear to represent superior oblique muscle overaction in the normal eye. If the surgeon is misled and performs superior oblique tenotomy on the normal eye, thereby converting a unilateral superior oblique palsy to a bilateral one, disabling torsional diplopia can result.

In the unusually severe case with a vertical deviation greater than 35Δ in primary position, 3-muscle surgery usually is required. In this situation, most surgeons would favor recession of the overacting antagonist inferior oblique muscle, ipsilateral superior oblique tendon tuck, and either ipsilateral superior rectus recession or contralateral inferior rectus recession, as dictated by forced duction test results.

Whatever the approach, it is important to avoid overcorrection of a long-standing unilateral superior oblique muscle paralysis in adult patients. Overcorrection will be aggravated with time and can cause disabling diplopia resembling the original problem.

Bilateral superior oblique muscle paralysis

Bilateral superior oblique muscle paralysis requires surgery on both eyes, graded for unequal severity. Bilateral inferior oblique muscle weakening is appropriate but may not be completely effective. Other options are the Harada-Ito procedure and those used for unilateral palsy. When inferior rectus muscle recession is employed, care is required to avoid postoperative retraction of the lower eyelid margin (see Chapter 12).

The Harada-Ito procedure is preferred in cases with predominantly torsional complaints. This operation involves displacement of the anterior portions of the superior oblique tendons to a location adjacent to the upper edge of the lateral rectus muscle, about 8 mm posterior to that muscle's insertion. The procedure, which can be done with adjustable sutures, corrects the deficient intorsion but not the vertical deviation in primary position. The effect tends to lessen with time.

Helveston EM, Mora JS, Lipsky SN, et al. Surgical treatment of superior oblique palsy. *Trans Am Ophthalmol Soc.* 1996;94:315–334.

Nishimura JK, Rosenbaum AL. The long-term torsion effect of the adjustable Harada-Ito procedure. *J AAPOS.* 2002;6(3):141–144.

Siatkowski RM. Third, fourth, and sixth nerve palsies. *Focal Points: Clinical Modules for Ophthalmologists.* San Francisco: American Academy of Ophthalmology; 1996, module 8.

Inferior Oblique Muscle Paralysis

Whether inferior oblique muscle paralysis actually exists has been questioned. It is difficult to understand how a selective lesion of the branch of the inferior division of cranial nerve (CN) III that specifically serves the inferior oblique muscle might occur. It has been suggested recently that at least some cases, especially those with an associated history of head trauma or with additional neurologic findings, are a form of skew deviation even if the diagnosis of inferior oblique muscle palsy is supported by results of the 3-step test (Fig 10-5). Other cases are thought to be explained by demonstrable abnormalities of the muscle.

In inferior oblique muscle paralysis, the hypotropic eye should be incyclotorted; in skew deviation, the hypotropic eye is seen to be excyclotorted, a finding incompatible with the former diagnosis. These phenomena are analogous to those described earlier for superior oblique paralysis. When the 3-step test results are not clear, such cases may represent asymmetric or unilateral primary superior oblique muscle overaction with secondary underaction of the inferior oblique muscle.

Donahue SP, Lavin PJ, Mohney B, Hamed L. Skew deviation and inferior oblique palsy. *Am J Ophthalmol.* 2001;132(5):751–756.

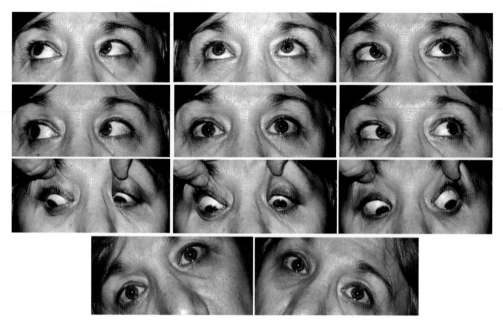

Figure 10-5 Right inferior oblique muscle palsy. Small left hypertropia in primary position, increasing in left gaze and in left head tilt, the 3-step pattern consistent with this diagnosis. This patient had no abnormal neurologic findings. Note convergence in straight upgaze, an important point of differentiation from Brown syndrome. *(Courtesy of Edward L. Raab, MD.)*

Clinical Features

As with Brown syndrome (see Chapter 11), elevation is deficient in the adducted position of the eye. The features that distinguish Brown syndrome from inferior oblique muscle paralysis are listed in Table 10-1.

Management

Indications for treatment of inferior oblique muscle paralysis are abnormal head position, vertical deviation in primary position, and diplopia. Management consists of either ipsilateral superior oblique muscle or contralateral superior rectus muscle weakening. The former procedure will aggravate the existing excyclotorsion of the hypotropic eye if an undetected skew deviation is the true underlying abnormality.

Table 10-1 Comparison of Inferior Oblique Muscle Paralysis and Brown Syndrome

	Inferior Oblique Muscle Paralysis	Brown Syndrome
Forced ductions	Negative	Positive
Strabismus pattern	A pattern	V pattern
Superior oblique muscle overaction	Usually present	None or minimal

Monocular Elevation Deficiency (Double Elevator Palsy)

Although the term *double elevator palsy* implies a paralysis of the inferior oblique and superior rectus muscles of the same eye, it has become an umbrella term for any strabismus manifesting deficient elevation in all horizontal orientations of the eye. Because this motility pattern is well known to be caused by restriction to elevation as well as by weakness of 1 or both elevator muscles, "double elevator palsy" is a misnomer as an inclusive term and has been replaced by *monocular elevation deficiency*.

Clinical Features

In monocular elevation deficiency, there is hypotropia of the involved eye that increases in upgaze, a chin-up position with fusion in downgaze, and ptosis or pseudoptosis (Fig 10-6). An element of true ptosis is present in 50% of patients. If any other feature of third cranial

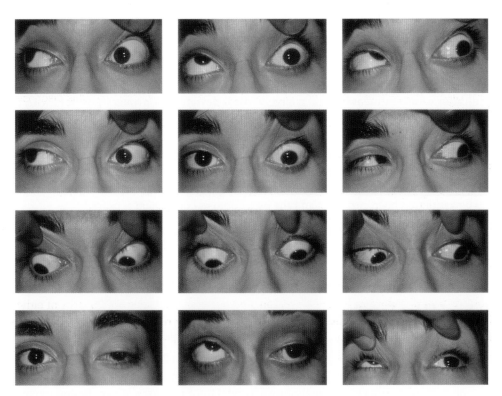

Figure 10-6 Monocular elevation deficiency of the left eye. **Top row,** No voluntary elevation of the left eye above horizontal. **Second row,** Hypotropia of the left eye across the fields of gaze. **Third row,** Depression of the left eye is unaffected. **Bottom left,** Ptosis (true and pseudo-) of the left upper eyelid during fixation with the right eye, persisting during fixation with the left eye **(bottom center).** [In the top 3 rows, the left upper eyelid is elevated manually.] **Bottom center,** Also shows the marked secondary overelevation of the right eye during fixation with the left eye. **Bottom right,** A partial Bell phenomenon, with the left eye elevating above the horizontal on forced eyelid closure.

nerve paralysis is present, that condition should be suspected rather than monocular elevation deficiency.

Three types of monocular elevation deficiency are found:

1. restriction
   - positive forced duction for elevation
   - normal elevation force generation and elevation saccadic velocity (no muscle paralysis)
   - often an extra or deeper lower eyelid fold on attempted upgaze
   - poor or absent Bell phenomenon
2. elevator muscle weakness
   - free forced ductions
   - reduced elevation force generation and saccadic velocity
   - Bell phenomenon often preserved (indicating a supranuclear cause)
3. combination
   - positive forced duction for elevation
   - reduced force generation and saccadic velocity for elevation

Management

Indications for treatment include a large vertical deviation in primary position, with or without ptosis, and an abnormal chin-up head position. If restriction originating from below the eye is present, the inferior rectus muscle should be recessed, if possible using a technique that allows adjustment of the muscle. If there is no restriction, the medial rectus and the lateral rectus muscles can be transposed toward the superior rectus muscle *(Knapp procedure)*. Upper eyelid surgery for ptosis should be deferred until after the vertical deviation has been corrected and the pseudoptosis component removed.

Rose LV, Elder JE. Management of congenital elevation deficiency due to congenital third nerve palsy and monocular elevation deficiency. *Clin Experiment Ophthalmol.* 2007;35(9): 840–846.

Orbital Floor Fractures

For a discussion of the anatomical features of the bony orbit, see BCSC Section 2, *Fundamentals and Principles of Ophthalmology,* and BCSC Section 7, *Orbit, Eyelids, and Lacrimal System,* the latter also dealing with the management of orbital floor fractures.

Blunt facial trauma is the usual cause of orbital floor fractures. When the rim remains intact, this is termed *blowout fracture.* Orbital floor fracture is considered to be caused by an acute increase in intraorbital pressure from direct impact that closes the orbital entrance, or by compression of the rim, which results in buckling of the floor. Orbital floor fracture can be part of more extensive fractures of the orbit and midface. In some cases, the mechanism causing floor fractures extends to include the medial wall as well and restricts horizontal rotation.

Injury to the inferior rectus muscle or to its nerve, with resulting weakness, may be caused by hemorrhage or ischemia, in addition to restriction. It can occur either at the time of orbital floor fracture or during repair of the fracture. The discussion in this chapter focuses on the implications for subsequent impaired motility.

Orbital roof fractures are discussed in Chapter 30.

Clinical Features

Hypoesthesia in the cutaneous distribution of the infraorbital nerve, especially after local swelling has subsided, is an ancillary sign of orbital fracture.

In the presence of limited elevation (Fig 10-7), a positive forced duction test indicates the presence of restriction. When the entrapment involves the more anterior portion of the orbital floor or when there is associated injury to the inferior rectus muscle, there can also be restriction to depression. Bradycardia, heart block, nausea, or syncope can occur as a vagal response to entrapment. Saccadic velocity and force generation testing help determine whether the eye is further limited in movement because of weak muscle action. Orbital computed tomography and high-resolution, multipositional magnetic resonance imaging are useful to reveal the presence and extent of the fracture.

Some authors have described a special presentation termed the "white-eyed blowout fracture." It is characterized by marked vertical motility restriction in both directions despite minimal soft tissue findings; this restriction is due to entrapment of the inferior rectus muscle either beneath a trapdoor fracture or, in the case of children, in a linear opening caused by flexion deformity of the floor. Early surgery, rather than observation, is required to minimize permanent muscle and nerve damage.

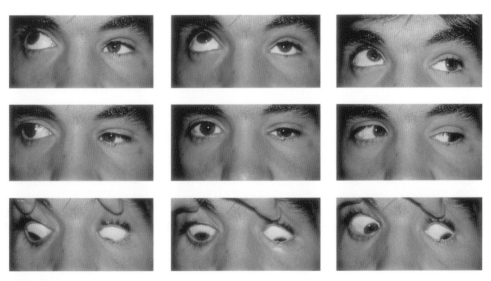

Figure 10-7 Old left orbital fracture with inferior rectus muscle entrapment. Note limitation of elevation of the left eye and pseudoptosis from enophthalmos. The eyelids are elevated manually in the bottom row.

Criden MR, Ellis FJ. Linear nondisplaced orbital fractures with muscle entrapment. *J AAPOS.* 2007;11(2):142–147.

Jordan DR, Allen LH, White J, Harvey J, Pashby R, Esmaeli B. Intervention within days for some orbital floor fractures: the white-eyed blowout. *Ophthal Plast Reconstr Surg.* 1998;14(6): 379–390.

Ortube MC, Rosenbaum AL, Goldberg RA, Demer JL. Orbital imaging demonstrates occult blowout fracture in complex strabismus. *J AAPOS.* 2004;8(3):264–273.

Management

A complete ophthalmic examination should be done to detect associated ocular injury (see Chapter 30).

There are several approaches to the management of orbital floor fractures. Some clinicians advocate exploration in all cases, irrespective of forced duction test results. The justification for this approach is that, especially with large bony defects, orbital contents can progressively herniate into the adjacent maxillary sinus, resulting in disfiguring enophthalmos. Others recommend waiting, from a few days to 2 weeks, for orbital ecchymosis to subside; the main indication to operate for these surgeons is evidence of restriction. A few ophthalmologists would not repair the fracture and deal only with any subsequent strabismus. Diplopia in the immediate postinjury stage is to be expected and is not necessarily an indication for urgent intervention.

The initial management of inferior rectus muscle weakness without entrapment is observation, because the weakness may reverse with time. If complete recovery does not take place within 6 months of the injury and if there is at least a moderate degree of active force, resection of the affected muscle combined with recession of the ipsilateral superior rectus muscle can be performed. Use of an adjustable suture as part of the recession procedure is a valuable addition when possible. Alternatively, a recession of the contralateral inferior rectus muscle with or without the addition of a posterior fixation suture can be used to limit that eye in downgaze and match the duction deficiency of the injured eye. This approach is known as *fixation duress* and is particularly useful when diplopia occurs in the reading position but no deviation is present in primary position. Transposition of the ipsilateral medial and lateral rectus muscles to the inferior rectus muscle (inverse Knapp procedure) is necessary for treatment of complete inferior rectus muscle palsy.

Whether or not there has been prior orbital surgery to release entrapped tissues, partial restriction persists in many cases even though imaging studies may show that there is no residual entrapment. For strabismus correction under these circumstances, the patient is assessed in the usual fashion, with emphasis on analysis of any limited rotations. If restrictions cannot be overcome, surgery on the uninvolved eye to create fixation duress, as described above, can be combined with whichever procedure is appropriate to correct the primary position.

Bansagi ZC, Meyer DR. Internal orbital fractures in the pediatric age group: characterization and management. *Ophthalmology.* 2000;107(5):829–836.

Burnstine MA. Clinical recommendations for repair of isolated orbital floor fractures: an evidence-based analysis. *Ophthalmology.* 2002;109(7):1207–1211.

CHAPTER **11**

Special Forms of Strabismus

The BCSC *Master Index* and BCSC Section 5, *Neuro-Ophthalmology,* should be consulted for additional discussion of several entities covered in this chapter.

Duane Syndrome

Duane syndrome presents in several ways, all of which are characterized by anomalous co-contraction of the medial and lateral rectus muscles, producing retraction of the globe in actual or attempted adduction. Horizontal eye movement can be limited to various degrees of severity in both abduction and adduction. A 1–2 mm vertical slippage of a tight lateral rectus muscle, which has been demonstrated by magnetic resonance imaging (MRI) studies, has been proposed as the cause of the upshoot or downshoot that often occurs when the affected eye is innervated to adduct. An alternative theory, based on questionable electromyographic evidence, is that anomalous vertical rectus muscle activity is responsible for upshoots and downshoots, but this is not widely credited.

Although most affected patients have Duane syndrome alone, many associated systemic defects have been observed, such as Goldenhar syndrome (hemifacial microsomia, ocular dermoids, ear anomalies, preauricular skin tags, and eyelid colobomas) and Wildervanck syndrome (sensorineural hearing loss, Klippel-Feil anomaly with fused cervical vertebrae). A defect in development occurring in the fourth week of gestation appears to be the cause of Duane syndrome, according to studies of patients prenatally exposed to thalidomide. The condition is considered one entity in a class termed *congenital cranial dysinnervation disorders,* which also includes the Möbius and congenital fibrosis syndromes, both discussed later in this chapter.

Most cases of Duane syndrome are sporadic, but about 5%–10% show autosomal dominant inheritance. Instances of linkage to more generalized disorders have been reported. Discordance in monozygotic twins raises the possibility that the intrauterine environment may be important in the development of Duane syndrome. A higher prevalence in females is reported in most series, and there is a predilection for the left eye.

In most anatomical and imaging studies, the nucleus of the sixth cranial nerve is absent and an aberrant branch of the third cranial nerve innervates the lateral rectus muscle. Results of electromyographic studies have been consistent with this finding. Although Duane syndrome is considered an innervational anomaly, tight and broadly inserted medial rectus muscles and fibrotic lateral rectus muscles, with corresponding forced duction abnormalities, are often encountered at surgery.

Engle EC. The genetic basis of complex strabismus. *Pediatr Res.* 2006;59(3):343–348.

Engle EC. Oculomotility disorders arising from disruptions in brainstem motor neuron development. *Arch Neurol.* 2007;64(5):633–637.

Traboulsi EI. Congenital cranial dysinnervation disorders and more. *J AAPOS.* 2007;11(3): 215–217.

Clinical Features

The most widely used classification of Duane syndrome defines 3 groups, although these may represent differences only in severity of the limited horizontal rotations: type 1 refers to poor abduction, frequently with primary position esotropia (Fig 11-1); type 2 refers to poor adduction and exotropia (Fig 11-2); and type 3 refers to poor abduction and adduction, with esotropia, exotropia, or no primary position deviation (Fig 11-3). About 15% of cases are bilateral; the type need not be the same in each eye.

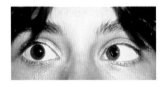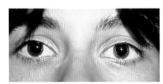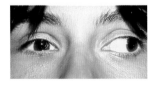

Figure 11-1 Type 1 Duane syndrome with esotropia, left eye, showing limitation of abduction, almost full adduction, and retraction of the globe on adduction. **Extreme right,** Compensatory left face turn. *(Courtesy of Edward L. Raab, MD.)*

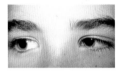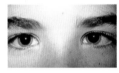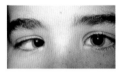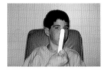

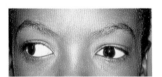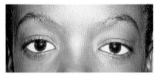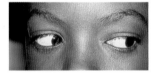

Figure 11-2 Type 2 Duane syndrome, left eye. **Top row,** Full abduction and marked limitation of adduction. **Bottom row,** Variable up- or downshoot of the left eye with extreme right gaze effort. The typical primary position exotropia is not present in this patient. *(Courtesy of Edward L. Raab, MD.)*

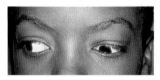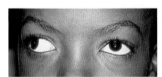

Figure 11-3 Type 3 Duane syndrome, right eye. Severe limitation of abduction and adduction, with palpebral fissure narrowing even though adduction cannot be accomplished. No deviation in primary position. *(Courtesy of Edward L. Raab, MD.)*

Type 1 Duane syndrome is the most common form (50%–80% in several series). Affected individuals or their caregivers often incorrectly believe that what is actually the normal eye is turning in excessively, not realizing that the involved eye is not abducting. Observation of globe retraction on adduction obviates a neurologic investigation for a sixth cranial nerve paralysis, although retraction can be difficult to appreciate in an infant. Another indicator pointing away from sixth cranial nerve paralysis is the lack of correspondence between the absent or typically modest primary position esotropia and the usually profound abduction deficit (a comparison useful in ruling out paralysis in other entities as well). A further point of differentiation is that, even in esotropic Duane syndrome, a small-angle exotropia frequently is present in gaze to the side opposite the affected eye, a finding not present in lateral rectus muscle paralysis.

Alexandrakis G, Saunders RA. Duane retraction syndrome. *Ophthalmol Clin North Am.* 2001; 14(3):407–417.

Raab EL. Clinical features of Duane's syndrome. *J Pediatr Ophthalmol Strabismus.* 1986;23(2): 64–68.

Management

No surgical approach will normalize rotations. Surgery is reserved for cases with a primary position deviation, a face turn, marked globe retraction, or large upshoots or downshoots. Many patients with Duane syndrome have some position of gaze in which the eyes are properly aligned, allowing the development of binocular vision. One goal of surgery is to centralize and expand the field of single binocular vision.

For type 1 Duane syndrome, recession of the medial rectus muscle on the involved side has been the most often used procedure to correct the primary position deviation and eliminate the face turn. Adding recession of the opposite medial rectus has been recommended for deviations over 20Δ in primary position. Abduction is not improved by these operations. Primary position overcorrection by medial rectus recession can occur, as can exotropia when the involved eye is adducted. Recession of the lateral rectus muscle of the uninvolved eye can offset this effect.

Because of the likelihood that globe retraction will worsen, most surgeons do not favor resection of the lateral rectus muscle for type 1 Duane syndrome, although there are occasional exceptions. Partial or full transposition of the vertical rectus muscles with posterior scleral fixation, as described by Foster, has been found helpful to improve abduction.

The recommended surgery for type 2 Duane syndrome is comparable to that for type 1: recession of the lateral rectus on the involved side for small deviations and of both lateral recti for large deviations, with avoidance of resection of the medial rectus muscle.

Patients with type 3 Duane syndrome often have straight eyes in or near the primary position and little, if any, head turn. Severe globe retraction may be helped by recession of both the medial and the lateral rectus muscles, which also may benefit the induced anomalous vertical excursion. Additional suggested procedures for the upshoot or downshoot are splitting the lateral rectus muscle in a Y configuration, a posterior fixation procedure on this muscle, and, more recently, disinsertion of the lateral rectus muscle and reattachment to the lateral wall of the orbit.

Foster RS. Vertical muscle transposition augmented with lateral fixation. *J AAPOS*. 1997;1(1): 20–30.

Jampolsky A. Duane syndrome. In: Rosenbaum AL, Santiago AP, eds. *Clinical Strabismus Management: Principles and Surgical Techniques*. Philadelphia: Saunders; 1999:325–346.

Rao VB, Helveston EM, Sahare P. Treatment of upshoot and downshoot in Duane syndrome by recession and Y-splitting of the lateral rectus muscle. *J AAPOS*. 2003;7(6):389–395.

Rosenbaum AL. Costenbader Lecture. The efficacy of rectus muscle transposition surgery in esotropic Duane syndrome and VI nerve palsy. *J AAPOS*. 2004;8(5):409–419.

Brown Syndrome

Though included in most lists of vertical deviations, Brown syndrome is best considered as a special form of strabismus. The characteristic restriction of elevation in adduction was originally thought to be caused by shortening of the supposed sheath of the superior oblique tendon. It is now attributed to various abnormalities of the tendon–trochlea complex (see Chapter 2), and recent evidence indicates that structural problems within the orbit but remote from the superior oblique tendon, including lateral rectus pulley instability, can give an identical clinical picture ("pseudo–Brown syndrome").

Most cases are congenital. Prominent causes of the acquired form include trauma in the region of the trochlea and systemic inflammatory conditions. The latter often result in intermittent Brown syndrome, which may resolve spontaneously. Sinusitis has also led to Brown syndrome; thus, patients with an acute-onset presentation of Brown syndrome of undetermined cause should undergo CT of the orbits and paranasal sinuses to investigate this possibility. The condition is bilateral in approximately 10% of cases. Resolution of congenital Brown syndrome has been thought unusual, but a recent report describes improvement in 75% of cases.

Bhola R, Rosenbaum AL, Ortube MC, Demer JL. High-resolution magnetic resonance imaging demonstrates varied anatomic abnormalities in Brown syndrome. *J AAPOS*. 2005;9(5): 438–448.

Dawson E, Barry J, Lee J. Spontaneous resolution in patients with congenital Brown syndrome. *J AAPOS*. 2009;13(2):116–118.

Clinical Features

Well-recognized clinical features of Brown syndrome include deficient elevation in adduction that improves in abduction but often not completely (Fig 11-4). Several findings differentiate Brown syndrome from inferior oblique muscle paralysis (see Chapter 10, Table 10-1).

An unequivocally positive forced duction test demonstrating restricted passive elevation in adduction is essential for the diagnosis. Retropulsion of the globe during this determination stretches the superior oblique tendon and accentuates the restriction, in contrast to restrictions involving the inferior rectus muscle or its surrounding tissues, in which the limitation of passive elevation is accentuated by forceps-induced proptosis of the eye rather than by retropulsion.

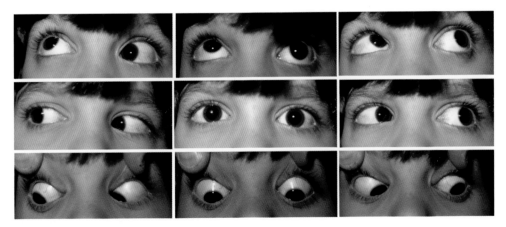

Figure 11-4 Brown syndrome, left eye. No elevation of the left eye when adducted. Left eye is depressed instead. Elevation is also severely limited in straight-up gaze and moderately so even in up-and-left gaze. The characteristic divergence in straight-up gaze should be noted. *(Courtesy of Edward L. Raab, MD.)*

Attempts at straight-ahead elevation usually cause divergence (V pattern). This finding is an important difference from inferior oblique muscle paralysis. In adduction, the palpebral fissure widens and a downshoot of the involved eye on gaze to the opposite side occurs in severe cases; it can be distinguished from that of superior oblique muscle overaction because downshoot in the latter condition occurs less abruptly as adduction is increased. In mild Brown syndrome, no hypotropia is present in primary position. Severe Brown syndrome cases have both a downshoot in adduction and a primary gaze hypotropia, often accompanied by a chin-up head posture and sometimes by a face turn away from the affected eye. Moderate cases show findings between these extremes.

Plager DA. Traction testing in superior oblique palsy. *J Pediatr Ophthalmol Strabismus.* 1990; 27(3):136–140.

Management

Observation alone is appropriate for mild Brown syndrome. When Brown syndrome is associated with rheumatoid arthritis or other systemic inflammatory diseases, resolution may occur as systemic treatment brings the underlying disease into remission or when corticosteroids are injected near the trochlea.

Surgery is indicated for more severe cases. Harold Brown's original advocacy of sheathectomy has been abandoned in favor of ipsilateral superior oblique tenotomy nasal to the superior rectus muscle. However, iatrogenic superior oblique muscle palsy frequently occurs after this procedure. The occurrence rate of this sequel can be reduced by careful handling of the intermuscular septum during tenotomy; by an inert spacer sewn to the cut ends of the superior oblique tendon (see Chapter 12); or by controlling the gap between the cut ends with an adjustable suture. Using either of these procedures, the surgeon should repair the intermuscular septum to prevent contact of the spacer or suture with nearby structures and therefore avoid a downgaze restriction due to adhesions to the nasal quadrant of the globe. To further reduce the consequences of superior oblique muscle palsy after tenotomy, some surgeons perform simultaneous ipsilateral inferior oblique muscle weakening. Partial (80%) tenectomy of the posterior portion of the tendon is efficacious and avoids the complication of superior oblique muscle palsy.

Velez FG, Velez G, Thacker N. Superior oblique posterior tenectomy in patients with Brown syndrome with small deviations in the primary position. *J AAPOS*. 2006;10(3):214–219.

Wright KW. Brown's syndrome: diagnosis and management. *Trans Am Ophthalmol Soc*. 1999;97: 1023–1109.

Third Cranial Nerve Paralysis

Third cranial (oculomotor) nerve paralysis in children can be congenital (40%–50%) or can be caused by conditions such as trauma, inflammation, viral infection, and migraine; it can also occur following inoculations and (infrequently) from neoplastic lesions. In adults, the usual causes are intracranial aneurysm, microvascular infarction, diabetes, inflammation, trauma, infection, or tumor. See BCSC Section 5, *Neuro-Ophthalmology,* for detailed discussion of the causes and manifestations of third cranial nerve paralysis. This section is concerned primarily with the principles of treatment of the disturbed motility.

Clinical Features

The location of the lesion along the central and peripheral pathway of the third cranial nerve determines the presenting features. Complete external (ie, pupil sparing) paralysis results in limited adduction, elevation, and depression of the eye, causing exotropia and often hypotropia. These findings would be expected because the remaining unopposed muscles are the lateral rectus (abductor) and the superior oblique (abductor and depressor), unless the cause of the paralysis involves the nerves supplying these muscles as well. Upper eyelid ptosis usually is present, often with a pseudoptosis component due to the depressed position of the involved eye (Fig 11-5). The clinical findings and treatment may be complicated by misdirection (aberrant regeneration) of the damaged nerve, presenting as anomalous eyelid elevation, pupil constriction, or vertical excursion of the globe—any or all of which can occur on attempted rotation into the field of action of the extraocular muscles supplied by the injured nerve. A miotic pupil is sometimes seen in congenital cases, irrespective of whether there is aberrant regeneration. Affected adults complain of diplopia unless the involved eye is occluded by ptosis or other means.

Management

Except in congenital cases, it is advisable to wait 3–6 months for any spontaneous recovery before surgical correction is planned. Patients with at least partial recovery are much better candidates for good functional and cosmetic results. Because the visual system is still developing in pediatric patients, amblyopia is a common finding that must be treated aggressively.

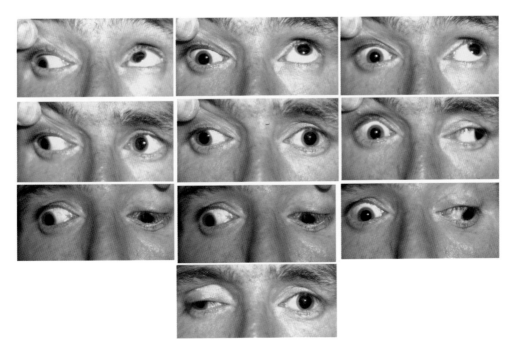

Figure 11-5 Third cranial nerve paralysis, right eye, with ptosis *(bottom)* and limited adduction, elevation, and depression (upper eyelid elevated manually in top 3 rows). *(Courtesy of Edward L. Raab, MD.)*

Elevation of the upper eyelid and incomplete realignment without useful single binocular fields may reinforce the incapacitating diplopia in adult patients with previously good binocular visual function. Prism adaptation testing has shown that adult patients who can achieve single binocular vision with prisms of any power prior to surgery are most likely to do well. The occurrence rate of diplopia in patients younger than 8 years is low because of the ability of the young binocular visual system to suppress conflicting visual information.

Third cranial nerve paralysis presents difficult surgical challenges because multiple extraocular muscles as well as the levator are involved. Replacing all of the lost rotational forces on the globe is impossible; therefore, the goal of surgery is adequate alignment for binocular function in primary position and in slight downgaze for reading.

Planning the appropriate surgical procedure is dictated by the number and condition of the involved muscles and the presence of noticeable paradoxical rotations. Frequently, a large recession-resection procedure on the horizontal rectus muscles to correct the exo-deviation, with supraplacement of both to correct the hypotropia, is effective, especially with incomplete paralysis. Large lateral rectus muscle recession combined with fixation of the globe to the nasal orbital periosteum is one suggested approach for complete palsy. Maximum inactivation of the lateral rectus muscle can be obtained by disinsertion and reattachment to the lateral orbital periosteum. Some surgeons correct hypotropia with superior oblique tenotomy. Transfer of the superior oblique tendon to the upper nasal quadrant of the globe also has been employed; however, anomalous eye movements can result from this procedure. Most surgeons reserve correction of ptosis for a subsequent procedure, which allows for a more accurate assessment.

Aoki K, Sakaue T, Kubota N, Maruo T. Outcome of surgery for bilateral third nerve palsy. *Jpn J Ophthalmol.* 2002;46(5):540–547.

Mudgil AV, Repka MX. Ophthalmologic outcome after third cranial nerve palsy or paresis in childhood. *J AAPOS.* 1999;3(1):2–8.

Schumacher-Feero LA, Yoo KW, Solari FM, Biglan AW. Third cranial nerve palsy in children. *Am J Ophthalmol.* 1999;128(2):216–221.

Siatkowski RM. Third, fourth, and sixth nerve palsies. *Focal Points: Clinical Modules for Ophthalmologists.* San Francisco: American Academy of Ophthalmology; 1996, module 8.

Sixth Cranial Nerve Paralysis

Paralysis of the sixth cranial (abducens) nerve is less common in children than in adults. A prominent cause of this entity in childhood occurs in association with viral infections. In this setting, recovery is usually prompt, but the condition can be recurrent. See BCSC Section 5, *Neuro-Ophthalmology,* for additional discussion.

Clinical Features

The causes and features of sixth cranial nerve paralysis are discussed in Chapter 7. Findings distinguishing this entity from Duane syndrome include the absence of upshoots or downshoots and of retraction of the globe on adduction, and the presence of esotropia in primary position that is commensurate with the usually severe limitation of abduction (Fig 11-6), which is not seen in Duane syndrome. Limitation of abduction resulting from medial wall orbital fractures will give a positive forced duction test result (if it is possible to perform this test), and in most cases there will be a clear history of facial trauma. Analysis of the limited rotations is described in Chapter 6.

Management

Spontaneous resolution may occur in more than half of patients with traumatic paralysis, particularly if it is unilateral. Injection of botulinum toxin into the antagonist medial rectus muscle may align the eye by temporarily paralyzing the medial rectus muscle (see

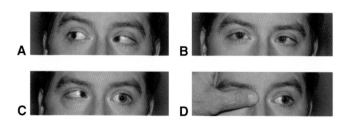

Figure 11-6 Sixth cranial nerve paralysis, left eye. **A,** Right gaze. **B,** Esotropia in primary position. **C,** Limited abduction, left eye. **D,** Still incomplete but further abduction of left eye when fixating, a finding important in the plan for surgical correction. *(Courtesy of Edward L. Raab, MD.)*

Chapter 13). Botulinum treatment has not been shown to be helpful in improving the rate of recovery.

Surgery is indicated when spontaneous resolution does not take place after 6 months or more of follow-up. In patients with some lateral rectus muscle function, a large recession of the antagonist medial rectus muscle, combined with resection of the lateral rectus muscle, often is a successful first operation. In cases of total paralysis, muscle transposition procedures usually are required.

Holmes JM, Beck RW, Kip KE, Droste PJ, Leske DA. Botulinum toxin treatment versus conservative management in acute traumatic sixth nerve palsy or paresis. *J AAPOS*. 2000;4(3): 145–149.

Thyroid Eye Disease

Thyroid eye disease affects the eye and the orbit in a variety of ways. This condition is discussed in several other volumes of the BCSC as *thyroid ophthalmopathy* or *thyroid-associated orbitopathy* (consult the *Master Index*). Additional terms for this entity include *thyroid orbitopathy, thyroid-related immune orbitopathy,* and *Graves disease.* Only motility disturbances are covered in this volume.

Edema, inflammation, and fibrosis of the extraocular muscles due to lymphocytic infiltration occur in this disease. Not only do these restrict motility, but the massively enlarged muscles can cause compressive optic neuropathy. Detection of muscle enlargement by orbital ultrasonography, CT, or MRI helps confirm the diagnosis.

The myopathy is not caused by thyroid dysfunction. Rather, both conditions probably result from a common autoimmune disease. Some patients also have myasthenia gravis (discussed later in this chapter), complicating the clinical findings. An association between thyroid eye disease and smoking has recently become apparent.

Clinical Features

The muscles affected, in decreasing order of severity and frequency, are the inferior rectus, medial rectus, superior rectus, and lateral rectus. The condition most often is bilateral and asymmetric. Forced duction test results are almost always positive in 1 or more directions.

The patient presents most often with some degree of upper eyelid retraction, proptosis, hypotropia, and esotropia (Fig 11-7). Thyroid eye disease is a common cause of acquired vertical deviation in adults, especially females, but is rare in children.

Management

Diplopia and abnormal head position are the principal indications for strabismus surgery. The operation may eliminate diplopia in primary gaze but rarely restores normal motility because of the restrictive myopathy, the need for very large recessions to allow the eye to be in primary position, and the ongoing underlying disease.

Stability of the strabismus measurements is desirable before surgery is performed; waiting for at least 6 months is recommended. In the meantime, prisms may alleviate

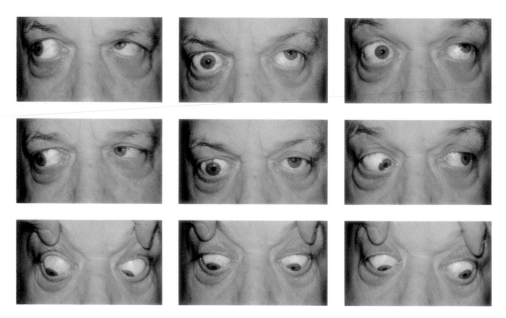

Figure 11-7 Thyroid eye disease. Note right upper eyelid retraction and restrictive right hypotropia with very limited elevation. Other rotations are not affected.

diplopia. Performance of surgery before stability is achieved in patients with severe head positions has been studied. The results were favorable, although half of the patients required further surgery.

Recession of the affected muscles is the preferred surgical treatment. Strengthening procedures usually worsen restriction. Adjustable sutures can be helpful in these difficult cases. Slight initial undercorrection is desirable, because late progressive overcorrection is common, especially with large inferior rectus muscle recessions. Limited depression of the eyes after inferior rectus muscle recessions can interfere with bifocal use by patients. Proptosis can become worse after extraocular muscle recessions.

If the need for orbital decompression is foreseeable, it is usually preferable to postpone strabismus surgery until decompression has been accomplished. Likewise, eyelid surgery usually is postponed because upper eyelid retraction may be improved when the patient no longer strains to elevate the eye.

Large recessions of very tight inferior rectus muscles can also cause lower eyelid retraction severe enough to require subsequent correction. Severing the lower eyelid retractors as part of the strabismus surgery has led to some success at preventing this complication. If necessary, a spacer of banked sclera or synthetic material can be placed to vertically lengthen the lower lid tarsus (see also Chapter 12).

Cockerham KP, Kennerdel JS. Thyroid-associated orbitopathy. *Focal Points: Clinical Modules for Ophthalmologists.* San Francisco: American Academy of Ophthalmology; 1997, module 1.

Mills MD, Coats DK, Donahue SP, Wheeler DT; American Academy of Ophthalmology. Strabismus surgery for adults: a report by the American Academy of Ophthalmology. *Ophthalmology.* 2004;111(6):1255–1262.

Thomas SM, Cruz OA. Comparison of two different surgical techniques for the treatment of strabismus in dysthyroid ophthalmopathy. *J AAPOS.* 2007;11(3):258–261.

Chronic Progressive External Ophthalmoplegia

Clinical Features

Chronic progressive external ophthalmoplegia (CPEO) usually begins in childhood with ptosis and slowly progresses to total paralysis of the eyelids and extraocular muscles. CPEO may be sporadic or familial. Although a true pigmentary retinal dystrophy usually is absent, constricted fields and electrodiagnostic abnormalities can occur. Defects in mitochondrial DNA have been found in some patients. *Kearns-Sayre syndrome* consists of retinal pigmentary changes, CPEO, and cardiomyopathy (especially heart block).

See BCSC Section 2, *Fundamentals and Principles of Ophthalmology*, Section 5, *Neuro-Ophthalmology*, and Section 12, *Retina and Vitreous*, for additional information on these and other mitochondrial disorders.

Management

It is important to ensure that the patient's cardiac status is evaluated, because life-threatening arrhythmias can occur in Kearns-Sayre syndrome. Treatment options for the ocular motility disorder are limited. Cautious surgical elevation (suspension) of the upper eyelids can lessen a severe chin-up head position.

Myasthenia Gravis

Onset of myasthenia gravis in childhood is uncommon. A transient neonatal form, caused by the placental transfer of acetylcholine receptor antibodies of mothers with myasthenia gravis, usually subsides rapidly. Another variety is not immune-mediated and exhibits a familial incidence.

The disease may be purely ocular but, in the most severe form, frequently occurs as part of a major systemic disorder, with other skeletal muscles involved as well, especially in patients who have not received immunosuppressive therapy. BCSC Section 5, *Neuro-Ophthalmology*, discusses both the ocular and the systemic aspects of myasthenia gravis in depth. Additional information is available on the website of the Myasthenia Gravis Foundation of America, Inc (www.myasthenia.org).

Clinical Features

The principal ocular manifestation is weakening of the extraocular muscles, including the levator muscle. Most cases (90%) have both ptosis and limited ocular rotations. The ocular signs can resemble any unilateral or bilateral ophthalmoplegia, even the extremely rare isolated inferior rectus muscle paralysis.

Affected muscles fatigue rapidly, so ptosis typically increases when the patient is required to look upward for 30 seconds. In the sleep test, ptosis often resolves after 20–30 minutes in a dark room with the eyelids closed. The presence of *Cogan twitch*, an overshoot of the eyelid when the patient looks straight ahead after looking down for several minutes, also is highly suggestive.

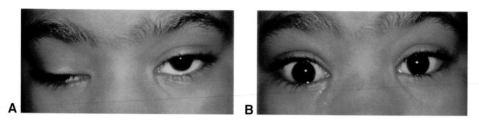

Figure 11-8 Myasthenia gravis. **A,** Bilateral ptosis (right more than left) with right hypotropia and exotropia. **B,** Following Tensilon injection, the eyes show orthophoria, normal eyelid position, and the lacrimation that frequently accompanies Tensilon injection.

External application of ice for 2–5 minutes improves function of the levator and other affected extraocular muscles, providing a rapid and reliable method of establishing this diagnosis without the need for drug administration.

The classic edrophonium (Tensilon) test can establish the diagnosis (Fig 11-8). Neostigmine (Prostigmin), an alternative, has the advantage of allowing more time to measure changes in alignment, as the effect of this agent begins later than that of edrophonium and is prolonged.

Electromyography shows decreased electrical activity of involved muscles after prolonged voluntary innervations, and increased activity (including saccadic velocity) after the administration of edrophonium or neostigmine. Documentation of abnormalities by single-fiber electromyography or the presence of circulating antiacetylcholine receptor or anti-MuSK protein antibodies is confirmatory, although a negative result does not rule out the presence of this disease.

Table 11-1 compares the features of thyroid eye disease with CPEO and myasthenia gravis.

Ellis FD, Hoyt CS, Ellis FJ, Jeffery AR, Sondhi N. Extraocular muscle responses to orbital cooling (ice test) for ocular myasthenia gravis diagnosis. *J AAPOS.* 2000;4(5):271–281.

Mullaney P, Vajsar J, Smith R, Buncic JR. The natural history and ophthalmic involvement in childhood myasthenia gravis at the Hospital for Sick Children. *Ophthalmology.* 2000;107(3):504–510.

Management

A full discussion of treatment of the various forms of myasthenia gravis is beyond the scope of this chapter. The ocular manifestations frequently are resistant to the usual systemic myasthenia treatment. When the ocular deviation has stabilized, standard eye muscle surgery can be helpful in restoring binocular function in at least some gaze positions. Ptosis occasionally requires upper eyelid surgery.

Congenital Fibrosis Syndrome

Congenital fibrosis syndrome is a group of rare congenital disorders in which extraocular muscle restriction is present and fibrous tissue replaces these muscles. Some forms have

Table 11-1 Differentiation of Conditions Producing Ptosis and Extraocular Muscular Involvement

	Thyroid Eye Disease	Chronic Progressive External Ophthalmoplegia (CPEO)	Myasthenia Gravis
Age	Any age	Any age	Any age
Muscle preferentially involved	Inferior rectus, medial rectus muscles	Levator, extraocular muscles	Levator, extraocular muscles
Fatiguability	No, unless coexistent myasthenia gravis	No	Yes
Response to Tensilon	No, unless coexistent myasthenia gravis	No	Yes
Other eye signs	External eye signs	Pigmentary retinopathy, optic neuropathy	No
Forced ductions	Restriction	Restriction if long-standing	Normal
Clinical course	May resolve or progress	Slowly progressive	Fluctuation; may have generalized weakness
Eyelids	Retraction	Ptosis	Ptosis
Diplopia	Yes	No	Yes
Other signs and symptoms	Tachycardia, arrhythmia, tremor, weight loss, diarrhea, heat intolerance	Heart block (manifestation of Kearns-Sayre syndrome)	Dysphagia, jaw weakness, limb weakness, dyspnea

been noted to be inherited, usually as an autosomal dominant trait but occasionally as an autosomal recessive, and involve developmental defects of cranial nerve nuclei and of the nerves themselves, resulting in dysinnervation and aberrant responses of the extraocular muscles. Congenital fibrosis syndrome is now included in the group of diseases termed *congenital cranial dysinnervation disorders.*

Heidary G, Engle EC, Hunter DG. Congenital fibrosis of the extraocular muscles. *Semin Ophthalmol.* 2008;23(1):3–8.

Clinical Features

There are several variations of this entity. Generalized fibrosis is the most severe form, affecting all the extraocular muscles of both eyes, including the levator muscle. Congenital unilateral fibrosis is nonfamilial.

Involvement of the inferior rectus muscle alone may be unilateral or bilateral and sporadic or familial. This condition is commonly inherited as an autosomal dominant trait.

Strabismus fixus involves the horizontal recti, usually the medial rectus muscles, causing severe esotropia. The condition usually is sporadic and can be acquired late.

Vertical retraction syndrome affects the superior rectus muscle, with inability to depress the eye.

Diagnosis of congenital fibrosis syndrome depends on finding limited voluntary motion, with restriction confirmed by forced duction testing. The congenital origin is an important distinction from thyroid eye disease.

Management

Surgery is difficult and requires release of the restricted muscles (ie, weakening procedures). Fibrosis of the adjacent tissues may be present as well. A good surgical result aligns the eyes in primary position, but full ocular rotations cannot be restored and the outcome is unpredictable.

> Yazdani A, Traboulsi EI. Classification and surgical management of patients with familial and sporadic forms of congenital fibrosis of the extraocular muscles. *Ophthalmology.* 2004; 111(5):1035–1042.

Möbius Syndrome

Clinical Features

Möbius (Moebius) syndrome (or "sequence"; see Chapter 14) is a rare condition characterized by the association of both sixth and seventh cranial nerve palsies, the latter causing masklike facies. Patients may also manifest gaze palsies that can be attributed to abnormalities in the pontine paramedian reticular formation or the sixth cranial nerve nucleus. Many patients also show limb, chest, and tongue defects, and some geneticists think that Möbius syndrome is one of a family of syndromes in which hypoplastic limb anomalies are associated with orofacial and cranial nerve defects. Poland syndrome (absent pectoralis muscle) is another variant.

The patient with Möbius syndrome has esotropia or straight eyes in primary position. Both abduction and adduction may be limited (Fig 11-9); in some patients, adduction is better with convergence than with versions, similar to a gaze paralysis. Some patients appear to have palpebral fissure changes on adduction, or vertical extraocular muscle involvement.

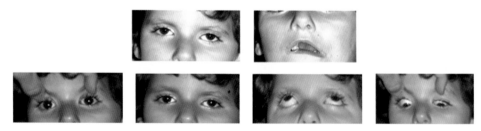

Figure 11-9 Möbius syndrome (sequence). **Top row, left,** Straight eyes in primary position; **right,** the patient cannot smile because of bilateral seventh cranial nerve palsy. **Bottom row,** Bilaterally absent adduction and severely limited abduction. Vertical movements are not affected. *(Courtesy of Edward L. Raab, MD.)*

Management

Medial rectus muscle recession has been advocated, but caution should be exercised in the presence of a significant limitation of adduction. Some surgeons have undertaken to improve abduction by vertical rectus muscle transposition procedures after medial rectus muscle restriction has been relieved.

Miller MT, Strömland K. The Möbius sequence: a relook. *J AAPOS*. 1999;3(4):199–208.

Esotropia Associated With High Myopia

In highly myopic patients, extremely increased axial length can result in stretching and slippage of the lateral rectus pulley and other supporting tissues, causing esotropia. Various surgical procedures have been devised to reinforce the defect by stabilizing the position of the lateral rectus muscle.

Rowe FJ, Noonan CP. Surgical treatment for progressive esotropia in the setting of high-axial myopia. *J AAPOS*. 2006;10(6):596–597.

Internuclear Ophthalmoplegia

The anatomical and functional features of the *medial longitudinal fasciculus (MLF)* are discussed in BCSC Section 5, *Neuro-Ophthalmology*. The MLF integrates the nuclei of the cranial nerves governing ocular motility and has major connections with the vestibular nuclei. An intact MLF is essential for the production of conjugate eye movements. Lesions of the MLF result in a typical pattern of disconjugate movement called *internuclear ophthalmoplegia*. Abnormalities of this pathway are seen frequently in patients with demyelinating disease, but they may also occur in patients who have had cerebrovascular accidents or brain tumors.

Clinical Features

The eye ipsilateral to the lesion adducts slowly and incompletely or not at all, whereas the abducting eye exhibits a characteristic horizontal nystagmus. Both eyes adduct normally on convergence. Skew deviation may be present, in addition to exotropia.

Management

If exotropia persists, medial rectus muscle resection and contralateral lateral rectus muscle recession (to limit exotropia in lateral gaze) can be helpful in eliminating diplopia, particularly in bilateral cases.

Ocular Motor Apraxia

Ocular motor apraxia, also known as *saccadic initiation failure,* is a rare supranuclear disorder of ocular motility, sometimes including strabismus. The congenital form may be familial, most commonly showing autosomal dominant inheritance.

This condition has been associated with premature birth and developmental delay. Bilateral lesions of the frontoparietal cortex, agenesis of the corpus callosum, hydrocephalus, and Joubert syndrome (abnormal eye movements, developmental delay, microcephaly, and retinal dysplasia, among several anomalies) also have been associated, as have type 3 Gaucher disease and ataxia-telangiectasia. Several case reports have identified mass lesions of the cerebellum that compress the rostral part of the brainstem, or hypoplasia of the cerebellar vermis. Neurodevelopmental evaluation and imaging of the brain are advisable for assessment of children with ocular motor apraxia, especially if there is an associated vertical apraxia.

Clinical Features

In ocular motor apraxia, there is inability to generate normal voluntary horizontal saccades. Instead, changes in horizontal fixation are made by a head thrust that overshoots the target, followed by a rotation of the head back in the opposite direction once fixation is established. The initial thrust serves to break fixation; an associated blink serves the same purpose. Vertical saccades and random eye movements are intact, but vestibular and optokinetic nystagmus are impaired. The head thrust may improve in late childhood.

The differential diagnosis of acquired ocular motor apraxia subsumes conditions that affect the generation of voluntary saccades, including metabolic and degenerative diseases such as Huntington chorea. (See also BCSC Section 5, *Neuro-Ophthalmology*.)

Le Ber I, Moreira MC, Rivaud-Péchoux S, et al. Cerebellar ataxia with oculomotor apraxia type 1: clinical and genetic studies. *Brain.* 2003;126(12):2761–2772.

Tusa RJ, Hove MT. Ocular and oculomotor signs in Joubert syndrome. *J Child Neurol.* 1999; 14(10):621–627.

Superior Oblique Myokymia

Superior oblique myokymia is a rare entity whose cause is poorly understood. There is some evidence that it is caused by aberrant regeneration of fourth cranial nerve fibers. Another suggested etiology is vascular compression of the nerve, which can be confirmed by MRI.

Clinical Features

In superior oblique myokymia, there are abnormal torsional movements of the eye that cause diplopia and monocular oscillopsia. Patients are usually otherwise neurologically normal. Recurrences may persist indefinitely.

Management

Treatment is not necessary if the patient is not disturbed by the visual symptoms. Various systemic medications (carbamazepine, phenytoin, propranolol, baclofen, gabapentin) and topical timolol have given inconsistent results but have been advocated as first-line treatment, since some patients will benefit, at least in the short term. Effective surgical treatment requires that the superior oblique muscle be disconnected from the globe by generous tenectomy. This can be expected to result in palsy and usually would require simultaneous inferior oblique muscle weakening.

Plager DA. Superior oblique palsy and superior oblique myokymia. In: Rosenbaum AL, Santiago AP, eds. *Clinical Strabismus Management: Principles and Surgical Techniques.* Philadelphia: Saunders; 1999:219–229.

Williams PE, Purvin VA, Kawasaki A. Superior oblique myokymia: efficacy of medical treatment. *J AAPOS.* 2007;11(3):254–257.

Other Settings for Strabismus

Refractive surgery that creates monovision (performed mainly in adults of presbyopic age; see BCSC Section 13, *Refractive Surgery*) to facilitate visual clarity at distance and near without optical aid can result in dissimilar sensory input to the 2 eyes sufficient to cause loss of motor control of the extraocular muscles and disruption of fusion in predisposed patients.

Holgado S, Toth CA, Freedman SF. Fixation switch and diplopia after full macular translocation surgery. *J AAPOS.* 2007;11(2):114–119.

Kushner BJ, Kowal L. Diplopia after refractive surgery: occurrence and prevention. *Arch Ophthalmol.* 2003;121(3):315–321.

Surgery for retinal detachment can lead to restricted rotations, because of scarring from necessary dissection of the extraocular muscles and the application of devices required to bring about reattachment. Corrective surgery can be extremely difficult, especially if removal of these elements is needed. The presence of a retinal surgeon for guidance during the strabismus correction is valuable. Macular translocation surgery can cause torsional diplopia and other binocular sensory disturbances.

Aqueous drainage devices for patients with glaucoma are another source of scarring and interference with ocular rotations. Treatment may require removal and relocation or substitution of the device, a dilemma if it has been functioning well.

The extraocular muscles can be damaged from retrobulbar injections, either by direct injury to the muscle or from a toxic effect of the injected material. Because of the usual placement of these injections, the vertical rectus muscles are the most vulnerable.

Injection of botulinum toxin into the eyelids can result in diffusion of this substance and a direct paralyzing effect on the extraocular muscles.

Laceration or inadvertent excision of an entire section of the medial rectus muscle has been described as one of several serious ocular and orbital complications of pterygium removal or endoscopic sinus surgery. Restoration of function can be an extremely difficult surgical challenge.

Bhatti MT, Stankiewicz JA. Ophthalmic complications of endoscopic sinus surgery. *Surv Ophthalmol.* 2003;48(4):389–402.

Roizen A, Ela-Dalman N, Velez FG, Coleman AL, Rosenbaum AL. Surgical treatment of strabismus secondary to glaucoma drainage device. *Arch Ophthalmol.* 2008;126(4):480–486.

Suh DW. Acquired esotropia in children and adults. *Focal Points: Clinical Modules for Ophthalmologists.* San Francisco: American Academy of Ophthalmology; 2003, module 10.

CHAPTER **12**

Surgery of the Extraocular Muscles

A thorough knowledge of the anatomy of the extraocular muscles and surrounding tissues and an understanding of their physiology are essential for the planning and execution of strabismus operations. The history and a detailed motility evaluation, as part of a complete ocular examination, provide the information necessary to plan the correct surgery. Evaluation, tailored to the type of case, may include sensory testing, forced ductions, active force generation, saccadic velocities, and diplopia or binocular vision fields. Preoperative planning should address the patient's and family's expectations, as well as risks and potential complications, especially if surgery on the only eye with good vision is considered.

Indications for Surgery

Surgery is performed to improve function, appearance, and well-being. It may relieve asthenopia (a sense of ocular fatigue) in patients with heterophorias or intermittent heterotropias, or may relieve the double vision that is often the complaint of patients with adult-onset strabismus. Alignment of the visual axes can establish or restore fusion and stereopsis, especially if the preoperative deviation is intermittent or of recent onset. Some patients require an abnormal head position to relieve diplopia or to improve vision (eg, with nystagmus and an eccentric null point; see Chapter 25). For these patients, surgical treatment may not only increase the field of binocular vision but also shift it to a more centered location. Correcting strabismus can be considered reconstructive rather than merely cosmetic.

Costello PA, Simon JW, Jia Y, Lininger LL. Acquired esotropia: subjective and objective outcomes. *J AAPOS*. 2001;5(3):193–197.

Mills MD, Coats DK, Donahue SP, Wheeler DT; American Academy of Ophthalmology. Strabismus surgery for adults: a report by the American Academy of Ophthalmology. *Ophthalmology*. 2004;111(6):1255–1262.

Planning Considerations

Visual Acuity

Most surgeons prefer to avoid surgery on the good eye whenever possible in patients with unimprovable severe vision loss in the other eye. When poor vision in a child is due to amblyopia, surgery is normally delayed until the vision reaches maximal improvement by appropriate therapy.

Incomitance

Deviations whose amounts vary in different gaze positions require modifications to make the postoperative alignment more nearly comitant.

Vertical incomitance of horizontal deviations

Horizontal deviations that change in magnitude in upgaze and downgaze are described as *A or V patterns;* these are discussed in Chapter 9.

Horizontal incomitance

When the esodeviation or exodeviation in left gaze is significantly different from that in right gaze, paralysis or restriction is suggested. In general, restrictive forces must be relieved for surgery to be effective, and the usual surgical amounts for a misalignment of a given size may no longer be applicable.

If there is no restriction to account for an incomitant deviation, the deviation is treated as if it were caused by a weak muscle, whether from neurologic, traumatic, or other causes. As a general consensus, most surgeons would approach this problem by weakening the direct antagonist or yoke muscle of the disadvantaged muscle (sometimes both) to equalize muscle forces as much as possible.

Lateral incomitance

It is thought that the surgeon's usual quantity of surgery for intermittent exotropia may result in overcorrection if the measurement in each side gaze is less than that in primary position by at least 10 prism diopters (Δ). If recession of the lateral rectus muscles is planned in these patients, it is thought that the amount of surgery on each side should be reduced by 1 mm. Some surgeons consider such alignment measurements to be an artifact.

Distance-near incomitance

Horizontal distance-near incomitance has classically suggested muscles to be operated on for horizontal deviations. Recent evidence suggests that it may be of minor importance.

Archer SM. The effect of medial versus lateral rectus muscle surgery on distance-near incomitance. *J AAPOS.* 2009;13(1):20–26.

Cyclovertical Strabismus

In many patients with cyclovertical strabismus, the deviation is different in right and left gaze and often between upgaze and downgaze on the side of the greater deviation. In general, surgery should be performed on those muscles whose field of action corresponds to the greatest vertical deviation. For example, in a patient with a right hypertropia that is greatest down and to the patient's left, the surgeon should strongly consider either strengthening the right superior oblique muscle or weakening the left inferior rectus muscle. If the right hypertropia is the same in left upgaze, straight left, and left downgaze, then any of the 4 muscles whose greatest vertical action is in left gaze may be chosen for surgery. In this example, the left superior rectus muscle or right superior oblique muscle could be strengthened, or the left inferior rectus muscle or right inferior oblique muscle could be weakened. Larger deviations may require surgery on more than 1 muscle.

Available operations and the timing of surgery are discussed in the chapters of this volume that deal with the various strabismus entities.

Prior Surgery

It is preferable to operate on muscles that have not undergone prior surgery. However, in cases with restriction resulting from prior surgery, reoperation on the involved muscle usually is necessary. If retinal detachment surgery may be the cause of the restriction, consultation with the patient's retinal surgeon about possible removal or manipulation of scleral explants is advisable.

Surgical Techniques for the Muscles and Tendons

The ophthalmologist should become familiar with the appropriate types of instruments, sutures, and needles used in strabismus surgery. Step-by-step descriptions of each surgical procedure are beyond the scope of this volume. The references that follow are among several in which this information can be found. See also Chapters 2 and 3 of this volume.

Coats DK, Olitsky SE, eds. *Strabismus Surgery and Its Complications.* Berlin: Springer; 2007.

Rosenbaum AL, Santiago AP, eds. *Clinical Strabismus Management: Principles and Surgical Techniques.* Philadelphia: Saunders; 1999.

Wright KW. *Color Atlas of Strabismus Surgery.* Irvine, CA: Wright; 2000.

Weakening Procedures

Table 12-1 defines various weakening procedures and describes when each is used.

"Hang-back" recession

Because the conventional rectus muscle recession technique involves passing the reinsertion sutures through thin sclera with the attendant risk of perforation, some surgeons prefer to suspend the recessed tendon by sutures that pass through the thicker stump of the original insertion. Although it is not known where the tendon reattaches to the sclera, there is empirical experience indicating that this method can be used reliably.

Rodrigues AC, Nelson LB. Long-term results of hang-back lateral rectus recession. *J Pediatr Ophthalmol Strabismus.* 2006;43(3):161–164.

Strengthening Procedures

Strengthening procedures do not actually give the operated muscles more strength. Rather, they provide a tightening effect that tends to offset the opposite action of the antagonist muscle. Surgeons usually use the *resection* technique for this purpose. It can be employed on any of the rectus muscles but is rarely used on the oblique muscles. A rectus muscle can also be tightened by *advancing* its insertion toward the limbus. This is an effective procedure when previous recession has resulted in an overcorrection.

Table 12-1 Weakening Procedures Used in Strabismus Surgery

Procedure	Used For
Myotomy: cutting across a muscle *Myectomy:* removing a portion of muscle }	Used by some surgeons to weaken the inferior oblique muscles
Marginal myotomy: cutting partway across a muscle, usually following a maximal recession	To weaken a rectus muscle further
Tenotomy: cutting across a tendon *Tenectomy:* removing a portion of tendon }	Both used routinely to weaken the superior oblique muscle; silicone spacers have been interposed by some surgeons to control the weakening effect
Recession: removal and reattachment of a muscle (rectus or oblique) so that its insertion is closer to its origin	The standard weakening procedure for rectus muscles
Denervation and extirpation: the ablation of the entire portion of the muscle, along with its nerve supply, within the Tenon capsule	Used only on severely or recurrently overacting inferior oblique muscles
Recession and anteriorization: movement of the muscle's insertion anterior to its original position	Used only on the inferior oblique muscle, to reduce its elevation function; particularly useful when an inferior oblique muscle overaction and dissociated vertical deviation (DVD) both exist
Posterior fixation suture (fadenoperation): attachment of a rectus muscle to the sclera 11–18 mm posterior to the insertion using a nonabsorbable suture; fixation to the muscle's pulley may be safer and equally effective	Used to weaken a muscle by decreasing its mechanical advantage; often used in conjunction with recession; sometimes used in DVD, nystagmus, high AC/A esotropia, and noncomitant strabismus

The anterior half of the superior oblique tendon may be advanced temporally and somewhat closer to the limbus, a procedure known as *Harada-Ito,* to reduce excyclotorsion in patients with superior oblique muscle paralysis. In an alternative procedure, the superior oblique tendon can be tucked to enhance its vertical and torsional effect. However, this may produce an iatrogenic Brown syndrome (see Chapter 11).

Adjustable Sutures

Some surgeons employ adjustable sutures to avoid an immediately obvious poor result or to increase the likelihood of success with 1 operation, but this modification does not ensure long-term satisfactory alignment, which depends on the potential for fusion, the establishment of focused and comparable retinal images in both eyes, and the effect of tonic and other innervational forces acting on the extraocular muscles. Surgery is completed using externalized sutures and slip knots so that the position of the muscle can be altered during the early postoperative days or within just a few hours. The latter method has been used successfully in children. However, a second general anesthesia is required.

Another alternative, used mainly in adults, is performance of surgery with the patient awake. Drugs that might affect ocular motility are avoided, and the patient's dynamic ocular motility and ocular alignment are observed and adjusted at the time of surgery. This technique is not appropriate for most patients with significant scarring, persons with thyroid eye disease, and almost all children.

Isenberg SJ, Abdarbashi P. Drift of ocular alignment following strabismus surgery. Part 1: using fixed scleral sutures. *Br J Ophthalmol.* 2009;93(4):439–442.

Isenberg SJ, Abdarbashi P. Drift of ocular alignment following strabismus surgery. Part 2: using adjustable sutures. *Br J Ophthalmol.* 2009;93(4):443–447.

Pull-Over (Stay) Sutures

A temporary suture is attached to the sclera at the limbus or under a rectus muscle insertion, brought out through the eyelids, and secured to periocular skin over a bolster to fix the eye in a selected position during postoperative healing. Some surgeons believe that this modification is particularly useful in cases with severely restricted rotations. Its disadvantages are that patients experience some discomfort and that the limbal attachment of the stay suture tends to be lost before the desired interval of 10–14 days after placement.

Transposition Procedures

Transposition procedures involve redirection of the paths of the extraocular muscles within the orbit. These procedures are employed most often for treatment of paralytic strabismus, small vertical A and V patterns, Duane syndrome, and monocular elevation deficiency. These conditions are discussed in Chapters 9 through 11. In specific circumstances, nonabsorbable sutures that secure the transposed muscles in their altered directions have been particularly useful in augmenting the surgical effect. Vertical deviations are an occasional complication of transposition, requiring additional operation.

Posterior Fixation

See the beginning of the Surgical Techniques section for a list of sources that describe the indications and conventional techniques for posterior fixation. A novel operation involving fixation to the pulley of a rectus muscle appears in the following reference.

Clark RA, Ariyasu R, Demer JL. Medial rectus pulley posterior fixation is as effective as scleral posterior fixation for acquired esotropia with a high AC/A ratio. *Am J Ophthalmol.* 2004; 137(6):1026–1033.

Guidelines for Strabismus Surgery

Any two surgeons are unlikely to perform a specific surgical procedure in exactly the same way. The amount of dissection, the measurement and placement of sutures in the muscle and sclera, and the location of the conjunctival incision will vary among surgeons, even when following the same quantity table. Nonetheless, the beginning surgeon will find the following guidelines a useful starting point for routine strabismus cases. Each surgeon must refine his or her approach by continually reviewing the results and adjusting the amounts of surgery to achieve the best possible outcomes.

Esodeviation and Exodeviation

Chapters 7 and 8 discuss esodeviations and exodeviations in detail.

Symmetric surgery

Well-known guidelines for medial rectus muscle recession and lateral rectus muscle resection for esodeviations are given in Table 12-2. Some surgeons advocate medial rectus muscle recessions of 7.0 mm for 60Δ–80Δ of esotropia; others avoid these large recessions and favor operating on 3 or 4 muscles for such deviations.

The surgical guidelines for exodeviation are listed in Table 12-3. Some surgeons employ bilateral lateral rectus muscle recessions of 9.0 mm or greater for deviations larger than 40Δ. Others prefer adding resection of 1 or both medial rectus muscles for larger-angle exotropias.

Most surgeons prefer recession over resection procedures as a first operation.

Monocular recession-resection procedures

The figures given in Tables 12-2 and 12-3 may be used in monocular recession-resection procedures, with the surgeon selecting the appropriate number of millimeters for each muscle. For example, for an esotropia of 30Δ, the surgeon would recess the medial rectus muscle 4.5 mm and resect the lateral rectus muscle 7.0 mm. For an exodeviation of 15Δ, the surgeon would recess the lateral rectus muscle 4.0 mm and resect the antagonist medial rectus muscle 3.0 mm. Monocular surgery for exotropia beyond these guidelines

Table 12-2 Surgery for Esodeviation

Angle of Esotropia	Recess MR OU	or	Resect LR OU
15Δ	3.0 mm		4.0 mm
20Δ	3.5 mm		5.0 mm
25Δ	4.0 mm		6.0 mm
30Δ	4.5 mm		7.0 mm
35Δ	5.0 mm		8.0 mm
40Δ	5.5 mm		9.0 mm
50Δ	6.0 mm		9.0 mm

Table 12-3 Surgery for Exodeviation

Angle of Exotropia	Recess LR OU	or	Resect MR OU
15Δ	4.0 mm		3.0 mm
20Δ	5.0 mm		4.0 mm
25Δ	6.0 mm		5.0 mm
30Δ	7.0 mm		6.0 mm
40Δ	8.0 mm		6.0 mm

(ie, ≥50Δ) is likely to result in a limited rotation, again suggesting that a 3- or 4-muscle procedure would be preferable if there is at least moderately good vision in each eye.

Value of immediate overcorrection in exodeviation

The surgical dosages listed in Table 12-3 for bilateral lateral rectus recessions tend to produce a small to moderate overcorrection of exotropia in the early postoperative period. Available evidence suggests that a temporary esotropia during the first few days or weeks after surgery yields the most favorable long-term result. Many patients have diplopia during the time they are esotropic, and younger children may develop monocular suppression or monofixational fusion. Patients or their caregivers should be advised of this possibility.

Raab EL, Parks MM. Recession of the lateral recti. Early and late postoperative alignments. *Arch Ophthalmol.* 1969;82(2):203–208.

Oblique Muscle Weakening Procedures

Weakening the inferior oblique muscle

Table 12-1 lists the various inferior oblique muscle weakening operations. The surgeon must be sure that the entire inferior oblique muscle is weakened, since the distal portion and the insertion can be anomalously duplicated.

In cases that show marked asymmetry of the overactions of the inferior oblique muscles and no superior oblique muscle paralysis, unilateral surgery only on the muscle with the more prominent overaction is often followed by a significant degree of overaction in the fellow eye. Therefore, some surgeons recommend bilateral inferior oblique weakening for asymmetric cases. A good symmetric result is the rule, and overcorrections are rare. However, inferior oblique muscles that are not overacting at all, even when there is overaction in the fellow eye, should not be weakened. There is no consensus on whether inferior oblique muscles with asymmetric overaction should be weakened equally. Bilateral 12-mm myectomy rather than recession or anterior transposition has been advocated as giving a symmetric result, without an overeffect even on the less dysfunctional inferior oblique muscle.

Secondary overaction of the inferior oblique muscle occurs in most patients who have superior oblique muscle paralysis. A weakening of that inferior oblique muscle could be expected to correct up to 15Δ of vertical deviation in primary position. The amount of vertical correction is roughly proportional to the degree of preoperative overaction (see Chapter 10).

Frequently, a weakening procedure is performed on each inferior oblique muscle for V-pattern strabismus. This is discussed in Chapter 9.

Awadein A, Gawdat G. Bilateral inferior oblique myectomy for asymmetric primary inferior oblique overaction. *J AAPOS.* 2008;12(6):560–564.

De Angelis D, Makar I, Kraft SP. Anatomic variations of the inferior oblique muscle: a potential cause of failed inferior oblique weakening surgery. *Am J Ophthalmol.* 1999;128(4):485–488.

Goldchmit M, Felberg S, Souza-Dias C. Unilateral anterior transposition of the inferior oblique muscle for correction of hypertropia in primary position. *J AAPOS.* 2003;7(4):241–243.

Stager DR. Costenbader Lecture. Anatomy and surgery of the inferior oblique muscle: recent findings. *J AAPOS.* 2001;5(4):203–208.

Weakening the superior oblique muscle

Procedures to weaken the superior oblique muscle include tenotomy; tenectomy; Z-lengthening; placement of a spacer (of silicone), fascia lata, or nonabsorbable suture loops between the cut edges of the tendon to functionally lengthen it; and recession. The purpose of spacers is to prevent an excessive gap between the cut edges, but they have the disadvantage of possible formation of adhesions, which can alter motility. Unilateral weakening of a superior oblique muscle is not commonly performed except as the treatment for Brown syndrome (see Chapter 10), or for an isolated inferior oblique muscle weakness, which is rare. Superior oblique muscle weakening can affect not only vertical alignment but also intorsion, creating an undesired excyclodeviation. Many ophthalmologists favor a tenotomy of just the posterior 75%–80% of the tendon, toward its distal end, to leave the torsional action, which is controlled by the most anterior tendon fibers, intact.

Bilateral weakening of the superior oblique muscle can be performed for A-pattern deviations and can be expected to cause an eso shift of up to 30Δ–40Δ in downgaze, a variable change in primary position, and almost no change in upgaze. In surgery on patients with normal binocularity, the possibility of creating diplopia from vertical or torsional strabismus must be considered (see Chapter 9).

Oblique Muscle Tightening (Strengthening) Procedures

Tightening the inferior oblique muscle

As mentioned previously, the actual effect of strengthening procedures is tightening of the muscle. Inferior oblique muscle tightening is performed very infrequently. To be effective, advancement of the inferior oblique muscle requires reinsertion more posteriorly and superiorly, which is technically difficult and exposes the macula to possible injury.

Tightening the superior oblique muscle

Tucking or plication of the tendon is employed where applicable (see Chapter 10). These procedures should be performed on the distal portion of the tendon to avoid producing an iatrogenic Brown syndrome. The Harada-Ito procedure is designed to primarily affect torsion.

Vertical Rectus Muscle Surgery for Hypotropia and Hypertropia

Comitant vertical deviations

For comitant vertical deviations, recession and resection of vertical rectus muscles is appropriate. Recessions generally are preferred as a first procedure. For comitant vertical deviations of less than 10Δ that accompany horizontal deviations, displacement of the reinsertions, in the same direction, by about one-half the tendon width (up or down, as appropriate) in a horizontal rectus muscle recession-resection procedure is sufficiently effective. Because of its effectiveness, this technique may be selected for the horizontal deviation instead of the usually preferred choice, symmetric surgery.

Dissociated vertical deviation

For the treatment of dissociated vertical deviation (DVD), recession of the superior rectus muscle, possibly on a "hang-back" suture (ie, without reattachment to sclera) of 6–10 mm, is effective. Bilateral, perhaps asymmetric, superior rectus muscle surgery is indicated whenever both eyes can fixate. If only one eye can fixate, unilateral surgery is possible. Some surgeons favor the *fadenoperation,* or posterior fixation suture, on the superior rectus muscle(s), often combined with recession. Resection of the inferior rectus muscle ranges from 4 mm for small-angle deviations to 8 mm for large angles. This procedure may inadvertently advance the lower eyelid margin upward, especially if careful dissection is not performed.

Moving the insertion of the inferior oblique muscles anteriorly to a point adjacent to the lateral border of the inferior rectus (anterior transposition) has been found effective in reducing or eliminating DVD, as well as severe inferior oblique overaction. This procedure is especially useful when a patient has both DVD and a component of inferior oblique overaction. (See also Chapter 10.) A special consideration should be mentioned: this is a powerful operation that can result in restricted elevation of the eye in abduction *(anti-elevation syndrome)* if reattachment of the lateral corner of the muscle is done at or anterior to the spiral of Tillaux.

The texts cited earlier in this chapter (see Surgical Techniques for the Muscles and Tendons) offer more specific guidance concerning selection of muscles and determination of the size of the recession or resection.

Elliott RL, Nankin SJ. Anterior transposition of the inferior oblique. *J Pediatr Ophthalmol Strabismus.* 1981;18(3):35–38.

Other Rectus Muscle Surgery

Vertical displacement of the horizontal rectus muscles for A and V patterns
See Chapter 9.

Surgery for paralysis of the third and sixth cranial nerves
Surgery for paralysis of the third and sixth cranial nerves is discussed in Chapter 11. It varies according to the degree of weakness of the affected muscles and the degree of contracture of their intact antagonists. Botulinum toxin injection is another option, but it is less often employed.

Transposition procedures
Transposition procedures involve the risk of anterior segment ischemia if antagonist muscle recession is added (see Anterior Segment Ischemia later in this chapter). Some surgeons prefer to isolate and preserve the anterior ciliary vessels. Options to be considered include augmenting the effect of the transposition by resecting the transposed muscles or by employing the Foster modification.

Brooks SE. Transposition procedures. *Focal Points: Clinical Modules for Ophthalmologists.* San Francisco: American Academy of Ophthalmology; 2001, module 10.

Foster RS. Vertical muscle transposition augmented with lateral fixation. *J AAPOS.* 1997;1(1): 20–30.

McKeown CA, Lambert HM, Shore JW. Preservation of the anterior ciliary vessels during extraocular muscle surgery. *Ophthalmology.* 1989;96(4):498–506.

Surgery for motor nystagmus

Rectus muscle procedures are employed to improve head position for null point motor nystagmus. See Chapter 25.

Approaches to the Extraocular Muscles

Fornix Incision

The fornix incision is made in either the superior or (more frequently) the inferior quadrants. The incision is located on bulbar conjunctiva, not actually in the fornix, 1–2 mm to the limbal side of the cul-de-sac, so that bleeding is minimized. The incision is made parallel to the fornix and is approximately 8–10 mm in length.

Bare sclera is exposed by incising the Tenon capsule deep to the conjunctival incision. Using this bare scleral exposure, the surgeon engages the muscle with a succession of muscle hooks. The conjunctival incision is pulled over the hook that has passed under the muscle belly. All 6 extraocular muscles can be explored, if necessary, through an inferotemporal and a superonasal conjunctival incision.

When properly placed, the 2-plane incision can be self-closed at the end of the operation by gently massaging the tissues into the fornix, with the edges of the incision splinted by the overlying eyelid. Some surgeons prefer to close the incision with conjunctival sutures, especially when 2 contiguous incisions become connected, as occasionally happens.

Parks MM. Fornix incision for horizontal rectus muscle surgery. *Am J Ophthalmol.* 1968;65(6): 907–915.

Limbal or Peritomy Incision

The fused layer of conjunctiva and Tenon capsule is cleanly severed from the limbus for about 120°. A short radial incision is made at each end of the peritomy so that the combined conjunctiva/Tenon capsule flap can be retracted to expose the muscle for surgery. At the completion of surgery, the flap is reattached, without tension, close to its original position with a single suture at each extremity. If the conjunctiva is scarred from prior surgery and is tight, closure should be accomplished by leaving a recessed forward edge.

von Noorden GK. The limbal approach to surgery of the rectus muscles. *Arch Ophthalmol.* 1968;80(1):94–97.

Complications of Strabismus Surgery

Chapter 2 discusses important anatomical considerations that should be understood thoroughly in order to avoid or minimize several of the complications discussed here.

Unsatisfactory Alignment

Unsatisfactory postoperative alignment is perhaps better characterized as one of several possible outcomes of strabismus surgery—albeit a disappointing one—rather than as a complication. Alignment in the immediate postoperative period, whether or not satisfactory, may not be permanent. Among the reasons for this unpredictability are poor fusion, poor vision, and contracture of scar tissue. Reoperations are often necessary.

Refractive Changes

Changes in refractive error are most common when strabismus surgery is performed on 2 rectus muscles of 1 eye. An induced astigmatism of low magnitude usually resolves within a few months.

Preslan MW, Cioffi G, Min YI. Refractive error changes following strabismus surgery. *J Pediatr Ophthalmol Strabismus.* 1992;29(5):300–304.

Diplopia

Diplopia occasionally follows strabismus surgery in older children and especially in adults. Surgery can move the image of the fixation object in the deviating eye out of a suppression scotoma. In the several months following surgery, various responses are possible:

- Fusion of the 2 images can occur.
- A new suppression scotoma may form, corresponding to the new angle of alignment. If the initial strabismus was acquired before age 10 years, the ability to suppress generally is well developed.
- Diplopia may persist.

Prolonged postoperative diplopia is uncommon. However, if strabismus was first acquired in adulthood, diplopia that was symptomatic before surgery is likely to persist unless comitant alignment and fusion are regained. Prisms that compensate the deviation may be helpful in preoperatively assessing the fusion potential and the risk of bothersome postoperative diplopia.

Patients with unequal visual acuities can frequently be taught to ignore the dimmer, more blurred image. Further treatment is indicated for patients whose symptomatic diplopia persists more than 4–6 weeks following surgery, especially if it is severe and in the primary position. If vision is equal or nearly so, temporary prisms should be tried and, if necessary, oriented to correct both vertical and horizontal deviations. The prism power can be changed periodically to address any residual diplopia. If this approach fails, additional surgery or botulinum toxin injection (see Chapter 13) is a consideration.

Kushner BJ. Intractable diplopia after strabismus surgery in adults. *Arch Ophthalmol.* 2002; 120(11):1498–1504.

Perforation of the Sclera

A needle may perforate into the suprachoroidal space or through the choroid and retina during reattachment of a muscle. In most cases, this results in only a small chorioretinal scar, with no effect on vision. Most perforations are unrecognized unless specifically looked for by ophthalmoscopy. If vitreous escapes through the perforation site, many surgeons apply immediate local cryotherapy or laser therapy. Topical antibiotics generally are given during the immediate postoperative period, even when vitreous has not escaped. Repeated follow-up ophthalmoscopy is an appropriate precaution.

Perforation can lead to endophthalmitis, a detailed discussion of which is found in BCSC Section 9, *Intraocular Inflammation and Uveitis.*

Awad AH, Mullaney PB, Al-Hazmi A, et al. Recognized globe perforation during strabismus surgery: incidence, risk factors, and sequelae. *J AAPOS.* 2000;4(3):150–153.

Dang Y, Racu C, Isenberg SJ. Scleral penetrations and perforations in strabismus surgery and associated risk factors. *J AAPOS.* 2004;8(4):325–331.

Postoperative Infections

Intraocular infection is uncommon following strabismus surgery. Some patients develop mild conjunctivitis, which may be caused by allergy to suture material or postoperative medications, as well as by infectious agents. Preseptal cellulitis and orbital cellulitis with proptosis, eyelid swelling, chemosis, and fever are rare complications (Fig 12-1). These conditions usually develop 2–3 days after surgery and generally respond well to systemic antibiotics. Patients should be warned of the signs and symptoms of orbital cellulitis and endophthalmitis prior to release from the surgical facility so they will seek emergency consultation if necessary.

Recchia FM, Baumal CR, Sivalingam A, Kleiner R, Duker JS, Vrabec TR. Endophthalmitis after pediatric strabismus surgery. *Arch Ophthalmol.* 2000;118(7):939–944.

Foreign-Body Granuloma and Allergic Reaction

A foreign-body granuloma occasionally develops after extraocular muscle surgery, usually at the muscle's reattachment site. The granuloma is characterized by a localized elevated, hyperemic, slightly tender mass (Fig 12-2). It may respond to topical corticosteroids. Surgical excision is necessary if the granuloma persists. Reactions to suture materials are infrequent today because gut suture is now used rarely (Fig 12-3).

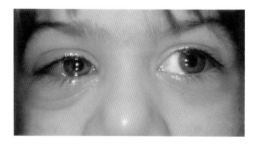

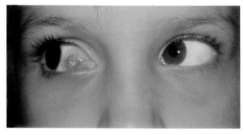

Figure 12-1 Orbital cellulitis, right eye, 2 days after bilateral recession of lateral rectus muscles.

Figure 12-2 Severe postoperative granuloma over the right medial rectus persisting 1 year after medial rectus recessions.

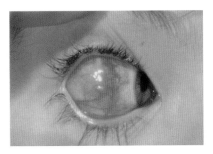

Figure 12-3 Allergic reaction to chromic gut.

Conjunctival Inclusion Cyst

A noninflamed subconjunctival translucent mass may appear if conjunctival epithelium is buried during muscle reattachment or closure of the incision (Fig 12-4). Occasionally, this resolves spontaneously. Topical steroids may be helpful, although persistent cases may require surgical excision.

Conjunctival Scarring

Satisfaction from improved alignment may occasionally be overshadowed by unsightly scarring of the conjunctiva and the Tenon capsule. The tissues remain hyperemic and salmon-pink instead of returning to their usual whiteness. This complication may result from the following factors:

- *Advancement of thickened Tenon capsule too close to the limbus.* In resection procedures, pulling the muscle forward may advance the Tenon capsule. The undesirable result is exaggerated in reoperations, when the Tenon capsule around and anterior to the insertion may be hypertrophied.
- *Advancement of the plica semilunaris.* In surgery on the medial rectus muscle using the limbal approach, the surgeon may mistake the plica semilunaris for a conjunctival edge and incorporate it into the closure. Though not strictly a conjunctival scar, the advanced plica, now pulled forward and hypertrophied, retains its fleshy color (Fig 12-5).

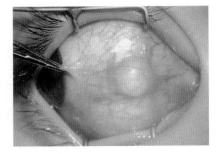

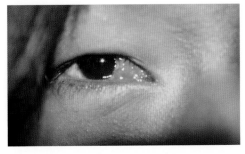

Figure 12-4 Postoperative conjunctival epithelial inclusion cyst following right medial rectus recession.

Figure 12-5 Hypertrophy involving the plica semilunaris. *(Courtesy of Scott Olitsky, MD.)*

Adherence Syndrome

Tears in the Tenon capsule with prolapse of orbital fat into the sub–Tenon space can cause formation of a fibrofatty scar that may restrict motility. If recognized at the time of surgery, the prolapsed fat can be excised and the rent closed with absorbable sutures. Meticulous surgical technique usually prevents this serious complication.

Dellen

The term *dellen* (*delle*, singular) refers to shallow depressions and corneal thinning just anterior to the limbus; these occur when raised abnormal bulbar conjunctiva prevents the eyelid from adequately resurfacing the cornea with tear fluid during blinking (Fig 12-6). Dellen are more apt to occur when the limbal approach to muscle surgery is used. They usually heal eventually. Artificial tears or lubricants may be needed until the chemosis subsides. If there is discomfort, patching of the eye may be helpful initially.

Anterior Segment Ischemia

Most of the blood supply to the anterior segment of the eye comes through the anterior ciliary arteries that travel in the 4 rectus muscles. Simultaneous surgery on 3 of these rectus muscles, or even 2 of them in patients with poor blood flow, may lead to anterior segment ischemia. The earliest signs of this complication are cells and flare in the anterior chamber. More severe cases are characterized by corneal epithelial edema, folds in Descemet's membrane, and irregular pupil (Fig 12-7). This complication may lead to anterior segment necrosis and phthisis bulbi. No universally agreed upon treatment exists for anterior segment ischemia. Because the signs of anterior segment ischemia are similar to those of typical uveitis, most ophthalmologists elect to treat with topical, subconjunctival, or systemic corticosteroids, although there is no firm evidence for this approach.

It is possible to recess or resect a rectus muscle while sparing its anterior ciliary vessels. Though difficult and time-consuming, this technique may be indicated in high-risk

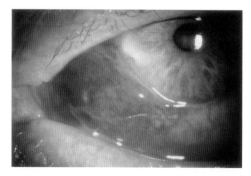

Figure 12-6 Corneal delle subsequent to postoperative subconjunctival hemorrhage.

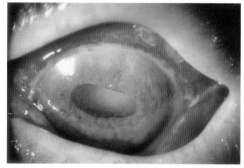

Figure 12-7 Superotemporal segmental anterior segment ischemia after simultaneous superior rectus muscle and lateral rectus muscle surgery following scleral buckling procedure.

cases. It is not clear whether staging surgeries, with an interval of several months between surgeries, is helpful.

Rosenbaum AL, Santiago AP. *Clinical Strabismus Management: Principles and Surgical Techniques.* Philadelphia: Saunders; 1999.

Change in Eyelid Position

Change in the position of the eyelids is most likely to occur with surgery on the vertical rectus muscles. Pulling the inferior rectus muscle forward, as in a resection, advances the lower eyelid upward; recessing this muscle pulls the lower eyelid down, exposing bare sclera below the lower limbus (Fig 12-8). Surgery on the superior rectus muscle is somewhat less likely to affect upper eyelid position.

Eyelid position changes can be obviated somewhat by careful dissection. In general, all intermuscular septum and fascial connections of the operated vertical rectus muscle must be severed at least 12–15 mm posterior to the muscle insertion, although doing this is contrary to the view of many surgeons that there should be minimal disturbance of the Tenon capsule. Release of the lower eyelid retractors or advancement of the capsulo-palpebral head are helpful to prevent lower eyelid retraction after inferior rectus muscle recession.

Kim DB, Meyer DR, Simon JW. Retractor lysis as prophylaxis for lower lid retraction following inferior rectus recession. *J Pediatr Ophthalmol Strabismus.* 2002;39(4):198–202.

Lost and Slipped Muscles

A rectus muscle that sustains trauma or that slips out of the sutures or instruments while not attached to the globe during operation can become inaccessible posteriorly in the orbit. This consequence is most severe when it involves the medial rectus muscle, since it is the most difficult to recover. A lost muscle does not reattach to the globe but instead retracts through the Tenon capsule. The surgeon should immediately attempt to find the lost muscle, if possible with the assistance of a surgeon experienced in this potentially complex surgery. Malleable retractors and a headlight are helpful. Minimal manipulation should be employed to bring into view the anatomical site through which the muscle and its sheath normally penetrate the Tenon capsule, where, it is hoped, the distal end of the

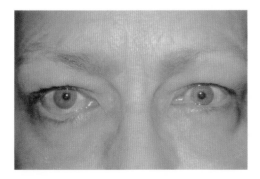

Figure 12-8 Patient with left hypertropia. Postoperative photograph after recession of the right inferior rectus muscle, which pulled the right lower eyelid down, and resection of the left inferior rectus muscle, which pulled the left lower eyelid up.

muscle can be observed and captured. If inspection does not reliably indicate that the muscle has been identified, sudden bradycardia when traction is exerted can often be confirmatory. In the case of the medial rectus muscle, recovery by a transnasal endoscopic approach through the ethmoid sinus or employing a medial orbitotomy can be useful alternatives. Transposition surgery may be required if the lost muscle is not found, although anterior segment ischemia may be a risk. Where to reattach the recovered muscle depends on several factors in the particular case and is largely a matter of judgment.

Slipped muscle is the result of inadequate suturing. The muscle recedes posteriorly within its capsule during the postoperative period. Clinically, the patient manifests a weakness of that muscle, with limited rotations and possibly decreased saccades in its field of action (Fig 12-9). Surgery should be performed as soon as possible in order to secure the muscle before further retraction and contracture take place. Slippage can be prevented by full-thickness lock bites, to include muscle tissue and not merely capsule, prior to disinsertion. In reoperations for strabismus with deficient rotations, slippage or "stretched scar" should be suspected and the involved muscles explored.

Lenart TD, Lambert SR. Slipped and lost extraocular muscles. *Ophthalmol Clin N Am.* 2001;14(3):433–442.

Ludwig IH, Chow AY. Scar remodeling after strabismus surgery. *J AAPOS.* 2000;4(6):326–333.

Sebastian RT, Marsh IB. Adjustment of the surgical nomogram for surgery on slipped extraocular muscles. *J AAPOS.* 2006;10(6):573–576.

Anesthesia for Extraocular Muscle Surgery

Methods

In cooperative patients, topical anesthetic drops (eg, tetracaine 0.5%, proparacaine 0.5%) alone are effective for most steps in an extraocular muscle surgical procedure. Lid blocks are not necessary if the eyelid speculum is not spread to the point of causing pain. Topical anesthesia is not effective for control of the pain produced by pulling on or against a restricted muscle or for cases in which exposure is difficult.

Both local infiltration (peribulbar) and retrobulbar anesthesia make most extraocular muscle procedures pain-free and should be considered in adults for whom general anesthesia may pose an undue hazard. The administration of a short-acting hypnotic by an anesthesiologist just before retrobulbar injection greatly improves patient comfort. Because

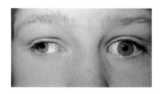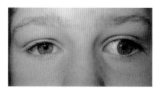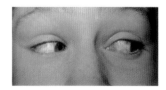

Figure 12-9 Slipped left medial rectus muscle. **Left,** Gaze right shows inability to adduct left eye. **Middle,** Exotropia in primary position. **Right,** Gaze left shows full abduction. Note left palpebral fissure is wider than right.

injected anesthetics may influence alignment during the first few hours after surgery, suture adjustment is best delayed for at least half a day.

General anesthesia is necessary for children and is frequently used for adults as well, particularly those requiring bilateral surgery. Neuromuscular blocking agents such as succinylcholine, which are administered to facilitate intubation for general anesthesia, can temporarily affect the results of a traction test. Nondepolarizing agents, which do not present this disadvantage, can be employed instead. In recent years, laryngeal mask airways, which avoid the need for intubation, have been in more common use.

Postoperative Nausea and Vomiting

Nausea and vomiting formerly were common following eye muscle surgery. They now occur less frequently with the use of newer anesthetic agents and ancillary drugs such as droperidol, metoclopramide (Reglan), diphenhydramine (Benadryl), ondansetron (Zofran), and propofol.

Kovac AL. Management of postoperative nausea and vomiting in children. *Paediatr Drugs.* 2007;9(1):47–69.

Oculocardiac Reflex

The oculocardiac reflex is a slowing of the heart rate caused by traction on the extraocular muscles, particularly the medial rectus muscle. In its most severe form, the reflex can produce asystole. The surgeon should be aware of the possibility of inducing the oculocardiac reflex when manipulating a muscle and should be prepared to release tension if the heart rate drops excessively. Intravenous atropine and other agents can protect against this reflex.

Malignant Hyperthermia

Malignant hyperthermia (MH) may be triggered by many inhalational anesthetics and by the muscle relaxant succinylcholine. MH is a defect of calcium binding by the sarcoplasmic reticulum of skeletal muscle. Unbound intracellular calcium increases, stimulating muscle contracture. As this increased metabolism outstrips oxygen delivery, anaerobic metabolism develops with lactate production and massive acidosis. The earliest sign is unexplained elevation of end-tidal carbon dioxide concentration. In its fully developed form, MH is characterized by extreme heat production, resulting from the hypermetabolic state, in which cell breakdown, with loss of potassium and myoglobin, occurs.

MH can occur sporadically or be dominantly inherited with incomplete penetrance. Disorders associated with MH include strabismus, myopathies, ptosis, and other musculoskeletal abnormalities. The prevalence is variously reported as between 1:6000 and 1:60,000 and is thought to be higher in children, although it occurs in all age groups. The mortality rate has decreased substantially with modern treatment. When personal or family history is suggestive of MH, susceptibility testing is warranted. If testing is not available, nontriggering anesthetic agents should be used and the patient treated as MH susceptible. Muscle biopsy with in vitro halothane and caffeine contraction testing are the most specific laboratory methods to confirm the presence of MH.

Clinical picture

The surgeon should be aware of the manifestations of possible MH. Tachycardia and other arrhythmias can occur, as well as unstable blood pressure. Other early signs include tachypnea, sweating, muscle rigidity, blotchy discoloration of the skin, cyanosis, and dark urine.

Onset may be manifested during the induction of anesthesia by trismus caused by masseter muscle spasm, but the significance of masseter spasm is controversial since most of these patients do not develop MH. Later signs are a rise in temperature, respiratory and metabolic acidosis, hyperkalemia, hypercalcemia, myoglobinuria and renal failure, skeletal muscle swelling, heart failure, disseminated intravascular coagulation, and cardiac arrest.

Treatment

Malignant hyperthermia can be fatal if diagnosis and treatment are delayed. As soon as the diagnosis is made, surgery should be terminated, even if incomplete. Treatment is in the province of the anesthesiologist rather than of the ophthalmologist. The protocol for this treatment and contact information for the MH hotline appear in BCSC Section 1, *Update on General Medicine.*

CHAPTER 13

Chemodenervation Treatment of Strabismus and Blepharospasm Using Botulinum Toxin

Pharmacology and Mechanism of Action

Botox (purified botulinum toxin type A) is a protein drug produced from the bacterium *Clostridium botulinum*. This agent paralyzes muscles by blocking the release of acetylcholine at the neuromuscular junction. Following injection, botulinum toxin is bound and internalized in 24–48 hours within local motor nerve terminals, where it remains for many weeks to interfere with the release of acetylcholine. Paralysis of the injected muscle begins within 2–4 days after injection and lasts clinically for at least 5–8 weeks in the extraocular muscle and for 3 or more months in the orbicularis muscle. An extraocular muscle lengthens while it is paralyzed by botulinum, and its antagonist contracts. These changes may produce long-term improvement in the alignment of the eyes.

Indications, Techniques, and Results

When used to treat patients with strabismus or blepharospasm, the toxin is injected directly, using a small-gauge needle, into selected extraocular muscles or into the orbicularis muscle. Injections into the orbicularis muscle can be performed without the need for special equipment. In adults, injections into the extraocular muscles are performed with the use of a portable electromyographic device. Injections in children may require general anesthesia.

Botulinum toxin is very effective in the treatment of essential blepharospasm. Repeated injections every 2–3 months are usually required. Botulinum toxin may also be injected into the levator muscle to induce ptosis in patients with corneal disease, providing a temporary protective effect.

Clinical trials using botulinum for the treatment of strabismus have shown this agent to be most effective in the following conditions:

- small- to moderate-angle esotropia and exotropia (<40Δ)
- postoperative residual strabismus (2–8 weeks following surgery or later)

163

- acute paralytic strabismus (especially sixth cranial nerve palsy), to eliminate diplopia while the palsy recovers
- cyclic esotropia
- active thyroid eye disease (Graves disease) or inflamed or prephthisical eyes, when surgery is inappropriate
- as a supplement to medial rectus recessions in large-angle infantile esotropia

Multiple injections may be required, particularly in adults. As with surgical treatment, results are best when there is fusion to stabilize the alignment. Botulinum injection is usually not effective in patients with large deviations, restrictive or mechanical strabismus (trauma, chronic thyroid eye disease), or secondary strabismus wherein a muscle has been overrecessed. Injection is ineffective in A and V patterns, dissociated vertical deviations, oblique muscle disorders, and chronic paralytic strabismus. The long-term recovery rate for patients with acute sixth cranial nerve paralysis treated with observation alone is similar to that of patients who receive botulinum.

Complications

The most common adverse effects of ocular botulinum treatment are ptosis, incomplete eyelid closure, dry eye, and induced vertical strabismus. These complications are usually temporary, resolving after several weeks. Rare complications include scleral perforation, retrobulbar hemorrhage, pupillary dilation, and permanent diplopia. Systemic botulism has been reported in animals and humans following massive injections of large muscle groups, but this has not been encountered in ophthalmology.

Coté TR, Mohan AK, Polder JA, Walton MK, Braun MM. Botulinum toxin type A injections: adverse events reported to the US Food and Drug Administration in therapeutic and cosmetic cases. *J Am Acad Dermatol.* 2005;53(3):407–415.

Crouch ER. Use of botulinum toxin in strabismus. *Curr Opin Ophthalmol.* 2006;17(5):435–440.

Dutton JJ, Fowler AM. Botulinum toxin in ophthalmology. *Surv Ophthalmol.* 2007;52(1): 13–31.

Gardner R, Dawson EL, Adams GG, Lee JP. Long-term management of strabismus with multiple repeated injections of botulinum toxin. *J AAPOS.* 2008;12(6):569–575.

PART II

Pediatric Ophthalmology

CHAPTER 14

Growth and Development of the Eye

Normal Growth and Development

The human eye undergoes dramatic anatomical and physiologic development throughout infancy and early childhood (Table 14-1). Ophthalmologists caring for children should be familiar with the normal growth and development of the pediatric eye, since departures from the norm may indicate pathology. See also BCSC Section 2, *Fundamentals and Principles of Ophthalmology*.

Dimensions of the Eye

Most of the growth of the eye takes place in the first year of life. The change in the axial length of the eye occurs in 3 phases (Fig 14-1). The first phase is a rapid period of growth

Table 14-1 Dimensions of Newborn and Adult Eyes

	Newborn	Adult
Axial length (mm)	15–17	23
Corneal horizontal diameter (mm)	9.5–10.5	12
Radius of corneal curvature (mm)	6.6–7.4	7.4–8.4

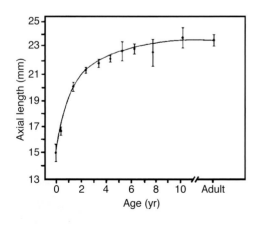

Figure 14-1 Axial length plotted with respect to age. *Dots* represent mean values for age group indicated; *bars* represent standard deviations. *(Figures 14-1 to 14-3 reproduced by permission from Gordon RA, Donzis PB. Refractive development of the human eye.* Arch Ophthalmol. *1985;103(6):785–789. © 1985, American Medical Association.)*

in the first 6 months of life during which the axial length increases by approximately 4 mm. During the second (age 2–5 years) and third (age 5–13 years) phases, growth slows; only about 1 mm of growth is added during each of these phases.

Similarly, the cornea grows rapidly over the first several months of life (Fig 14-2). Keratometry values change markedly in the first year of life, starting at approximately 52 D at birth, flattening to 46 D by 6 months, and reaching their adult power of 42–44 D by age 12. The average corneal horizontal diameter is 9.5–10.5 mm in newborns, increasing to 12 mm in adulthood; most of this change occurs in the first year of life. Mild corneal clouding can be normal in newborns and is expected in premature infants; it resolves as the cornea gradually thins from an average central thickness of 0.96 mm at birth to 0.52 mm at 6 months.

The power of the pediatric lens decreases dramatically over the first several years of life, an important fact to consider with intraocular lens (IOL) implantation in children undergoing cataract extraction in infancy and early childhood. Figure 14-3 shows the theoretical power of the pediatric lens at a given age, based on IOL power calculations performed with the modified SRK formula, which uses pediatric keratometry and axial length values.

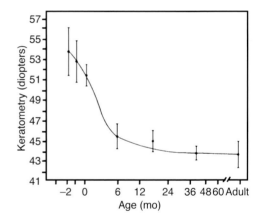

Figure 14-2 Keratometry values plotted with respect to age on a logarithmic scale. The negative number represents months of prematurity; *dots* represent mean value for age group indicated; and *bars*, standard deviations.

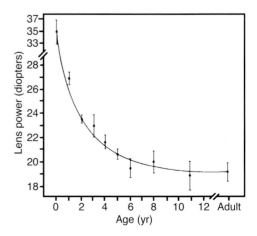

Figure 14-3 Mean values *(dots)* and standard deviations *(bars)* for calculated lens power as determined by modified SRK formula, plotted with respect to age.

Refractive State

The refractive state of the eye changes as the eye's axial length increases and the cornea and lens flatten. In general, infants are hyperopic at birth, become slightly more hyperopic until age 7, and then experience a myopic shift toward plano until the eye reaches its adult dimensions, usually by about age 16 (Fig 14-4). Changes in refractive error vary widely, but if myopia presents before age 10, there is a higher risk of eventual progression to myopia of 6 D or greater. Astigmatism is common in infants and often regresses.

The term *emmetropization* refers to the process in the developing eye in which the refractive power of the anterior segment and the axial length of the eye adjust to reach emmetropia. The loss of astigmatism that many infants experience and the loss of hyperopia that children experience after 6–8 years of age are likely examples of emmetropization. Studies with several animal species have revealed that imposing hyperopia or myopia with spectacle lenses on the infant eye produces compensatory changes in axial growth that eliminate the imposed refractive error.

Kee CS, Hung LF, Qiao-Grider Y, Roorda A, Smith EL 3rd. Effects of optically imposed astigmatism on emmetropization in infant monkeys. *Invest Ophthalmol Vis Sci.* 2004;45(6):1647–1659.

Orbit and Ocular Adnexa

During infancy and childhood, the orbital volume increases, the shape of the orbital opening becomes less circular and more like a horizontal oval, the lacrimal fossa becomes more superficial, and the angle formed by the axes of the 2 orbits assumes a less divergent position.

The palpebral fissure measures approximately 18 mm horizontally and 8 mm vertically at birth and changes very little during the first year of life, but a rapid increase in palpebral fissure length occurs during the first decade, causing the round infant eye to acquire an elliptical adult shape.

Although the development of the nasolacrimal duct is complete in most infants, a substantial number of infants show clinical evidence of nasolacrimal duct (NLD) obstruction. Spontaneous resolution of NLD obstruction is seen in 75%–90% of cases by 1 year of age.

Iris, Pupil, and Anterior Chamber

Most iris color changes occur over the first 6 to 12 months of life, as pigment accumulates in the iris stroma and melanocytes, but iris pigmentation may continue. Compared with

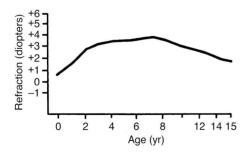

Figure 14-4 Change in mean refractive error as a function of age. *(Reproduced with permission from Wright KW, Spiegel PH, eds.* Pediatric Ophthalmology and Strabismus. *2nd ed. New York: Springer-Verlag: 2003:49.)*

the adult pupil, the infant pupil is relatively small, but a pupil size smaller than 1.8 mm or greater than 5.4 mm is suggestive of an abnormality. A pupillary light response is expected to be present in infants of 31 or more weeks' gestational age. At birth, the iris insertion is near the level of the scleral spur, but during the first year of life, the lens and ciliary body migrate posteriorly, resulting in the formation of the angle recess.

Intraocular Pressure

Intraocular pressure determination in infants can be difficult, and normal pressures vary depending on the method used to obtain them. Nevertheless, normal intraocular pressure is lower in infants than in adults, and a pressure of greater than 21 mm Hg should be considered abnormal. Increased central corneal thickness may falsely elevate intraocular pressure.

Extraocular Muscle Anatomy and Physiology

The rectus muscles of infants are smaller than those of adults; muscle insertions on average are 2.3–3 mm narrower in infants than in adults; and the tendons are thinner. In newborns, the distance from the rectus muscle insertion to the limbus is roughly 2 mm less than that in adults; by 6 months of age, it is 1 mm less; and at 20 months, it is similar to that in adults. Posteriorly, the topographic anatomy of neonates differs substantially from that of adults and older children; enlargement of the posterior segment occurs during the first 2 years of life, resulting in a separation of 4–5 mm between the superior and inferior oblique insertions and migration of the inferior oblique insertion temporally.

Development of extraocular muscle function continues after birth. Vestibular-driven eye movements are present as early as 34 weeks' gestational age. Conjugate horizontal gaze is present at birth, but vertical gaze may not be fully functional until 6 months of age. About two-thirds of young infants have intermittent strabismus in infancy, but most will have straight eyes by 2–3 months of age. Accommodation and fusional convergence are usually present by 3 months.

Retina

The macula is poorly developed at birth but changes rapidly until about age 4 years. Most notable are changes in macular pigmentation, annular ring, foveal light reflex, and cone photoreceptor differentiation. Improvement in visual acuity with growth is attributed to 3 processes: differentiation of cone photoreceptors, reduction in the diameter of the rod-free zone, and an increase in foveal cone density. Retinal vascularization proceeds in a centrifugal manner, starting at the optic disc and reaching the temporal ora serrata by 40 weeks' gestational age.

Visual Acuity and Stereoacuity

Two major methods are used to quantitate visual acuity in preverbal infants and toddlers: *preferential looking (PL)* and *visually evoked potential (VEP)*.

One type of preferential looking test is the Teller acuity card procedure. This test allows the examiner to measure visual acuity by observing the child's response to a series of rectangular cards on which alternating black and white stripes are printed (on 1 side only) on a gray background. Stripe width decreases on successive cards. The examiner presents the cards to the patient, one at a time, and observes the child's eye movements to determine whether the stripes were seen. Seeing the narrower stripes denotes better vision (see Chapter 5, Fig 5-1).

A special form of VEP, a sweep VEP, can also assess vision in nonverbal patients. VEP shows improvement of vision from about 20/400 in infancy to 20/20 by age 6–7 months. However, PL studies estimate the vision of a newborn infant to be 20/600, improving to 20/120 by age 3 months and to 20/60 by 6 months. Acuity of 20/20 is not reached with PL testing until age 3–5 years. The discrepancy between these 2 methods may relate to the higher cortical processing required for PL compared to VEP. Stereoacuity reaches 60 sec arc by about age 5–6 months.

Clifford-Donaldson CE, Haynes BM, Dobson V. Teller Acuity Card norms with and without use of a testing stage. *J AAPOS.* 2006;10(6):547–551.

Eustis HS, Guthrie ME. Postnatal development. In: Wright KW, Spiegel PH, eds. *Pediatric Ophthalmology and Strabismus.* 2nd ed. New York: Springer-Verlag; 2003:39–53.

Abnormal Growth and Development

Major congenital anomalies occur in 2%–3% of live births. Causes include chromosomal anomalies, multifactorial disorders, environmental agents, and idiopathic etiologies. Regardless of etiology, from a developmental point of view, congenital anomalies may be organized into the following categories (examples are given in parentheses):

- *agenesis:* developmental failure (anophthalmos)
- *hypoplasia:* developmental arrest (optic nerve hypoplasia)
- *hyperplasia:* developmental excess (distichiasis)
- failure to divide or canalize (congenital NLD obstruction)
- *dysraphia:* failure to fuse (choroidal coloboma)
- persistence of vestigial structures (persistent fetal vasculature)

A *malformation* implies a morphologic defect present from the onset of development or from a very early stage. A disturbance to a group of cells in a single developmental field may cause multiple malformations. Multiple etiologies may result in similar field defects and patterns of malformation. A single structural defect or factor can lead to a cascade, or domino effect, of secondary anomalies called a *sequence.* The Pierre Robin group of anomalies (cleft palate, glossoptosis, micrognathia, respiratory problems) may represent a sequence caused by abnormal descent of the tongue and is seen in many syndromes (such as Stickler and fetal alcohol) and chromosomal anomalies. A *syndrome* is a recognizable and consistent pattern of multiple malformations known to have a specific cause, which is usually a mutation of a single gene, a chromosome alteration, or an environmental agent. An *association* represents defects known to occur together in a statistically significant number of patients, such as the CHARGE association (ocular *c*oloboma, *h*eart defects, choanal *a*tresia, mental *r*etardation, and *g*enitourinary and *e*ar anomalies). An association may represent a variety of yet-unidentified causes. Two or more minor anomalies in combination significantly increase the chance of an associated major malformation.

Jones KL. *Smith's Recognizable Patterns of Human Malformation.* 6th ed. Philadelphia: Elsevier Saunders; 2006.

CHAPTER **15**

Orbital Dysmorphology and Eyelid Disorders

Orbital and eyelid malformations can be isolated conditions or features of a syndrome; therefore, systematic evaluation of the orbit is an essential part of the clinical evaluation of a dysmorphic infant. Morphologic measurements of the orbit can be performed with transparent rulers or calipers and compared to normal reference measures (Fig 15-1). Alternatively, indices such as the Farcas canthal index, defined by the inner to outer intercanthal ratio × 10, can be used. Hypotelorism and hypertelorism are defined as having a canthal index greater than 42 and less than 38, respectively. It is important to consider ethnic variations.

Terminology and Associations of Abnormal Interocular Distance

Hypotelorism

Hypotelorism is characterized by a reduced distance between the medial walls of orbits with reduced inner and outer canthal distances. The finding is associated with over 60 syndromes. Hypotelorism can be the result of skull malformation or a failure in brain development.

Hypertelorism

Orbital hypertelorism refers to lateralization of the entire orbit. *Ocular hypertelorism* is defined as an increase in both the inner and the outer intercanthal distances. Clinically, interpupillary distance is the best parameter of this anomaly. Hypertelorism occurs in over 550 disorders and is thought to be caused by early ossification of the lesser wing of the sphenoid, which fixes the orbits in the fetal position; by failure of development of the nasal capsule, which allows the primitive brain to protrude, as in frontal encephalocele; or by a disturbance in the development of the skull base, as in craniosynostosis syndromes.

Exorbitism

Some clinicians define exorbitism as prominent eyes due to shallow orbits; others define it as an increased angle of divergence of the orbital walls.

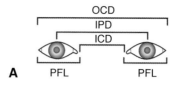

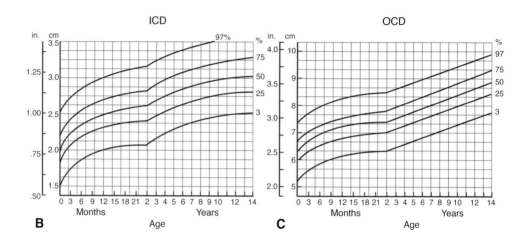

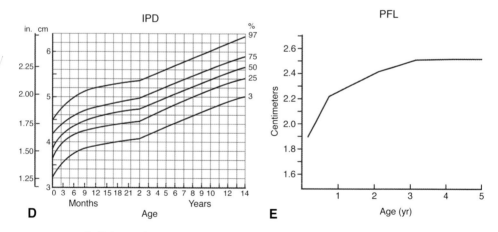

Figure 15-1 **A,** Schematic representation of measurements involved in the evaluation of the orbital region. *OCD* = outer canthal distance; *ICD* = inner canthal distance; *IPD* = interpupillary distance; *PFL* = palpebral fissure length. **B,** ICD measurements according to age. **C,** OCD measurements according to age. **D,** IPD measurements according to age. **E,** Normal PFL measurements according to age. *(Modified with permission from Dollfus H, Verloes A. Dysmorphology and the orbital region: a practical clinical approach. Surv Ophthalmol. 2004;49(6):549.)*

Telecanthus

Telecanthus is a condition characterized by an increased distance between the inner can-thi. It is considered primary if the interpupillary measurement is normal and secondary if it is greater than normal. Telecanthus is common in many syndromes.

Dystopia Canthorum

Dystopia canthorum is specific for Waardenburg syndrome type 1. It is described as lateral displacement of both the inner canthi and the lacrimal puncta such that an imaginary vertical line drawn connecting the upper and lower puncta crosses the cornea (Fig 15-2).

> Dollfus H, Verloes A. Dysmorphology and the orbital region: a practical clinical approach. *Surv Ophthalmol.* 2004;49(6):547–561.

Eyelid Disorders

Congenital eyelid disorders can result from abnormal differentiation of the eyelids and adnexa, developmental arrest, intrauterine environmental insults, and other unknown factors. Examples of these groups are discussed below. See also BCSC Section 2, *Fundamentals and Principles of Ophthalmology,* and Section 7, *Orbit, Eyelids, and Lacrimal System.*

Cryptophthalmos

Cryptophthalmos, a rare condition, results from failure of differentiation of eyelid structures. The skin passes uninterrupted from the forehead over the eye to the cheek and blends in with the cornea of the eye, which is usually malformed (Fig 15-3). Fraser syndrome is an autosomal recessive disorder that is characterized by partial syndactyly and genitourinary anomalies; it may include cryptophthalmos and other ocular malformations.

Congenital Coloboma of the Eyelid

Congenital coloboma usually involves the upper eyelid and can range from a small notch to the absence of the entire length of the eyelid, which can be fused to the globe (Fig 15-4). Eyelid colobomas are commonly associated with Goldenhar syndrome. The eye of an infant with a congenital coloboma should be observed for exposure keratopathy. Surgical closure of the eyelid defect is eventually required in most cases.

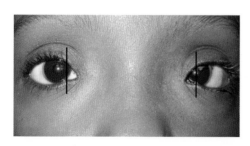

Figure 15-2 Dystopia canthorum in a patient with Waardenburg syndrome. Notice that the vertical lines drawn through the puncta intersect the cornea. *(Courtesy of Amy Hutchinson, MD.)*

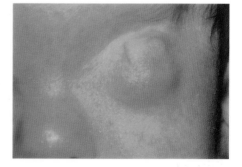

Figure 15-3 Cryptophthalmos, left eye.

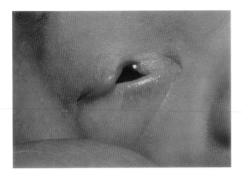

Figure 15-4 Congenital eyelid coloboma, right eye. The eyelid is fused to the globe.

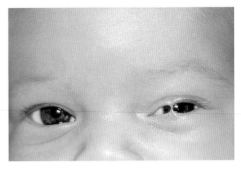

Figure 15-5 Ankyloblepharon. The eyelid margins are fused by a fine strand. The eyelids were easily separated with blunt Westcott scissors in the office without anesthesia. *(Courtesy of Amy Hutchinson, MD.)*

Ankyloblepharon

Fusion of part or all of the eyelid margins is known as ankyloblepharon. This condition may be dominantly inherited. A variant is *ankyloblepharon filiforme adnatum,* in which the eyelid margins are connected by fine strands (Fig 15-5). Treatment is surgical.

Congenital Ectropion

Congenital ectropion is a disorder characterized by eversion of the eyelid margin that usually involves the lower eyelid secondary to a vertical deficiency of the skin. A lateral tarsorrhaphy may be needed for mild cases. More severe cases may require a skin flap or graft.

Congenital Entropion

Congenital entropion is a rare abnormality in which an eyelid inversion is noted at birth. Unlike epiblepharon, it does not resolve spontaneously. Surgery should be performed when corneal integrity is threatened.

Epiblepharon

Epiblepharon is a congenital anomaly characterized by a horizontal fold of skin adjacent to either the upper or lower eyelid—most commonly, the lower eyelid—that may turn the lashes inward against the cornea. The child's cornea often tolerates this condition surprisingly well, and in the first few years of life, epiblepharon usually resolves spontaneously. Severe cases require surgical repair.

Congenital Tarsal Kink

The origin of congenital tarsal kink is unknown, but a child with this condition is born with the upper eyelid bent back and open. The upper tarsal plate often has an actual 180° fold. As with large congenital colobomas, the cornea may be exposed and traumatized by the bent edge, resulting in ulceration. Minor defects can be managed by manually unfolding the tarsus and taping the eyelid shut with a pressure dressing for 1–2 days. More severe cases require surgical incision of the tarsal plate or even excision of a V-shaped wedge from the inner surface to permit unfolding.

Distichiasis

A partial or complete accessory row of eyelashes growing out of or slightly posterior to the meibomian gland orifices is known as distichiasis. The abnormal lashes tend to be thinner, shorter, softer, and less pigmented than normal cilia and are therefore often well tolerated. Treatment is indicated if the patient is symptomatic or if corneal irritation is evident (Fig 15-6).

Trichotillomania

Trichotillomania is characterized by the pulling out of one's hair, frequently including the eyebrows and cilia. It is discussed in further detail in BCSC Section 7, *Orbit, Eyelids, and Lacrimal System.*

Euryblepharon

Enlargement of the lateral part of the palpebral aperture with downward displacement of the temporal half of the lower eyelid is known as euryblepharon. This condition gives the appearance of a very wide palpebral fissure or a droopy lower eyelid.

Epicanthus

Epicanthus, a crescent-shaped fold of skin running vertically between the eyelids and overlying the inner canthus, is shown in Figure 15-7. There are 4 types of epicanthus:

1. *epicanthus tarsalis:* fold is most prominent in the upper eyelid
2. *epicanthus inversus:* fold is most prominent in the lower eyelid
3. *epicanthus palpebralis:* fold is equally distributed in the upper and lower eyelids
4. *epicanthus supraciliaris:* fold arises from the eyebrow and terminates over the lacrimal sac

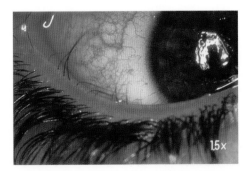

Figure 15-6 Distichiasis. An accessory row of eyelashes exits from the meibomian gland orifices. *(Reproduced by permission from Byrnes GA, Wilson ME. Congenital distichiasis. Arch Ophthalmol. 1991;109(12):1752–1753. ©1991, American Medical Association.)*

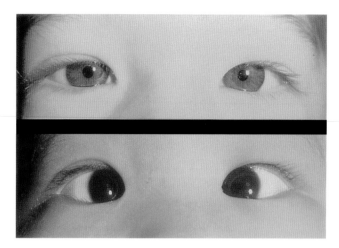

Figure 15-7 Epicanthus, bilateral. **Top,** Epicanthus tarsalis. **Bottom,** Epicanthus palpebralis. *(Reproduced by permission from Crouch E. The Child's Eye: Strabismus and Amblyopia. Slide script. San Francisco: American Academy of Ophthalmology; 1982.)*

Epicanthus may be associated with blepharophimosis or ptosis, or it may be an isolated finding. Surgical correction is only occasionally required.

Palpebral Fissure Slants

In the normal eye, the eyelids are generally positioned so that the lateral canthus is about 1 mm higher than the medial canthus. Slight upward or downward slanting of palpebral fissures normally occurs on a familial basis or in groups such as people of Asian descent. However, certain craniofacial syndromes frequently cause palpebral fissures to have a characteristic upward or downward (eg, Treacher Collins syndrome) slant (see Chapter 28, Fig 28-10).

Blepharophimosis Syndrome

Blepharophimosis syndrome consists of blepharophimosis, epicanthus inversus, telecanthus, and ptosis; it may occur as an isolated or autosomal dominant disorder. The palpebral fissures are shortened horizontally and vertically *(blepharophimosis)*, with poor levator function and no eyelid fold (Fig 15-8). The horizontal palpebral fissure length, normally 25–30 mm, is reduced to 18–22 mm in these patients. Repair of the ptosis, usually with frontalis suspension procedures, may be needed early in life. Because the epicanthus and telecanthus may improve with age, repair of these defects is often delayed.

Ptosis

Ptosis (blepharoptosis) describes eyelid droop; the condition can be congenital or acquired (Table 15-1). Congenital ptosis may be familial. Anisometropic astigmatism may be associated with ptosis and is the most common cause of amblyopia in these patients. Astigmatism often persists after eyelid surgery.

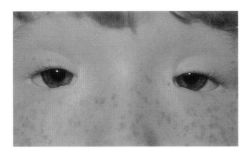

Figure 15-8 Blepharophimosis syndrome: blepharophimosis, epicanthus inversus, telecanthus, and ptosis.

Table 15-1 Classification of Ptosis

Pseudoptosis

Congenital ptosis

Acquired ptosis
   Myogenic
      Myasthenia gravis
      Progressive external ophthalmoplegia
   Neurogenic
      Horner syndrome
      Third cranial nerve palsy
   Mechanical

Evaluation of ptosis requires documentation of the presence or absence of the upper eyelid fold, as well as measurements of the amount of ptosis and of the degree of levator muscle function. The severity of the ptosis is determined by measuring the palpebral fissure height and the margin–reflex distance (MRD). The MRD is the distance from the margin of the upper eyelid to the corneal light reflex, when the eye is in primary gaze. Levator function is measured by determining the distance the upper eyelid moves from downgaze to upgaze, while the effect of the frontalis muscle is blocked by pressure from the examiner's fingers. Both tear function and corneal sensitivity should be evaluated because exposure and drying may occur after surgical repair. If the Bell phenomenon is poor, the cornea can decompensate quickly after ptosis repair. A photograph of the patient is desirable for documentation. It is also important to determine whether the globe is microphthalmic or whether a hypotropia is present, as either of these conditions may produce a pseudoptosis.

Correction of ptosis in a child can often be delayed until the patient is several years old, although a compensatory chin-up head posturing may justify earlier surgery. Though rarely encountered, a completely closed eyelid must be elevated early in infancy to avoid occlusion amblyopia. Surgical techniques include levator resection, tucking of the levator aponeurosis, and eyelid suspension anchored into the frontalis muscle. When levator function is less than 4 mm, frontalis suspension surgery is usually performed. Some surgeons prefer autogenous fascia lata for frontalis suspension surgery. However, others report good results with silicone rods or human donor fascia lata. Autogenous fascia cannot be obtained until the patient is 3 or 4 years old. One study reported a 50% recurrence rate by 8–10 postoperative years when human donor fascia lata was used.

Marcus Gunn Jaw-Winking

Marcus Gunn jaw-winking syndrome is the result of a congenital trigemino-oculomotor synkinesis of the jaw and levator muscles. The ptotic eyelid elevates with opening of the mouth or movement of the jaw to the contralateral side. Testing for this condition in an infant may be performed by having the child suck on a bottle or pacifier. Treatment requires disinserting the levator muscle of the affected eyelid and performing a frontalis lid suspension. This procedure may also be performed on the normal eyelid to achieve a symmetrical appearance in downgaze.

Meyer DR. Congenital ptosis. *Focal Points: Clinical Modules for Ophthalmologists.* San Francisco: American Academy of Ophthalmology; 2001, module 2.

CHAPTER 16

Infectious and Allergic Ocular Diseases

Intrauterine and Perinatal Infections of the Eye

Maternally transmitted congenital infections cause ocular damage in 3 ways:

1. through direct action of the infecting agent, which damages tissue
2. through a teratogenic effect resulting in malformation
3. through a delayed reactivation of the agent after birth, with inflammation that damages developed tissue

These infections can cause ongoing tissue damage; therefore, long-term evaluation is required to determine their full impact. Most perinatal disorders have an exceedingly broad spectrum of clinical presentation, ranging from silent disease to life-threatening tissue and organ damage. Only the common types of congenital infections are included in this chapter. They can be remembered by the acronym TORCHES: *to*xoplasmosis; *r*ubella; *c*ytomegalic inclusion disease; *h*erpesviruses, including *E*pstein-Barr; *s*yphilis.

Toxoplasmosis

The etiologic agent of toxoplasmosis, *Toxoplasma gondii*, is an obligate intracellular parasite. Cats are the definitive host, wherein the parasite resides in the intestinal mucosa in the form of an oocyst. Once excreted into the environment, the oocyst can be ingested by many animals, including humans. Humans can also acquire the disease secondarily by ingesting undercooked infected meat or contaminated drinking water.

The ingested cyst has a predilection for muscle, including the heart, and neural tissue, including the retinas. Encysted organisms can remain dormant indefinitely, or the cyst can rupture, releasing hundreds of thousands of *tachyzoites*, the proliferative phase of the protozoan. The stimulus for local reactivation of an infected cyst is unknown.

Systemic infection in humans is common and usually goes undiagnosed. Symptoms may include fever, lymphadenopathy, and sore throat. The percentage of antibody titer–positive persons in the United States increases with age, with an overall prevalence of 23%. Previously, apparently acquired *Toxoplasma* retinitis was thought to represent reactivation of a congenital infection; however, recent evidence suggests that most of these patients are infected postnatally.

Toxoplasmosis can be acquired congenitally via transplacental transmission from an infected mother to the fetus. Congenital infection can result in varying degrees of retinitis, hepatosplenomegaly, intracranial calcifications, microcephaly, and developmental delay.

Ocular manifestations include retinitis, sometimes with associated choroiditis, iritis, and anterior uveitis (Fig 16-1). The active area of retinal inflammation is usually thickened and cream-colored with an overlying vitritis. The area may be at the edge of an old flat atrophic scar, frequently in the macular area, or adjacent to the scar (a so-called satellite lesion).

The diagnosis of toxoplasmosis is primarily clinical, based on the characteristic retinal lesions. It can be supported by a positive enzyme-linked immunosorbent assay (ELISA) for *Toxoplasma* antibody. Any positivity, even undiluted, is significant, but the rate of false-positive results is very high. Lack of antibody essentially rules out the diagnosis. Because maternal IgM does not cross the placenta, finding toxoplasma-specific IgM in the infant serum is diagnostic of congenital infection in the infant.

Ocular inflammation from reactivated toxoplasmosis does not require treatment unless it threatens vision. Vision can be compromised by the location of the reactivation adjacent to the macula or optic nerve or by significant vitritis. If the lesion is in the periphery of the eye and does not affect vision, it will likely quiet on its own in 1–2 months. Although the benefit of treatment has not been proven, most practitioners recommend treatment if the macula or optic nerve is involved or if massive vitritis threatens vision. Systemic treatment involves the use of 1 or more antimicrobial drugs with or without oral corticosteroids. The most commonly used antimicrobials are pyrimethamine and sulfadiazine. Steroids should never be used alone without antimicrobial coverage.

In the setting of maternal *Toxoplasma* infection, prenatal treatment and treatment during the infant's first year of life appear to decrease the risk of poor visual outcomes. In congenitally infected children, new lesions may occur in the second decade of life; therefore, serial monitoring of these patients is needed.

For additional details on drug therapy for toxoplasmosis, see BCSC Section 9, *Intraocular Inflammation and Uveitis.*

Brézin AP, Thulliez P, Couvreur J, Nobré R, McLeod R, Mets MB. Ophthalmic outcomes after prenatal and postnatal treatment of congenital toxoplasmosis. *Am J Ophthalmol.* 2003;135(6): 779–784.

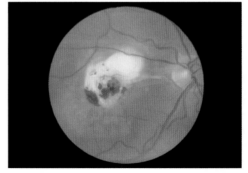

Figure 16-1 Toxoplasmosis, right eye.

Holland GN. Ocular toxoplasmosis: a global reassessment. Part I: epidemiology and course of disease. *Am J Ophthalmol.* 2003;136(6):973–988.

Holland GN, Lewis KG. An update on current practices in the management of ocular toxoplasmosis. *Am J Ophthalmol.* 2002;134(1):102–114.

Phan L, Kasza K, Jalbrzikowski J, et al. Longitudinal study of new eye lesions in treated congenital toxoplasmosis. *Ophthalmology.* 2008;115(3):553–559.

Rubella

Congenital rubella (German measles) syndrome is a well-defined combination of ocular, otologic, and cardiac abnormalities, along with microcephaly and variable developmental delay. Described in 1941 by ophthalmologist Norman Gregg, the rubella virus was the first virus recognized as a teratogenic agent. The syndrome is caused by transplacental transmission of the rubella virus from an infected mother. The incidence of congenital rubella syndrome has decreased markedly in North America since widespread vaccination of children was instituted in the late 1960s, although rubella remains a cause of infant morbidity and mortality in less-developed countries. Humans are the only known host.

Ocular abnormalities from rubella include a peculiar nuclear cataract that is sometimes floating in a liquefied lens cortex, glaucoma, microphthalmos, and retinopathy varying from a subtle salt-and-pepper appearance to pseudoretinitis pigmentosa (Fig 16-2).

Diagnosis is based on the characteristic clinical picture as described and is supported by serologic testing. The virus itself can be isolated from pharyngeal swabs and from the lens contents at the time of cataract surgery.

Lensectomy usually is required (see Chapter 21), although infected eyes are prone to postoperative inflammation and subsequent secondary membrane formation. Topical steroids and mydriatics should be used aggressively.

In adults, rubella has been identified as a probable causative agent of Fuchs heterochromic iridocyclitis.

Gregg NM. Congenital cataract following German measles in the mother. *Trans Ophthalmol Soc Aust.* 1941;3:35–46.

Quentin CD, Reiber H. Fuchs heterochromic cyclitis: rubella virus antibodies and genome in aqueous humor. *Am J Ophthalmol.* 2004;138(1):46–54.

Vijayalakshmi P, Srivastava MK, Poornima B, Nirmalan P. Visual outcome of cataract surgery in children with congenital rubella syndrome. *J AAPOS.* 2003;7(2):91–95.

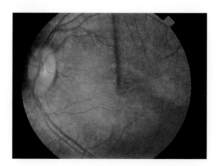

Figure 16-2 Fundus photograph of a 6-year-old with rubella syndrome (ERG normal).

Wolff SM. The ocular manifestations of congenital rubella: a prospective study of 328 cases of congenital rubella. *J Pediatr Ophthalmol.* 1973;10:101–141.

Cytomegalic Inclusion Disease

Cytomegalovirus (CMV) is a member of the herpesvirus family. CMV can cause a variety of human disease manifestations, both congenital and acquired, although symptomatic acquired infections occur almost exclusively in immunocompromised persons. Over 80% of adults in developed countries have antibodies to the virus.

Congenital infection with CMV, or *cytomegalic inclusion disease,* is the most common congenital infection in humans, occurring in approximately 1% of infants, although over 90% of these remain asymptomatic. Transmission to the newborn can occur transplacentally, from contact with an infected birth canal during delivery, or from infected breast milk or maternal secretions. Congenital CMV disease is characterized by fever, jaundice, hematologic abnormalities, deafness, microcephaly, and periventricular calcifications.

Ophthalmic manifestations of congenital CMV infection occur primarily in infants with systemic symptoms and include retinochoroiditis, optic nerve anomalies, microphthalmos, cataract, and uveitis (Fig 16-3). The retinochoroiditis usually presents with bilateral focal involvement consisting of areas of retinal pigment epithelium atrophy and whitish opacities mixed with retinal hemorrhages. The retinitis can be progressive.

CMV retinitis can be acquired in children who are immunocompromised (most frequently by HIV/AIDS, or following organ transplantation or chemotherapy). The retinitis is a diffuse retinal necrosis with areas of retinal thickening and whitening, hemorrhages, and venous sheathing. Vitritis may also be present.

Diagnosis is based on the clinical presentation in acquired disease and supplemented by serologic testing for antibodies to CMV in congenital infection. In infected infants, the virus can be recovered from bodily secretions through cell culture techniques.

Infants with severe systemic or sight-threatening disease are usually treated with ganciclovir. Medications available for treatment of older immunocompromised children include ganciclovir, valganciclovir, foscarnet, cidofovir, and fomivirsen. Intraocular ganciclovir implants have not been extensively studied in children.

Baumal CR, Levin AV, Read SE. Cytomegalovirus retinitis in immunosuppressed children. *Am J Ophthalmol.* 1999;127(5):550–558.

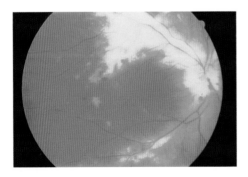 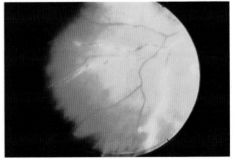

Figure 16-3 Active CMV retinochoroiditis in a premature infant, right eye.

Coats DK, Demmler GJ, Paysse EA, Du LT, Libby C. Ophthalmologic findings in children with congenital cytomegalovirus infection. *J AAPOS.* 2000;4(2):110–116.

Malley DS, Barone R, Heinemann MH. Treatment of bilateral cytomegalovirus retinitis with sustained-release ganciclovir implants in a child. *Am J Ophthalmol.* 1996;122(5):731–732.

Schleiss MR. Congenital cytomegalovirus infection: update on management strategies. *Curr Treat Options Neurol.* 2008;10(3):186–192.

Herpes Simplex Infection

Herpes simplex virus (HSV) is a member of the herpesvirus family that includes 2 types of simplex virus (HSV-1 and HSV-2), herpes zoster, Epstein-Barr virus, and CMV. HSV-1 typically affects the eyes, skin, and mouth region and is transmitted by close personal contact. HSV-2 is typically associated with genital infection through venereal transmission and is responsible for most neonatal infections.

Congenital infection is usually acquired during passage through an infected birth canal. The neonatal infection is confined to the central nervous system, skin, oral cavity, and eyes in one-third of cases. It commonly manifests with vesicular skin lesions, ulcerative mouth sores, and keratoconjunctivitis. Disseminated disease occurs in two-thirds of cases and can involve the liver, adrenal glands, and lungs. Eye involvement in congenital infection can include conjunctivitis, keratitis, retinochoroiditis, and cataracts. Keratitis can be epithelial or stromal. Retinal involvement can be severe, including massive exudates and retinal necrosis. Affected infants are treated with systemic acyclovir. The mortality rate from disseminated disease is significant, and survivors usually have permanent impairment.

Arvin AM, Whitley RJ, Gutierrez KM. Herpes simplex virus infections. In: Remington JS, Klein JO, eds. *Infectious Diseases of the Fetus and Newborn Infant.* 6th ed. Philadelphia: Elsevier Saunders; 2006.

Syphilis

Syphilis is caused by the spirochete *Treponema pallidum,* and sexual contact is the usual route of transmission. Fetal infection occurs following maternal spirochetemia. The longer the mother has had syphilis, the lower the risk of transmitting the disease to her child. If the mother has contracted primary or secondary disease, about half of her offspring will be infected. In cases of untreated late maternal syphilis (the most common form), approximately 70% of infants are healthy.

Signs and symptoms of congenital syphilis include premature births of unexplained cause, large placenta, persistent rhinitis, intractable rash, unexplained jaundice, hepatosplenomegaly, pneumonia, anemia, generalized lymphadenopathy, and metaphyseal abnormalities or periostitis on radiographs. Congenitally acquired infection can lead to neonatal death. Early eye involvement in congenital syphilis is rare.

Chorioretinitis appears as a salt-and-pepper granularity of the fundus in some infants. An appearance of pseudoretinitis pigmentosa may ensue; rarely, anterior uveitis, glaucoma, or both may develop. In other cases, symptoms may not appear until late childhood or adolescence. Widely spaced, peg-shaped teeth; eighth nerve deafness; and interstitial keratitis constitute the *Hutchinson triad.* Other manifestations include saddle nose, short maxilla, and linear scars around body orifices. Bilateral interstitial keratitis is the classic ophthalmic finding in older children and adults, occurring in approximately 10% of patients.

A diagnosis of congenital syphilis is confirmed by identification of *T pallidum* by dark-field microscopy. The disease can be presumptively diagnosed by the combination of a positive VDRL (Venereal Disease Research Laboratory) test result and 1 or more of the following:

- evidence of congenital syphilis on physical examination
- characteristic changes of the long bones on radiographic examination
- a positive result on VDRL testing of cerebrospinal fluid
- otherwise unexplained elevation of cerebrospinal fluid protein or cell count
- quantitative nontreponemal serologic titer 4 times greater than the mother's
- a positive FTA-ABS (fluorescent treponemal antibody absorption) test result

Congenital syphilis in neonates is treated with intravenous aqueous crystalline penicillin G. Serologic tests are repeated at 2 to 4, 6, and 12 months after the conclusion of treatment, or until results become nonreactive or the titer has decreased fourfold. Persistent positive titers or a positive cerebrospinal fluid VDRL test result at 6 months should prompt retreatment.

Ingall D, Sanchez P, Baker CJ. Syphilis. In: Remington JS, Klein JO, eds. *Infectious Diseases of the Fetus and Newborn Infant.* 6th ed. Philadelphia: Elsevier Saunders; 2006.

Lymphocytic Choriomeningitis

Lymphocytic choriomeningitis virus (LCMV) is an arenavirus that is transmitted by exposure to infected rodents. Infants with congenital LCMV infection present with central nervous system abnormalities, including hydrocephaly, microcephaly, intracranial calcifications, and mental retardation. Chorioretinal scars, which may involve the entire macula, have been described in several patients, including some with no neurologic abnormalities. The appearance of these scars is similar to that of scars seen in patients with toxoplasmosis. The diagnosis of LCMV infection should be considered in infants with chorioretinal scars when results of tests for more common etiologies, such as toxoplasmosis, are negative. Elevated LCMV antibody titers support the diagnosis.

Mets MB, Barton LL, Khan AS, Ksiazek TG. Lymphocytic choriomeningitis virus: an underdiagnosed cause of congenital chorioretinitis. *Am J Ophthalmol.* 2000;130(2):209–215.

Ophthalmia Neonatorum

Ophthalmia neonatorum refers to conjunctivitis occurring in the first month of life. This condition is caused by a number of different agents, including bacterial, viral, and chemical agents. Widespread effective prophylaxis has diminished its morbidity to very low levels in industrialized countries, but ophthalmia neonatorum remains a significant cause of ocular morbidity, blindness, and even death in medically underserved areas around the world.

Etiology

Worldwide, the incidence of ophthalmia neonatorum is high in areas with high rates of sexually transmitted disease. Incidence ranges from 0.1% in highly developed countries with effective prenatal care to 10% in areas such as East Africa.

The organism usually infects the infant through direct contact during passage through the birth canal. Infections are known to ascend to the uterus so that even infants delivered via cesarean can be infected. This possibility is enhanced by prolonged rupture of membranes at the time of delivery.

Most Important Agents

Neisseria

The most serious form of ophthalmia neonatorum is caused by *Neisseria gonorrhoeae*. Onset is typically in the first 3–4 days of life but may be delayed for up to 3 weeks. Although some cases may present with mild conjunctival hyperemia and discharge, severe cases have marked chemosis, copious discharge, and potentially rapid corneal ulceration and perforation of the eye (Fig 16-4). Systemic infection can cause sepsis, meningitis, and arthritis.

Gram stain of the conjunctival exudate showing gram-negative intracellular diplococci allows a presumptive diagnosis of *N gonorrhoeae* infection, and treatment should be started immediately. Ophthalmia neonatorum from *Neisseria meningitidis* has also been reported. The 2 *Neisseria* organisms cannot be differentiated by Gram stain. Definitive diagnosis is based on culture of the conjunctival discharge. Affected infants should be tested for concomitant infection with HIV, *Chlamydia,* and syphilis.

Treatment of gonococcal ophthalmia neonatorum includes systemic ceftriaxone and topical irrigation with saline. Topical antibiotics may be indicated if there is corneal involvement.

Chlamydia

The agent responsible for *Chlamydia trachomatis* (called *trachoma-inclusion conjunctivitis,* or *TRIC*) is an obligate intracellular organism.

Onset of conjunctivitis in the infant usually occurs around 1 week of age, although onset may be earlier, especially in cases with premature rupture of membranes. Eye

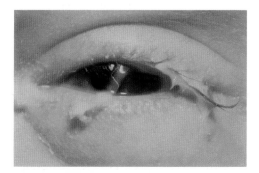

Figure 16-4   *Neisseria gonorrhoeae* conjunctivitis.

infection is characterized by mild swelling, hyperemia, and a papillary reaction with mini-mal to moderate discharge. Rare severe cases can be accompanied by more copious dis-charge and pseudomembrane formation. A follicular conjunctival reaction typical of adult inclusion conjunctivitis can occur after about 1 month of age.

The gold standard for diagnosis is culture of conjunctival scrapings. Because the agents are obligate intracellular organisms, the culture material must include epithelial cells. Nu-cleic acid amplification testing (eg, polymerase chain reaction) is more sensitive than cul-ture. Direct fluorescent antibody tests and enzyme immunoassays are also available.

Systemic treatment of neonatal chlamydial disease is indicated because of the risk of pneumonia. The treatment of choice is oral erythromycin, 50 mg/kg per day in 4 divided doses for 14 days. Topical treatment is not effective. As is done with other venereally trans-mitted diseases, public health authorities should be contacted to initiate evaluation and treatment of other maternal contacts.

Herpes simplex

Infection with herpes simplex virus (HSV) is a rarer form of ophthalmia neonatorum. It typically presents later than infection with *N gonorrhoeae* or *C trachomatis,* frequently in the second week of life. See the discussion of congenital HSV infection earlier in this chapter.

Chemical conjunctivitis

Chemical conjunctivitis refers to a mild, self-limited irritation and redness of the con-junctiva occurring in the first 24 hours after instillation of silver nitrate, a preparation used for prophylaxis of ophthalmia neonatorum. These symptoms can suggest the onset of conjunctivitis in the newborn, but the condition will improve spontaneously by the second day.

Prophylaxis for Ophthalmia Neonatorum

In 1880, Credé introduced the concept of widespread prophylaxis for gonorrheal ophthal-mia neonatorum with 2% silver nitrate. Silver nitrate prophylaxis significantly reduced the incidence of gonorrheal conjunctivitis and is still used in some places today. Silver nitrate is not effective against TRIC and therefore has been supplanted by agents effective against *Gonococcus* and TRIC, such as erythromycin and tetracycline ointments.

Povidone-iodine drops were shown to be effective and less toxic when compared with erythromycin or silver nitrate ointment in a clinical trial in Kenya. This agent may be particularly useful in developing countries because of its low cost and ease of application.

Isenberg SJ, Apt L, Wood M. A controlled trial of povidone-iodine as prophylaxis against oph-thalmia neonatorum. *N Engl J Med.* 1995;332(9):562–566.

Conjunctivitis

Common causes of conjunctival inflammation, or red eye, in infants and children are listed in Table 16-1. Most cases of acute conjunctivitis in children are bacterial; a viral eti-ology has been found in 20%–40% of cases. BCSC Section 8, *External Disease and Cornea,* discusses conjunctivitis in detail.

Table 16-1 Causes of Conjunctival Inflammation in Children

Infectious conjunctivitis	Trauma
Bacterial	Foreign body
Viral	Drug, toxin, or chemical reaction
Chlamydial	Nasolacrimal duct obstruction
Blepharitis	Iritis
Allergic conjunctivitis	Episcleritis or scleritis

Common clinical findings in children with infectious conjunctivitis are burning, stinging, foreign-body sensation, ocular discharge, and matting of the eyelids. Symptoms and signs may present unilaterally or bilaterally. The character of the discharge, which can provide some diagnostic help, may be serous, mucopurulent, or purulent. Purulent discharge suggests a polymorphonuclear response to a bacterial infection, mucopurulence suggests a viral or chlamydial infection, and a serous or watery discharge suggests a viral or allergic reaction.

Bacterial Conjunctivitis

The most common causes of bacterial conjunctivitis in school-aged children are *Streptococcus pneumoniae,* some *Haemophilus* species, and *Moraxella.* The incidence of infection from *Haemophilus* has dropped in recent years because of widespread immunization. Older children with bacterial conjunctivitis present with unilateral or bilateral conjunctival hyperemia, discharge, morning eyelid crusting, and ocular irritation. In clinical practice, culture to identify the offending agent usually is not necessary. If untreated, symptoms will be self-limited but may last up to 2 weeks. A broad-spectrum topical ophthalmic drop or ointment should shorten the course to a few days. Medications that are usually effective include sulfacetamide; trimethoprim-polymyxin B; gentamicin or tobramycin; erythromycin ointment; third-generation fluoroquinolones such as ciprofloxacin; newer, fourth-generation fluoroquinolones such as moxifloxacin and gatifloxacin; and azithromycin. Advantages of the newer medications include the more rapid effectiveness of fourth-generation fluoroquinolones and the simplified dosing regimen of azithromycin, but the newer drugs are considerably more expensive.

More severe forms of bacterial conjunctivitis accompanied by copious discharge suggest infection with more virulent organisms, including *N gonorrhoeae, N meningitidis,* or various *Streptococcus, Staphylococcus,* or *Haemophilus* species. In such cases, Gram stain and culture can be used to identify the specific offending organisms.

Although infection with *N gonorrhoeae* in children usually is associated with ophthalmia neonatorum from passage through an infected birth canal, older children who are sexually active or victims of sexual abuse can contract this infection. Patients with *N meningitidis* conjunctivitis require systemic treatment because of the high risk of meningitis. Gonorrheal conjunctivitis is further discussed in BCSC Section 8, *External Disease and Cornea.*

Parinaud oculoglandular syndrome

Parinaud oculoglandular syndrome (POS) manifests as a unilateral granulomatous conjunctivitis associated with preauricular and submandibular adenopathy. The adenopathy

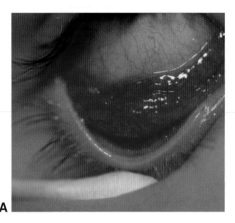 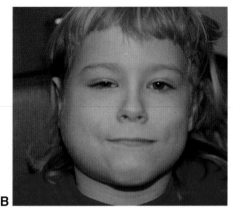

A   B

Figure 16-5 Parinaud oculoglandular syndrome. **A,** Marked follicular reaction in lower fornix. **B,** Massive submandibular lymph node enlargement on affected right side. *(Courtesy of David A. Plager, MD.)*

can be very marked (Fig 16-5). Cat-scratch disease is the most common cause of POS. Other causative organisms include *Mycobacterium tuberculosis, Mycobacterium leprae, Francisella tularensis, Yersinia pseudotuberculosis, T pallidum,* and *C trachomatis.*

Cat-scratch disease is usually associated with a scratch from a young kitten, although a cat bite and perhaps even touching the eye with a hand that has been licked by an infected kitten can cause the disease. The etiologic agent, which is endemic in cats, is *Bartonella henselae,* a pleomorphic gram-negative bacillus.

Diagnosis is made on clinical grounds and supported by a compatible history of exposure to cats. An immunofluorescent assay directed at *B henselae* is available.

Treatment can be supportive in mild cases because the disease is self-limited and is not known to cause corneal complications. In more severe cases, systemic antibiotics may be considered, although an optimal treatment has not been identified.

Trachoma

Except in areas of the South and on Native American reservations, trachoma is uncommon in the United States. Most cases are mild. Clinical manifestations include acute purulent conjunctivitis, follicles, papillary hypertrophy, vascularization of the cornea, and progressive cicatricial changes of the cornea and conjunctiva. Diagnosis is made from corneal scrapings, which reveal cytoplasmic inclusion bodies. Expressed follicular material demonstrates large macrophages and lymphoblasts. Treatment includes topical or systemic sulfonamides (or both), erythromycin, and tetracyclines.

Viral Conjunctivitis

Most viral conjunctivitis is caused by adenovirus, a DNA virus that can cause a range of human diseases, including upper respiratory tract infection, gastroenteritis, and conjunctivitis. Some serotypes (types 18, 19, and 37) are associated with epidemic keratoconjunctivitis, others with pharyngoconjunctival fever (types 3 and 7), acute hemorrhagic conjunctivitis (types 11 and 21), or an acute follicular conjunctivitis (types 1, 2, 3, 4, 7, and 10).

Epidemic keratoconjunctivitis

Epidemic keratoconjunctivitis is a highly contagious conjunctivitis that tends to occur in epidemic outbreaks. This infection is an acute follicular conjunctivitis that is usually unilateral at onset and associated with preauricular lymphadenopathy. Initial complaints are foreign-body sensation and periorbital pain. A diffuse superficial keratitis is followed by focal epithelial lesions that stain. After 11–15 days, subepithelial opacities begin to form under the focal epithelial infiltrates. The epithelial component fades by day 30, but the subepithelial opacities may linger for up to 2 years. In severe infections, particularly in infants, a conjunctival membrane and marked swelling of the eyelids occur and must be differentiated from orbital or preseptal cellulitis (discussed later under Orbital and Adnexal Infections).

The infection is easily transmitted. Infected children may need to be kept out of school or day care for up to 2 weeks. Medical personnel who become infected should be excluded from ophthalmic examination areas for at least 2 weeks, and isolation areas should be designated for examination of patients known or suspected to have adenoviral infections.

Diagnosis is usually made on clinical grounds but can be confirmed in the office by rapid immunochromatographic testing. The organism can be recovered from the eyes and throat for 2 weeks after onset, demonstrating that patients are infectious during this period. Complications include persistent subepithelial opacities and conjunctival scar formation. Treatment is supportive. Topical steroids administered 3 to 4 times daily may be used judiciously to decrease symptoms in severe cases, but such agents may prolong the time to full recovery. Steroid use in adenovirus infections is seldom indicated in children. Artificial tears and cold compresses can provide symptomatic relief.

Pharyngoconjunctival fever

Pharyngoconjunctival fever presents with conjunctival hyperemia and frequently with subconjunctival hemorrhage, edema, epiphora, and eyelid swelling, accompanied by sore throat and fever. Within a few days, a follicular conjunctival reaction and preauricular adenopathy develop. Pharyngoconjunctival fever is caused by an adenovirus, usually type 3 or 7. Symptoms may last for 2 weeks or more. No topical or systemic treatment alters the course of the disease.

Herpes simplex virus conjunctivitis

Herpes simplex virus (HSV) conjunctivitis can occur as a primary or secondary infection and typically presents with ocular redness, discomfort, foreign-body sensation, watery discharge, and preauricular adenopathy. HSV conjunctivitis is more commonly unilateral. Typical herpetic eyelid vesicles help identify the cause of the conjunctivitis, but they are not always present. Bulbar conjunctival ulceration, though rare, is highly suggestive of HSV infection.

Most cases of primary eye involvement are caused by HSV-1 and are associated with gingivostomatitis or recurrent orolabial infection (cold sores). HSV-2 is associated with

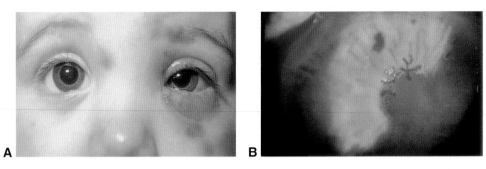

Figure 16-6 Herpes simplex. **A,** Vesicular lesions, left eyelid. **B,** Dendritic keratitis demonstrated by stain with rose bengal solution.

genital infection and is the more common cause of neonatal eye infections. Recurrent disease is characterized by dendritiform or geographic keratitis (Fig 16-6).

Diagnosis is usually made based on characteristic clinical findings. Epithelial disease is marked by epithelial vesicles and dendritic ulcers. In atypical or questionable cases, culture, ELISA, or polymerase chain reaction (PCR) testing can be used to confirm the diagnosis.

Treatment of pure conjunctival disease does not seem to alter the course of disease. Treatment is indicated when the cornea is involved. Oral acyclovir has been shown to be effective for treating herpetic epithelial keratitis and for reducing the rate of recurrences when used prophylactically.

Corneal involvement can be treated with debridement of the infected area, in addition to topical drops. See BCSC Section 8, *External Disease and Cornea*, for more discussion of the various forms of corneal disease and their treatment.

Schwartz GS, Holland EJ. Oral acyclovir for the management of herpes simplex virus keratitis in children. *Ophthalmology.* 2000;107(2):278–282.

Varicella and zoster

Varicella (chickenpox) is a contagious viral exanthem of childhood that causes fever and vesicular eruptions of skin and mucous membranes. The cause is varicella-zoster (VZV), a herpes family virus. Varicella vaccine is very effective in preventing severe disease, but children exposed to VZV may develop mild symptoms. Clinical manifestations of primary VZV infection include fever and characteristic skin lesions. Ocular involvement is usually mild and self-limited. Conjunctival vesicles or ulcerations and internal ophthalmoplegia can occur. The cornea may be involved with a dendritic ulcer, opacification, punctate epithelial keratitis, or interstitial keratitis. Anterior uveitis can be seen but is usually mild and resolves without treatment.

Treatment of the conjunctivitis is symptomatic. Topical steroids are contraindicated except for late nonulcerative interstitial keratitis. Topical antibiotics may prevent secondary infection. Intravenous or oral acyclovir may be considered in the treatment of immunocompromised children with varicella but should be administered under the direction of a pediatrician.

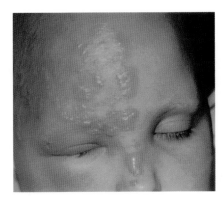

Figure 16-7 Herpes zoster.

Reactivation of latent VZV from dorsal root and cranial nerve ganglia results in herpes zoster. Vesicular lesions may erupt on the periorbital skin with subsequent ocular involvement (Fig 16-7). Ocular involvement is most likely if the nasociliary branch of cranial nerve VI is affected. Keratitis and anterior uveitis can result.

Treatment of herpes zoster includes the use of topical steroids for severe iritis. Systemic treatment with antivirals (famciclovir, valacyclovir, acyclovir) may be indicated in immunocompromised patients. Early treatment of young children with herpes zoster, unlike that of adults, has not been shown to be effective.

Infectious mononucleosis

Infectious mononucleosis is caused by Epstein-Barr virus. The disease usually occurs between ages 15 and 30 years and is benign and self-limited. Findings include fever, widespread lymphadenopathy, pharyngitis, hepatic involvement, and the presence of atypical lymphocytes and heterophil antibodies in the circulating blood. Conjunctivitis occurs in a very high percentage of cases. Nummular keratitis may also be seen. Treatment is supportive, including bed rest, antipyretics, analgesics, and cool compresses to the eyes.

Molluscum contagiosum

Molluscum contagiosum is caused by a DNA pox virus and presents most commonly as numerous umbilicated skin lesions in the periocular region (Fig 16-8A). Lesions on or near the eyelid margin can release viral particles onto the conjunctival surface, resulting in a follicular conjunctivitis (Fig 16-8B). The lesions tend to be self-limited, but those causing conjunctivitis, in particular, should be treated by incising and debriding the central core from each lesion. For young children, this usually requires general anesthesia.

Blepharitis

Though less common in children than in adults, blepharitis is a common cause of chronic conjunctivitis in children. The signs and symptoms in children are similar to those in adults, including ocular irritation, morning crusting, eyelid margin erythema, and meibomian gland obstipation. Intermittent blurred vision may be present because of tear film

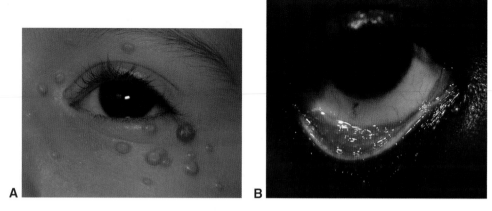

Figure 16-8 Molluscum contagiosum. **A,** Eyelid lesions. **B,** Secondary follicular conjunctivitis. *(Part A courtesy of Edward L. Raab, MD; part B courtesy of Gregg T. Lueder, MD.)*

instability. Inferior keratitis may develop in more severe cases. Initial treatment includes warm compresses and eyelid scrubs with baby shampoo. Flaxseed oil supplementation may benefit some patients. Persistent cases may benefit from a course of oral antibiotics. Erythromycin is most commonly used in young children to avoid the potential dental staining associated with use of tetracycline. Judicious use of topical steroids may be indicated in patients with corneal disease.

Jones SM, Weinstein JM, Cumberland P, Klein N, Nischal KK. Visual outcome and corneal changes in children with chronic blepharokeratoconjunctivitis. *Ophthalmology.* 2007;114(12): 2271–2280.

Orbital and Adnexal Infections

Orbital cellulitis and preseptal cellulitis are both usually more rapidly progressive and more severe in children than in adults. See also BCSC Section 7, *Orbit, Eyelids, and Lacrimal System.*

Preseptal Cellulitis

Preseptal cellulitis, a common infection in children, is an inflammatory process involving the tissues anterior to the orbital septum (see Chapter 2, Fig 2-5). Eyelid edema may extend into the eyebrow and forehead. The periorbital skin becomes taut and inflamed, and edema may appear on the contralateral eyelids. Proptosis is not a feature of preseptal cellulitis, and the globe remains uninflamed. Full ocular motility and absence of pain on eye movement help distinguish preseptal from orbital cellulitis.

Preseptal cellulitis can occur in 1 of 3 ways. Posttraumatic cellulitis occurs following puncture, laceration, or abrasion of the eyelid skin. In these cases, organisms found on the skin, such as *Staphylococcus* or *Streptococcus* species, are most commonly responsible for the infection.

The second cause of preseptal cellulitis is severe conjunctivitis such as epidemic kera-toconjunctivitis or skin infection such as impetigo or herpes zoster.

The third mechanism for preseptal cellulitis tends to occur in young children and is sec-ondary to upper respiratory tract or sinus infection or to unknown cause. Until the 1990s, *H influenzae* was the most common causative agent. The incidence has dropped markedly since widespread use of Hib vaccine began in the early 1990s but may increase because of greater parental noncompliance with vaccination recommendations. *S pneumoniae* and other streptococcal infections and *S aureus* are currently the most common causes.

Children with nonsevere preseptal infections who are not systemically ill can be treated as outpatients with oral antibiotics. Broad-spectrum drugs effective against the most common pathogens, such as cephalosporins or ampicillin-clavulanic acid combina-tion, are usually effective. Patients require careful follow-up, particularly because of the increasing prevalence of methicillin-resistant *S aureus,* which should be considered in patients who do not improve with treatment.

If the child is younger than 1 year or has signs of systemic illness such as sepsis or meningeal involvement, hospitalization—for appropriate cultures, imaging of the sinuses and orbits, and intravenous (IV) antibiotics—is appropriate.

Orbital Cellulitis

Orbital cellulitis is an infection of the orbit that involves the tissues posterior to the orbital septum. Orbital cellulitis is most commonly associated with ethmoid or frontal sinusitis. It can also occur following penetrating injuries of the orbit.

The etiologic agents most commonly responsible for orbital cellulitis vary with age. In general, children younger than 9 years have infections caused by a single aerobic patho-gen. Children older than 9 years may have complex infections with multiple pathogens, both aerobic and anaerobic. *S aureus* and gram-negative bacilli are most common in the neonate. In older children and adults, *S aureus, S pyogenes, S pneumoniae,* and various anaerobic species are common pathogens. Gram-negative organisms are found primarily in immunosuppressed patients.

Early signs and symptoms of orbital cellulitis include lethargy, fever, eyelid edema, rhinorrhea, headache, orbital pain, and tenderness on palpation. The nasal mucosa be-comes hyperemic, with a purulent nasal discharge. Increased venous congestion may cause elevated intraocular pressure. Proptosis and limited ocular movement suggest or-bital involvement. In general, children with orbital cellulitis present with more systemic manifestations than children of similar age with preseptal involvement only.

The differential diagnosis of orbital cellulitis includes inflammatory pseudotumor, benign orbital tumors such as lymphangioma and hemangioma, and malignant tumors such as rhabdomyosarcoma, leukemia, and metastatic disease.

Paranasal sinusitis is the most common cause of bacterial orbital cellulitis (Fig 16-9). In children younger than 10 years, the ethmoid sinuses are most frequently involved. If orbital cellulitis is suspected, orbital imaging is indicated to confirm orbital involvement, to document the presence and extent of sinusitis and subperiosteal abscess (Fig 16-10), and to rule out a foreign body in a patient with a history of trauma.

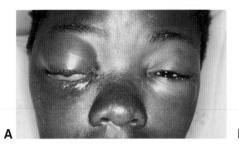
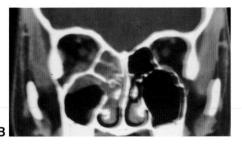

A   **B**

Figure 16-9   Orbital cellulitis with proptosis **(A)** secondary to sinusitis **(B)**. *(Courtesy of Jane Edmond, MD.)*

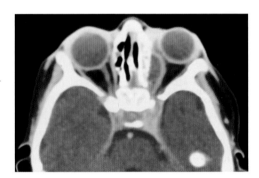

Figure 16-10   Axial CT showing a medial sub-periosteal abscess of the right orbit associated with ethmoid sinusitis. *(Courtesy of Jane Edmond, MD.)*

It is crucial to distinguish orbital cellulitis from preseptal cellulitis because the former requires hospitalization and treatment with IV broad-spectrum antibiotics. Choice of IV antibiotic should be based on the most likely pathogens until results from nasal, nasopharyngeal, or blood cultures are known.

If associated sinusitis or subperiosteal abscess is present, pediatric otolaryngologists should be consulted. The patient should be observed closely for signs of visual compromise. Many subperiosteal abscesses in children younger than 9 years will resolve with medical management. Emergency drainage of a subperiosteal abscess is indicated for a patient of any age with either of the following: evidence of optic nerve compromise (decreasing vision, relative afferent pupillary defect) and an enlarging subperiosteal abscess; or an abscess that does not resolve within 48–72 hours of administration of antibiotics. Intraconal orbital abscesses are much less common than subperiosteal abscesses in children and require urgent surgical drainage.

Complications of orbital cellulitis include cavernous sinus thrombosis or intracranial extension (subdural or brain abscesses, meningitis, periosteal abscess), which may result in death. Cavernous sinus thrombosis can be difficult to distinguish from simple orbital cellulitis. Paralysis of eye movement in cavernous sinus thrombosis is often out of proportion to the degree of proptosis. Pain on motion and tenderness to palpation are absent. Decreased sensation along the maxillary division of cranial nerve V (trigeminal) supports the diagnosis. Bilateral involvement is virtually diagnostic of cavernous sinus thrombosis.

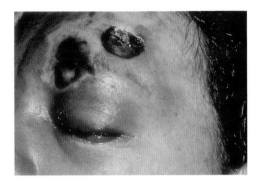

Figure 16-11 Mucormycosis, left orbit.

Other complications of orbital cellulitis include corneal exposure with secondary ulcerative keratitis, neurotrophic keratitis, secondary glaucoma, septic uveitis or retinitis, exudative retinal detachment, optic nerve edema, inflammatory neuritis, infectious neuritis, central retinal artery occlusion, and panophthalmitis.

Garcia GH, Harris GJ. Criteria for nonsurgical management of subperiosteal abscess of the orbit: analysis of outcomes 1988–1998. *Ophthalmology.* 2000;107(8):1454–1458.

Related conditions

Maxillary osteomyelitis is a rare condition of early infancy. Infection spreads from the nose into the tooth buds, with unilateral erythema and edema of the eyelids, cheek, and nose. Infection may spread and cause orbital cellulitis.

Fungal orbital cellulitis (mucormycosis) occurs most frequently in patients with ketoacidosis or severe immunosuppression. The infection causes thrombosing vasculitis with ischemic necrosis of involved tissue (Fig 16-11). Cranial nerves often are involved, and extension into the central nervous system is common. Smears and biopsy of the involved tissues reveal the fungal organisms. Treatment includes debridement of necrotic and infected tissue plus administration of amphotericin.

Ocular Allergy

Allergic ocular disease is a common problem in children, often associated with asthma, allergic rhinitis, and atopic dermatitis. Marked itching and bilateral conjunctival inflammation of a chronic, recurrent, and possibly seasonal nature are hallmarks of external ocular disease of allergic origin. Other signs and symptoms may be nonspecific and include tearing, stinging, burning, and photophobia.

Three specific types of ocular allergy are discussed in this section: seasonal allergic conjunctivitis, vernal keratoconjunctivitis, and atopic keratoconjunctivitis. All have some element of type I hypersensitivity reaction caused by the interaction between an allergen and specific IgE antibodies on the surface of mast cells in the conjunctiva. This interaction results in the initiation of a cascade of biochemical events involved in mediation of the allergic response and includes prostaglandins and leukotrienes. Among the mediators released as a result of these interactions is histamine, which is known to cause much of the itching, vasodilation, and edema that are characteristic of the ocular allergic response.

Seasonal Allergic Conjunctivitis

Seasonal allergic conjunctivitis is a common clinical entity, affecting approximately 40 million people living in the United States, including many children. As the name implies, it is a seasonal affliction, occurring in the spring and fall and triggered by environmental contact with specific airborne allergens such as pollens from grasses, flowers, weeds, and trees. Conjunctival scrapings reveal eosinophils, a finding that is almost diagnostic of an allergic response. Patients typically present with reddened, watery eyes, boggy-appearing conjunctiva, and complaints of itchy eyes. Lower-lid ecchymoses termed *allergic shiners* are common. Perennial allergic conjunctivitis is a related, though usually milder and less seasonal, form of type I hypersensitivity reaction to more ubiquitous household allergens, such as dust mites and dander from domestic pets.

Treatment of all allergic conjunctivitis is fundamentally similar to treatment of other allergy-related disorders. The most effective treatment is to remove the offending allergens from the patient's environment. Unfortunately, such attempts at removal frequently fall short of what is required to adequately alleviate the patient's symptoms.

Medical treatment can be systemic or topical, although oral medications may be less effective at relieving specific ocular symptoms (Table 16-2). Children often tolerate oral medications better because of their aversion to eyedrops.

Topical medications include mast-cell stabilizers, H_1-receptor blockers, vasoconstrictors, anti-inflammatory agents, or combinations thereof (Table 16-3). Mast-cell stabilizers are often effective, but they must be used for a few days before an effect is seen. Topical steroid drops used in pulsed doses can be effective in reducing severe allergic ocular symptoms, but patients must be closely monitored for steroid adverse effects, including glaucoma and cataracts.

Vernal Keratoconjunctivitis

Vernal keratoconjunctivitis (VKC) shows evidence of a mast cell/lymphocyte–mediated allergic response. This condition most commonly affects males in the first 2 decades of life and, like seasonal allergic conjunctivitis, usually occurs in the spring and fall. It occurs in 2 forms—palpebral and bulbar—depending on which conjunctival surface is most affected.

Clinically, the palpebral form of VKC preferentially affects the tarsal conjunctiva of the upper eyelid (Fig 16-12). Changes in the lower eyelid are rare and slight. In the early

---

Table 16-2 Oral Antihistamines

Cetirizine hydrochloride (Zyrtec)
Fexofenadine hydrochloride (Allegra)
Loratadine (Claritin, Alavert)

Table 16-3 Topical Drops for Treatment of Allergic Eye Disorders

Over-the-counter antihistamines/vasoconstrictors
Naphazoline/pheniramine (Naphcon-A, Opcon-A)
Naphazoline/antazoline (Vasocon-A)
Mast-cell stabilizers
Cromolyn sodium 4% (Crolom, Opticrom)
Lodoxamide tromethamine 0.1% (Alomide)
H_1-receptor antagonists
Emedastine difumarate 0.05% (Emadine)
Levocabastine hydrochloride 0.05% (Livostin)
Drops with both mast-cell stabilizer and H_1-blocking activity ± NSAID
Ketotifen fumarate 0.025% (Zaditor)
Olopatadine hydrochloride 0.1% (Patanol)
Nedocromil sodium 2% (Alocril)
Pemirolast potassium 0.1% (Alamast)
Azelastine hydrochloride (Optivar)
Steroids
Fluoromethalone 1%/0.25% (FML/FML-F)
Prednisolone acetate 1%/0.12% (Pred Forte/Pred Mild)
Rimexolone 1% (Vexol)
Loteprednol etabonate 0.5%/0.2% (Lotemax, Alrex)
Medrysone 1% (HMS)
Nonsteroidal anti-inflammatory drug (NSAID)
Ketorolac 0.5% (Acular)

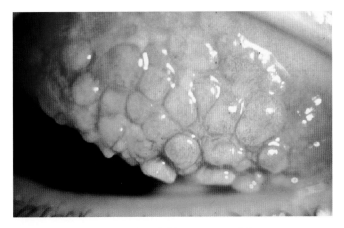

Figure 16-12 Palpebral vernal keratoconjunctivitis, upper eyelid. *(Courtesy of Ken K. Nischal, FRCOphth.)*

stages, the eye may be diffusely injected, with little discharge, and the conjunctiva appears milky. The most prominent features are photophobia and intense itching. There may be no progression beyond this stage. However, papillae may multiply, covering the tarsal area with a mosaic of flat papules. The conjunctiva is then covered with a milky veil. The discharge is characteristically thick, ropy, and dirty white.

The limbal, or bulbar, form of VKC is also bilateral and seasonal. Intense itching is the most constant clinical feature. The earliest changes are thickening and opacification of the conjunctiva at the limbus, usually most marked at the upper margin of the cornea. The discrete limbal nodules that appear in this thickened conjunctiva are gray, jellylike, elevated lumps with vascular cores. A whitish center may occur in the raised lesion filled with eosinophils and epithelioid cells. The complex is called a *Horner-Trantas dot.* The limbal nodules may increase in number and become confluent. They persist as long as the seasonal exacerbation of the disease lasts.

The cornea can become involved with punctate epithelial erosions, especially superiorly. Corneal involvement can progress to a large confluent area of epithelial defect, typically in the upper half of the cornea, called a *shield ulcer.* The ulcer is sterile and clinically looks like an ovoid corneal abrasion.

Treatment of VKC is usually less effective than that of seasonal allergic conjunctivitis. Eyedrops combining a mast-cell stabilizer and an H_1-receptor blocker may be used initially. Topical cyclosporine is often effective in more-severe cases. Supratarsal injection of corticosteroids may be used in patients with refractory palpebral VKC.

Atopic Keratoconjunctivitis

Atopic keratoconjunctivitis (AKC) has elements of a variety of immune responses, including type I hypersensitivity and cell-mediated response. This condition is relatively rare in children and tends to present in males from the late teens to the sixth decade of life. AKC is not seasonal and occurs in atopic persons with a tendency to develop hypersensitivity reactions such as atopic dermatitis, eczema, and asthma. Chronic inflammation of the eyelids is usually apparent. In AKC, unlike in VKC, the inferior palpebral conjunctiva is usually involved with papillae and scarring. Other ocular involvement is common, including punctate corneal erosions and cataracts. Treatment of AKC is similar to that used for seasonal allergic conjunctivitis, although more aggressive topical or systemic therapy may be necessary for patients with severe disease (see also BCSC Section 8, *External Disease and Cornea*).

Stevens-Johnson Syndrome

Stevens-Johnson syndrome (erythema multiforme) is an acute inflammatory polymorphic disease affecting skin and mucous membranes. All ages may be affected, and the incidence is equal in both sexes. This is a severe disease with a 5%–15% mortality rate. Ocular involvement, which occurs in as many as half of patients, varies from a mild mucopurulent conjunctivitis to severe perforating corneal ulcers. Blindness occasionally occurs in patients with severe late-phase corneal complications, such as ulceration, vascularization, and perforation.

Stevens-Johnson syndrome has been associated with various bacterial, viral, mycotic, and protozoal infections. Vaccines, collagen diseases, and many drugs have also been implicated. The pathogenesis consists of angiitis leading to erythematous lesions that become edematous or bullous and darken, leaving concentric rings in a target shape. When bullae are present, they are subepidermal and without acantholysis.

Clinical manifestations range from mild to severe. A prodrome of chills is followed by pharyngitis, headache, tachypnea, and tachycardia. In several days, bullous mucosal

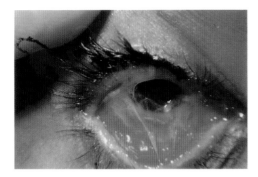

Figure 16-13 Stevens-Johnson syndrome. Early involvement of conjunctiva, right eye.

lesions develop, especially in the oropharynx. These lesions rupture and ulcerate and become covered by gray-white membranes and a hemorrhagic crust.

Ocular involvement in Stevens-Johnson syndrome begins with edema, erythema, and crusting of the eyelids. The palpebral conjunctiva becomes hyperemic, and distinct vesicles or bullae may occur. In many instances, a concomitant conjunctivitis appears that is characterized by watery discharge with mucoid strands (Fig 16-13). Secondary infection, most commonly with *Staphylococcus* species, may develop. In severe cases, a membranous or pseudomembranous conjunctivitis may result from coalescence of fibrin and necrotic cellular debris. Symblepharon formation may occur with severe pseudomembranous conjunctivitis. Primary corneal involvement and iritis are rare ocular manifestations of Stevens-Johnson syndrome.

Late ocular complications occur in approximately 20% of patients and include structural anomalies of eyelid position (ectropion and entropion), trichiasis, and symblepharon. Dry eye syndrome may also result from deficiencies in the tear film—either in the aqueous layer, from scarring of lacrimal duct orifices, or, more commonly, in the mucin layer, from destruction of the conjunctival goblet cells.

Early intervention is important in preventing the late ocular complications of Stevens-Johnson syndrome. Systemic therapy with corticosteroids is controversial. Antiviral treatment for cases associated with herpes simplex infection may be required. A discussion of systemic treatment is beyond the scope of this book. A dermatologist and pediatric infectious disease expert should be consulted.

Local measures should be instituted early in the course of the disease. Ocular lubrication with artificial tears and ointments (preferably preservative-free) should be applied regularly. Under topical anesthesia, the superior and inferior fornices should be inspected and debrided daily. A glass rod can be used for symblepharon lysis, although this may be ineffective. A symblepharon ring can be useful in severe cases in cooperative patients. Surveillance cultures for microbial infection should be taken as needed. Amniotic membrane grafting may be considered in patients with advanced disease. See also BCSC Section 8, *External Disease and Cornea.*

Kawasaki Disease

Kawasaki disease, also known as *mucocutaneous lymph node syndrome,* is a febrile illness primarily affecting children younger than 5 years. The cause is unknown. Abnormalities include unexplainable fever lasting 5 or more days; bilateral conjunctival injection; mucous membrane changes of injected or fissured lips, injected pharynx, or "strawberry tongue"; extremity changes involving erythema of the palms or soles, edema of the hands or feet, or generalized or periungual desquamation; rash; and cervical lymphadenopathy. The most significant complication of Kawasaki disease is coronary artery aneurysm. Coronary artery evaluation by 2-dimensional echocardiography is therefore indicated.

Anterior uveitis during the acute phase of the illness is common but generally self-limited. Conjunctival scarring can occur, and bilateral retinal ischemia has been observed histopathologically.

Treatment is mainly supportive, and aspirin is considered the drug of choice. Corticosteroid therapy is contraindicated because of its association with an increased rate of coronary artery aneurysm formation.

Blatt AN, Vogler L, Tychsen L. Incomplete presentations in a series of 37 children with Kawasaki disease: the role of the pediatric ophthalmologist. *J Pediatr Ophthalmol Strabismus.* 1996;33(2):114–119.

CHAPTER 17

The Lacrimal Drainage System

The pertinent developmental and anatomical features of the lacrimal drainage system are described in BCSC Section 2, *Fundamentals and Principles of Ophthalmology,* and BCSC Section 7, *Orbit, Eyelids, and Lacrimal System.*

Two points about the lacrimal drainage system deserve emphasis:

- The upper and lower puncta are normally positioned so as to contact the surface of the eye. This contact facilitates entry of the tear strip fluid into the drainage system. Malposition of the puncta will prevent this and cause epiphora without blockage. The position and patency of the puncta should be evaluated in a patient with suspected lacrimal obstruction before the conclusion is reached that epiphora indicates obstruction.
- While lacrimal obstruction occurs most often in patients aged 0–12 months, tearing in an infant can be an important sign of primary congenital (infantile) glaucoma. The examiner should always consider this possibility in any infant showing excessive tearing. Other external indications of glaucoma are photophobia, corneal clouding with or without enlargement, and breaks in Descemet's membrane (see Chapter 20).

Developmental Anomalies

Atresia or Stenosis of the Lacrimal Puncta or Canaliculi

Atresia of the lacrimal puncta or canaliculi results from failure of the upper end of the developing lacrimal structures to canalize. There is overflow of clear tears; mucopurulent discharge, while present, is not seen to the degree typical of an obstruction of the lacrimal duct. Children with Down syndrome have a higher rate of canalicular stenosis and narrow ducts than of distal membranous obstruction.

A thin punctal membrane can obstruct a well-developed canalicular system. The site is easily identified in such cases, and perforating the membrane with a needle or fine probe, followed by dilation, usually is curative. If this is not successful, more elaborate surgery is required, ranging from an incisional punctoplasty combined with silicone intubation to conjunctivodacryocystorhinostomy.

Coats DK, McCreery KM, Plager DA, Bohra L, Kim DS, Paysse EA. Nasolacrimal outflow drainage anomalies in Down's syndrome. *Ophthalmology.* 2003;110(7):1437–1441.

Supernumerary Puncta

Supernumary puncta occasionally occur nasal to the normal opening; typically, they do not disturb tear drainage and require no treatment.

Congenital Lacrimal Fistula

A congenital lacrimal fistula is an epithelial-lined tract extending from the common canaliculus or lacrimal sac to the overlying skin surface. Discharge from the fistula often is associated with nasolacrimal duct (NLD) obstruction and may cease after the lower drainage system becomes patent. Persistence of discharge despite adequate drainage requires surgical excision of the entire fistulous tract.

Dacryocele

Congenital dacryocele *(dacryocystocele)* of the lacrimal sac occurs when a distal blockage causes distention of the sac that also kinks and closes off the entrance to it of the common canaliculus, preventing decompression by retrograde discharge of accumulated secretions through massage or blinking action. Involvement occasionally is bilateral.

Clinical Features

Dacryocele presents as a bluish swelling just below and nasal to the medial canthus (Fig 17-1). There is the possibility of confusion with hemangioma, dermoid cyst, or encephalocele. However, hemangiomas typically do not present at birth, often increase in size when the infant is held in a head-down position, and are generally less firm to the touch. Dermoid cysts and encephaloceles present most often above the medial canthal tendon, in contrast to dacryoceles.

Associated nasal mucocele (bulging of mucosa at the lower end of the NLD into the nasal cavity) can significantly compromise the airway. Nasal endoscopy facilitates inspection of the nasal passages for the presence of this condition. This finding also can be seen with obstruction that does not result in a dacryocele. If the condition does not resolve

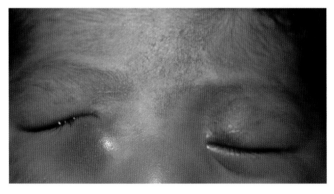

Figure 17-1 Congenital dacryocele, right eye, in a newborn infant. Note typical location and bluish discoloration of the overlying skin. *(Courtesy of Edward L. Raab, MD.)*

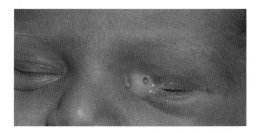

Figure 17-2 Dacryocele decompressed by digital massage. *(Courtesy of Edward L. Raab, MD.)*

spontaneously, infection with obvious local inflammatory changes usually develops within the first few weeks of life.

Management

A dacryocele sometimes can be decompressed by careful digital massage (Fig 17-2). There is controversy about treatment prior to any evidence of infection. At any sign of progression to dacryocystitis (diffuse erythema and swelling of the overlying skin and in the eyelids), most pediatricians would employ systemic antibiotics, because of concern for infection in these very young infants. If dacryocystitis shows no improvement within a few days of initiation of systemic antibiotics, decompression of the sac usually is necessary. This can be accomplished initially by gently passing a probe or lacrimal cannula through a canaliculus into the distended sac, to interrupt the valvelike action of the sac on the common canalicular entrance and allow the contents to reflux externally.

Permanent relief requires elimination of associated NLD obstruction, for which probing should be performed when the inflammation has substantially decreased. If present, an associated nasal mucocele can be marsupialized to improve drainage into the nose. Decompression of an infected dacryocele via a skin incision should be avoided because of the danger of creating a persistent fistulous tract.

Becker BB. The treatment of congenital dacryocystocele. *Am J Ophthalmol.* 2006;142(5):835–838.

Lueder GT. Endoscopic treatment of intranasal abnormalities associated with nasolacrimal duct obstruction. *J AAPOS.* 2004;8(2):128–132.

Schnall BM, Christian CJ. Conservative treatment of congenital dacryocele. *J Pediatr Ophthalmol Strabismus.* 1996;33(5):219–222.

Nasolacrimal Duct Obstruction

Nasolacrimal duct obstruction is the more typical nonemergency obstruction to drainage and occurs in about 5% of full-term newborns. Usually, a thin mucosal membrane at the lower end of the NLD is the cause. Signs of obstruction become manifest as early as age 1 month in 80%–90% of such cases.

Clinical Features

The most severe cases of NLD obstruction resemble congenital dacryocele in showing a distended lacrimal sac that can be seen and palpated beneath the skin, just inferior to the

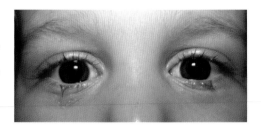

Figure 17-3 Bilateral nasolacrimal duct obstruction. Wetness and mucus accumulation without evidence of inflammation. *(Courtesy of Edward L. Raab, MD.)*

medial canthal tendon. Unlike with congenital dacryocele, digital pressure usually results in retrograde discharge of mucopurulent material. Milder cases with low-grade chronic inflammation typically present with epiphora and a mucoid or mucopurulent discharge (Fig 17-3). The severity of these manifestations may vary from day to day. Imaging studies such as dacryocystography are impractical in most instances. Applying fluorescein solution to the tear film and noting significant retention after 5–10 minutes and failure of dye to appear in the nose or pharynx after 10–15 minutes can confirm the blockage. Culture of the discharge typically indicates the presence of multiple strains of bacteria, but this information ordinarily is not necessary for clinical management. Bilateral involvement is common.

The differential diagnosis of NLD obstruction, in addition to primary congenital glaucoma and other entities with glaucoma in infancy, includes conjunctivitis, in which the lacrimal sac is not enlarged to palpation and there is no reflux of fluid or retention of fluorescein; epiblepharon, in which tearing can be caused by cilia rubbing against the cornea; and blepharitis, characterized by dry crusting on the eyelid margins.

Nonsurgical Management

The most important initial measure is digital massage of the lacrimal sac. Instillation of topical antibiotics several times per day over a period of 1–2 weeks may clear the secondary infection but should be considered adjunctive treatment that does not address the underlying problem. The antimicrobial agent should cover a broad spectrum of bacteria.

Massage serves 2 purposes: it empties the sac, reducing the opportunity for bacterial growth; and it applies hydrostatic pressure to the obstruction that occasionally opens the duct and permanently relieves the condition. To create sufficient pressure to accomplish the latter goal, it is preferable to compress the sac while occluding the canaliculi. The child's caregiver is instructed to place a finger above the medial canthus and then firmly press and slide the finger downward.

Surgical Management

The timing of surgery for congenital NLD obstruction is controversial, since this condition resolves spontaneously with conservative management in many cases. Published series have shown clearing without probing in approximately 70% of patients by age 1 year. Recent studies have shown that although extensive delay is not the treatment of choice, cases with membranous obstruction persisting after the first year of life have success rates with simple probing comparable to those of younger infants.

Early probing (ie, before age 1 year) reduces the duration of bothersome symptoms, the burden of conservative management, and the potential for chronic infection. However, delaying probing beyond age 1 year may avoid surgery altogether, despite the classic view that the rate of spontaneous resolution is significantly reduced by chronic infection. A small proportion of newborns with congenital NLD obstruction have anatomical variants that are unlikely to resolve spontaneously or be relieved by simple probing.

Surgical procedures for NLD obstruction are also discussed in BCSC Section 7, *Orbit, Eyelids, and Lacrimal System*.

Pediatric Eye Disease Investigator Group; Repka MX, Chandler DL, Beck RW, et al. Primary treatment of nasolacrimal duct obstruction with probing in children younger than 4 years. *Ophthalmology.* 2008;115(3):577–584.

Probing

Probing must be done with care, since the tarsal plate does not extend into the portion of the eyelid containing the canaliculi, which consequently are easily torn. Probing can be done in the office under topical anesthesia with the infant securely immobilized, avoiding general anesthesia and the trouble and expense of even brief hospitalization. Probing under general anesthesia in the operating room setting gives increased control and provides the additional advantages of allowing evaluation and treatment of an obstructing inferior turbinate or an intranasal mucocele and of employing balloon dilation or intubation if indicated.

Describing the technique used in probing is difficult as much of the procedure involves the sense of touch rather than sight and must be experienced. The surgeon dilates the upper or lower punctum and canaliculus and proceeds directly to probing or attempts to relieve the obstruction by irrigating a small amount of saline under no more than moderate pressure from a syringe attached to a blunt-tipped cannula introduced into the lacrimal sac; if irrigation is not successful at relieving the obstruction, inability to irrigate will at least confirm it.

Even if irrigation is successful, the surgeon should proceed with probing. A Bowman probe (usually #0 or #1; finer probes are too flexible, and the "feel" of their placement is less precise) is advanced along the canaliculus toward the sac. The surgeon should sense easy passage of the probe through the canaliculus; if this is not the case, gradually increasing force should be applied to clear what is probably a canalicular stenosis or obstruction. However, extreme force should be avoided to minimize possible injury to this structure.

When the probe tip encounters the nasal wall of the bony lacrimal fossa and overlying sac tissue, the probe is very slightly backed off the nasal wall and pivoted so that it is directed downward toward the floor of the nose. Lateral traction on the lower eyelid should be discontinued while the probe is pivoted. If there is distal membranous obstruction, as the probe advances through the NLD, a sudden decrease in resistance is felt when the obstruction is overcome. Many surgeons confirm the presence of the probe tip in the nose by introducing a second probe underneath the inferior turbinate and observing movement of the first probe as the second probe rubs directly against it (Fig 17-4). Alternatively, direct inspection with a nasal speculum and headlamp or with a nasal endoscope can determine the precise position of the probe. The degree of force to exert against an obstruction is a matter of judgment that is, again, based on experience.

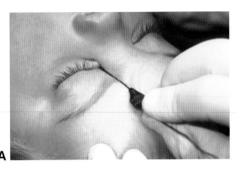
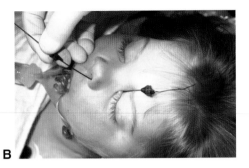

A **B**

Figure 17-4 Probing for lacrimal obstruction. **A,** Probe advancing through the lacrimal sac and nasolacrimal duct, in this instance via the lower canaliculus. **B,** Instrument introduced into the nose beneath the inferior turbinate confirms the presence of the probe tip in the nose by direct contact. *(Courtesy of Edward L. Raab, MD.)*

Minor bleeding from the nose or into the tears sometimes occurs but requires no treatment. Some surgeons recommend that massage over the lacrimal sac be continued for 1–2 weeks. Optional postoperative medications include antibiotic drops, corticosteroid drops, or both 2 to 4 times per day for up to 2 weeks. Phenylephrine 1/8% nose drops can be used concurrently for 3–5 days to promote tear drainage by minimizing edema of the nasal mucosa. Because transient bacteremia can occur after probing, systemic antibiotic prophylaxis should be considered for the patient with congenital heart disease.

Resolution of signs after probing may not occur until 1 week or more after discontinuation of postoperative treatment. Recurrence after unsuccessful probing usually is evident within 2 months. If the initial attempt to relieve congenital NLD obstruction with probing is unsuccessful, repeating the procedure may be sufficient. The success rate of properly performed initial probing for congenital NLD obstruction exceeds 90% in infants up to 15 months old. Simple probing first performed after age 24 months fails to relieve symptoms in as many as one-third of cases in some series, not necessarily because of inability to relieve the obstruction, but because of recurrent closure caused by scarring from prolonged inflammation or by diffuse stenosis of the bony lacrimal canal.

A common undesired outcome of probing is creation of a false passage into the nose, either from faulty manipulation of the probe or because of anatomical variations. The usual consequence of false passage is simply postoperative persistence of symptoms, but damage to the tissue lining the canaliculus or NLD can cause scarring that increases the difficulty of subsequent efforts to relieve obstruction. Significant complications of probing are otherwise rare.

In some cases, mild epiphora still occurs occasionally, particularly outdoors in cold weather or in conjunction with an upper respiratory tract infection. This epiphora probably is attributable to a patent but narrow lacrimal drainage channel that becomes occluded when the nasal mucosa swells. Usually no additional treatment is required.

Infracture of the inferior turbinate

Infracture is accomplished by placing a small periosteal elevator beneath the turbinate or by grasping it with a hemostat, then rotating the instrument inward. Some surgeons routinely perform this procedure at the initial probing, irrespective of the nature of the obstruction or the difficulty encountered. The value of turbinate fracture with mere membranous obstructions is debatable. Most reserve this procedure for use when firm resistance is felt as the advancing probe approaches the lowest portion of the bony nasolacrimal canal, or for subsequent procedures after initial probing fails.

Balloon dilation

In recent years, an inflatable balloon integrated on a probe has become a popular method for dilating a lacrimal drainage system that appears to be blocked by scarring or constriction rather than merely by a distal membrane (Fig 17-5). Some surgeons routinely perform this procedure in all previously untreated cases, and many observers think that this method increases the success rate of delayed treatment at any age.

The technique also can be employed as an adjunct to intubation (see the following section). It probably is not valuable in cases with a prominent bony abnormality. Although the original proponents of this procedure advocated prolonged pretreatment and posttreatment use of systemic antibiotics and corticosteroids, most ophthalmologists do not employ these measures.

Lueder GT. Balloon catheter dilation for treatment of older children with nasolacrimal duct obstruction. *Arch Ophthalmol.* 2002;120(12):1685–1688.

Pediatric Eye Disease Investigator Group; Repka MX, Melia BM, Beck RW, et al. Primary treatment of nasolacrimal duct obstruction with balloon catheter dilation in children younger than 4 years of age. *J AAPOS.* 2008;12(5):451–455.

Intubation

Intubation of the lacrimal system usually is recommended when 1 or more simple probings or balloon dilations have failed. However, it has been employed as primary treatment over a broad age range of pediatric patients.

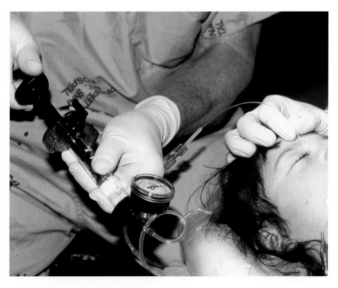

Figure 17-5 Balloon dilation. Probe positioned in the nasolacrimal duct. The surgeon inflates the balloon. *(Courtesy of Edward L. Raab, MD.)*

In one commonly used technique, once the probe with its attached silicone tubing is passed into the nose, the probe tip is engaged with a specially configured hook and withdrawn from the nares, bringing the tubing with it. This can be a difficult step to carry out. Both the upper and lower canaliculi are intubated, leaving a small loop of tubing between the puncta. A variation of the procedure employs a probe of a different design, which is said to facilitate recovery of the threaded stenting material from the nose, but not in all instances. A variety of measures is employed to secure the ends of the tubing in the nose, such as placing knots in the tubing, passing the tubing through a bolster, or suturing the tubes to the lateral nasal wall to prevent retrograde entry into the NLD.

Parents should be cautioned about the possibility of canalicular lacerations from the presence of bicanalicular tubing. When they occur, early removal is necessary. Occasionally, the tubing becomes dislodged and protrudes excessively out of the nose or the puncta. In such situations, attempts should be made to reposition the tubing. A tube laterally displaced at the puncta sometimes can be repositioned by rethreading, although usually it must be removed.

Ideally, the silicone tubing should be left in place for 3–6 months, but shorter periods can be successful. The technique to be used for tube removal depends on the age of the patient, the measure employed to secure the tubing, and the position of the tube (in place or partially dislodged).

An alternative intubation method involves intubation via one canaliculus only. The supposed advantages of this method are ease of insertion and removal of the tube and easily achieved fixation in the intended location. There have been reports of corneal abrasions with this technique.

Crawford JS. Intubation of the lacrimal system. *Ophthal Plast Reconstr Surg.* 1989;5(4):261–265.

Goldstein SM, Goldstein JB, Katowitz JA. Comparison of monocanalicular stenting and balloon dacryoplasty in secondary treatment of congenital nasolacrimal duct obstruction after failed primary probing. *Ophthal Plast Reconstr Surg.* 2004;20(5):352–357.

Pe MR, Langford JD, Linberg JV, Schwartz TL, Sondhi N. Ritleng intubation system for treatment of congenital nasolacrimal duct obstruction. *Arch Ophthalmol.* 1998;116(3):387–391.

Pediatric Eye Disease Investigator Group; Repka MX, Melia BM, Beck RW, et al. Primary treatment of nasolacrimal duct obstruction with nasolacrimal duct intubation in children younger than 4 years of age. *J AAPOS.* 2008;12(5):445–450.

Dacryocystorhinostomy

Dacryocystorhinostomy is a final option when the procedures described in the preceding sections cannot be accomplished or when obstruction persists or recurs. The decision of when to perform the procedure is affected by the severity of the signs and symptoms of obstruction.

BCSC Section 7, *Orbit, Eyelids, and Lacrimal System,* also discusses the procedures described in this chapter.

CHAPTER **18**

Diseases of the Cornea and Anterior Segment

This chapter discusses disorders of the cornea and anterior segment whose onset is during infancy and childhood. To better understand these developmental anomalies, readers will find it helpful to be familiar with the embryology of the eye. See BCSC Section 2, *Fundamentals and Principles of Ophthalmology*, for a discussion of this topic.

Congenital Corneal Anomalies

Abnormalities of Corneal Size and Shape

In the newborn, the normal horizontal corneal diameter is 9.5–10.5 mm. The average 12-mm adult corneal diameter is attained by age 2 years. Abnormalities of corneal size and shape in childhood include simple megalocornea, keratoglobus, keratoconus, and microcornea. (See also the discussion of congenital anomalies in BCSC Section 8, *External Disease and Cornea*.)

Megalocornea

Megalocornea is a nonprogressive enlargement of the cornea, with the diameter being 13 mm or greater. Megalocornea is a rare, usually bilateral, congenital condition. Inheritance is typically X-linked, so that 90% of affected patients are male. The condition is usually not associated with an elevated intraocular pressure and must be differentiated from infantile glaucoma. Megalocornea is generally an isolated finding but may be associated with lens subluxation, iris hypoplasia, iris transillumination, and ectopic pupils (anterior megalophthalmos).

Keratoglobus

Keratoglobus is the result of a cornea that is thinner than normal and arcs higher over the iris, creating a deeper than normal anterior chamber. Spontaneous breaks in Descemet's membrane may produce acute corneal edema, and the cornea is easily ruptured by minor blunt trauma. Patients with keratoglobus should be advised to routinely wear protective lenses. This rare autosomal recessive disorder may occur in Ehlers-Danlos type VI syndrome, which is characterized by generalized thinning and anterior bulging of the cornea; hyperextensible joints; blue sclera; and gradual, progressive neurosensory hearing loss.

Keratoconus

The central or paracentral cornea in keratoconus undergoes progressive thinning and bulging, so that the cornea takes on the shape of a cone. Keratoconus may present and progress during the adolescent years. It can occur with Down syndrome, atopic diseases, and chronic eye rubbing. Keratoconus may be familial.

Microcornea

Microcornea is usually defined as a corneal diameter less than 9 mm in the newborn and less than 10 mm after 2 years of age (Fig 18-1). Even if both corneal diameters are within the normal range for age, if 1 cornea is significantly smaller than the other, it is usually abnormal. Microcornea may be inherited in an autosomal dominant manner, especially in the oculodentodigital dysplasia syndrome, or it may appear sporadically. Microcornea can accompany many other abnormalities of the eye, including cataracts, colobomas, high myopia, or persistent fetal vasculature (also known as *persistent hyperplastic primary vitreous,* or *PHPV*). Microcornea may occur with nanophthalmos, a disorder in which the entire eye is smaller than normal without other major structural abnormalities.

Peripheral Developmental Abnormalities: Anterior Segment Dysgenesis

The spectrum of developmental anomalies that is known as anterior segment dysgenesis is sometimes called *mesenchymal dysgenesis* and was previously known as *anterior chamber cleavage syndrome* or *mesectodermal dysgenesis*. It has also been described as *anterior segment developmental anomalies (ASDA)*.

Posterior embryotoxon

Posterior embryotoxon, also called a *prominent Schwalbe line,* is a central thickening and displacement of the Schwalbe line. This anomaly is visible with the slit lamp as an irregular white line just concentric with and anterior to the limbus (Fig 18-2). Gonioscopically, the condition appears as a continuous or broken ridge protruding into the anterior chamber. There may be pigmented spots on the internal surface of the ridge. This anomaly is most often associated with Axenfeld-Rieger syndrome but is also found in arteriohepatic dysplasia (Alagille syndrome) and velocardiofacial syndrome (22q deletion) and may be an isolated finding in 15% of normal patients.

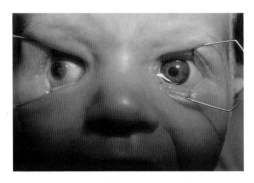

Figure 18-1 Microcornea, right eye.

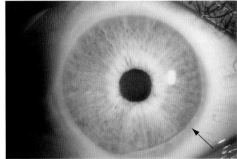

Figure 18-2 Posterior embryotoxon *(arrow)* in Axenfeld-Rieger syndrome.

Axenfeld-Rieger syndrome

Axenfeld-Rieger syndrome represents a spectrum of developmental disorders character-ized by an anteriorly displaced Schwalbe line (posterior embryotoxon), with attached iris strands, iris hypoplasia, and anterior chamber dysgenesis; progression to glaucoma occurs during childhood or adulthood in 50% of cases (Figs 18-3, 18-4, 18-5). The conditions, previously called *Axenfeld anomaly, Rieger anomaly, Rieger syndrome, iridogoniodysgenesis anomaly and syndrome, iris hypoplasia,* and *familial glaucoma iridogoniodysplasia,* all

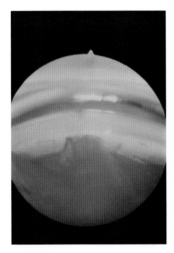

Figure 18-3   Gonioscopic view in Axenfeld-Rieger syndrome.

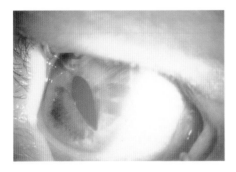
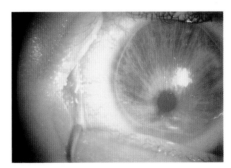

Figure 18-4   Axenfeld-Rieger syndrome, bilateral.

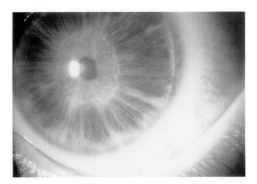

Figure 18-5   Iridogoniodysgenesis. *(Courtesy of Jane D. Kivlin, MD.)*

have genotypic and phenotypic overlap and are now considered a single entity known as *Axenfeld-Rieger syndrome*. With the identification of several causative genes and loci for these disorders, it is now known that there are cases in which the same ocular appearance is caused by different genes, and others in which very different ocular presentations, which previously would have been classified as distinct conditions (Peters anomaly, Rieger anomaly, or primary glaucoma, for example), are caused by the same mutated gene.

Axenfeld-Rieger syndrome may include a smooth, cryptless iris surface and a high iris insertion, sometimes accompanied by iris transillumination. Iris hypoplasia can range from mild stromal thinning to marked atrophy with hole formation, corectopia, and ectropion uveae. The severity of the iris hypoplasia may be so great as to mimic aniridia. Posterior embryotoxon, megalocornea (secondary to glaucoma), or microcornea may occur. Most important, glaucoma develops in 50% of cases. Associated nonocular abnormalities include small teeth, which may also be reduced in number; redundant periumbilical skin; hypospadias; and anomalies in the region of the pituitary gland.

Autosomal dominant inheritance is most common. Mutations in the *PITX2* gene on band 4q25 have been identified. This is a paired homeobox gene that regulates expansion of other genes during embryonic development. Patients with mutations of *PITX2* have been reported with phenotypes of aniridia, Peters anomaly, Rieger anomaly, and Axenfeld anomaly. The nonocular findings are actually more consistent and should be sought with any of these ocular phenotypes. Mutations in the forkhead transcription factor gene *FOXC1* (formerly called *FKHL7*) also cause Axenfeld-Rieger syndrome, with features such as autosomal dominant iris hypoplasia, juvenile glaucoma, Rieger anomaly and syndrome, posterior embryotoxon, Peters anomaly, and primary congenital glaucoma. *FOXC1* is also expressed in the heart, and some patients have cardiac valve abnormalities.

Alward WL. Axenfeld-Rieger syndrome in the age of molecular genetics. *Am J Ophthalmol.* 2000;130(1):107–115.

Khan AO, Aldahmesh MA, Al-Amri A. Heterozygous FOXC1 mutation (M161K) associated with congenital glaucoma and aniridia in an infant and a milder phenotype in her mother. *Ophthalmic Genet.* 2008;29(2):67–71.

Lines MA, Kozlowski K, Walter MA. Molecular genetics of Axenfeld-Rieger malformations. *Hum Mol Genet.* 2002;11(10):1177–1184.

Perveen R, Lloyd IC, Clayton-Smith J, et al. Phenotypic variability and asymmetry of Rieger syndrome associated with PITX2 mutations. *Invest Ophthalmol Vis Sci.* 2000;41(9):2456–2460.

Central Corneal Developmental Abnormalities

The primary abnormality of central corneal developmental abnormalities is a localized loss or attenuation of the corneal endothelium or Descemet's membrane, which is usually associated with an overlying stromal and epithelial opacity. The mnemonic "STUMPED" is helpful for remembering the differential diagnosis for congenital corneal opacities: *s*clerocornea, *t*ears in Descemet's membrane (usually forceps or congenital glaucoma), *u*lcers, *m*etabolic (eg, mucopolysaccharidosis), *P*eters anomaly, *e*dema (congenital hereditary endothelial dystrophy [CHED], posterior polymorphous dystrophy [PPMD], glaucoma), *d*ermoid.

An alternative way to remember this differential diagnosis would be recognizing that all central corneal opacities can be classified as primary or secondary:

- primary: CHED; congenital hereditary stromal dystrophy (CHSD); dermoids
- secondary: iatrogenic (forceps or amniocentesis injury); trabeculodysgenesis (congenital glaucoma); iridodysgenesis (iridocorneal adhesion leading to type I Peters anomaly); keratodysgenesis (keratolenticular adhesion resulting in type II Peters anomaly or sclerocornea phenotype); metabolic; corneal ulcers

Posterior corneal depression

Posterior corneal depression (central posterior keratoconus), a discrete posterior corneal indentation, is detected as an abnormal red reflex during examination with a retinoscope or direct ophthalmoscope. This condition can also be diagnosed with the slit lamp by moving the beam across the defect to discern the increased convexity of the posterior corneal surface. Pigment deposits may sometimes appear on the border of the posterior defect. The anterior curvature of the cornea is normal. This defect usually causes irregular astigmatism and can result in amblyopia if the refractive error is not corrected.

Peters anomaly

Peters anomaly is a posterior corneal defect with an overlying stromal opacity, often accompanied by adherent iris strands. Some observers have noted that the stromal opacity decreases with time. Lysis of adherent iris strands has been reported to improve corneal clarity in other cases. The size and density of the opacity can range from a faint stromal opacity to a dense opaque central leukoma. In severe cases, the central leukoma may be vascularized and protrude above the level of the cornea. The strands from the iris to the borders of this defect vary in number and density. A more severe variety of this condition involves adherence of the lens to the cornea at the site of the central defect (Fig 18-6). Peters anomaly is the result of many defects, including—but not limited to—the genetic Axenfeld-Rieger syndrome (discussed earlier) and nongenetic conditions such as congenital rubella.

Bilateral Peters anomaly is often associated with a syndrome. When associated with microphthalmia and reddish linear skin lesions, Peters anomaly may be part of a syndrome

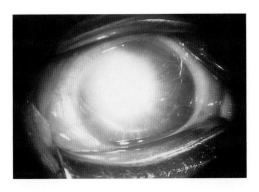

Figure 18-6 Peters anomaly.

called *microphthalmia with linear skin defects (MLS)*, which includes life-threatening cardiac arrhythmias. Bilateral cases warrant complete genetic and systemic workup. Unilateral cases are usually isolated.

Doward W, Perveen R, Lloyd IC, Ridgway AE, Wilson L, Black GC. A mutation in the RIEG1 gene associated with Peters' anomaly. *J Med Genet.* 1999;36(2):152–155.

Hanson IM, Fletcher JM, Jordan T, et al. Mutations at the PAX6 locus are found in heterogeneous anterior segment malformations including Peters' anomaly. *Nat Genet.* 1994;6(2):168–173.

Infantile Corneal Opacities

In addition to Peters anomaly, discussed in the previous section, there are other possible infantile corneal opacities to be considered in a differential diagnosis. These are listed in Table 18-1.

Sclerocornea

Sclerocornea is a congenital disorder in which the cornea is opaque and resembles the sclera, making the limbus indistinct. The central cornea is clearer than the periphery in

Table 18-1 Differential Diagnosis of Infantile Corneal Opacities

Entity	Location and Description of Opacity	Other Signs	Method of Diagnosis
Sclerocornea	Peripheral opacity, clearest centrally; unilateral or bilateral	Flat cornea	Inspection
Forceps injury	Central opacity; unilateral	Breaks in Descemet's membrane	History
Posterior corneal defects	Central opacity; unilateral or bilateral	Iris adherence to cornea; posterior keratoconus	Inspection
Mucopolysaccharidosis, mucolipidosis	Diffuse opacity; bilateral	Smooth epithelium	Conjunctival biopsy; biochemical testing
Congenital hereditary stromal dystrophy (CHSD)	Diffuse opacity; bilateral	Stromal opacities, normal thickness, normal epithelium	Autosomal dominant; examine family members
Congenital hereditary endothelial dystrophy (CHED)	Diffuse opacity; bilateral	Thickened cornea	Inspection
Infantile glaucoma	Diffuse opacity; unilateral or bilateral	Enlarged cornea; breaks in Descemet's membrane	Elevated intraocular pressure
Dermoid	Inferotemporal opacity; unilateral; elevated; surface hair; keratinized	Associated with Goldenhar syndrome	Inspection

nearly all cases, in contradistinction to Peters anomaly, in which the periphery is generally clearer. Severe cases show no increased corneal curvature and no apparent scleral sulcus. Sclerocornea is often associated with other ocular or systemic abnormalities.

Tears, Breaks, or Ruptures of Descemet's Membrane

Injuries to Descemet's membrane may be caused by forceps trauma to the eye during delivery. Rupture of Descemet's membrane leads to stromal and sometimes epithelial edema. Other signs of trauma are frequently apparent on the child's head. In most cases, the stromal and epithelial edema regresses, but the edges of the broken Descemet's membrane persist indefinitely and can be seen as ridges protruding slightly from the posterior corneal surface. Amblyopia may result from the corneal opacity. The anisometropic astigmatism induced by the trauma can cause severe amblyopia even if the corneal haze resolves quickly. Postnatal examinations are recommended, as optical correction and patching may be required.

Lambert SR, Drack AV, Hutchinson AK. Longitudinal changes in the refractive errors of children with tears in Descemet's membrane following forceps injuries. *J AAPOS.* 2004;8(4): 368–370.

Mucopolysaccharidosis and Mucolipidosis

For a discussion of the varied systemic findings and ultrastructural abnormalities of the lysosomal disorders mucopolysaccharidosis and mucolipidosis, see Table 29-1 in this volume; BCSC Section 8, *External Disease and Cornea;* and BCSC Section 12, *Retina and Vitreous.* Corneal haze may be present in early life in 3 of these disorders: by age 6 months in mucopolysaccharidosis I H *(Hurler syndrome)* (see also Chapter 29, Fig 29-1); by age 12–24 months in mucopolysaccharidosis I S *(Scheie syndrome);* and as early as age 6 weeks in mucopolysaccharidosis IV *(Morquio syndrome).* Enzymatic and DNA analyses usually can identify the metabolic defect. Conjunctival biopsies show abnormal cytoplasmic inclusions on electron microscopy.

Congenital Hereditary Endothelial Dystrophy

Congenital hereditary endothelial dystrophy (CHED) is an uncommon corneal dystrophy with onset at birth or shortly thereafter. The cornea is diffusely and uniformly edematous because of a defect of the corneal endothelium and Descemet's membrane. The edema involves both the stroma and the epithelium. The hallmark of CHED is increased corneal thickness. The appearance of the cornea is similar to that in congenital glaucoma but without increased corneal diameter and elevated intraocular pressure. CHED can be inherited in an autosomal dominant or autosomal recessive manner. The dominant and recessive forms are caused by different genes. The dominant form maps to the same genetic locus as posterior polymorphous dystrophy on pericentromeric chromosome 20. The autosomal recessive form is located on another locus of chromosome 20.

Hand CK, Harmon DL, Kennedy SM, Fitzsimon JS, Collum LM, Parfrey NA. Localization of the gene for autosomal recessive congenital hereditary endothelial dystrophy (CHED2) to chromosome 20 by homozygosity mapping. *Genomics.* 1999;61(1):1–4.

Dermoids

A corneal dermoid is a choristoma composed of fibrofatty tissue covered by keratinized epithelium. Dermoids sometimes contain hair follicles, sebaceous glands, and sweat glands. Dermoids can be up to 8–10 mm in diameter and usually straddle the limbus. They may extend into the corneal stroma and adjacent sclera but seldom occupy the full thickness of either cornea or sclera. Most dermoids are on the inferior temporal limbus. Many produce a lipoid infiltration of the corneal stroma at their leading edge.

Limbal dermoids are often seen with Goldenhar syndrome (see Chapter 28). They are sometimes continuous with subconjunctival lipodermoids that involve the upper outer quadrant of the eye and extend into the orbit under the lateral aspect of the upper eyelid. Large dermoids can cover the visual axis; small dermoids can produce anisometropic astigmatism with secondary amblyopia. Surgical excision may result in scarring and astigmatism, which can also lead to amblyopia. Although excision will not eliminate the pre-existing astigmatism, surgery may be useful for treating very elevated lesions (Fig 18-7).

Congenital or Infantile Glaucoma

Glaucoma in an infant can make the cornea edematous, cloudy, and enlarged. Chapter 20 discusses pediatric glaucoma in more detail.

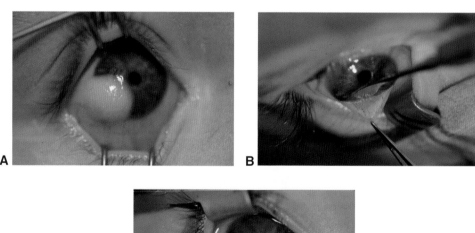

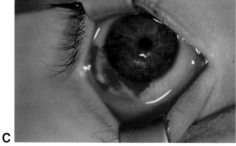

Figure 18-7 Limbal dermoid before **(A),** during **(B),** and after **(C)** surgical excision. Although the cornea will likely heal with a scar, the scar will be less irritating and noticeable than the original dermoid. *(Courtesy of David A. Plager, MD.)*

Congenital Hereditary Stromal Dystrophy

Congenital hereditary stromal dystrophy (CHSD) is a very rare congenital stationary opacification of the cornea transmitted in an autosomal dominant manner. A flaky or feathery clouding of the stroma, which is of normal thickness, is covered by a smooth, normal epithelium. These features are in contrast with those of CHED, which has a thickened stroma and epithelial edema.

Corneal Ulcers

Corneal ulcers are rare and may be due to herpes simplex keratitis or other infection (bacterial, fungal). Occasionally, corneal anesthesia may lead to a neurotrophic ulcer.

Amniocentesis

Trauma from amniocentesis is a rare cause of unilateral corneal opacification in a newborn.

Treatment of Corneal Opacities

The treatment of congenital corneal opacities is difficult and often visually unrewarding. If bilateral dense opacities are present, keratoplasty should be considered for 1 eye as soon as possible so that deprivation amblyopia can be avoided. If the opacity is unilateral, the decision is more difficult. Keratoplasty should be undertaken only if the family and the physicians involved in the care of the child are prepared for the significant commitment of time and effort needed to deal with corneal graft rejection, which often occurs in children, as well as with amblyopia. The team should include ophthalmologists skilled in the management of pediatric corneal surgery, pediatric glaucoma, amblyopia, and strabismus. Contact lens expertise is important for fitting infants with small eyes and large refractive errors. Repeated examinations under anesthesia are often required, and infectious keratitis may occur. An optical iridectomy may be used as an alternative in the treatment of a central corneal opacity.

Although there is ample evidence that deprivation amblyopia must be reversed before the age of 3 months to achieve excellent vision, it may be appropriate, in some cases of Peters anomaly, to delay corneal transplantation until the child is older. One study found better final vision in patients treated at about the age of 1 year as opposed to age 3 months because there was less graft rejection in older children, who ultimately had a clearer cornea. However, very few patients in either group achieved good vision.

Other modalities, such as lamellar keratoplasty, Descemet membrane–stripping keratoplasty (DSEK), or laser procedures, may be indicated in some cases, but there are few data for children.

Cosar CB, Laibson PR, Cohen EJ, Rapuano CJ. Topical cyclosporine in pediatric keratoplasty. *Eye Contact Lens.* 2003;29(2):103–107.

Yang LL, Lambert SR, Lynn MJ, Stulting RD. Long-term results of corneal graft survival in infants and children with Peters anomaly. *Ophthalmology.* 1999;106(4):833–848.

Systemic Diseases With Corneal Manifestations in Childhood

The mucopolysaccharidoses are discussed in a previous section. Several of the mucopolysaccharidoses may involve deposits in the cornea, leading to some degree of clinical corneal clouding.

Cystinosis

Cystinosis, a metabolic disease characterized by elevated levels of cystine within the cell, is rare. French-speaking Canada has the highest incidence in the world. Cystine crystals are deposited in various places throughout the body. The major presenting symptoms of the infantile form of cystinosis are failure to thrive; rickets; and progressive renal failure, collectively resulting in *Fanconi syndrome.* The ocular findings of cystinosis are pathognomonic. Iridescent elongated corneal crystals appear at approximately age 1 year, first in the peripheral part of the cornea and the anterior part of the stroma. These crystals are also present in the uvea and can be seen with the slit lamp on the surface of the iris (Fig 18-8). Severe photophobia can make a slit-lamp examination almost impossible without anesthesia. Cystine can be found in conjunctival biopsy specimens, although diagnosis is typically made with a blood test. As survival has improved, reports of angle-closure glaucoma have increased because of plateau iris–like syndrome secondary to crystal deposition in the ciliary processes and ciliary body. Oral cysteamine has been shown to help the systemic problems but not the corneal crystal deposition. Topical cysteamine may be applied every 1–2 hours, but it has an unpleasant odor and is difficult to obtain; however, it can markedly reduce crystal deposition in the cornea.

Kaiser-Kupfer MI, Fujikawa L, Kuwabara T, Jain S, Gahl WA. Removal of corneal crystals by topical cysteamine in nephropathic cystinosis. *N Engl J Med.* 1987;316(13):775–779.

Khan AO, Latimer B. Successful use of topical cysteamine formulated from the oral preparation in a child with keratopathy secondary to cystinosis. *Am J Ophthalmol.* 2004;138(4):674–675.

Mungan N, Nischal KK, Héon E, MacKeen L, Balfe JW, Levin AV. Ultrasound biomicroscopy of the eye in cystinosis. *Arch Ophthalmol.* 2000;118(10):1329–1333.

Hepatolenticular Degeneration

Hepatolenticular degeneration *(Wilson disease),* an autosomal recessive inborn error of metabolism, results in excess copper deposition in the liver, kidneys, and basal ganglia

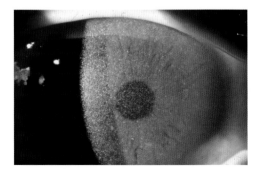

Figure 18-8 Cystinosis with corneal involvement. *(Courtesy of Gregg T. Lueder, MD.)*

of the brain, leading to cirrhosis, renal tubular damage, and a Parkinson-like disorder of motor function. The characteristic copper-colored Kayser-Fleischer ring is limited to Descemet's membrane and is thus separated from the limbus. The ring can be several millimeters in width. It may resolve with treatment. Because it can develop fairly late, laboratory tests for serum copper and ceruloplasmin are better than an eye examination for early diagnosis.

Congenital Syphilis

Interstitial keratitis may occur in the first decade of life secondary to congenital syphilis. The keratitis presents as a rapidly progressive corneal edema followed by abnormal vascularization in the deep stroma adjacent to Descemet's membrane. Intense vascularization may give the cornea a salmon-pink color—hence the term *salmon patch*. Blood flow through these vessels gradually ceases over several weeks to several months, leaving empty "ghost" vessels in the corneal stroma. Immune-mediated uveitis, arthritis, and hearing loss may also develop and recur even after syphilis treatment. Immunosuppression may be needed to decrease sequelae.

Familial Dysautonomia

Familial dysautonomia *(Riley-Day syndrome),* a complex autosomal recessive condition, occurs largely in children of Eastern European Jewish (Ashkenazi) descent. It is characterized by autonomic dysfunction, relative insensitivity to pain, temperature instability, and absence of the fungiform papillae of the tongue. Exposure keratitis and corneal ulcers with secondary opacification are frequent problems because of abnormal lacrimation and decreased corneal sensitivity. Failure to respond with a wheal and flare to the intradermal injection of 1:1000 histamine solution is characteristic of this condition. Treatment includes artificial tears and tarsorrhaphy. The gene for familial dysautonomia has been mapped to chromosome arm 9q.

Blumenfeld A, Slaugenhaupt SA, Liebert CB, et al. Precise genetic mapping and haplotype analysis of the familial dysautonomia gene on human chromosome 9q31. *Am J Hum Genet.* 1999;64(4):1110–1118.

CHAPTER 19

Iris Abnormalities

Dyscoria

The term *dyscoria* refers to an abnormality of the shape of the pupil and is usually reserved for congenital malformations. Acquired inflammatory conditions can lead to posterior synechiae, which can also produce a misshapen pupil. Colobomatous iris defects produce a dyscoric pupil. Iris hypoplasia, especially if sectorial, can produce dyscoria as well as corectopia (discussed later in the chapter). Slitlike pupils have been described in the Axenfeld-Rieger syndrome (see Chapter 18, Fig 18-4), in ectopia lentis et pupillae (see the discussion of these disorders later in the chapter), and, rarely, as an isolated condition with normal visual acuity. Some patients with congenital cataracts have an associated microcoria. Microcoria or irregular pupil can also develop with progressive fibrosis of the plaque in persistent fetal vasculature (PFV).

Aniridia

Aniridia is a panocular, bilateral disorder. The term *aniridia* is a misnomer, because at least a rudimentary iris is always present. Variation in the degree of iris formation ranges from almost total absence to only mild hypoplasia, the latter of which can be confused with Axenfeld-Rieger syndrome. In addition to iris involvement, foveal hypoplasia is usually present, with nystagmus and visual acuity less than 20/100. Glaucoma, optic nerve hypoplasia, and cataracts are common. Corneal opacification often develops later in childhood and may lead to progressive deterioration of visual acuity. The cornea appears to develop a pannus, which gradually encroaches on central vision. The condition is due to a stem cell deficiency and therefore should be treated with keratolimbal allograft stem cell transplantation rather than corneal transplantation.

The typical presentation of aniridia is an infant with nystagmus who appears to have absent irides or dilated, unresponsive pupils. Photophobia may also be present. Examination findings commonly include small anterior polar cataracts, at times with attached persistent pupillary membrane strands (Fig 19-1).

A defect in the *PAX6* gene on band 11p13 is the cause of aniridia, which can be sporadic or familial. The familial form is autosomal dominant with complete penetrance but variable expressivity. There are reports of autosomal dominant pedigrees in which patients have severe glaucoma but normal maculae and good central vision. Two-thirds of all aniridic children have affected parents. The *PAX6* gene is the master control gene for

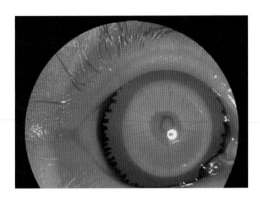

Figure 19-1 Aniridia in an infant. Both the ciliary processes and the edge of the lens are visible. Also present are persistent pupillary membrane fibers and a small central anterior polar cataract.

eye morphogenesis. This gene is probably involved in the complex inductive interactions between the optic cup, surface ectoderm, and neural crest during formation of the iris and other ocular structures. Many different mutations of the *PAX6* gene have been reported. It is likely that they cause aniridia by reducing the amount of functional PAX6 protein. See also BCSC Section 2, *Fundamentals and Principles of Ophthalmology,* for additional discussion of aniridia.

Sporadic aniridia is associated with Wilms tumor (nephroblastoma) in as many as one-third of cases. When associated with aniridia, Wilms tumor is diagnosed before patients reach age 5 in 80% of cases. The combination of aniridia and Wilms tumor represents a contiguous gene syndrome in which the adjacent *PAX6* and Wilms tumor *(WT1)* genes are both deleted. Some deletions create the WAGR complex of Wilms tumor, aniridia, genitourinary malformations, and mental retardation. All children with sporadic aniridia should undergo chromosomal deletion analysis to exclude the possibility of Wilms tumor formation. Positive results necessitate consultation with an oncologist along with repeated abdominal ultrasonographic and clinical examinations. Because of reports of Wilms tumor in patients with familial aniridia, these patients should also undergo chromosomal analysis.

Holland EJ, Djalilian AR, Schwartz GS. Management of aniridic keratopathy with keratolimbal allograft: a limbal stem cell transplantation technique. *Ophthalmology.* 2003;110(1): 125–130.

Coloboma of the Iris

Iris colobomas are classified as "typical" if they occur in the inferonasal quadrant and can thus be explained by failure of the embryonic fissure to close in the fifth week of gestation. With a typical iris coloboma, the pupil is shaped like a lightbulb, keyhole, or inverted teardrop (Fig 19-2). Typical colobomas may involve any or all of the following: the ciliary body, choroid, retina, optic nerve. These colobomas are part of a continuum that extends to microphthalmos and anophthalmos. Nystagmus is present if both optic nerves or both maculae are involved. Isolated colobomatous microphthalmia may be inherited as an autosomal dominant trait in approximately 20% of cases. Parents of an affected child may

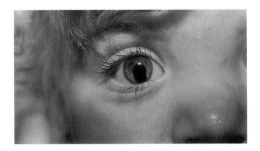

Figure 19-2 Typical iris coloboma, right eye.

have small, previously undetected chorioretinal or iris defects in an inferonasal location, so careful examination of family members is indicated.

Atypical iris colobomas occur in areas other than the inferonasal quadrant and are not usually associated with more posterior uveal colobomas. These colobomas probably result from fibrovascular remnants of the anterior hyaloid system and pupillary membrane.

Any child with a coloboma and at least 1 other organ system abnormality should undergo karyotypic analysis with extended banding.

Onwochei BC, Simon JW, Bateman JB, Couture KC, Mir E. Ocular colobomata. *Surv Ophthalmol.* 2000;45(3):175–194.

Iris Nodules

Lisch Nodules

Lisch nodules are melanocytic hamartomas commonly associated with neurofibromatosis 1 (NF1). These nodules are raised and usually tan in color but can vary significantly in appearance (Fig 19-3). (See also Chapter 27.) The incidence of Lisch nodules in NF1 increases with age, being approximately 10 times the patient's age (up to 9 years). For example, by age 8 years, Lisch nodules are present in approximately 80% of patients. Lisch nodules tend to be distributed more in the lower iris than in other areas, leading some authors to propose that exposure to sunlight may play a role.

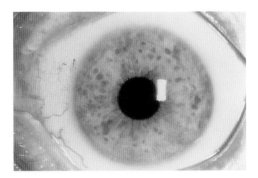

Figure 19-3 Lisch nodules in neurofibromatosis type 1.

Juvenile Xanthogranuloma

Juvenile xanthogranuloma is primarily a cutaneous disorder with a predilection for the head and face. Vascular iris lesions may occur as discrete yellowish or reddish nodules or as diffuse infiltration causing heterochromia. Spontaneous hyphema can occur. (See also Chapter 26.)

Iris Mamillations

Iris mamillations may be unilateral or bilateral. They appear as numerous, diffuse, tiny pigmented nodules on the surface of the iris (Fig 19-4). They are more common in darkly pigmented eyes and are usually of the same color as the iris. They may be bilateral, autosomal dominant, and isolated, or associated with oculodermal melanocytosis or phakomatosis pigmentovascularis type IIb (nevus flammeus with persistent aberrant Mongolian spots). They have also been reported in cases of ciliary body tumor and choroidal melanoma. Iris mamillations must be differentiated from Lisch nodules; the mamillations are usually dark brown, smooth, uniformly distributed, and equal in size or slightly larger near the pupil. The incidence of iris mamillations in NF1 is increased, but they are not diagnostic, as are Lisch nodules.

Primary Iris Cysts

Cysts of Iris Pigment Epithelium

Spontaneous cysts of the iris pigment epithelium result from a separation of the 2 layers of epithelium anywhere between the pupil and ciliary body (Fig 19-5). Clinically, these cysts tend to be stable and rarely cause ocular complications. They are usually not diagnosed until the teenage years.

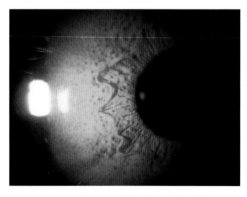

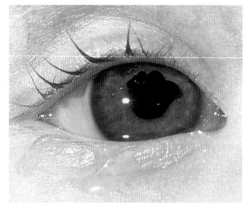

Figure 19-4 Iris mamillations. Nodules are diffuse and are the same color as the iris, as opposed to Lisch nodules, which are lighter or darker than the surrounding iris. *(Courtesy of Arlene Drack, MD.)*

Figure 19-5 Cysts of the pigmented epithelium of the iris.

Central (Pupillary) Cysts

Pigment epithelial cysts at the pupillary border are sometimes hereditary. They are usually diagnosed in infancy. They may enlarge slowly but generally remain asymptomatic and rarely require treatment. Rupture of these cysts can result in iris flocculi. Potent cholinesterase-inhibiting eyedrops such as phospholine iodide may produce similar pupillary cysts, especially in young phakic people. Discontinuation of the drug or concomitant administration of phenylephrine generally results in improvement.

Cysts of Iris Stroma

Primary iris stromal cysts are often diagnosed in infancy. They are most likely caused by sequestration of epithelium during embryologic development. The epithelium-lined stromal cysts usually contain goblet cells, and they may enlarge, causing obstruction of the visual axis, glaucoma, corneal decompensation, or iritis from cyst leakage. Numerous treatment modalities have been described, including cyst aspiration and photocoagulation or photodisruption, but the sudden release of cystic contents may result in transient iritis and glaucoma. Because of inherent complications or frequent cyst recurrences with other methods, surgical excision may be the preferred treatment method. Iris stromal cysts account for approximately 16% of childhood iris cysts. The visual prognosis is guarded.

Secondary Iris Cysts

Secondary iris cysts have been reported in childhood after trauma and associated with tumor or iris nevus.

Shields JA, Shields CL, Lois N, Mercado N. Iris cysts in children: classification, incidence, and management. The 1998 Torrence A Makley Jr Lecture. *Br J Ophthalmol.* 1999;83(3):334–338.

Brushfield Spots

Focal areas of iris stromal hyperplasia surrounded by relative hypoplasia occur in up to 90% of patients with Down syndrome, in whom these areas are known as *Brushfield spots.* These are hypopigmented spots. Essentially identical areas, known as *Wofflin nodules,* occur in 24% of patients who do not have Down syndrome. Neither condition is pathologic.

Pediatric Iris Heterochromia

The differential diagnosis of pediatric iris heterochromia is extensive. Causes can be classified on the basis of whether the condition is congenital or acquired and whether the affected eye is hypopigmented or hyperpigmented (Fig 19-6; Table 19-1). Trauma, chronic iridocyclitis, intraocular surgery, and use of topical prostaglandin analogues are important causes of acquired hyperpigmented heterochromia in children. Whether congenital or acquired, hypopigmented heterochromia, if associated with a more miotic pupil on the ipsilateral side, should prompt a workup for Horner syndrome (see Chapter 6). This may be related to a benign entity, such as shoulder dystocia at birth or previous neck-thoracic

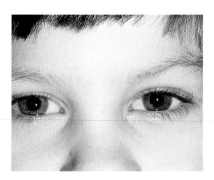

Figure 19-6 Heterochromia iridis. The left iris has become darker after developing a traumatic cataract. *(Courtesy of John W. Simon, MD.)*

Table 19-1 Pediatric Heterochromia Iridis

Hypochromic heterochromia
    Horner syndrome (congenital or early in life)
    Incontinentia pigmenti (rare)
    Fuchs heterochromia
    Waardenburg-Klein syndrome
    Nonpigmented tumors
    Hypomelanosis of Ito
Hyperchromic heterochromia
    Oculodermal melanocytosis (associated with glaucoma in nonwhite adults)
    Pigmented tumors
    Siderosis
    Iris ectropion syndrome
    Extensive rubeosis

Modified from Roy FH. *Ocular Differential Diagnosis*. 3rd ed. Philadelphia: Lea & Febiger; 1984.

surgery, or a life-threatening one, such as neuroblastoma along the sympathetic chain. (See BCSC Section 5, *Neuro-Ophthalmology*.)

Persistent Pupillary Membranes

Persistent pupillary membranes are the most common developmental abnormality of the iris. They are present in approximately 95% of newborns, and trace remnants are common in older children and adults. Persistent pupillary membranes are rarely of any visual significance. However, if especially prominent, they can adhere to the anterior lens capsule, causing a small anterior polar cataract. They may also be associated with various other anterior segment abnormalities (Fig 19-7). See the discussion of posterior synechiae at the end of this chapter.

Abnormalities in the Size, Shape, or Location of the Pupil

Congenital Miosis

Congenital miosis, or *microcoria,* may represent an absence or malformation of the dilator pupillae muscle. Congenital miosis can also occur secondary to contracture of fibrous

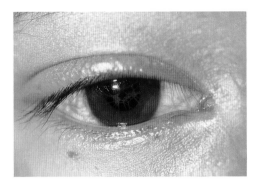

Figure 19-7 Persistent pupillary membrane. Uncorrected visual acuity is 20/40.

material on the pupil margin from remnants of the tunica vasculosa lentis or neural crest cell anomalies. The condition may be unilateral or bilateral and sporadic or hereditary. Severe cases require surgical pupilloplasty.

The pupil diameter rarely exceeds 2 mm, is often eccentric, and reacts poorly to mydriatic drops. Some patients with eccentric microcoria also have lens subluxation and are therefore part of the spectrum of *ectopia lentis et pupillae*. Congenital miosis may be associated with microcornea, cataract, megalocornea, iris atrophy, iris transillumination, myopia, and glaucoma. Congenital miosis can also be seen with congenital rubella syndrome and hereditary ataxia and in 20% of patients with Lowe oculocerebrorenal syndrome.

Congenital Mydriasis

Congenitally dilated and fixed pupils with normal-appearing irides have been reported under the names *familial iridoplegia* and *congenital bilateral mydriasis*. Iris sphincter trauma, pharmacologic mydriasis, and acquired neurologic disease affecting the parasympathetic innervation to the pupil must also be considered. Many cases of congenital mydriasis may fall within the aniridia spectrum, especially if the central iris structures from the collarette to the pupillary sphincter are absent. Congenital heart defects may be associated.

Anisocoria

An inequality in the diameters of the 2 pupils is called *anisocoria*. For a detailed discussion of anisocoria and the following conditions, see BCSC Section 5, *Neuro-Ophthalmology.*

Physiologic anisocoria

Physiologic anisocoria is a common cause of a difference in size between the 2 pupils. This difference is usually less than 1 mm and can vary from day to day in an individual. There is no significant change in the inequality when the patient is in dim light or bright light.

Adie tonic pupil

Features of an Adie pupil include an anisocoria that is greater in bright light and a pupil that is sluggishly and segmentally responsive to light and more responsive to near effort. Greater than normal constriction of a suspected Adie (larger) pupil in response to dilute pilocarpine is diagnostic. Possible etiologic causes in children include varicella-zoster.

Horner syndrome

A lesion at any location along the oculosympathetic pathway may lead to Horner syndrome. Affected patients demonstrate an anisocoria that is greater in dim light and a small degree of ptosis secondary to paralysis of the Müller muscle. Congenital cases show iris heterochromia, with the affected iris being lighter in color. However, the defect may not be seen in infants at the time of initial presentation, because time is required for the heterochromia to develop.

The diagnosis of Horner syndrome can be confirmed with the use of topical cocaine or apraclonidine drops. Apraclonidine causes reversal of the anisocoria with dilation of the affected (smaller) pupil and no effect on the normal pupil. This agent should be used with caution in young children, as it may cause excessive sedation due to its central nervous system side effects. Additional pharmacologic testing may not be needed in the presence of the above clinical findings.

Horner syndrome in children may be due to trauma, surgery, or the presence of neuroblastoma affecting the sympathetic chain in the chest. For children with acquired Horner syndrome but no history of trauma or surgery that could explain the anisocoria, evaluation should include imaging studies of the brain, neck, and chest. The value of measuring catecholamine excretion has been questioned because some patients with catecholamine measurements that are not abnormal have been found to have neuroblastomas.

Koc F, Kavuncu S, Kansu T, Acaroglu G, Firat E. The sensitivity and specificity of 0.5% apraclonidine in the diagnosis of oculosympathetic paresis. *Br J Ophthalmol.* 2005;89(11): 1442–1444.

Mahoney NR, Liu GT, Menacker SJ, Wilson MC, Hogarty MD, Maris JM. Pediatric Horner syndrome: etiologies and roles of imaging and urine studies to detect neuroblastoma and other responsible mass lesions. *Am J Ophthalmol.* 2006;142(4):651–659.

Corectopia

Corectopia refers to displacement of the pupil. Normally, the pupil is situated about 0.5 mm inferonasally from the center of the iris. Minor deviations up to 1.0 mm are usually cosmetically insignificant and should probably not be considered abnormal. Sector iris hypoplasia or other colobomatous lesions can lead to corectopia, and isolated non-colobomatous autosomal dominant corectopia has also been reported. More commonly, however, corectopia is associated with lens subluxation, and this combination is called *ectopia lentis et pupillae.* The condition is almost always bilateral, with the pupils and lenses displaced in opposite directions (see also Chapter 21).

The pupils may be oval or slit-shaped, and they often dilate poorly. Iris transillumination may occur, and microspherophakia has been reported.

Progressive corectopia can be associated with the Axenfeld-Rieger spectrum as well as iridocorneal endothelial (ICE) syndrome. Visual acuity may be good, even with eccentric pupils.

Polycoria and Pseudopolycoria

True polycoria, which must by definition include a sphincter mechanism in each pupil, is very rare. The vast majority of accessory iris openings can be classified as *pseudopolycoria.*

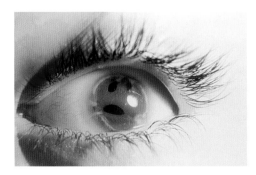

Figure 19-8 Pseudopolycoria that is secondary to Axenfeld-Rieger syndrome. *(Courtesy of John W. Simon, MD.)*

These iris holes may be congenital or may develop in response to progressive corectopia and iris hypoplasia in Axenfeld-Rieger syndrome or ICE syndrome (Fig 19-8). Pseudopolycoria can also result from trauma, surgery, or persistent pupillary membranes.

Congenital Iris Ectropion

Ectropion of the posterior pigment epithelium onto the anterior surface of the iris is called *ectropion uveae* in much of the literature. This term is a misnomer, however, because the iris posterior epithelium is derived from neural ectoderm and is not considered part of the uvea. This iris ectropion can occur as an acquired tractional abnormality, often associated with rubeosis iridis, or as a congenital nonprogressive abnormality. The combination of unilateral congenital iris ectropion; a glassy smooth, cryptless iris surface; a high iris insertion; dysgenesis of the drainage angle; and glaucoma has been called *congenital iris ectropion syndrome*. In some cases, congenital iris ectropion has been associated with neurofibromatosis and has been reported more rarely with facial hemihypertrophy and Prader-Willi syndrome.

Iris Transillumination

In albinism, iris transillumination results from the absence of pigmentation in the posterior epithelial layers. Also, iris hypoplasia can lead to iris transillumination, especially as part of Axenfeld-Rieger or ICE syndrome. In addition, iris transillumination has been reported in Marfan syndrome, ectopia lentis et pupillae, and microcoria. Patchy areas of transillumination can also be seen after trauma, surgery, or uveitis. Scattered iris transillumination defects may also be a normal variant in people with very lightly pigmented irides. Diffuse iris transillumination is characteristic of albinism.

Posterior Synechiae

Congenital adhesions between the iris margin and the lens capsule may occur in association with cataracts, aniridia, intrauterine inflammation, or other developmental abnormalities. These adhesions can also be isolated, benign remnants of the tunica vasculosa lentis. Acquired posterior synechiae secondary to iridocyclitis occur more frequently.

CHAPTER **20**

Pediatric Glaucomas

Pediatric glaucomas constitute a heterogeneous group of diseases that may result from an intrinsic disease or structural abnormality of the aqueous outflow pathways (primary glaucoma) or from abnormalities affecting other regions of the eye (secondary glaucoma). A variety of systemic abnormalities are also associated with pediatric glaucoma.

Genetics

Primary congenital glaucoma usually occurs sporadically, but it may be inherited as an autosomal recessive trait. One gene, *CYP1B1*, on band 2p21, has been shown to cause primary congenital glaucoma. Populations in which consanguinity is common have a higher incidence of congenital glaucoma, especially those in which the carrier rate of the *CYP1B1* gene is high. Two other locations, *GLC3B* on 1p36 and *GLC3C* on 14q24.3, have also been identified.

Juvenile-onset glaucoma is inherited as an autosomal dominant trait and has been linked to the *GLC1A TIGR/myocilin* gene *(MYOC)*, a gene also known to be responsible for some adult open-angle glaucomas.

The neurocristopathy/anterior segment dysgenesis syndromes (eg, Axenfeld-Rieger) are inherited in an autosomal dominant fashion. Mutations causing these disorders have been linked to *PITX2* on band 4q25 and *FOXC1* on 6p25. Defects in the *PAX6* gene can cause aniridia (see further discussion later in the chapter).

When no family history of congenital glaucoma exists, the chance of an affected parent having an affected child is approximately 2%. Primary congenital glaucoma does not appear to be associated with adult primary open-angle glaucoma.

Hewitt AW, MacKinnon JR, Giubilato A, Elder JE, Craig JE, Mackey DA. Familial transmission risk of infantile glaucoma in Australia. *Ophthalmic Genet.* 2006;27(3):93–97.

Primary Congenital Glaucoma

Primary congenital glaucoma (PCG) is also commonly called *congenital,* or *infantile, glaucoma.* The incidence of PCG varies with different populations, ranging from 1 in 2500 to 1 in 22,000. PCG results in blindness in 2%–15% of cases. Visual acuity is worse than 20/50 in at least 50% of cases. This condition is bilateral in about two-thirds of patients and occurs more frequently in males (65%) than in females (35%).

Although diagnosis is made in only 25% of affected infants at birth, disease onset occurs within the first year of life in more than 80% of cases. If this disease presents later in childhood (after about age 5 years), it is considered *primary juvenile open-angle glaucoma,* a disease that appears to have a different genetic origin (see the preceding section) and that often responds to the same treatment used for adult open-angle glaucoma (see BCSC Section 10, *Glaucoma*).

Pathophysiology

The basic pathologic defect in PCG remains controversial. Barkan originally proposed a thin, imperforate membrane that covered the anterior chamber angle and blocked aqueous outflow; however, the site of obstruction is now thought to be the trabecular meshwork itself. This disease probably represents a developmental abnormality of anterior chamber tissue derived from neural crest cells, with the anomaly occurring during late embryologic development.

Clinical Manifestations and Diagnosis

Primary congenital glaucoma usually presents in the neonatal or infantile period with a combination of signs and symptoms. Epiphora, photophobia, and blepharospasm constitute the classic clinical triad of PCG. Other signs include clouding and enlargement of the cornea (Fig 20-1).

Corneal edema results from elevated intraocular pressure (IOP) and may be gradual or sudden in onset. Corneal edema is often the presenting sign in infants younger than 3 months. Microcystic edema initially involves the corneal epithelium but later extends also to the stroma, often accompanied by 1 or more curvilinear breaks in Descemet's membrane *(Haab striae).* Although edema may resolve with IOP reduction, a scar will remain permanently at the site of Haab striae. Photophobia, epiphora, and blepharospasm result from the glare and epithelial abnormalities associated with corneal edema and opacification.

Corneal enlargement occurs with gradual stretching of the cornea as a result of elevated IOP. The normal newborn has a horizontal corneal diameter of 9.5–10.5 mm; a diameter of greater than 11.5 mm is suggestive of glaucoma. By age 1 year, normal corneal diameter is 10.0–11.5 mm; a diameter greater than 12.5 mm suggests abnormality. Glaucoma should be suspected in any child with a corneal diameter greater than 13.0 mm.

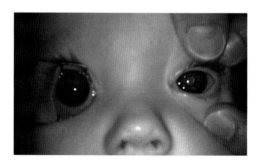

Figure 20-1 Congenital glaucoma, right eye. Cornea is enlarged and cloudy. *(Courtesy of Gregg T. Lueder, MD.)*

The signs and symptoms described for PCG can also occur in infants with other forms of glaucoma in which elevated IOP is present, because elevated IOP produces the same effects. Nonglaucomatous conditions may also cause some of the signs and symptoms seen in PCG (Table 20-1) (see also BCSC Section 10, *Glaucoma*).

Diagnostic examination

A full ophthalmic examination of every child suspected of glaucoma is imperative. Vision is usually poorer in the affected eye in unilateral cases and may be poor in both eyes when glaucoma is bilateral. The child's ability to fix and follow and the presence of nystagmus should be noted. Refraction, when possible, often reveals myopia and astigmatism from eye enlargement and corneal irregularity.

Corneal inspection   The cornea should be examined for size, clarity, and Haab striae. Careful measurement may reveal even a 0.5-mm difference in corneal diameter between the eyes. Haab striae are best seen against the red reflex after pupil dilation (Fig 20-2).

Table 20-1 Differential Diagnosis of Signs in Primary Congenital Glaucoma

Conditions sharing signs of epiphora and red eye
Conjunctivitis
Congenital nasolacrimal duct obstruction
Corneal epithelial defect/abrasion
Ocular inflammation (uveitis, trauma)
Conditions sharing signs of corneal edema or opacification
Corneal dystrophy
  Congenital hereditary endothelial dystrophy
  Posterior polymorphous dystrophy
Obstetric birth trauma with Descemet's tears
Storage disease
  Mucopolysaccharidoses
  Cystinosis
Congenital anomalies
  Sclerocornea
  Peters anomaly
Keratitis
  Maternal rubella keratitis
  Herpetic
  Phlyctenular
Idiopathic (diagnosis of exclusion only)
Conditions sharing sign of corneal enlargement
Axial myopia
Megalocornea
Conditions sharing sign of optic nerve cupping (real or apparent)
Physiologic optic nerve cupping
Optic nerve coloboma
Optic atrophy
Optic nerve hypoplasia
Optic nerve malformation

Reproduced with modification from Buckley EG. Primary congenital open angle glaucoma. In: Epstein DL, Allingham RR, Schuman JS, eds. *Chandler and Grant's Glaucoma*. 4th ed. Baltimore: Williams & Wilkins; 1997:598–608.

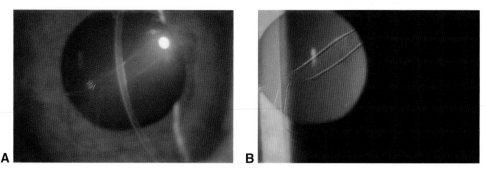

Figure 20-2 **A,** Breaks in Descemet's membrane (Haab striae), right eye. **B,** Retroillumination, same eye.

Tonometry and intraocular pressure IOP is best measured using topical anesthesia in a cooperative child. If the child is struggling, the IOP may be falsely elevated. It is unpredictably altered (usually lowered) when systemic sedatives and anesthetics are administered. A useful technique is to bring the child in slightly hungry and then bottle-feed at the time of pressure measurement. The Tono-Pen and Perkins tonometers are most commonly used for infants and young children. Goldmann applanation readings can be taken when a child is old enough to cooperate.

The normal IOP in infants and young children is lower than the normal IOP of adults; mean IOP is between 10 and 12 mm Hg in newborns, and it reaches approximately 14 mm Hg by age 7–8 years. In PCG, IOP commonly ranges between 30 and 40 mm Hg, and it is usually greater than 20 mm Hg even under anesthesia. Asymmetric IOP readings in a quiet or anesthetized child should raise suspicion of glaucoma in the eye with the higher IOP.

Central corneal thickness Portable pachymeters may be used to measure central corneal thickness (CCT), which is typically increased in infants with glaucoma. The CCT affects the IOP measurement, but there are not enough data at present to quantify these effects.

> Freedman SF. Central corneal thickness in children—does it help or hinder our evaluation of eyes at risk for glaucoma? *J AAPOS.* 2008;12(1):1–2.

Anterior segment examination The portable slit lamp allows detailed inspection of the anterior segment. An abnormally deep anterior chamber and relative peripheral iris stromal hypoplasia are common findings in PCG.

Gonioscopy provides important information regarding the mechanism of glaucoma. It is best performed with the use of a goniolens and a portable slit lamp or loupes. The anterior chamber angle of a normal infant (Fig 20-3A) differs from that of an adult in the following ways:

- The trabecular meshwork is more lightly pigmented.
- The Schwalbe line is often less distinct.
- The uveal meshwork is translucent so that the junction between the scleral spur and ciliary body band is often not well seen.

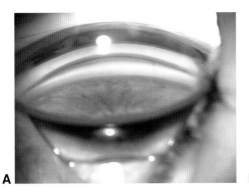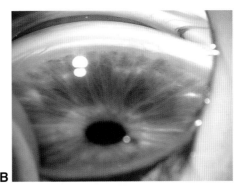

A B

Figure 20-3 **A,** Normal gonioscopic angle in young infant. **B,** Typical appearance of infant angle with congenital glaucoma. *(Courtesy of David A. Plager, MD.)*

In congenital glaucoma, the iris often shows an insertion more anterior than that of the normal angle, and the translucency of the uveal meshwork is altered, making the ciliary body band, trabecular meshwork, and scleral spur indistinct. (The membrane described by Barkan may indeed be these translucent uveal meshwork cells.) The scalloped border of the iris pigmented epithelium is often unusually prominent, especially when peripheral iris stromal hypoplasia is present (Fig 20-3B). In contrast, the angle usually appears normal in juvenile open-angle glaucoma.

Optic nerve examination The optic nerve, when visible, usually shows an increased cup–disc ratio. The pattern of generalized enlargement of the optic cup seen in very young patients with glaucoma has been attributed to stretching of the optic canal and backward bowing of the lamina cribrosa (Fig 20-4). In most cases of PCG, the cup–disc ratio exceeds 0.3; in contrast, most normal newborn eyes show a cup–disc ratio of less than 0.3. Cup–disc asymmetry greater than 0.2 between the 2 eyes is also suspicious for glaucoma on the more cupped side. In young children, reversal of optic nerve cupping may occur after successful surgery and lowering of IOP.

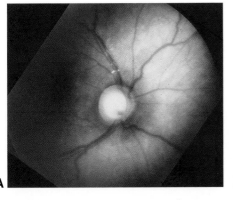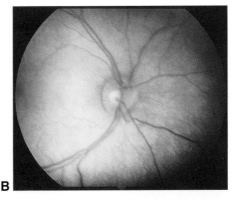

A B

Figure 20-4 Optic nerve changes after treatment for congenital glaucoma. **A,** Preoperative enlarged optic disc cup. **B,** Resolution of disc cupping after pressure is reduced by goniotomy. *(Courtesy of Sharon Freedman, MD.)*

Axial length   Serial measurement of axial length is useful to monitor disease progression in infant eyes. Excessive growth in an eye, especially when compared to the fellow eye, can be an indicator that the IOP control in the eye is not adequate.

Natural History

In almost all cases of untreated PCG, the disease progresses to blindness. The cornea becomes irreversibly opacified and may vascularize. It may continue to enlarge through the first 2–3 years of life, reaching a diameter of up to 16–17 mm. As the entire eye enlarges, pseudoproptosis and an "ox eye" appearance *(buphthalmos)* may result. Scleral thinning and myopic fundus changes may occur, and spontaneous lens dislocation can result. Optic nerve damage progresses, leading to complete blindness.

Secondary Pediatric Glaucomas

All other types of glaucomas are considered secondary glaucomas—caused by other ocular anomalies or secondarily associated with systemic conditions or trauma. Some of the more common secondary glaucomas are discussed in the following sections.

Secondary to Ocular Anomalies

Aniridia

Aniridia is a bilateral, congenital condition characterized by complete or nearly complete absence of the iris. Glaucoma occurs frequently in this disorder. The features of aniridia are discussed in Chapter 19.

Anterior segment developmental anomalies

Anterior segment developmental anomalies (also referred to as *anterior segment dysgenesis*) include *Axenfeld-Rieger anomaly/syndrome, Peters anomaly,* and *sclerocornea.* This spectrum of disorders involves abnormalities in the development of the anterior segment. Glaucoma occurs in over 50% of patients with these disorders. See Chapter 18 for further discussion.

Secondary to Systemic Disease

Sturge-Weber syndrome

Sturge-Weber syndrome (SWS), also known as *encephalotrigeminal angiomatosis,* is a phakomatosis that includes a port-wine stain *(nevus flammeus)* of the face, intracranial calcifications, and glaucoma. The presence of port-wine stains on the eyelids, particularly if both the upper and lower eyelids are involved, is associated with glaucoma. The glaucoma may occur in the absence of other manifestations of SWS.

Neurofibromatosis

Glaucoma associated with neurofibromatosis 1 (NF1) can be bilateral or unilateral. See Chapter 27 for a discussion of NF1.

Lowe syndrome

Lowe syndrome (oculocerebrorenal syndrome) is an X-linked disorder that presents with coexistent glaucoma and bilateral disciform cataracts. Children with Lowe syndrome have progressive renal tubular dysfunction and mental retardation.

Secondary Mechanical Glaucomas

Glaucoma can also be caused by mechanical factors obscuring or obstructing aqueous outflow. These include

- *lens-associated disorders:* Marfan syndrome, homocystinuria, Weill-Marchesani, microspherophakia
- *posterior segment abnormalities:* persistent fetal vasculature (PFV); retinopathy of prematurity (ROP); familial exudative vitreoretinopathy (FEVR); retinal, iris, or ciliary body tumors
- *topiramate (Topamax):* This medication, which is used to control seizures, can cause an acute, usually bilateral, secondary angle-closure glaucoma due to ciliary effusion. Peripheral iridectomy is not effective for treatment of this angle closure, but cessation of the medication is.

Other Secondary Glaucomas

In children, as in adults, glaucoma may also develop secondary to corticosteroid use, uveitis, or ocular trauma.

Aphakic Glaucoma

Aphakic glaucoma is a common cause of secondary glaucoma in childhood. The incidence of open-angle aphakic glaucoma after removal of congenital cataracts varies from 15% to 50% or higher. Aphakic glaucoma most commonly develops several years after cataract surgery, although it can occur within weeks to months of surgery and remains a lifelong risk. Consequently, these patients require regular ophthalmic examination.

The mechanism for aphakic glaucoma is uncertain. The angle is usually open on gonioscopy; the outflow channels are compromised by some combination of abnormal development of the anterior chamber angle, early surgery, and perhaps susceptibility of the infant eye to surgically induced inflammation, loss of lens support, or vitreous factors. The children at highest risk of developing aphakic glaucoma are those who have surgery during infancy, and the risk appears highest in patients with microcornea. Because most children with these cataracts have surgery in early infancy, it is uncertain whether the age at surgery is an independent risk factor.

Pseudophakic glaucoma in children has been reported less frequently than aphakic glaucoma, but this may be due to selection bias, in that children selected for intraocular lens placement have largely been those at lower risk for glaucoma.

Acute or subacute angle closure with iris bombé is a rare form of aphakic glaucoma. Although it usually occurs soon after surgery, onset can be delayed by a year or more. The diagnosis should be apparent with a slit lamp, but this may be difficult in young children.

Treatment consists of anterior vitrectomy to relieve the pupillary block, often with surgical iridectomy and goniosynechialysis.

Asrani S, Freedman S, Hasselblad V, et al. Does primary intraocular lens implantation prevent "aphakic" glaucoma in children? *J AAPOS.* 2000;4(1):33–39.

Chak M, Rahi JS; British Congenital Cataract Interest Group. Incidence of and factors associated with glaucoma after surgery for congenital cataract: findings from the British Congenital Cataract Study. *Ophthalmology.* 2008;115(6):1013–1018.

Wallace DK, Plager DA. Corneal diameter in childhood aphakic glaucoma. *J Pediatr Ophthalmol Strabismus.* 1996;33(5):230–234.

Treatment

In terms of treatment, there are essentially 2 types of glaucomas in childhood: (1) primary congenital (infantile) glaucoma and (2) everything else. PCG is usually effectively treated with angle surgery (goniotomy or trabeculotomy). Although angle surgery may be used in some secondary pediatric glaucomas—most notably Axenfeld-Rieger syndrome, Sturge-Weber, and aniridia—the outcome of such surgery in these entities is usually less successful. The treatment of most secondary glaucomas in childhood is similar to that of open-angle or secondary glaucomas in adults. Medical treatment may be attempted prior to surgery.

Surgical Therapy

Surgical intervention is the treatment of choice for PCG presenting in infancy and early childhood. BCSC Section 10, *Glaucoma,* also covers the procedures discussed in this chapter.

Angle surgery is the preferred initial surgical intervention in these cases. In a *goniotomy,* an incision is made, under direct gonioscopic visualization, across the trabecular meshwork (Fig 20-5). In a *trabeculotomy,* an external approach is used to identify, cannulate, and then connect the Schlemm canal with the anterior chamber through incision of the trabecular meshwork from outside the anterior chamber. A modification of

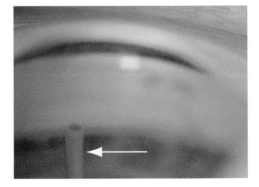

Figure 20-5 Goniotomy needle *(arrow)* with its tip in the trabecular meshwork. *(Courtesy of Edward L. Raab, MD.)*

this technique uses a 6-0 Prolene suture to cannulate and open the Schlemm canal for its entire 360° circumference in 1 surgery. If the cornea is clear, either a goniotomy or a trabeculotomy can be performed at the surgeon's discretion. If the view through the cornea is compromised, trabeculotomy or combined trabeculotomy-trabeculectomy can be performed.

In approximately 80% of infants with PCG presenting from 3 months to 1 year of age, IOP is controlled with 1 or 2 angle surgeries. If the first procedure is not sufficient, at least 1 additional angle surgery is performed before a different procedure is used.

For children in whom angle surgery is not successful or is not indicated (many secondary glaucomas), and medical therapy is inadequate, additional options are available, including trabeculectomy with or without antimetabolite therapy (eg, mitomycin C [MMC]), glaucoma implant procedures, or cycloablative procedures.

Trabeculectomy with the use of MMC is successful in approximately 50%–95% of children. The reported success rates vary considerably with the characteristics of the patient and the eye and usually decrease with increasing follow-up length. Patients younger than 1 year and those who are aphakic are more prone to failure. Although the success rate of trabeculectomy can be increased with the use of antimetabolites such as MMC, the long-term risk of bleb leaks, breakdown, and infection also increases. These complications have made some surgeons more reticent about using MMC-augmented trabeculectomy.

The reported success rate of glaucoma implant surgery with the Molteno, Baerveldt, and Ahmed implants has varied between 54% and approximately 80%–85%. Although most of these children must remain on adjunctive topical medical therapy to control IOP after surgery, their blebs are thicker and may be less prone to leaking and infection than those of patients undergoing MMC-augmented trabeculectomy. Potential complications include shunt failure, tube erosion and migration, corneal touch, cataract, restrictive strabismus, and endophthalmitis.

Cycloablation using the Nd:YAG laser, the diode laser, or cyclocryotherapy is generally reserved for resistant cases or those not amenable to the intraocular surgeries noted earlier. These techniques decrease ciliary body production of aqueous humor. *Cyclocryotherapy* (freezing the ciliary processes through the sclera) has a reported success rate of about 33%, and the complication rate is high. Repeated applications are often necessary, and the risk of phthisis and blindness is significant (approximately 10%). *Transscleral laser cycloablation* with the Nd:YAG or the diode laser has a lower risk of complications. The short-term success rate is about 50%. Patients usually require more than 1 treatment.

Endoscopic cyclophotocoagulation (ECP) has been used in both adults and children with difficult glaucomas. In ECP, a microendoscope is used to apply laser energy to the ciliary processes under direct observation (Fig 20-6). Up to 50% success rates have been reported; the rate is higher with repeated applications. Although this is an intraocular procedure, the complication rates have been lower than those observed with some of the less-controlled external cyclodestructive procedures. Use of the microendoscope is especially advantageous in eyes with abnormal anterior segment anatomy, including those with previous unsuccessful laser or cryoablative procedures. Some studies have shown especially encouraging results for aphakic glaucoma.

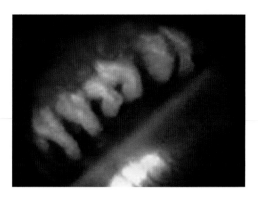

Figure 20-6 Endoscopic view of ciliary processes during endoscopic cyclophotocoagulation. The white structure at bottom right of the photo is the lens. *(Courtesy of Endo Optiks, Little Silver, NJ.)*

Carter BC, Plager DA, Neely DE, Sprunger DT, Sondhi N, Roberts GJ. Endoscopic diode laser cyclophotocoagulation in the management of aphakic and pseudophakic glaucoma in children. *J AAPOS.* 2007;11(1):34–40.

O'Malley Schotthoefer E, Yanovitch TL, Freedman SF. Aqueous drainage device surgery in refractory pediatric glaucomas: I. Long-term outcomes. *J AAPOS.* 2008;12(1):33–39.

Medical Therapy

See also BCSC Section 10, *Glaucoma.*

Topical medications

Topical beta-blocker therapy has been used in children for more than 30 years. It usually lowers IOP 20%–30%. Beta-blockers currently available for use in the United States include timolol maleate (Timoptic, Timoptic XE), betaxolol hydrochloride (Betoptic S), levobunolol (Betagan), timolol hemihydrate (Betimol), metipranolol (OptiPranolol), and carteolol (Ocupress). The major risks of this therapy are respiratory distress caused by apnea or bronchospasm and bradycardia, which occurs mostly in very young infants and in children with a history of bronchospasm. Betaxolol is a cardioselective B1 antagonist with fewer pulmonary and systemic side effects, although its pressure-lowering effect may be less than that of the nonselective agents. Timolol (or its equivalent) or betaxolol is usually used at 0.25% strength twice a day for initial therapy. Nasolacrimal occlusion at the time of drop placement may increase the efficacy of the drug and decrease its systemic side effects.

The *topical carbonic anhydrase inhibitors (CAIs)* dorzolamide 2% (Trusopt) and brinzolamide 1% (Azopt) are available as solutions. Studies using topical CAIs 3 times a day indicate that the drugs can be effective in children, although they produce a smaller reduction in IOP (<15%). There is no increased utility in using a topical CAI in a child already taking an oral CAI.

A *combined beta antagonist-CAI* (Cosopt) combines timolol and dorzolamide in a single eyedrop. It has been used effectively when administered twice daily in children requiring dual therapy for IOP control.

Prostaglandin analogues latanoprost 0.005% (Xalatan) and travoprost 0.004% (Travatan) and a prostamide bimatoprost 0.03% (Lumigan) have shown effectiveness in some pediatric patients. Side effects include increased iris pigmentation and eyelash growth. These medications are not recommended for patients with uveitic glaucoma.

Miotics such as pilocarpine (Pilopine gel and Ocusert) and echothiophate (Phospholine Iodide) are rarely used in children, although Phospholine Iodide may be effective in the treatment of aphakic glaucoma. *Adrenergic agents* such as epinephrine or dipivefrin (Propine) are not usually effective in children. The α_2-adrenergic agonist apraclonidine (Iopidine) may be useful for short-term IOP reduction, but it has a high incidence of tachyphylaxis and allergy in young children. The α_2-adrenergic agonist brimonidine (Alphagan) effectively reduces IOP in some cases of pediatric glaucoma, but this agent can produce profound systemic adverse effects in infants and small children (including lethargy, hypotonia, hypothermia, and serious central nervous system depression) and therefore is contraindicated in children younger than 2 years.

Oral medications

Carbonic anhydrase inhibitors (acetazolamide [Diamox], methazolamide [Neptazane]) may be used effectively in children, particularly to delay the need for surgery. The usefulness of oral CAIs may be limited by systemic adverse effects, including weight loss, lethargy, and metabolic acidosis.

See BCSC Section 10, *Glaucoma,* for a more detailed discussion of agents used in the medical treatment of glaucoma.

Coppens G, Stalmans I, Zeyen T, Casteels I. The safety and efficacy of glaucoma medications in the pediatric population. *J Pediatr Ophthalmol Strabismus.* 2009;46(1):12–18.

Prognosis and Follow-Up

If PCG presents at birth, the prognosis for IOP control and visual preservation is poor, with at least half of these patients becoming legally blind. With a corneal diameter greater than 14 mm at diagnosis, the visual prognosis is similarly poor. Up to 80%–90% of cases in the "favorable prognostic group" (onset 3–12 months) can be controlled with angle surgery. The remaining 10%–20% of these cases, and many of the remaining cases of primary and secondary glaucomas, often present a lifelong challenge.

Vision loss in childhood glaucoma is multifactorial. It may result not only from corneal scarring and opacification or optic nerve damage but also from significant myopic astigmatism and associated anisometropic and strabismic amblyopia, especially in unilateral cases. Myopia results from axial enlargement of the eye in the setting of high IOP; astigmatism may result from unequal expansion of the anterior segment or corneal scarring. Careful treatment of refractive errors and amblyopia is needed to optimize outcomes.

All cases of childhood glaucoma, as well as suspected but unconfirmed glaucoma, require diligent follow-up. After any given surgical intervention or change in medical therapy, control of IOP should be assessed within a few weeks. Examination under sedation or anesthesia is often necessary for accurate assessment. The IOP should be considered not as an isolated finding but rather in conjunction with other measurements obtained from the examination, including refractive error (measured serially), corneal diameter, axial length, and cup–disc ratio. If the IOP is less than 20 mm Hg under anesthesia but clinical evidence shows persistent corneal edema or enlargement, progressive optic nerve cupping, or myopic progression, further intervention should be pursued despite the IOP reading. In contrast, IOP of about 20 mm Hg in a young child who shows evidence of clinical improvement may be followed carefully in the short term without any other intervention.

Long-term follow-up of children with glaucoma is important. Even those patients who do well initially after angle surgery can experience relapse years later, with elevated IOP and subsequent vision loss. Though helpful in following disease progression in older children, visual fields are rarely reliable in children younger than 6–8 years. Optic nerve photographs should be taken whenever possible; these can be helpful for comparison during later examinations.

Walton DS, Katsavounidou G. Newborn primary congenital glaucoma: 2005 update. *J Pediatr Ophthalmol Strabismus.* 2005;42(6):333–341.

Childhood Cataracts and Other Pediatric Lens Disorders

Disorders of the pediatric lens include, in addition to cataract, abnormalities in shape, size, location, and development. Such abnormalities constitute a significant source of visual impairment in children. The incidence is approximately 6:10,000 infants. Pediatric lens abnormalities must be treated promptly to avoid lifelong vision loss. BCSC Section 11, *Lens and Cataract,* also covers conditions and procedures discussed in this chapter.

Pediatric Cataracts

Congenital cataracts are responsible for nearly 10% of all vision loss in children worldwide, and it is estimated that 1 in 250 newborns has some form of cataract. Cataracts in children can be

- isolated or part of a systemic condition
- congenital or acquired
- inherited or sporadic
- unilateral or bilateral
- partial or complete
- stable or progressive

Systemic Implications

Cataracts in children can be isolated or can be associated with many conditions, including chromosomal abnormalities, systemic syndromes and diseases, or congenital infection, as well as external factors such as trauma or radiation. In almost all cases of cataract associated with systemic disease, the cataracts are bilateral (although not all bilateral cataracts are associated with systemic disease). See Table 21-1.

Cataracts can also be associated with other ocular anomalies, including persistent fetal vasculature, coloboma, anterior segment dysgenesis, aniridia, and retinal disorders.

Onset

Pediatric cataracts can be congenital or acquired. Lens opacities that are visually significant prior to the development of the fixation reflex—that is, before 2–3 months of age—have

Table 21-1 Etiology of Pediatric Cataracts

Bilateral cataracts
Idiopathic
Familial (hereditary), usually autosomal dominant
Chromosomal abnormality
   Trisomy-21 (Down), -18 (Edward), -13 (Patau)
   Other translocations, deletions, and duplications
Craniofacial syndromes
   Hallermann-Streiff, Rubenstein-Taybi, Smith-Lemli-Opitz, others
Musculoskeletal
   Conradi, Albright, myotonic dystrophy
Renal
   Lowe, Alport
Metabolic
   Galactosemia, Fabry, Wilson, mannosidosis, diabetes mellitus
Maternal infection (TORCH diseases)
   Rubella
   Cytomegalovirus
   Varicella
   Syphilis
   Toxoplasmosis
Ocular anomalies
   Aniridia
   Anterior segment dysgenesis syndrome
Iatrogenic
   Corticosteroids
   Radiation (may also be unilateral)
Unilateral cataracts
Idiopathic
Ocular anomalies
   Persistent fetal vasculature (PFV)
   Anterior segment dysgenesis
   Traumatic (rule out child abuse)

much more potential impact on the child's visual development than those acquired later. In general, the earlier the onset, the more amblyogenic the cataract will be.

Inheritance

Most hereditary cataracts are autosomal dominant, and they are always bilateral. X-linked and autosomal recessive inheritance may also occur (Table 21-2).

Laterality

Pediatric cataracts can be unilateral or bilateral, although significant asymmetry can be present in bilateral cases.

Morphology

Cataracts can involve the entire lens (total or complete cataract) or can involve only part of the lens structure. The location in the lens and morphology of the cataract provide a great

Table 21-2 Hereditary Factors in Pediatric Cataracts

Type	OMIM Number	Gene/Gene Map
Aculeiform	115700	2q33-q35
Anterior polar 1 (CTAA1)	115650	14q24-qter
Anterior polar 2 (CTAA2)	601202	17p13
Cerulean type I (CCA1)	115660	17q24
Cerulean type II (CCA2)	601547	CRYBB2/22q
Congenital total	302200	Xp
Autosomal dominant		CRYAA/21q22.3
Coppock-like (CCL)		CRYGA/2q33-q35
Marner type (CAM)	116800	16q22.1
Posterior polar (CPP)	116600	1pter-p36.1
Volkmann type	115665	1p36
Dominant, zonular pulverulent (CZP3)	601885	GJA3/13q11-q12
Lamellar, zonular pulverulent (CZP1), Coppock (CAE)	116200	GJA8/1q21.1
Zonular with sutural opacities (CCZS)	600881	17q11-q12

Reproduced with permission from Traboulsi EI, ed. *A Compendium of Inherited Disorders and the Eye.* New York: Oxford University Press; 2005.

Table 21-3 Pediatric Cataracts: Selected Typical Cataract Appearances

Cataract Morphology	Diagnosis	Other Possible Findings
Spokelike	Fabry syndrome	Corneal whorls
	Mannosidosis	Hepatosplenomegaly
Vacuoles	Diabetes	Blood glucose level increased
Multicolor	Hypoparathyroidism	Decreased serum calcium
flecks	Myotonic dystrophy	Characteristic facial features, tonic "grip"
Green "sunflower"	Wilson disease	Kayser-Fleischer corneal ring
Thin disciform	Lowe syndrome	Hypotonia, glaucoma

deal of information about its onset, etiology, laterality, and prognosis (Table 21-3). The clinically most common and important morphologies of partial cataracts are discussed in the following sections.

Anterior polar cataract

Anterior polar cataracts (APCs) are common and usually less than 3 mm in diameter, appearing as small white dots in the center of the anterior lens capsule (Fig 21-1). They are congenital, usually sporadic, and can be bilateral or unilateral. They are usually nonprogressive and not visually significant. However, anisometropia is common, so careful refraction is indicated.

Nuclear cataract

Nuclear cataracts are opacities that involve the center, or nucleus, of the lens. They are typically approximately 3 mm in diameter, but the irregularity of lens fibers can extend peripherally. Density is variable. These opacities tend to be stable but can progress in density and can become slightly larger in size. They can be unilateral or bilateral, inherited or sporadic. They are congenital but may not be significantly dense at birth (Fig 21-2). Eyes

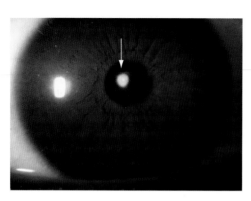

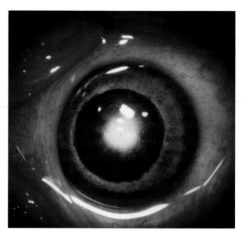

Figure 21-1 Anterior polar cataract *(arrow).* *(Courtesy of Gregg T. Lueder, MD.)*

Figure 21-2 Nuclear cataract. *(Courtesy of Marshal M. Parks, MD.)*

with nuclear cataracts may be smaller than normal and are at increased risk for developing glaucoma later in childhood.

Lamellar cataract

Lamellar, or *zonular,* cataracts are identified by their discrete, round (lenticular) shape and affect 1 or more of the "rings" in the developing lens cortex. The opacities are larger in diameter than nuclear cataracts, being typically 5 mm or more. Lamellar opacities are usually acquired but can be inherited. They can be unilateral or bilateral. These eyes are normal in size and corneal diameter (Fig 21-3).

Because onset is usually after the child's fixation reflex has been established, the visual prognosis following surgery is better than that for cataracts with earlier onset.

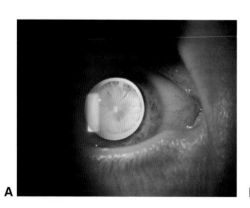

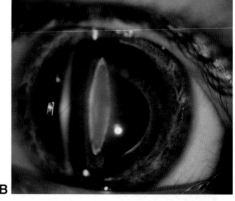

A

B

Figure 21-3 Lamellar cataract. **A,** Retroillumination shows size of the lamellar opacity. **B,** Slit-lamp view shows lamellar opacity surrounding clear nucleus. *(Courtesy of David A. Plager, MD.)*

Posterior lenticonus/lentiglobus

Posterior lenticonus/lentiglobus is caused by thinning of the central posterior capsule. This thinning initially causes an "oil droplet" appearance on red reflex examination. With time, as the outpouching of the lens progresses, the cortical fibers stretch and gradually opacify. This process can take many years, but if the capsule tears, rapid total opacification of the lens can occur (Fig 21-4).

Posterior lenticonus opacities are almost always unilateral, and the affected eye is equal in size to the unaffected eye. These opacities are not typically inherited, and although the weakness in the posterior capsule may be congenital, the cataract usually does not form until later and therefore behaves like an acquired cataract. Visual prognosis after surgery can be favorable.

Posterior subcapsular cataract

Posterior subcapsular cataracts (PSCs) are less common in children than in adults. When present, PSCs are usually acquired and bilateral; they also tend to be progressive. Secondary causes for the cataracts include steroids, uveitis, retinal abnormalities, and radiation exposure. PSCs can be seen with neurofibromatosis type 2 and may be the first observable manifestation of this disorder.

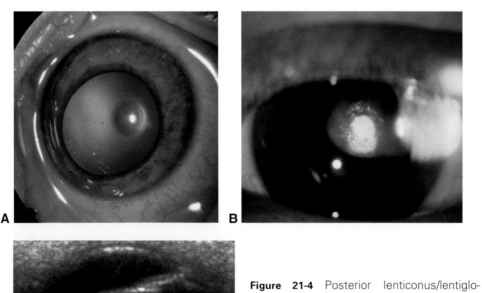

A

B

C

Figure 21-4 Posterior lenticonus/lentiglobus. **A,** Early central clear defect in posterior capsule and **(B)** early opacification of central defect. **C,** Ultrasound biomicroscopy of advanced posterior lenticonus. *(Part A courtesy of Edward L. Raab, MD; part B, David A. Plager, MD; part C, Ken K. Nischal, FRCOphth.)*

See Table 21-4 for a summary of characteristics of select cataract morphologies.

Miscellaneous

Some other, less common cataract morphologies are illustrated in Figure 21-5.

Persistent Fetal Vasculature

Persistent fetal vasculature (PFV) results from failure of the fetal hyaloid vascular complex to regress and is a common cause of cataract in infancy. Historically, this entity has been referred to as *persistent hyperplastic primary vitreous (PHPV)*, but in recent years the more anatomically accurate term *persistent fetal vasculature* has been preferred. Clinically, there is a retrolental membrane of varying size and density attached to the posterior lens surface. The membrane can be small and centrally located or may extend out to attach to the ciliary processes for 360° (Fig 21-6).

Like nuclear cataracts, PFV is congenital; these eyes are nearly always microphthalmic (microcornea) to some degree (if a PFV eye is not smaller than the fellow, normal eye, be suspicious of elevated IOP and secondary enlargement of the eye). PFV is almost always unilateral. The persistent hyaloid vessel may connect the retrolental membrane to the optic nerve, but often the vessel regresses, leaving only the membrane. In severe cases, the lens may be pushed forward, flattening the anterior chamber and causing secondary glaucoma. The glaucoma can occur acutely because of rapid total opacification and swelling of the lens that develop over a few days, or it may develop gradually over years. PFV may be associated with retinal abnormalities, which may adversely affect the visual prognosis. See also Chapter 23.

Evaluation

All newborns should have screening eye examinations, including an evaluation of the red reflexes. The red reflex test is best performed in a darkened room and involves shining a bright direct ophthalmoscope into both eyes simultaneously from a distance of 1–2 ft. This test can be used for routine ocular screening by nurses, pediatricians, and family

Table 21-4 Characteristics of Specific Pediatric Cataract Morphologies

	Congenital or Acquired	Inherited or Sporadic	Unilateral or Bilateral	Stable or Progressive	Microphthalmic
Anterior polar	Congenital	Sporadic	Either	Stable	No
Nuclear	Congenital	Either	Either	Stable	Some
Lamellar	Acquired	Either	Bilateral	Either	No
Posterior lenticonus	Acquired	Sporadic	Unilateral	Progressive	No
PFV	Congenital	Sporadic	Unilateral	Stable	Yes
PSC	Acquired	Sporadic	Bilateral	Progressive	No

PFV = persistent fetal vasculature; PSC = posterior subcapsular.

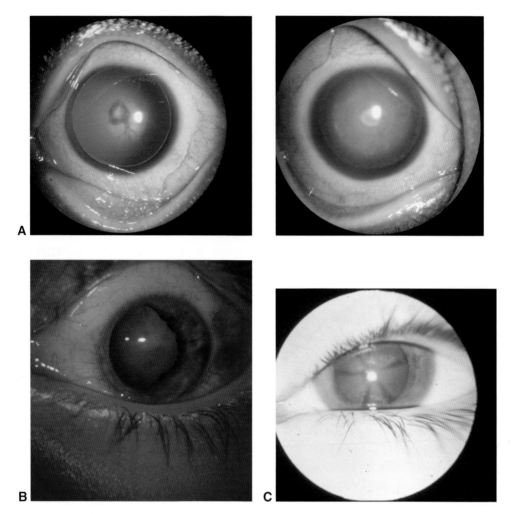

Figure 21-5 Miscellaneous cataracts in childhood. **A,** Aniridia, mild *(left)* and advanced *(right)*. **B,** Traumatic. **C,** Starfish cataract. *(Courtesy of David A. Plager, MD.)*

practitioners. Retinoscopy through the child's undilated pupil is helpful for assessing the potential visual significance of an axial lens opacity in a preverbal child. Any central opacity or surrounding cortical distortion greater than 3 mm can be assumed to be visually significant.

History

In addition to a family history, a detailed history of the child's growth, development, and systemic disorders should be elicited. A slit-lamp examination of immediate family members can reveal previously undiagnosed lens opacities that are visually insignificant, but that may indicate an inherited cause for the child's cataracts.

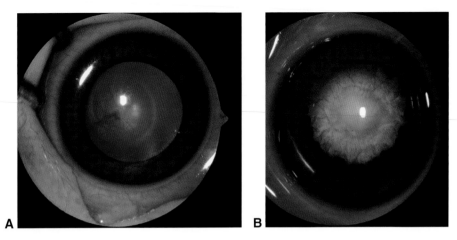

Figure 21-6 Persistent fetal vasculature (PFV; formerly, *persistent hyperplastic primary vitreous*). **A,** Mild variant with central retrolental membrane. **B,** Severe PFV variant with traction on ciliary processes. *(Courtesy of David A. Plager, MD.)*

Visual Function

The mere presence of a cataract does not imply that surgery to remove it is indicated. That determination requires assessment of the visual significance of the lens opacity.

In infants younger than 2 months, a normal fixation reflex is not developed, and therefore its absence in an infant with a cataract is not necessarily abnormal. In general, anterior capsule opacities are not visually significant unless they occlude the entire pupil, blocking out the red reflex. Central or posterior lens opacities of sufficient density that are greater than 3 mm in diameter are usually visually significant. Opacities that have a significant area of surrounding normal red reflex and opacities that have clear areas within them may allow for good visual development in infancy. Strabismus in unilateral cataract and nystagmus in bilateral cataracts indicate that the opacities are visually significant. Although these signs may also indicate that the optimal time for treatment is past, surgery may still result in significant improvement.

In preverbal children older than 2 months, standard clinical assessment of fixation behavior, fixation preference, and objection to occlusion provide additional evidence of the visual significance of the cataract(s). For bilateral cataracts, an assessment of the child's visual behavior, along with the family's observations of the child at home, helps determine the level of visual function. Special tests such as preferential looking cards and visually evoked potentials can provide additional quantitative information.

Ocular Examination

A slit-lamp examination can help to classify the morphology of the cataract and to examine any associated abnormalities of the cornea, iris, lens, and anterior chamber. A portable handheld slit lamp is very helpful for examining infants and young children.

If the cataract allows some view of the posterior segment, careful examination of the optic nerve head, retina, and fovea should be performed. If no view is present, B-scan ultrasonography can help assess the posterior segment; however, the presence of retinal or optic nerve abnormalities cannot be definitively ruled out until the optic nerve head, retina, and fovea are examined directly.

Workup

Unilateral cataracts are not usually associated with occult systemic or metabolic disease, and laboratory tests are not warranted. In contrast, bilateral cataracts may be associated with many systemic and metabolic diseases (Fig 21-7). If a positive family history

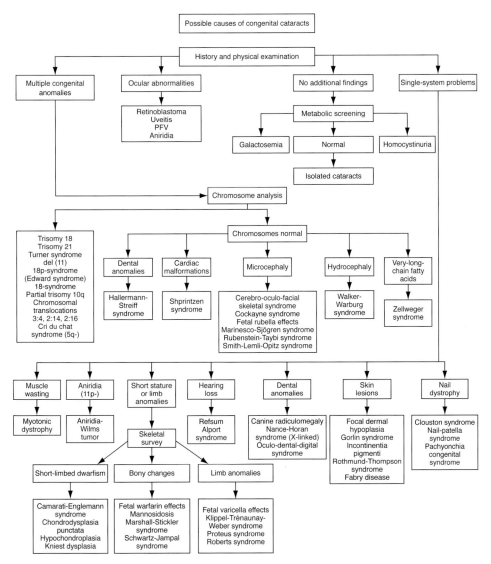

Figure 21-7   Causes of congenital cataracts. *PFV* = persistent fetal vasculature. *(Adapted from Buckley EG. Pediatric cataracts. In: Parrish R, ed.* Bascom Palmer Eye Institute's Atlas of Ophthalmology. *Philadelphia: Current Medicine; 2000.)*

Table 21-5 Evaluation of Pediatric Cataracts

Family history (autosomal dominant or X-linked)
Pediatric physical examination
Ocular examination including
  Corneal diameter
  Iris configuration
  Anterior chamber depth
  Lens position
  Cataract morphology
  Posterior segment
    Rule out posterior mass.
    Rule out retinal detachment.
    Rule out optic nerve stalk to lens.
  Intraocular pressure
Laboratory studies
  Bilateral cataracts
    Disorders of galactose metabolism: urine for reducing substance; galactose 1-phosphate
      uridyltransferase; galactokinase
    Infectious diseases: TORCH and varicella titers, VDRL
    Metabolic diseases: urine for amino acids; serum calcium, phosphorus, and glucose; serum
      ferritin

of isolated infantile or childhood cataracts can be elicited or examination of the parents' lenses shows congenital lens opacities (and there are no associated systemic diseases to explain their cataracts), a systemic and laboratory evaluation is not necessary. A basic laboratory evaluation for bilateral cataracts of unknown etiology in apparently healthy children is outlined in Table 21-5.

Any further workup should be directed by other systemic abnormalities. Evaluation by a geneticist may be helpful for determining whether there are associated disorders and for counseling the patient's family regarding recurrence risks.

Surgery

Once a decision has been made to remove the cataract(s), the next issues to be resolved are when to perform surgery and whether to implant an intraocular lens (IOL). In general, the younger the child, the greater the urgency in removing the cataract, because of the risk of amblyopia. For optimal visual development in newborns and young infants, a visually significant unilateral congenital cataract should be detected and removed before age 6 weeks, and visually significant bilateral congenital cataracts should be removed before age 10 weeks.

Birch EE, Stager DR. The critical period for surgical treatment of dense congenital unilateral cataract. *Invest Ophthalmol Vis Sci.* 1996;37(8):1532–1538.

Lambert SR, Lynn MJ, Reeves R, Plager DA, Buckley EG, Wilson ME. Is there a latent period for the surgical treatment of children with dense bilateral congenital cataracts? *J AAPOS.* 2006;10(1):30–36.

In older children with bilateral cataracts, surgery should be suggested when the level of visual function interferes with the child's visual needs. Although children with vision in the 20/70 range may function relatively well in early grade school, they are still at risk for amblyopia, and surgery should be considered if the vision decreases to 20/40 or less. During the teenaged years, cataract surgery may be indicated to meet the visual requirements for obtaining a driver's license. For unilateral cataracts in older children, cataract surgery is suggested for vision that cannot be improved past the 20/40 range with optical treatment and amblyopia therapy. In older children, glare testing may also be useful to assess decreased vision, particularly in patients with lamellar or posterior subscapsular cataracts.

The choice of optical device for correction of aphakia depends primarily on the age of the patient and the laterality of the cataracts. For children aged 1–2 years and older, IOL implantation has gained widespread acceptance, and numerous studies have documented the safety and efficacy of this procedure. In infants, the use of IOLs is controversial because of a higher incidence of complications and the rapid shift in refractive error during the first 1–2 years of life. A multicenter randomized controlled clinical trial, the Infant Aphakia Treatment Study, is currently under way to assess IOL implantation in infants.

Wilson ME, Trivedi RH. Multicenter randomized controlled clinical trial in pediatric cataract surgery: efficacy and effectiveness. *Am J Ophthalmol.* 2007;144(4):616–617.

Management of the Anterior Capsule

To allow access to the lens nucleus and cortex during cataract surgery, a *capsulorrhexis* is performed. The tearing characteristics of the pediatric capsule are significantly different from those of the adult capsule; thus, modifications of techniques for lens removal used in adults are usually necessary to minimize the risk of inadvertent extension of the tear. The toughness and elasticity of the capsule are greatest in younger patients, especially infants. Continuous curvilinear capsulorrhexis, which is the creation of a continuous circular tear in the anterior capsule, is more difficult in infants. The pulling force should be directed closer to 90° from the direction of intended tear, and the capsule should be regrasped frequently to maintain optimal control over the direction of tear. The use of a 2-incision push-pull technique may be helpful (Fig 21-8). An alternative to capsulorrhexis in infants is vitrectorhexis, the creation of an anterior capsule opening using a vitrectomy instrument. In children with opaque capsules, visibility can be enhanced by the application of trypan blue ophthalmic solution 0.06% (Vision Blue, Dutch Ophthalmic, USA, Kingston, NH).

Hamada S, Low S, Walters BC, Nischal KK. Five-year experience of the 2-incision push-pull technique for anterior and posterior capsulorrhexis in pediatric cataract surgery. *Ophthalmology.* 2006;113(8):1309–1314.

Wilson ME Jr, Trivedi RH, Bartholomew LR, Pershing S. Comparison of anterior vitrectorhexis and continuous curvilinear capsulorhexis in pediatric cataract and intraocular lens implantation surgery: a 10-year analysis. *J AAPOS.* 2007;11(5):443–446.

Lensectomy Without Intraocular Lens Implantation

In children who will be left aphakic, lensectomy is performed through a small limbal or pars plana incision with a vitreous-cutting instrument. Irrigation can be provided by an

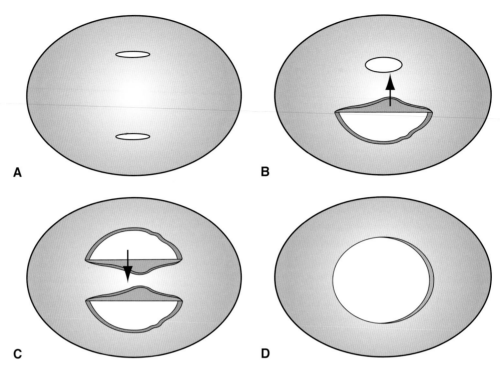

Figure 21-8 In young children, the capsule is very elastic, and the 2-incision push-pull rhexis technique can be achieved by creating 2 small linear incisions in the superior and inferior lens capsule **(A)** and grasping the center of the flap of the superior incision **(B)**; pushing to the center of the pupil will result in a semicircular tear **(B)**. This is extended to halfway between the 2 initial stab incisions **(B)**. **C,** The flap of the inferior stab incision is then grasped and pulled to the center of the pupil, forming another semicircular tear. **D,** The semicircular tears are joined to form a complete, continuous curvilinear capsulorrhexis. *(Redrawn with permission from Hamada S, Low S, Walters BC, Nischal KK. Five-year experience of the 2-incision push-pull technique for anterior and posterior capsulorrhexis in pediatric cataract surgery. Ophthalmology. 2006;113(8):1309–1314.)*

integrated infusion sleeve or by a separate cannula. Lens cortex and nucleus are generally soft in children of all ages; ultrasonic phacoemulsification is not required (Fig 21-9A). It is important to remove all cortical material because of the propensity of pediatric lens epithelial cells to reproliferate. Tough, fibrotic plaques, such as those encountered in some severe PFV cases, may require manual excision of the plaques with intraocular scissors and forceps. A large, round anterior capsulectomy is performed either before or after complete cortical removal.

Because posterior capsule opacification occurs rapidly in young children, a controlled posterior capsulectomy and anterior vitrectomy should be performed at the time of surgery, particularly in infants (Fig 21-9B). This technique allows for rapid, permanent establishment of a clear visual axis for retinoscopy and prompt fitting and monitoring of aphakic optical correction. Sufficient peripheral capsular remnants should be left, if possible, to facilitate secondary posterior chamber IOL implantation at a later date.

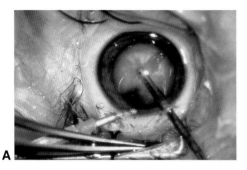 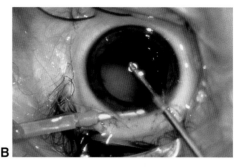

Figure 21-9 **A,** After anterior capsulotomy or vitrectorhexis, both the nucleus and the surrounding cortex are aspirated. Complete cortical removal is important because remaining pediatric lens fibers will quickly reproliferate, causing opacification and adhesions. **B,** After lens removal, a posterior capsulectomy and limited anterior vitrectomy are necessary to minimize the development of recurrent pupillary membranes, iris capsular adhesions, and posterior membranes. A rim of capsule should be left to support possible secondary intraocular lens implant in the future. *(Courtesy of Edward G. Buckley, MD.)*

Lensectomy With Intraocular Lens Implantation

If an IOL is going to be placed at the time of cataract extraction, 2 basic techniques can be used for the lensectomy, depending on whether the posterior capsule will be left intact. Many pediatric cataract surgeons leave the posterior capsule intact if the child is approaching the age when a Nd:YAG capsulotomy could be performed without anesthesia (usually 5–6 years of age and older). Studies have shown that pediatric capsules in the postinfant years will opacify in 18–24 months after surgery on average, although considerable variation can occur.

Technique with posterior capsule intact

In children older than 5–6 years, the technique leaving the posterior capsule intact is similar to that described earlier for a lensectomy (see the section Lensectomy Without Intraocular Lens Implantation).

After the cortex is aspirated, the clear corneal or scleral tunnel incision is enlarged to allow placement of the IOL. Single-piece acrylic foldable lenses, which can be placed through a 3-mm incision, have become popular among pediatric cataract surgeons, although some prefer to use larger single-piece polymethylmethacrylate (PMMA) lenses. Placement of the IOL in the capsular bag is desirous, but sulcus fixation is an acceptable alternative. The surgeon should remove all viscoelastic material to prevent postoperative IOP spikes, especially because it can be difficult to measure IOP in the early postoperative period in young children. Closure of 3-mm clear cornea incisions with 10-0 absorbable suture has been shown to be safe and astigmatically neutral in children.

Bradfield YS, Plager DA, Neely DE, Sprunger DT, Sondhi N. Astigmatism after small-incision clear corneal cataract extraction and intraocular lens implantation in children. *J Cataract Refract Surg.* 2004;30(9):1948–1952.

Technique for primary posterior capsulectomy

In children younger than 3–4 years or in older children who are unlikely to cooperate for a Nd:YAG capsulotomy while awake, a primary posterior capsulectomy with vitrectomy should generally be performed at the time of cataract/IOL surgery. The posterior capsulectomy/vitrectomy can be performed either before or after IOL placement.

Posterior capsulectomy/vitrectomy before IOL placement   After lensectomy, the vitrector settings should be set to the low-suction, high-cutting rate appropriate for vitreous surgery, and a posterior capsulectomy or posterior capsulorrhexis with anterior vitrectomy is performed. The anterior incision is enlarged to an appropriate size for the IOL, and the lens is implanted in the capsular bag, if possible, or in the ciliary sulcus, as an alternative. The surgeon must take care to ensure that the capsulotomy does not extend, the IOL does not go through the posterior opening, and vitreous does not become incorporated with the IOL or anterior chamber.

Posterior capsulectomy/vitrectomy after IOL placement   Some pediatric cataract surgeons prefer to place the IOL in the capsular bag, close the anterior incision, and approach the posterior capsule through the pars plana. Irrigation can be maintained through the same anterior infusion cannula used during lensectomy. A small conjunctival opening is made over the pars plana, and a sclerotomy is made with an MVR blade 2.5–3.0 mm posterior to the limbus. This provides good access to the posterior capsule, and a wide anterior vitrectomy can be performed.

> Wilson ME, Trivedi RH, Pandey SK. *Pediatric Cataract Surgery: Techniques, Complications, and Management.* Philadelphia: Lippincott Williams & Wilkins; 2005.

Intraocular Lens Implantation

Because the child's eye continues to elongate throughout the first decade of life and beyond, the selection of an appropriate IOL power is complicated. Power calculations in infants and young children may be unpredictable due to several factors, including widely variable growth of the eye, difficulty obtaining accurate keratometry and axial eye length measurements, and the use of power formulas that were developed for adults rather than children. Studies have shown that the refractive error of aphakic children undergoes a variable myopic shift of approximately 7–8 D from age 1 to age 10, with a wide standard deviation. This would suggest that if a child is made emmetropic at age 1 with an IOL, refraction at age 10 would be expected to be up to –8 D or greater (refractive change below age 1 year is even more unpredictable). This approach assumes that presence of an IOL does not alter this normal aphakic growth curve, an assumption that may not be valid based on both animal and early human studies.

Lens implantation in children requires a compromise that accounts for the age of the child and the target refraction at the time of surgery. There are 2 approaches to this situation. Some surgeons implant IOLs with powers that are expected to be required in adulthood, allowing the child to grow into the power selection of the lens. Thus, the child is undercorrected and requires hyperopic spectacles of decreasing powers until the teenaged years. Other surgeons aim for emmetropia at the time of lens implantation, especially in unilateral cases, believing that this approach may decrease the risk of amblyopia and facilitate development of binocular function by decreasing anisometropia. These children can be expected to become progressively more myopic with time and eventually may require a secondary procedure in order to eliminate the increasing anisometropia.

Eibschitz-Tsimhoni M, Archer SM, Del Monte MA. Intraocular lens power calculation in children. *Surv Ophthalmol.* 2007;52(5):474–482.

Neely DE, Plager DA, Borger SM, Golub RL. Accuracy of intraocular lens calculations in infants and children undergoing cataract surgery. *J AAPOS.* 2005;9(2):160–165.

Intraocular lens material

Both single-piece PMMA and foldable acrylic lenses have been widely used in pediatric cataract surgery in recent years. Many studies have shown them to be well tolerated. Silicone lenses have not been well studied in children.

Postoperative Care

Medical therapy

If all cortical material is adequately removed, postoperative inflammation in children without a lens implant is usually mild. Postoperative topical antibiotics, steroids, and cycloplegics are commonly used for a few weeks. Topical steroids need to be used much more aggressively in children if an IOL is placed. Some surgeons prescribe oral steroids, especially in very young children and children with heavily pigmented irides.

Amblyopia management

Amblyopia therapy should begin as soon as possible after surgery. For patients who become aphakic, corrective lenses—in general, contact lenses for unilateral or bilateral aphakia, spectacles for bilateral aphakia—can be dispensed within 1 week of surgery.

For infants with bilateral aphakia, spectacles are the safest and simplest method of correction available. They can be easily changed to accommodate the refractive shifts that occur with growth. Until the child can use a bifocal lens, the power selected should make the child myopic, because most of an infant's visual activity occurs at near.

For infants with monocular aphakia, contact lenses are the most popular method of correction, and they may also be used in bilateral patients. Some advantages of contact lenses are that power changes are relatively easy, and some lenses can be worn for extended periods. The disadvantages of contact lenses include easy displacement by eye rubbing, the expense of replacement, and the risk of corneal ulceration. Aphakic spectacles are occasionally used in infants with monocular cataracts who are unable to tolerate contact lenses, but these spectacles are suboptimal owing to the amblyogenic effect induced by the highly asymmetric lenses. Secondary IOL implantation for aphakic infants can be performed at a later age.

Patching of the better eye is frequently indicated in cases of unilateral cataracts or asymmetric bilateral cataracts. The amount of patching should be titrated to the degree of amblyopia and the age of the child. Part-time occlusion in the neonatal period may allow stimulation of binocular vision and may help prevent associated strabismus.

Complications

Complications after lens extraction are different in children than in adults. Retinal detachments, macular edema, and corneal abnormalities are rare in children. The incidence of postoperative infections and bleeding is similar in adults and in children. The risk of glaucoma is increased in children who have surgery in infancy, and glaucoma often develops many years after lens extraction. See Chapter 20 for a discussion of aphakic and pseudophakic glaucoma.

Visual Outcome After Cataract Extraction

Good visual outcome after cataract surgery depends on many factors, including age of onset and type of cataract, the timing of surgery, optical correction, and treatment of amblyopia. For dense unilateral congenital cataracts, visual acuity is best in patients who undergo surgery before 6 weeks of age and who adhere to amblyopia treatment. Early surgery by itself does not ensure a good outcome. Optimal visual acuity requires careful postoperative management to treat amblyopia. Conversely, even when congenital cataracts are detected late (after age 4 months), cataract removal combined with a strong postoperative vision rehabilitation program can achieve good vision in some eyes.

Structural or Positional Lens Abnormalities

Congenital Aphakia

Congenital aphakia, the absence of the lens at birth, is rare. This condition is usually associated with a markedly abnormal eye.

Spherophakia

A lens that is spherical and smaller than a normal lens is called *spherophakic*. This condition is usually bilateral. The lens may dislocate, causing secondary glaucoma (Fig 21-10).

Coloboma

A lens coloboma (a misnomer) involves flattening or notching of the lens periphery (Fig 21-11). A lens coloboma can be associated with a coloboma of the iris, optic nerve, or

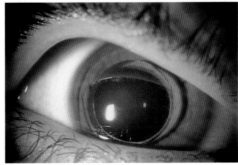

Figure 21-10 Spherophakia with lens dislocation into anterior chamber, left eye.

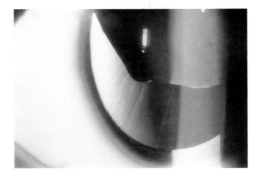

Figure 21-11 Lens equator flattening (with dislocation), which may be referred to as *lens coloboma.*

retina, which is caused by the abnormal closure of the embryonic fissure. Lens colobomas are usually located inferonasally. Zonular fibers are typically absent in the colobomatous area, resulting in a flattening of the lens at that location without any dislocation. In more significant colobomatous defects, lens dislocations may occur superiorly and temporally. Most colobomatous lenses do not worsen progressively.

Dislocated Lenses in Children

When the lens is not in its normal anatomical position, it is said to be *dislocated, subluxed, subluxated, luxed, luxated,* or *ectopic.* Luxed or luxated lenses are completely detached from the ciliary body and can be loose in the posterior chamber or vitreous (Fig 21-12) or can prolapse to the anterior chamber. The amount of dislocation can vary from only slight displacement with minimal *iridodonesis* (tremulousness of the iris) to severe displacement, with the periphery of the lens totally out of the pupillary margin. Lens dislocation can be familial or sporadic or be associated with multisystem disease or an inborn error of metabolism (Table 21-6). Lens dislocation can occur with trauma, although this is not common and usually involves a significant injury to the eye. Spontaneous lens dislocation has been reported rarely both in aniridia and in buphthalmos associated with congenital glaucoma.

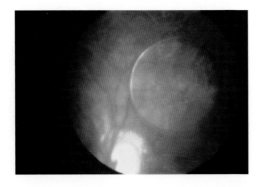

Figure 21-12 Lens dislocation into vitreous.

Table 21-6 Subluxated Lenses

Systemic conditions	Ocular conditions
Marfan syndrome	Aniridia
Homocystinuria	Iris coloboma
Weill-Marchesani syndrome	Trauma
Sulfite oxidase deficiency	Hereditary ectopia lentis
Syphilis	Congenital glaucoma
Ehlers-Danlos syndrome	

Simple Ectopia Lentis

Simple ectopia lentis is usually bilateral and symmetric, with upward and temporal lens displacement. Autosomal dominant inheritance is most common. The onset may be congenital or occur later. Glaucoma is common in the late-onset type.

Ectopia Lentis et Pupillae

Ectopia lentis et pupillae is a rare autosomal recessive condition. It consists of bilateral displacement of the pupil, usually inferotemporally, with lens dislocation in the opposite direction (Fig 21-13A). Affected patients have microspherophakia, miosis, and poor pupillary dilation with mydriatics. Ectopia lentis et pupillae may be the result of membranes extending from a posterior origin to attach to the proximal pupil margin (Fig 21-13B). These membranes cause traction of the iris toward the membranes (resulting in the iris abnormality) and disruption of the zonules (resulting in lens subluxation in the opposite direction). Some family members may have only subluxation without the pupillary displacement. The condition is nonprogressive.

Byles DB, Nischal KK, Cheng H. Ectopia lentis et pupillae. A hypothesis revisited. *Ophthalmology.* 1998;105(7):1331–1336.

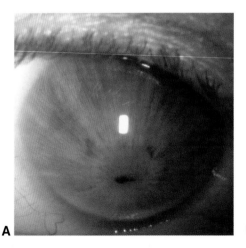 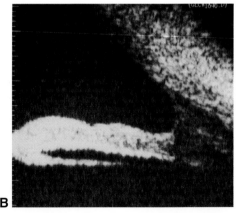

A   B

Figure 21-13 **A,** Ectopia lentis et pupillae. **B,** 50-MHz ultrasonographic scan showing membrane posterior to iris attaching at pupil margin. *(Reproduced with permission from Byles DB, Nischal KK, Cheng H. Ectopia lentis et pupillae. A hypothesis revisited. Ophthalmology. 1998;105(7):1331–1336.)*

Marfan Syndrome

Marfan syndrome is the systemic disease most commonly associated with dislocated lenses. The syndrome consists of abnormalities of the cardiovascular, musculoskeletal, and ocular systems. It is inherited as an autosomal dominant trait, but family history is negative in 15% of cases. Marfan syndrome is caused by mutations in the fibrillin gene on chromosome 15, which is the major constituent of extracellular microfibrils. Affected patients are characteristically tall, with long limbs and fingers *(arachnodactyly);* loose, flexible joints; scoliosis; and chest deformities. Cardiovascular abnormalities are a source of significant mortality and manifest as enlargement of the aortic root, dilation of the descending aorta, dissecting aneurysm, and floppy mitral valve. The life expectancy of patients with Marfan syndrome is about half that of the normal population.

Ocular abnormalities occur in over 80% of affected patients, with lens dislocation being the most common. In approximately 75% of cases, the lens is upwardly dislocated. Typically, the zonules that are visible are intact and unbroken, in contradistinction to the broken zonules seen in homocystinuria. Examination of the iris usually shows iridodonesis and may reveal transillumination defects that are more marked near the iris base. The pupil is small and dilates poorly. The corneal curvature is often decreased. The axial length is increased, and the patients are usually myopic. Retinal detachment can occur spontaneously, commonly in the second and third decades of life.

Homocystinuria

Homocystinuria is a rare autosomal recessive condition that occurs in approximately 1 in 100,000 births. The classic form is caused by an abnormality in the enzyme cystathionine β-synthase, although it can be caused by other enzyme defects. This abnormality causes homocystine to accumulate in the plasma and be excreted in the urine.

The clinical manifestations of homocystinuria vary markedly, affecting the eye, skeletal system, central nervous system, and vascular system. Most of the abnormalities develop after birth and become progressively worse with age. The skeletal features are similar to those of Marfan syndrome. Affected patients are usually tall, with osteoporosis, scoliosis, and chest deformities. Central nervous system abnormalities occur in approximately 50% of patients, with mental retardation and seizures being the most common.

Vascular complications are common and secondary to thrombotic disease, which affects large or medium-sized arteries and veins anywhere in the body. Partial or complete vascular obstruction is present in various organs, and hypertension, cardiac murmurs, and cardiomegaly are common. Anesthesia carries a higher risk for patients with homocystinuria because of thromboembolic phenomena, and therefore this disorder should be identified before patients undergo general anesthesia.

The main ocular finding is lens dislocation (frequently downward, although the direction of subluxation is not invariable or diagnostic), which typically occurs between the ages of 3 and 10 years. The lenses may dislocate into the anterior chamber, a finding suggestive of homocystinuria (Fig 21-14).

Diagnosis is confirmed by the detection of disulfides, including homocystine, in the urine. The medical management of homocystinuria is directed toward normalizing the biochemical abnormality. Dietary management (low methionine and high cystine) has

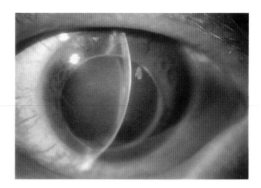

Figure 21-14 Homocystinuria. The lens may dislocate into the anterior chamber with acute pupillary block glaucoma.

been attempted, and coenzyme supplements (pyridoxine or vitamin B_6) decrease systemic problems in about 50% of cases.

Weill-Marchesani Syndrome

Patients with Weill-Marchesani syndrome can be thought of as clinical opposites of patients with Marfan syndrome in that the former are characteristically short, with short fingers and limbs, while the latter are characteristically tall and may display arachnodactyly. Inheritance can be autosomal dominant or recessive. The lenses are also small and nearly round *(microspherophakia)*. With time, the lens dislocates anteriorly and pupillary block glaucoma may occur. Because of this, prophylactic laser peripheral iridectomy has been recommended, although lensectomy may be required.

Sulfite Oxidase Deficiency

Sulfite oxidase deficiency (molybdenum cofactor deficiency) is a very rare hereditary disorder of sulfur metabolism manifested by severe neurologic disorders and ectopia lentis. The enzyme deficiency interferes with conversion of sulfite to sulfate, resulting in increased urine excretion of sulfite. The diagnosis can be confirmed by the absence of sulfite oxidase activity in skin fibroblasts. Neurologic abnormalities include infantile hemiplegia, choreoathetosis, and seizures. Irreversible brain damage and death usually occur by age 5.

Treatment

Optical correction

Optical correction of the refractive error caused by lens dislocation is often difficult. With mild subluxation, the patient may be only myopic and corrected visual function may be good. More severe amounts of dislocation cause optical distortion because the patient is looking through the far peripheral part of the lens. Because the resultant myopic astigmatism is difficult to measure accurately by retinoscopy or automated refractometry, visual acuity using an aphakic correction may be superior. Predilation and postdilation refractions are often helpful in deciding on the best choice. If satisfactory visual function cannot be obtained or if visual function worsens, lens removal should be considered.

Surgery

Subluxated lenses can be removed either from the anterior segment through a limbal incision or through the pars plana. In most circumstances, complete lensectomy is indicated. Postoperative vision rehabilitation can be achieved with the use of contact lenses or glasses, and postoperative visual results are quite good. The use of sutured IOLs is not recommended because of the high rate of suture breakage. Caution should be exercised in patients with Marfan syndrome because there is an increased risk of retinal detachment, which may occur years after surgery.

Buckley EG. Safety of transscleral-sutured intraocular lenses in children. *J AAPOS.* 2008;12(5): 431–439.

CHAPTER 22

Uveitis in the Pediatric Age Group

Pediatric uveitis is relatively uncommon, occurring in only 5% of all cases of uveitis seen in tertiary care centers. However, when this condition does occur in the pediatric age group, the diagnosis and treatment of these patients present many challenges. Children may not verbalize symptoms until the disease is advanced, and therapeutic options may be limited by the potential side effects of medications. This chapter discusses the features of uveitis occurring in children. See BCSC Section 9, *Intraocular Inflammation and Uveitis,* for a more detailed description of the clinical features and mechanisms of inflammation of the conditions mentioned here.

Classification

As in adults, uveitis in children can be classified by several methods, including anatomical location (anterior, intermediate, posterior, panuveitis); pathology (granulomatous, non-granulomatous); course (acute, chronic, recurrent); or etiology (traumatic, immunologic, infectious, masquerade syndromes, idiopathic; exogenous or endogenous). Anatomical location can be helpful in determining etiology (Table 22-1). Traditionally, posterior uveitis has been thought to account for 40%–50% of uveitis cases in children; anterior uveitis, 30%–40%; intermediate uveitis, approximately 20%; and panuveitis, less than 10%. These percentages are based on studies published by tertiary care centers. In contrast, recent population-based studies suggest that the majority of children with uveitis have disease that is restricted to the anterior segment. Nevertheless, posterior uveitis probably accounts for a greater proportion of uveitis cases in children than it does in adults.

Anterior Uveitis

Juvenile Idiopathic Arthritis

Nomenclature
Ophthalmologists may be confused by the different terminology used for chronic childhood arthritis. In Europe, the disease is referred to as *juvenile chronic arthritis,* and the criteria of the European League of Associations of Rheumatology (EULAR) are used. In the United States, the criteria of the American College of Rheumatology (ACR) are employed, and the disease is referred to as *juvenile rheumatoid arthritis.* The primary differences between the EULAR and ACR criteria are the duration of joint symptoms necessary for the

Table 22-1 Differential Diagnosis of Uveitis

Anterior uveitis
Juvenile idiopathic arthritis
Trauma
Sarcoidosis
Herpes and other viruses
Syphilis
Lyme disease
Fuchs heterochromic iridocyclitis
Kawasaki syndrome
Tubulointerstitial nephritis and uveitis syndrome
Behçet syndrome
Orbital pseudotumor
Idiopathic
Intermediate uveitis
Pars planitis
Sarcoidosis
Tuberculosis
Juvenile xanthogranuloma
Lyme disease
Idiopathic
Posterior uveitis and panuveitis
Toxoplasmosis
Toxocariasis
Herpes, rubella, rubeola, measles
Histoplasmosis
Syphilis
Sympathetic ophthalmia
Sarcoidosis
Bartonella
Candida albicans
Lyme disease
Familial juvenile systemic granulomatosis (Blau syndrome)
Diffuse unilateral subacute neuroretinitis (DUSN)
Tuberculosis
Vogt-Koyanagi-Harada syndrome
Behçet syndrome
Idiopathic

diagnosis of arthritis and inclusion versus exclusion of certain disease conditions, such as juvenile ankylosing spondylitis and juvenile psoriatic arthritis.

Recently, a set of criteria was published by the International League of Associations of Rheumatology (ILAR), which includes all idiopathic childhood arthritides under the name *juvenile idiopathic arthritis (JIA)*. We have chosen to use the term *JIA* in this chapter. The 3 sets of criteria for childhood chronic arthritis are shown in Table 22-2, and the subtypes of JIA are listed in Table 22-3.

Occurrence of uveitis in JIA

Juvenile idiopathic arthritis is the most common identifiable etiology of childhood anterior uveitis. The categories of JIA (see Table 22-3) that are particularly important for uveitis

Table 22-2 **Comparison of the European League of Associations of Rheumatology (EULAR), American College of Rheumatology (ACR), and International League of Associations of Rheumatology (ILAR) Criteria for Diagnosis of JIA**

	EULAR	ACR	ILAR
Age of patients (years)	0–15	0–15	0–15
Disease duration	3 months	6 weeks	6 weeks
JAS, JpsA, IBD	Included	Excluded	Included

JIA = juvenile idiopathic arthritis; JAS = juvenile ankylosing spondylitis; JpsA = juvenile psoriatic arthritis; IBD = arthropathy associated with inflammatory bowel disease.

Modified with permission from Kotaniemi K, Savolainen A, Karma A, Aho K. Recent advances in uveitis of juvenile idiopathic arthritis. *Surv Ophthalmol.* 2003;48(5):489–502.

Table 22-3 **Subtypes of Juvenile Idiopathic Arthritis**

Disease Type
I Systemic arthritis
II Oligoarthritis
a. persistent
b. extended
III Polyarthritis, rheumatoid factor (RF)-negative
IV Polyarthritis, rheumatoid factor (RF)-positive
V Psoriatic arthritis
VI Enthesitis-related arthritis
VII Other forms of arthritis

Used with permission from Kotaniemi K, Savolainen A, Karma A, Aho K. Recent advances in uveitis of juvenile idiopathic arthritis. *Surv Ophthalmol.* 2003;48(5):489–502.

are oligoarthritis, rheumatoid factor (RF)-negative polyarthritis, psoriatic arthritis, and enthesitis-related arthritis. Uveitis almost never occurs in children with systemic arthritis and is very rare in those with RF-positive polyarthritis.

Oligoarthritis is the most frequent type of chronic arthritis in children in North America and Europe. Oligoarthritis occurs predominantly in young girls and is defined as a persistent arthritis lasting more than 6 weeks and affecting 4 or fewer joints during the first 6 months of the disease. Anterior uveitis or iritis is most likely to occur with this type of arthritis; anterior uveitis has been reported in 10%–30% of children with oligoarthritis and is usually diagnosed in the first 4 years of the disease. Laboratory markers include a high frequency of nonspecific low-titer antinuclear antibodies (ANA). RF is almost always absent. Human leukocyte antigen (HLA) associations include −A2, −DR5, −DR8, −DR11, and −DP2.1.

RF-negative polyarthritis probably represents a heterogeneous group of disorders. Children with this disorder have more than 4 inflamed joints during the first 6 months of the disease. It is more common in girls, and its mean age of onset is older than in children with oligoarthritis. Uveitis occurs in about 10% of these children. ANA-positivity may be present, but RF is absent. Strong HLA associations have not been consistently documented.

The pathogenesis of the anterior uveitis associated with JIA is unknown, although it is likely to have an immunologic basis. Correlation between the onset and course of the arthritis and uveitis is uncertain. Although 90% of patients with JIA who develop uveitis do so within 7 years of the onset of arthritis, this interval may be longer. Occasionally, uveitis is diagnosed before the onset of joint symptoms; these patients often have a poorer prognosis, although this may be the result of a delayed diagnosis because of the initial asymptomatic nature of this ocular inflammation. Other features associated with more aggressive uveitis include shorter interval between the onset of arthritis and uveitis, and severe uveitis at the first examination.

JIA-associated uveitis is usually bilateral and nongranulomatous with fine to medium-sized keratic precipitates, although a minority of children, especially African-American children, may have granulomatous precipitates. Chronic inflammation may produce band keratopathy, posterior synechiae, ciliary membrane formation, hypotony, cataract, glaucoma, and phthisis (Fig 22-1). Vitritis and macular edema occur infrequently. Because many patients are asymptomatic initially and the involved eye is often white and without obvious inflammation, the disease may be advanced at diagnosis.

Recognition of the importance of screening for uveitis in children with JIA has resulted in an improved prognosis for this disorder. However, visual impairment has been reported in up to 40% of children with JIA-associated uveitis, and blindness may occur in as many as 10% of affected eyes. Screening guidelines continue to undergo revision, but are generally based on 4 factors believed to predispose children with JIA to uveitis:

1. category of arthritis
2. age at onset of arthritis
3. presence of ANA-positivity
4. gender: females with JIA have a higher incidence of uveitis than do males

Table 22-4 outlines an eye examination schedule recommended by the American Academy of Pediatrics for children with JIA.

Other arthritic diseases of childhood may also be associated with uveitis. *Psoriatic arthritis* may resemble oligoarthritis or RF-negative polyarthritis and, for this reason, although it is uncommon, it is probably underdiagnosed. The diagnosis is suggested by the presence of arthritis and 2 of the following findings: nail pitting or onycholysis, dactylitis,

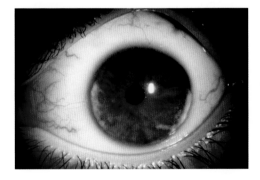

Figure 22-1 Slit-lamp photograph of a patient with JIA-associated uveitis. As is typical, the conjunctiva is "white." Band keratopathy is present. *(Courtesy of Amy Hutchinson, MD.)*

Table 22-4 Frequency of Ophthalmologic Examination in Patients With JIA

Type	ANA	Age at Onset, y	Duration of Disease, y	Risk Category	Eye Examination Frequency, mo
Oligoarthritis or polyarthritis	+	≤6	≤4	High	3
	+	≤6	>4	Moderate	6
	+	≤6	>7	Low	12
	+	>6	≤4	Moderate	6
	+	>6	>4	Low	12
	–	≤6	≤4	Moderate	6
	–	≤6	>4	Low	12
	–	>6	NA	Low	12
Systemic disease (fever, rash)	NA	NA	NA	Low	12

JIA = juvenile idiopathic arthritis; ANA = antinuclear antibodies; NA = not applicable.
Recommendations for follow-up continue through childhood and adolescence.

Modified from Cassidy J, Kivlin J, Lindsley C, Nocton J; Section on Rheumatology; Section on Ophthalmology. Ophthalmologic examinations in children with juvenile rheumatoid arthritis. *Pediatrics.* 2006;117(5):1844.

or a history of psoriasis in a first-degree relative. Insidious and chronic anterior uveitis, usually bilateral, is seen in 10% of affected children.

Enthesitis-related arthritis is a chronic arthritis that is associated with inflammation of entheses, which are the sites of attachment of the ligaments, tendons, fascia, and capsule to the bone. This form of childhood arthritis, which has also been referred to as *juvenile ankylosing spondylitis,* usually has its onset at age 8–10 years and is more common in males. The uveitis is acute, symptomatic, and unilateral, although both eyes may be affected at different times. Most patients are HLA-B27 positive, and many will eventually develop lumbosacral spine disease and sacroiliitis.

Cassidy J, Kivlin J, Lindsley C, Nocton J; Section on Rheumatology; Section on Ophthalmology. Ophthalmologic examinations in children with juvenile rheumatoid arthritis. *Pediatrics.* 2006;117(5):1843–1845.

Kotaniemi K, Savolainen A, Karma A, Aho K. Recent advances in uveitis of juvenile idiopathic arthritis. *Surv Ophthalmol.* 2003;48(5):489–502.

Smith JR, Rosenbaum JT. Immune-mediated systemic diseases associated with uveitis. *Focal Points: Clinical Modules for Ophthalmologists.* San Francisco: American Academy of Ophthalmology; 2003, module 11.

Tubulointerstitial Nephritis and Uveitis Syndrome

Tubulointerstitial nephritis and uveitis syndrome (TINU) may be associated with unexplained chronic or recurrent anterior uveitis in children. The renal disease is characterized by low-grade fever, fatigue, pallor, and weight loss. Elevated levels of β_2-microglobulin may be present in the urine. The uveitis is usually bilateral and may occur before, simultaneously with, or after the renal disease. The median age of onset of TINU is 15 years, and there is a 3:1 female-to-male ratio. Prognosis is generally good, although long-term follow-up is required because the inflammation may recur.

Mandeville JT, Levinson RD, Holland GN. The tubulointerstitial nephritis and uveitis syndrome. *Surv Ophthalmol.* 2001;46(3):195–208.

Orbital Pseudotumor

Unlike the adult form of this disorder, pediatric orbital pseudotumor may be associated with anterior uveitis. The iritis may be unilateral or bilateral. A persistent or recurrent uveitis in a child with an otherwise negative laboratory evaluation for iritis may be an indication for ultrasonography, computed tomography, or magnetic resonance imaging to investigate the possibility of orbital pseudotumor.

Bloom JN, Graviss ER, Byrne BJ. Orbital pseudotumor in the differential diagnosis of pediatric uveitis. *J Pediatr Ophthalmol Strabismus.* 1992;29(1):59–63.

Other Causes of Anterior Uveitis

Anterior uveitis may also be associated with a variety of infectious and noninfectious diseases—including herpes viruses, syphilis, sarcoidosis, Kawasaki syndrome, Fuchs heterochromic iridocyclitis, Lyme disease, and Behçet syndrome—and with trauma. These conditions are discussed in more detail in Chapter 16 and in BCSC Section 9, *Intraocular Inflammation and Uveitis.*

Intermediate Uveitis

The term *intermediate uveitis* is an anatomical-based description of the primary site of the ocular inflammation in this condition. The inflammation is localized in the vitreous base overlying the ciliary body, pars plana, and peripheral retina, as well as in the anterior vitreous. Intermediate uveitis accounts for 5%–15% of all cases of uveitis and about 25% of uveitis in the pediatric age group. It may occur with a variety of conditions in children, including sarcoidosis, Lyme disease, juvenile xanthogranuloma, and tuberculosis. Idiopathic disease, known as *pars planitis* (Fig 22-2), accounts for 85%–90% of cases. The distinction between pars planitis and intermediate uveitis is not always clear in common usage, and the 2 terms are often used interchangeably. The clinical features, diagnosis, and treatment of intermediate uveitis are discussed in BCSC Section 9, *Intraocular Inflammation and Uveitis.*

Posterior Uveitis

Toxoplasmosis

Toxoplasmosis is the most common cause of posterior uveitis in children. The diagnosis, clinical manifestations, and treatment of toxoplasmosis are discussed in Chapter 16.

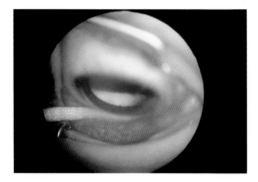

Figure 22-2 Intermediate uveitis with inferior snowbank formation, right eye.

Toxocariasis

Ocular toxocariasis is caused by the nematode larvae of a common intestinal parasite of dogs *(Toxocara canis)*. This disease primarily affects children, as it is contracted through the ingestion of ascarid ova in soil contaminated by dog feces. *Visceral larval migrans (VLM)* is an acute systemic infection produced by this organism and commonly occurs at approximately age 2 years. If symptomatic, it is associated with fever, cough, rashes, malaise, and anorexia. Laboratory testing reveals esosinophilia. VLM and ocular toxocariasis, for unknown reasons, seldom occur in the same patient.

Ocular toxocariasis is usually unilateral and is not associated with systemic illness or an elevated eosinophil count. The average age of onset is 7.5 years. Retinal findings include posterior pole granuloma, peripheral granuloma with macular traction (Fig 22-3), and endophthalmitis. There is often little external evidence of inflammation. Patients may present with leukocoria, strabismus, or decreased vision. These abnormalities are also found with retinoblastoma, which must be differentiated from ocular toxocariasis. Although ELISA titers for *Toxocara* have a high sensitivity and specificity and are useful in diagnosing this disease, a positive laboratory finding does not eliminate the possibility of retinoblastoma, as elevated titers may be found in a significant percentage of the general pediatric population.

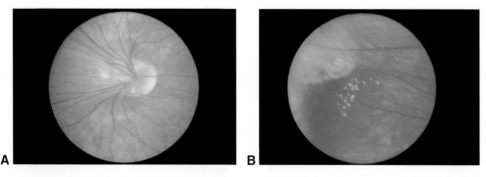

A   B

Figure 22-3 Toxocariasis, right eye. **A,** Distortion of posterior pole vessels. **B,** Peripheral granuloma.

Treatment includes observation of peripheral lesions, periocular or systemic steroids for posterior lesions and endophthalmitis, or surgical intervention to address retinal traction, cataract, glaucoma, or cyclitic membranes. Systemic antihelmintics are not useful in treating ocular toxocariasis, as the organism producing the inflammation is already dead. See also BCSC Section 9, *Intraocular Inflammation and Uveitis*.

Shields JA. Ocular toxocariasis. A review. *Surv Ophthalmol.* 1984;28(5):361–381.

Panuveitis

Sarcoidosis

Sarcoidosis may present differently in children than in adults. In young sarcoid patients (below age 5 years), the incidence of lung disease is less frequent, and the disease is more often characterized by arthritis and rash. Older children (between ages 8 and 15 years) have the pulmonary abnormalities and lymph node findings more commonly associated with the adult form of the disease. Both groups are at risk for uveitis. Although anterior uveitis (Fig 22-4) is the most common manifestation of ocular sarcoidosis in children, this disease can produce a panuveitis.

Diagnosis and treatment in children is similar to that in adults (see BCSC Section 9, *Intraocular Inflammation and Uveitis*), but serum angiotensin-converting enzyme (ACE) levels are normally higher in children and can be misleading when used to diagnose pediatric sarcoidosis. If this disorder is suspected, children should undergo careful rheumatologic evaluation for the systemic disease.

Shetty AK, Gedalia A. Sarcoidosis: a pediatric perspective. *Clin Pediatr.* 1998;37(12):707–717.

Familial Juvenile Systemic Granulomatosis

Familial juvenile systemic granulomatosis *(Blau syndrome)* is an autosomal dominantly inherited disease that includes granulomatous arthritis, uveitis associated with multifocal choroiditis, and vasculitic rash. The disease usually presents during childhood. It resembles sarcoidosis, but pulmonary involvement and adenopathy are absent. Chronic panuveitis associated with multifocal choroiditis is the most common ocular presentation, but uveitis may be limited to the anterior segment in some cases, and the disease is often misdiagnosed as JIA or sarcoidosis. Ocular complications, including cataract, glaucoma,

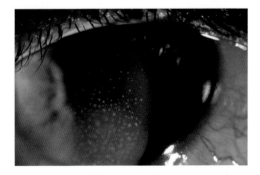

Figure 22-4 Keratic precipitates in sarcoidosis. *(Courtesy of Ken K. Nischal, FRCOphth.)*

band keratopathy, and vision loss, are common. A positive family history is helpful in determining the diagnosis. The gene for this disease is located on chromosome 16.

Latkany PA, Jabs DA, Smith JR, et al. Multifocal choroiditis in patients with familial juvenile systemic granulomatosis. *Am J Ophthalmol.* 2002;134(6):897–904.

Vogt-Koyanagi-Harada Syndrome

Vogt-Koyanagi-Harada syndrome is a chronic progressive bilateral panuveitis that is associated with exudative retinal detachments and may be accompanied by signs of meningeal irritation, auditory disturbances, and skin changes. It is rare in children, but is associated with a higher frequency of ocular complications such as cataract and glaucoma and with a poorer visual prognosis than in adults.

Tabbara KF, Chavis PS, Freeman WR. Vogt-Koyanagi-Harada syndrome in children compared to adults. *Acta Ophthalmol Scand.* 1998;76(6):723–726.

Other Causes of Posterior Uveitis and Panuveitis

Additional possible causes of posterior uveitis and panuveitis include herpes, rubella, rubeola, and measles viruses; syphilis; *Bartonella;* tuberculosis; Lyme disease; histoplasmosis; *Candida albicans;* sympathetic ophthalmia; and Behçet syndrome (see BCSC Section 9, *Intraocular Inflammation and Uveitis*).

Masquerade Syndromes

Other conditions can simulate pediatric uveitis. These masquerade syndromes are listed together with their diagnostic features in Table 22-5.

Diagnosis of Pediatric Uveitis

Establishing the correct diagnosis is the essential first step in managing a pediatric patient with uveitis, although some ophthalmologists prefer to postpone the workup of isolated anterior uveitis unless it is recurrent or unresponsive to initial therapy. Establishing an accurate diagnosis requires a detailed history, thorough ophthalmic examination, and selected laboratory tests. An examination under anesthesia may be needed if the child is not cooperative enough for an office evaluation. Laboratory investigations are chosen based on the suspected diagnoses (Table 22-6; also see Table 22-5).

Treatment of Pediatric Uveitis

The goal of uveitis treatment in children is to decrease the inflammation of the eye before complications occur and, if complications secondary to the uveitis do arise, to treat them without producing adverse side effects from the medical or surgical therapies. It is important to note that although cells in the anterior chamber indicate active inflammation, flare (protein) may chronically persist even after the inflammation has been successfully treated.

Table 22-5 Masquerade Syndromes

Disease	Age (Years)	Signs of Inflammation	Diagnostic Studies
Anterior segment			
Retinoblastoma	<15	Flare, cells, pseudohypopyon	Ultrasonography; CT
Leukemia	<15	Flare, cells, heterochromia	Bone marrow, peripheral blood smear
Intraocular foreign body	Any age	Flare, cells	X-ray, CT, ultrasonography
Malignant melanoma	Any age	Flare, cells	Fluorescein angiography, ultrasonography
Juvenile xanthogranuloma	<15	Flare, cells, hyphema	Examination of skin, iris biopsy
Peripheral retinal detachment	Any age	Flare, cells	Ophthalmoscopy
Posterior segment			
Retinitis pigmentosa	Any age	Cells in vitreous	ERG, EOG, visual fields
Reticulum cell sarcoma	15+	Vitreous exudate, retinal hemorrhage or exudates, retinal pigment epithelium infiltrates	Cytology study of aqueous and vitreous
Lymphoma	15+	Retinal hemorrhage or exudates, vitreous cells	Node biopsy, bone marrow, physical examination
Retinoblastoma	<15	Vitreous cells, retinal exudates	Ultrasonography, CT
Malignant melanoma	15+	Vitreous cells	Fluorescein angiography, ultrasonography
Multiple sclerosis	15+	Periphlebitis	Neurologic examination

CT = computed tomography; ERG = electroretinogram; EOG = electro-oculogram.

Infectious disease and malignancies producing uveitis should be identified and treated appropriately (see BCSC Section 9, *Intraocular Inflammation and Uveitis*). Medical and surgical treatment of noninfectious uveitis is discussed in the following sections.

Medical Management

Anterior segment inflammation is initially treated with topical corticosteroid and mydriatic/cycloplegic agents. Because topical corticosteroids do not penetrate well into the vitreous or posterior segment, sub-Tenon injections of a corticosteroid may be useful in the treatment of intermediate or posterior uveitis. Short courses of oral corticosteroids may be used, but long-term use should be avoided because of significant ocular and systemic side effects.

Glaucoma and cataract formation are 2 of the most serious ocular complications of corticosteroid therapy. In general, the more potent topical corticosteroids are those most likely to produce an increase in intraocular pressure. Periocular injections of corticosteroids can produce elevations in intraocular pressure for weeks to months after injection. Risks of long-term systemic corticosteroid use in children include growth retardation, osteoporosis and bone fractures, cushingoid appearance, diabetes, peptic ulcers, myopathy,

Table 22-6 Laboratory Tests for Various Types of Uveitis

Anterior
Complete blood count (leukemia)
Antinuclear antibody (JIA)
Serum lysozyme (sarcoidosis)
Serum protein electrophoresis (alpha$_2$ globulin fraction in sarcoidosis)
FTA-ABS (syphilis)
HLA-B27 (enthesitis-related arthritis or ankylosing spondylitis)
PCR, ELISA, IFA (Lyme disease)
Tuberculin skin test, chest x-ray (sarcoidosis, tuberculosis)
GI series (if ulcerative colitis or regional enteritis [Crohn disease] is suspected)
Angiotensin-converting enzyme (sarcoidosis)
Intermediate
Serum lysozyme (sarcoidosis)
FTA-ABS (syphilis)
Chest x-ray (sarcoidosis, tuberculosis)
Tuberculin skin test (tuberculosis)
Angiotensin-converting enzyme (sarcoidosis)
Posterior
PCR, ELISA (toxoplasmosis)
PCR, ELISA (toxocariasis)
Serum lysozyme (sarcoidosis)
FTA-ABS (syphilis)
PCR, blood cultures, viral cultures, or antibody levels if cytomegalovirus, herpes simplex
  (especially in a newborn), or rubella is suspected
PCR, ELISA, IFA (Lyme disease)
Angiotensin-converting enzyme (sarcoidosis)

hypertension, altered mental status, pseudotumor cerebri, and increased mortality from infection. Patients may also require increased doses of corticosteroids during times of stress to avoid an addisonian crisis.

Naproxen and tolmetin are 2 nonsteroidal anti-inflammatory drugs (NSAIDs) that are commonly used to treat arthritis in children and may have some efficacy in treating uveitis. Potential complications of NSAIDs include gastrointestinal irritation, renal toxicity, rashes, and central nervous system reactions.

Systemic immunosuppressive therapy may be beneficial in treating both uveitis and arthritis. It can sometimes reduce or eliminate the need for steroids. The therapy should be undertaken in cooperation with a pediatric specialist familiar with the use of immunosuppressive and immunomodulatory medications and their adverse effects.

Methotrexate is an antimetabolite that is commonly used to treat arthritis and uveitis in children. Less commonly used antimetabolites include azathioprine, mycophenolate mofetil, and leflunomide. These agents inhibit nucleic acid synthesis by a variety of mechanisms. Gastrointestinal disturbance is the most common adverse effect of methotrexate; this can be alleviated by concurrent oral folic acid administration or by switching to subcutaneous injections. Hepatic toxicity and interstitial pneumonitis are rare but serious complications.

Cyclosporine is a fungal metabolite with immunosuppressive effects. It may be used as monotherapy for uveitis or in combination with steroids and methotrexate. Renal toxicity is a significant limiting complication of this medication. Other possible adverse effects include hypertension, gingival hyperplasia, gastrointestinal disturbance, and neurologic symptoms.

Alkylating agents, including chlorambucil and cyclophosphamide, cause cross-linking of DNA and prevent cell replication. Because of their serious adverse effects, including bone marrow suppression, infection, infertility, and secondary malignancies, they are usually not used in children. However, they may be occasionally prescribed in the most severe cases threatening blindness.

A number of newer therapies have been used for the treatment of refractory uveitis, including the tumor necrosis factor (TNF) inhibitors infliximab, adalimumab, and etanercept. Other medications are under investigation, including daclizumab, a humanized murine anti–interleukin-2 receptor.

Children receiving immunosuppressive drugs should receive a yearly influenza vaccine and, if susceptible, varicella-zoster virus immunoglobulin if exposed to chickenpox. If the CD4$^+$ T-lymphocyte count is less than 200 cells per microliter, then *Pneumocystis carinii* prophylaxis should be considered. An infectious diseases specialist should be consulted regarding the use of live attenuated viral vaccines in children receiving high-dose corticosteroids or immunosuppressive drugs.

Agle LM, Vazquez-Cobian LB, Lehman TJ. Clinical trials in pediatric uveitis. *Curr Rheumatol Rep.* 2003;5(6):477–481.

Jabs DA, Rosenbaum JT, Foster CS, et al. Guidelines for the use of immunosuppressive drugs in patients with ocular inflammatory disorders: recommendations of an expert panel. *Am J Ophthalmol.* 2000;130(4):492–513.

Smith JR. Management of uveitis in pediatric patients: special considerations. *Paediatr Drugs.* 2002;4(3):183–189.

Surgical Treatment of Uveitis Complications

Band keratopathy can be treated by removal of corneal epithelium followed by calcium chelation with ethylenediaminetetraacetic acid (EDTA). Repeat treatments may be needed. Phototherapeutic keratectomy (PTK) has also been used to treat band keratopathy.

Cataract surgery for patients with uveitis can be complicated by hypotony, glaucoma, synechiae formation, cystoid macular edema, and retinal detachment. In patients with JIA, a combined lensectomy/vitrectomy appears to produce better results than cataract extraction alone. Uveitis must be aggressively treated so that it is under control both before and after surgery. Intraocular lens implantation in children with uveitis is controversial.

Glaucoma surgery may become necessary in children with uveitis. Many different techniques have been used, and long-term success rates vary. Standard trabeculectomy is associated with a high rate of failure due to scarring. Intraoperative application of mitomycin C may improve outcomes, but the risk of postoperative infection and bleb leaks over the life span of a child is a concern. Goniotomy or trabeculotomy may be effective in some children. The use of aqueous shunts is currently the most popular technique for surgical management of pediatric uveitic glaucoma.

Holland GN, Stiehm ER. Special considerations in the evaluation and management of uveitis in children. *Am J Ophthalmol.* 2003;135(6):867–878.

CHAPTER 23

Vitreous and Retinal Diseases and Disorders

Early-Onset Retinal Disease

Persistent Fetal Vasculature

Persistent fetal vasculature (PFV) is the more accurate term for the condition referred to for many years as *persistent hyperplastic primary vitreous (PHPV)*. This is the most common cause of a unilateral cataract and is typically an isolated, sporadic malformation of the eye. Bilateral cases may be associated with systemic or neurologic abnormalities and syndromes. Bilateral retinal folds, familial exudative vitreoretinopathy (FEVR), and Norrie disease may be phenocopies. The spectrum of severity is broad. Mild cases feature eyes with prominent hyaloid vessel remnants, large Mittendorf dots, and Bergmeister papillae (see Chapter 24). At the other end of the spectrum are microphthalmic eyes with dense retrolental plaques and a thick fibrous persistent hyaloid artery. The ciliary processes may be elongated and visible through the dilated pupil (classic for PFV), and prominent radial vessels are often noted on the iris surface (Fig 23-1). Varying degrees of lens opacification occur. The opacity usually consists of a retrolental plaque that is densest centrally and possibly contains cartilage and fibrovascular tissue. Congenital retinal nonattachment and optic nerve dysmorphism can also occur.

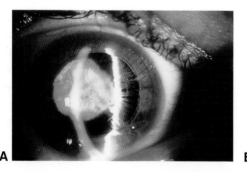 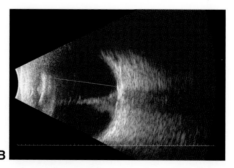

Figure 23-1 Persistent fetal vasculature (PFV; formerly called *persistent hyperplastic primary vitreous*). **A,** Elongated ciliary processes are adherent to lens. Note the dense fibrous plaque on the lens. **B,** Ultrasonogram of eye with PFV. Note the dense stalk arising from the optic nerve and attaching to the posterior lens. *(Part B courtesy of Edward L. Raab, MD.)*

The natural history of more severely affected untreated eyes is usually one of relentless progressive cataract formation and anterior chamber shallowing, resulting in angle-closure glaucoma. Retinal detachment, intraocular hemorrhage, and ciliary body detachment are other severe complications in PFV. The hemorrhages presumably originate in the fibrovascular membrane in the retrolental space. Affected eyes are typically smaller than the normal fellow eye, although this finding may be apparent only by ultrasonography or careful caliper measurement of the corneal diameters. It is important to document microphthalmos because retinoblastoma is rarely found in microphthalmic eyes, and retinoblastoma may be part of the initial differential diagnosis. The presence of a cataract is also evidence against the diagnosis of retinoblastoma, although lens opacities may develop in advanced cases.

Many eyes with PFV can be saved by early cataract surgery combined with membrane excision. In cases without significant posterior pole abnormalities, it is possible to obtain some degree of central vision, and occasionally excellent vision, only if early surgical intervention is followed by consistent contact lens wear, combined with carefully monitored, consistent patching of the uninvolved eye for amblyopia prevention and treatment. The visual prognosis depends on how extensively the retina is involved, whether glaucoma develops, and whether the patient adheres to the patching regimen.

Various surgical approaches to the management of PFV have been described. In most cases, the retrolenticular tissues can be removed by vitreous-cutting instruments and/or intraocular scissors, with intraocular cautery as necessary. Both limbal and pars plana approaches have been successfully employed. An anterior approach may decrease the chance of retinal detachment, as the pars plicata may be abnormally anterior. If the macula and optic nerve appear normal postoperatively, a vigorous effort should be made to correct aphakia optically and to patch, as would be done with a patient following unilateral cataract extraction. See also Chapter 21.

Goldberg MF. Persistent fetal vasculature (PFV): an integrated interpretation of signs and symptoms associated with persistent hyperplastic primary vitreous (PHPV). LIV Edward Jackson Memorial Lecture. *Am J Ophthalmol.* 1997;124(5):587–626.

Müllner-Eidenböck A, Amon M, Hauff W, Klebermass N, Abela C, Moser E. Surgery in unilateral congenital cataract caused by persistent fetal vasculature or minimal fetal vascular remnants: age-related findings and management challenges. *J Cataract Refract Surg.* 2004;30(3):611–619.

Retinopathy of Prematurity

Retinopathy of prematurity (ROP) is the current designation for what was previously called *retrolental fibroplasia (RLF)*. ROP includes the acute disease seen in the nursery and the cicatricial disease seen later.

Normally, retinal vascular development begins during week 16 of gestation. Mesenchymal tissue containing spindle cells is the source of retinal vessels. The mesenchyme grows centrifugally from the optic disc, reaching the nasal ora serrata in the eighth month of gestation and the temporal ora serrata up to 1–2 months later. Premature birth is a risk factor for ROP, in which normal retinal vascular development is altered and abnormal neovascularization may occur. The pathologic process may stop or reverse itself at any point, or the disease may eventually progress and lead to vitreoretinal traction and retinal detachment.

In the United States, ROP is rare in infants with a birth weight greater than 2000 g. Premature infants weighing less than 1500 g at birth are at risk for developing ROP, and the risk increases as gestational age and birth weight decrease. In the Early Treatment for Retinopathy of Prematurity (ETROP) Study, 68% of infants weighing less than 1251 g at birth developed ROP of any degree (stage 1 or greater, with stage 5 being the greatest). It was estimated that some degree of ROP occurred in 44% of infants with a birth weight of 1000–1250 g, in 76% of those with a birth weight of 751–999 g, and in 93% of those with a birth weight of 750 g or less.

> Good WV; Early Treatment for Retinopathy of Prematurity Cooperative Group. Final results of the Early Treatment for Retinopathy of Prematurity (ETROP) randomized trial. *Trans Am Ophthalmol Soc.* 2004;102:233–248.

In the 1950s, as more premature babies were surviving, it was noted that delivering high doses of supplemental oxygen to these babies was associated with ROP. This has been demonstrated in animal models as well. Curtailment of oxygen was attempted and did decrease rates of ROP; however, rates of death and cerebral palsy increased. As pulse oximetry became widespread, allowing better regulation of oxygen administration, low birth weight and gestational age became better predictors of ROP than did oxygen exposure, signifying the complex interaction of factors that cause disease development. Recent studies, using improved oxygenation monitors and avoidance of fluctuation in fraction of inspired oxygen, have shown a reduction in rate of severe ROP without increased morbidity or mortality.

Gestational age and birth weight are inversely correlated with the development of ROP. The amount of time in oxygen therapy is a strong correlate, but the level of oxygenation is a weaker one. Severe ROP is more prevalent in white newborns, especially males.

Other factors have also been examined for their role in ROP. The possibility of premature exposure to light as a factor was studied (LIGHT-ROP), but limiting light exposure was not found to decrease the incidence of ROP. Another study, Supplemental Therapeutic Oxygen for Prethreshold ROP (STOP-ROP), evaluated whether increasing oxygen saturation levels when prethreshold ROP was reached would prevent progression to severe ROP. No statistical difference was found between the high-oxygen group and the conventional oxygen group in terms of ROP progression, but the former had more pulmonary complications. Low levels of insulin-like growth factor I (IGF-I) are associated with an accumulation of vascular endothelial growth factor (VEGF) in the vitreous and an increase in ROP severity. This suggests that IGF-I supplementation could prevent severe ROP. Anti-angiogenic medications may have a role in ROP treatment in the future; currently, however, there is concern about their effect on the normally developing vasculature in other areas of the body. Some studies have shown that minimizing oxygen tension fluctuations and maintaining oxygen saturation levels at a lower level than was customary in early gestational infants can lower the incidence of ROP.

Currently, there is a rise in the incidence of ROP in developing countries, signaling the occurrence of an epidemic comparable to that which occurred in the United States and the United Kingdom in the 1940s and early 1950s. The affected infants in developing countries are larger and of older gestational age than infants in the United States who develop ROP, suggesting that screening criteria for ROP should be modified in developing countries.

Premature infants are at risk for other conditions, such as bronchopulmonary dysplasia, patent ductus arteriosus, intracranial hemorrhage, porencephalic cysts, periventricular leukomalacia, and cerebral palsy.

Sears JE, Pietz J, Sonnie C, Dolcini D, Hoppe G. A change in oxygen supplementation can decrease the incidence of retinopathy of prematurity. *Ophthalmology.* 2009;116(3):513–518.

Wallace DK. Retinopathy of prematurity. *Focal Points: Clinical Modules for Ophthalmologists.* San Francisco: American Academy of Ophthalmology; 2008, module 12.

Classification

Several classification systems have been created and later revised for ROP and are used for describing the disease and guiding treatment (cryotherapy or laser, or observation). The International Classification of ROP (ICROP) published in 1984 (a revised version was published in 2005) describes the disease by stage, zone, and extent. This classification functioned very well in the Cryotherapy for ROP (CRYO-ROP) Study and will probably persist for many years (Table 23-1; Figs 23-2 through 23-6). BCSC Section 12, *Retina and Vitreous,* also discusses this classification in detail.

Table 23-1 International Classification of Acute Stages of Retinopathy of Prematurity

Location—Zones II and III are based on convention rather than strict anatomy (see Figs 23-2, 23-8)
  Zone I (posterior pole)—Circle with radius of 30°, twice disc–macula distance
  Zone II—From edge of zone I to point tangential to nasal ora serrata and around to area near the temporal equator
  Zone III—Residual crescent anterior to zone II
Extent—Specified as hours of the clock as observer looks at each eye
Staging the disease
  Stage 0—Immature vascularization, no ROP
  Stage 1—Demarcation line (see Fig 23-3)
  Stage 2—Ridge, ± small tufts of fibrovascular proliferation (popcorns) (see Fig 23-4)
  Stage 3—Ridge with extraretinal fibrovascular proliferation (see Fig 23-5)
    • Mild fibrovascular proliferation
    • Moderate fibrovascular proliferation
    • Severe fibrovascular proliferation
  Stage 4—Subtotal retinal detachment (see Fig 23-6)
    A. Extrafoveal
    B. Retinal detachment including fovea
  Stage 5—Total retinal detachment
  Funnel: Anterior   Posterior
           Open   Open
           Narrow   Narrow
Plus disease—Plus (+) is added when vascular shunting is so marked that the veins are enlarged and the arteries tortuous in the posterior pole (see Fig 23-7).

Modified from the Committee for Classification of Retinopathy of Prematurity: an international classification of retinopathy of prematurity. *Arch Ophthalmol.* 1984;102(8):1130–1134.

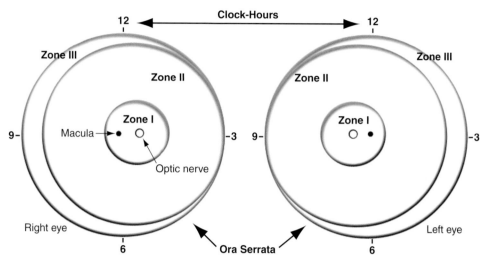

Figure 23-2 Scheme of retina of right eye and left eye showing zone borders and clock-hours employed to describe location and extent of retinopathy of prematurity. Diagrammatic representation of the potential total area of the premature retina, with zone I, the most posterior, symmetrically surrounding the optic nerve head, the earliest to develop. A larger retinal area is present temporally (laterally) than nasally (medially), representing zone III. Only zones I and II are present nasally. *(Reproduced by permission from the Committee for Classification of Retinopathy of Prematurity: an international classification of retinopathy of prematurity. Arch Ophthalmol. 1984;102(8):1131.)*

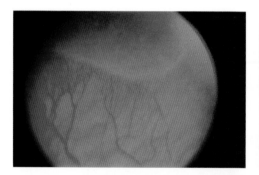

Figure 23-3 Stage 1 ROP. Demarcation line has no height. *(Reproduced courtesy of Oregon Health Sciences University Ophthalmic Photography Department.)*

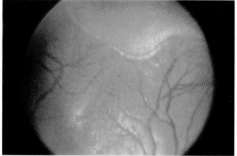

Figure 23-4 Stage 2 ROP. Demarcation height and width, creating a ridge. *(Reproduced courtesy of Oregon Health Sciences University Ophthalmic Photography Department and CRYO-ROP Cooperative Group.)*

Plus disease is defined by a standard photograph and refers to marked arteriolar tortuosity and venous engorgement of the posterior pole vasculature; it implies vascular shunting through the neovascularization and signifies severe disease (Fig 23-7). *Pre-plus* disease is abnormal dilation and tortuosity, but less than that seen in the standard photograph. A finding of pre-plus disease alerts the clinician to the need for close observation of the infant. The CRYO-ROP trial defined *threshold* disease as 5 contiguous or 8 total clock-hours of stage 3 ROP in zone I or II with plus disease (Fig 23-8). The ETROP trial

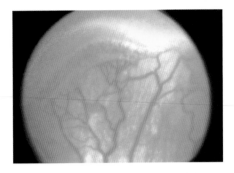

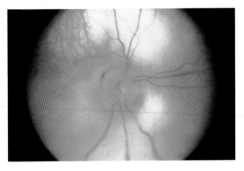

Figure 23-5 Stage 3 ROP. Ridge with extra-retinal fibrovascular proliferation. *(Reproduced by permission from Arch Ophthalmol. 1984;102(8):1134. ©1988 American Medical Association.)*

Figure 23-6 Stage 4 ROP. Subtotal retinal detachment. *(Reproduced by permission from Arch Ophthalmol. 1984;102(8):1132. ©1988 American Medical Association.)*

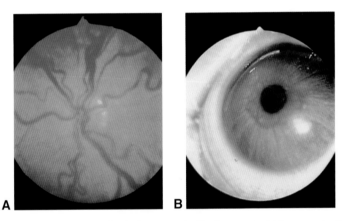

Figure 23-7 **A,** Plus disease, standard photograph. **B,** Congested iris vessels that can occur with severe plus disease.

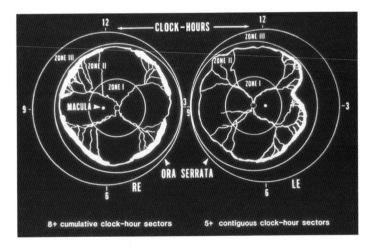

Figure 23-8 Diagram of threshold disease. *(Reprinted by permission of American Medical Association from Multicenter trial of cryotherapy for retinopathy of prematurity: preliminary results. Cryotherapy for Retinopathy of Prematurity Cooperative Group. Arch Ophthalmol. 1988;106:474.)*

Table 23-2 **Types of Prethreshold ROP**

Type 1 ROP
    Zone I, any stage with plus disease
    Zone I, stage 3 without plus disease
    Zone II, stage 2 or 3 with plus disease
Type 2 ROP
    Zone I, stage 1 or 2 without plus disease
    Zone II, stage 3 without plus disease

From Wallace DK. Retinopathy of prematurity. *Focal Points: Clinical Modules for Ophthalmologists.* San Francisco: American Academy of Ophthalmology; 2008, module 12:p 4.

further classified ROP into types 1 and 2, which are less than classic "threshold" disease and constitute *prethreshold* disease. These are listed in Table 23-2.

Management

Diagnosis   It has been recommended that a fundus examination be performed on infants who have a gestational age of 30 weeks or less; a birth weight of less than 1500 g; or a birth weight of 1500–2000 g with an oxygen supplementation requirement or an unstable course. The examination should be performed by a clinician trained in the diagnosis of this potentially blinding disease. The first examination should be done at 4 weeks to less than 5 weeks after birth or at a corrected gestational age of 30 to less than 31 weeks, whichever is later. These recommendations may change based on future data. The most current recommendations, created jointly by the American Academy of Pediatrics, the American Academy of Ophthalmology, and the American Association for Pediatric Ophthalmology and Strabismus, can be found on the website of the American Academy of Pediatrics (http://pediatrics.aappublications.org/cgi/content/full/pediatrics;117/2/572).

In the examination of premature infants, the recommended mydriatic solution to be used is Cyclomydril (0.2% cyclopentolate and 1.0% phenylephrine). Phenylephrine 10% (Neo-Synephrine) has the potential to cause hypertension. A nurse should be present for examinations in the neonatal intensive care unit because they are stressful for infants, and many of these patients experience apnea and bradycardia during examination. If an examination must be postponed, the postponement and medical reason should be documented in the patient's medical record.

Follow-up examinations should be done every 1–2 weeks thereafter until retinal vessels have grown normally into zone III or until the risk of developing ROP has passed (about 44–46 weeks postmenstrual age). If the normal blood vessels stop growing into the periphery of the retina or if ROP begins to develop, examinations are performed more frequently, either weekly or twice a week (Table 23-3). ROP can progress and then stabilize and regress; or it can progress, becoming severe, and require treatment.

Treatment   Treatment guidelines have been created based on the results of several multicenter ROP trials. These guidelines indicate which level of disease requires treatment (cryotherapy or laser, or observation) to prevent adverse visual sequelae. In the CRYO-ROP trial, cryotherapy was applied to the avascular peripheral retina when the eye met the criteria for threshold disease (Fig 23-9A). Treatment at threshold resulted in a 50% decrease in the rate of retinal detachment when compared to observation. In several later

Table 23-3 Recommended Follow-up Intervals When Plus Disease Is Absent

	Zone I	Zone II	Zone III
Stage 3	Laser treatment	≤1 week	≤1 week
Stage 2	≤1 week	1–2 weeks	2–3 weeks
Stage 1	≤1 week	2 weeks	2–3 weeks
No ROP—immature vascularization	1–2 weeks	2–3 weeks	2–3 weeks vs discontinue exams
Regressing ROP	1–2 weeks	2 weeks	2–3 weeks

From Wallace DK. Retinopathy of prematurity. *Focal Points: Clinical Modules for Ophthalmologists.* San Francisco: American Academy of Ophthalmology; 2008, module 12:p 5.

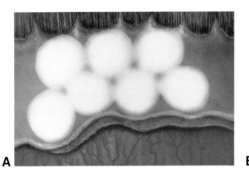 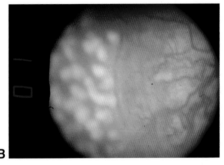

A B

Figure 23-9   A, Cryotherapy applied to the avascular retina. **B,** Laser photocoagulation applied to avascular retina. Note the thick band of neovascularization and plus disease. *(Part A reproduced by permission from* Arch Ophthalmol. *1988;106:474. ©1988 American Medical Association. Part B courtesy of Philip J. Ferrone, MD.)*

studies, laser was used following the same guidelines as those used in the CRYO-ROP trial and was shown to be equally effective in inducing the regression of the neovascularization and preventing adverse visual sequelae (Fig 23-9B). More recently, the ETROP trial found that earlier treatment at prethreshold resulted in better structural and visual outcomes when compared with conventional treatment at threshold. The median age at which eyes were treated for threshold disease in the CRYO-ROP Study was 36.9 weeks after conception; 90% of cases reached threshold between 33.6 and 42 weeks following conception. In the ETROP trial, the average age for treatment was 35.2 weeks following conception, with a range of 32–42 weeks. Based on ETROP, laser treatment is strongly considered for any eye with type 1 ROP. Eyes with type 2 ROP should be closely observed and, if there is progression to type 1 or threshold disease, treated.

Laser photocoagulation has largely replaced cryotherapy as the treatment of choice for ROP in the United States, although cryotherapy is still a valid form of treatment. Potential complications from laser treatment include an intense inflammatory response, hyphema, cataract, and glaucoma. Cataracts are often accompanied by hypotony, and the eye may be lost.

Sequelae and complications

One of the most common sequelae of advanced ROP, either treated or spontaneously re-solved, is myopia, which is often very severe. Retinal folds and dragging of the macula

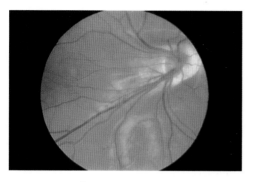

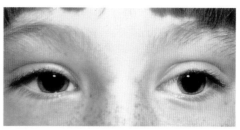

Figure 23-10 Posterior pole traction/dragging, a sequela of ROP, right eye. Central acuity is usually diminished in such eyes.

Figure 23-11 Pseudoexotropia in a fixating left eye in ROP. Patient has a positive angle kappa as a result of macular dragging.

can also occur, causing visual impairment (Fig 23-10). Amblyopia may be present as a result of high myopia, especially if asymmetric, or strabismus. Pseudostrabismus caused by dragging of the macula can occur, often giving the appearance of an exotropia as a result of a large positive angle kappa (Fig 23-11). Eyes that have undergone treatment may also experience late retinal detachments at the border of the treated and untreated retina. Therefore, a child who has had ROP requires periodic ophthalmic examinations beyond the newborn period. Other late changes associated with stage 5 ROP include microphthalmos, cataract, glaucoma, and phthisis bulbi.

When laser or cryotherapy has not prevented the progression of ROP to stage 4 or 5 (retinal detachment), scleral buckling and vitrectomy may be indicated. Anatomical success is as high as 83% in some studies, but visual results have been disappointing, particularly with stage 5 eyes. Even with successful treatment, several hundred babies are blinded by this disease in the United States yearly.

For areas underserved by trained specialists, a telemedicine approach to ROP screening has great potential.

Early Treatment for Retinopathy of Prematurity Cooperative Group. Revised indications for the treatment of retinopathy of prematurity: results of the early treatment for ROP randomized trial. *Arch Ophthalmol.* 2003;121(12):1684–1694.

Multicenter trial of cryotherapy for retinopathy of prematurity: Snellen visual acuity and structural outcome at 5½ years after randomization. Cryotherapy for Retinopathy of Prematurity Cooperative Group. *Arch Ophthalmol.* 1996;114(4):417–424.

Prenner JL, Capone A Jr, Trese MT. Visual outcomes after lens-sparing vitrectomy for stage 4A retinopathy of prematurity. *Ophthalmology.* 2004;111(12):2271–2273.

Coats Disease

The classic findings in Coats disease are yellow subretinal and intraretinal lipid exudates associated with retinal vascular abnormalities—most often telangiectasia, tortuosity, aneurysmal dilatations, and avascularity—with a variable clinical presentation, ranging from mild changes to total retinal detachment. Once the fovea is detached and the subretinal

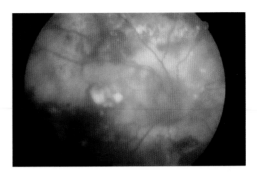

Figure 23-12 Coats disease. Affected right eye. Note extensive subretinal exudate and exudative retinal detachment.

exudate becomes organized, the prognosis for restoration of central vision is poor. See also BCSC Section 12, *Retina and Vitreous.*

Males are affected more frequently than females, and the condition is usually, but not always, unilateral. The average age at diagnosis is 6–8 years, but the disease has also been observed in infants (Fig 23-12). The most widely held theory for this is that the subretinal exudation originates from the leaking anomalous vessels. Hence, the diagnosis of Coats disease requires the presence of the abnormal retinal vessels, which occasionally are small and difficult to find. Fluorescein angioscopy and angiography may be helpful in demonstrating leakage from the telangiectatic vessels and in assessing the effectiveness of therapy.

The differential diagnostic possibilities include angiomatosis retinae, PFV, ROP, toxocariasis, metastatic retinitis, familial exudative vitreoretinopathy, Norrie disease, Eales disease, leukemia, and cavernous retinal hemangioma. Coats disease can mimic retinoblastoma. Calcium, detected by ultrasonography or CT scan, is frequently seen in retinoblastoma and is distinctly rare in Coats disease.

Treatment is directed at obliterating the abnormal vessels and includes cryotherapy or laser photocoagulation. The disease is stopped when the leaking vessels are destroyed. Eyes with progressive disease develop exudative retinal detachments and subretinal fibrosis. Recently, there have been reports of promising results with intravitreal bevacizumab and triamcinolone used as adjuncts to laser treatment.

The etiology of Coats disease is still unknown, but associations with various gene deletions have been reported. However, Coats disease is isolated in most cases.

Cahill M, O'Keefe M, Acheson R, Mulvihill A, Wallace D, Mooney D. Classification of the spectrum of Coats disease as subtypes of idiopathic retinal telangiectasias with exudation. *Acta Ophthalmol Scand.* 2001;79(6):596–602.

Cakir M, Cekiç O, Yilmaz OF. Combined intravitreal bevacizumab and triamcinolone injection in a child with Coats disease. *J AAPOS.* 2008;12(3):309–311.

Rubin MP, Mukai S. Coats disease. *Int Ophthalmol Clin.* 2008;48(2):149–158.

Hereditary Retinal Disease

Nystagmus is the most definitive presenting sign of a hereditary retinal disorder. The onset of nystagmus typically occurs between 8 and 12 weeks of age and indicates poor visual potential. Not all patients with hereditary retinal disease develop nystagmus (eg, those with less-severe retinal damage). Poor visual function may be the presenting abnormality in a young child, and school-aged children with retinal disease may present after a failed vision screening. Older children can be examined further with an electroretinogram (ERG), electro-oculogram (EOG), color vision testing, visual fields, and dark adaptation testing.

Table 23-4 outlines common causes of nystagmus in the first 3 months of life. Infectious diseases, optic nerve disorders, and congenital motor nystagmus are discussed in Chapters 16, 24, and 25, respectively. Hereditary retinal diseases with onset late in childhood are much like adult hereditary retinal diseases and are covered in depth in BCSC Section 12, *Retina and Vitreous*.

Leber Congenital Amaurosis

Leber congenital amaurosis (LCA) is a group of hereditary (usually autosomal recessive) retinal diseases that affect the rods and cones. LCA is characterized by severe vision loss noted in infancy, nystagmus, poorly reactive pupils, and an extinguished ERG. Vision ranges from 20/200 to bare light perception in most patients. Funduscopic appearance varies highly, often depending on the genotype, from a normal appearance, particularly in infancy; to pigment clumping in the retinal pigment epithelium (RPE); to one resembling classic retinitis pigmentosa, with bone spicules, attenuation of arterioles, and disc pallor. Other reported but less common fundus findings include extensive chorioretinal atrophy,

---

Table 23-4 Causes of Nystagmus in First 3 Months of Life

Primary sensory retinal abnormality
  Leber congenital amaurosis
  Achromatopsia
  Blue-cone monochromatism
  Congenital stationary night blindness (X-linked and autosomal recessive)
Vitreoretinal abnormality
  Retinopathy of prematurity, stage 4 or 5
  Norrie disease
  Familial exudative vitreoretinopathy
Foveal hypoplasia
  Associated with albinism
  Associated with aniridia
  Isolated
Optic nerve disorder (bilateral)
  Optic nerve hypoplasia
  Optic nerve coloboma
  Optic atrophy
Infectious disease
  Congenital toxoplasmosis
  Cytomegalovirus
  Rubella
  Syphilis
Congenital motor nystagmus
Generalized central nervous system disorder
  Aicardi syndrome
  Others

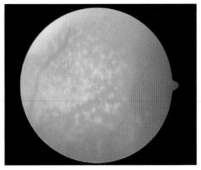

Figure 23-13 Leber congenital amaurosis, marbleized fundus type.

macular coloboma, white dots (similar to retinitis punctata albescens), marbleized retinal appearance, and disc edema (Fig 23-13). Histologic examination shows diffuse absence of photoreceptors.

Additional ocular manifestations include oculodigital reflex (eye poking), photoaversion, cataracts, keratoconus, and keratoglobus. High refractive errors, usually high hyperopia, are common.

There are several ocular entities that can mimic LCA because of their similar presentation: achromatopsia, congenital stationary night blindness, albinism, and optic nerve hypoplasia. LCA-like phenotypes can also be found in a number of systemic diseases. These diseases present similarly to LCA but do not manifest their systemic features until later in life, misleading the clinician initially. These diseases are Alström syndrome, Batten disease (neuronal ceroid-lipofuscinosis), Joubert syndrome, peroxisomal diseases (Zellweger disease, neonatal adrenoleukodystrophy, and infantile Refsum disease), and Senior-Loken syndrome.

Evaluation

An ERG is required to diagnose LCA. However, electroretinography can be technically difficult to perform in infants, and there is a maturation of the ERG response in the first year of life. Thus, an ERG can appear highly abnormal in an infant who will later develop a more normal response. It is often advisable either to delay the ERG until age 6 months or to repeat the ERG after this time. Sedation or general anesthesia may be required for ERG.

Genetic testing of LCA patients is also important and can be used to counsel the patient's family, confirm the diagnosis, distinguish LCA from other retinal diseases, and predict prognosis. A molecular diagnosis of LCA is hindered by the fact that the disease is very heterogeneous. Currently, there are 14 genetic mutations known to cause LCA, with the most frequently mutated genes being *CEP290* (15%), *GUCY2D* (12%), and *CRB1* (10%). Mutations cannot be identified in approximately 30% of cases.

Treatment

Gene therapy holds promise. A dog model of LCA due to mutations in the *RPE65* gene demonstrated that gene therapy using an adenovirus vector could restore some vision. In recent human trials, improvement in subjective and objective vision was shown after subretinal injections of the gene promoter attached to an adeno-associated viral particle.

den Hollander AI, Roepman R, Koenekoop RK, Cremers FPM. Leber congenital amaurosis: genes, proteins, and disease mechanisms. *Prog Retin Eye Res.* 2008;27(4):391–419.

Maguire AM, Simonelli F, Pierce EA, et al. Safety and efficacy of gene transfer for Leber's congenital amaurosis. *N Engl J Med.* 2008;358(21):2240–2248.

Achromatopsia

Achromatopsia can be difficult to distinguish initially from LCA, but infants with achromatopsia develop better visual functioning. Complete achromatopsia, also known as rod monochromatism, is a stationary autosomal recessive disorder in which patients have no color vision, poor central vision, nystagmus, and photophobia. The photophobia is actually a desire to avoid bright light rather than true pain or discomfort, and photophobia may be manifested by squinting or rapid fluttering of the eyelids in normal indoor illumination. Hemeralopia, the inability to see clearly in bright light (day blindness), occurs in these patients.

Findings on retinal examination are usually normal, with the possible exception of a decreased or absent foveal reflex. Color vision testing results are markedly abnormal, as is the ERG, which shows extinguished cone or photopic responses but normal rod responses.

To date, 3 autosomal recessive achromatopsia genes have been identified: *CNGA3*, *CNGB3*, and *GNAT2*. Other cone dystrophies causing early-onset vision impairment and nystagmus include *incomplete achromatopsia* and *blue-cone monochromacy*. In both disorders, patients have better vision than in complete achromatopsia. In incomplete achromatopsia, which is an autosomal recessive disorder, there is residual cone function. In blue-cone monochromacy, which is an X-linked disorder, function of the blue (short-wavelength) cones is retained; however, the photopic ERG is usually extinguished. Dark glasses or red glasses that exclude short wavelengths may help.

Michaelides M, Hunt DM, Moore AT. The cone dysfunction syndromes. *Br J Ophthalmol.* 2004:88(2):291–297.

Congenital Stationary Night Blindness

Congenital stationary night blindness (CSNB) refers to a group of nonprogressive retinal disorders characterized predominantly by abnormal function of the rod system. The condition may be X-linked (the most common form), autosomal recessive, or autosomal dominant.

CSNB, especially the autosomal recessive and X-linked forms, can present in early infancy with nystagmus and normal fundi. These forms are often also associated with myopia and decreased acuity in the range of 20/200. However, the range of vision in these patients is wide and, occasionally, patients have normal vision. The retina usually appears normal, although the optic nerve may show myopic tilt and temporal pallor. An ERG must be performed for diagnosis. The most common ERG pattern seen in CSNB is the "negative" dark-adapted ERG: a large a-wave and a reduced (negative) b-wave. Dark adaptation is abnormal in all patients with CSNB. Infants with CSNB may have a flat ERG until approximately 6 months of age, when it converts to the classic negative configuration.

Oguchi disease and *fundus albipunctatus* are forms of CSNB with abnormal fundi. In Oguchi disease, the fundus displays a yellow sheen after exposure to light; this sheen disappears following dark adaptation. In fundus albipunctatus, the retina develops yellow-white dots.

CSNB is also discussed in BCSC Section 12, *Retina and Vitreous.*

Foveal Hypoplasia

Foveal hypoplasia, or incomplete development of the fovea, is another cause of nystagmus in early infancy. This condition is most often associated with albinism or aniridia but may also be an isolated finding. The ophthalmoscopic appearance is of a decreased or absent foveal reflex with varying degrees of hypoplasia of the macula itself (patients with complete achromatopsia also show decreased foveal reflex). Foveal hypoplasia can be familial and may be related to a defect in the *PAX6* gene.

Aicardi Syndrome

Aicardi syndrome is an X-linked autosomal dominant disorder characterized by the clinical triad of widespread round or oval depigmented chorioretinal lacunae, infantile spasms, and agenesis of the corpus callosum (Fig 23-14). Colobomas and microphthalmos may also occur. Aicardi syndrome is typically lethal in males.

Aicardi J. Aicardi syndrome. *Brain Dev.* 2005;27(3):164–171.

Hereditary Macular Dystrophies

Macular abnormalities are seen in a number of hereditary disorders. The abnormality can be associated with a hereditary systemic disease (eg, the cherry-red spot seen in generalized gangliosidosis), or the abnormal macula can reflect a primary retinal disorder, such as Stargardt disease and Best vitelliform dystrophy.

Stargardt Disease

Stargardt disease (juvenile macular degeneration) is the most common hereditary macular dystrophy. It is usually autosomal recessive but may be autosomal dominant. It is

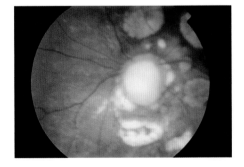

Figure 23-14 Aicardi syndrome. Fundus photograph showing disc and adjacent chorioretinal lacunae.

a bilateral, symmetric, progressive condition in which acuity levels off at approximately 20/70–20/100 but is variable, with some patients retaining better vision. Vision typically begins to deteriorate between ages 8 and 15 years.

The disease often progresses through stages. Initially, the fundus appears normal, even when vision is decreased; and the patient may be considered functional. The first ophthalmoscopic changes observed are loss of foveal reflex, followed by development of a characteristic macular bull's-eye atrophy with surrounding round or pisciform yellow flecks, which develop in the posterior pole at the level of the RPE (Fig 23-15). If the flecks are scattered throughout the fundus, the condition can be referred to as *fundus flavimaculatus*. Often, before development of the flecks, the macula will have an atrophic appearance due to diseased RPE, inducing a peculiar light-reflecting quality that has been described as beaten bronze. The "dark choroid" sign on fluorescein angiography is distinctive and helps confirm diagnosis of Stargardt disease. This phenomenon is due to the accumulation of lipofuscin-like pigment throughout the RPE, which blocks the choroidal fluorescein on fluorescein angiography and is present in 80% of patients with Stargardt disease.

ERG is often normal in the early stages of Stargardt disease but becomes abnormal as the disease progresses. Progressive cone–rod dystrophy may present like Stargardt disease in children but has a much worse prognosis, often resulting in very little vision. Repeated ERG and acuity measurements over the first year are recommended before a definitive diagnosis is made. Stargardt disease is caused by mutations in the retina-specific ATP-binding transporter gene *(ABCR)*. Gene therapy for Stargardt disease is being studied in animal models.

Rotenstreich Y, Fishman GA, Anderson RJ. Visual acuity loss and clinical observations in a large series of patients with Stargardt disease. *Ophthalmology.* 2003;110(6):1151–1158.

Best Disease

Best disease (juvenile-onset vitelliform macular dystrophy) is an autosomal dominant retinal disorder with variable penetrance and expressivity. Even though the EOG is always abnormal (Fig 23-16A), the retina may at first appear normal. The egg yolk–like or vitelliform stage begins between 4 and 10 years of age and is seen as a yellow-orange cystlike structure, usually in the macula, although the lesion may occur elsewhere and

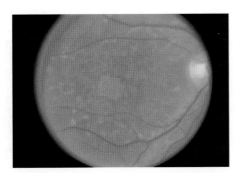

Figure 23-15 Stargardt disease. Note atrophic, beaten-metal appearance of macula. Early in the disease, usually at presentation, the macula appears normal.

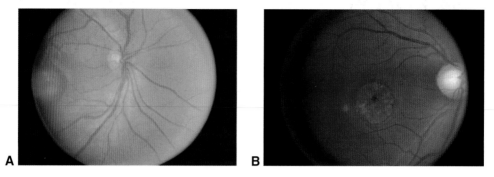

Figure 23-16 Best vitelliform dystrophy. **A,** Early disease, or "yolk" stage. **B,** Advanced disease, "scrambled egg" stage. *(Part B courtesy of Richard A. Lewis, MD.)*

can occasionally be multiple. It is usually 1.5–5.0 disc diameters in size. The egg yolk–like appearance is associated with good central vision. With time, the cystic material may become granular, giving rise to the "scrambled-egg" stage (Fig 23-16B). Typically, central vision remains good, often in the range of 20/30. The cyst may rupture and become partially resorbed, with formation of a pseudohypopyon from cystic contents. Twenty percent of patients develop subretinal neovascularization and serous detachment of the RPE, and subretinal hemorrhage may occur, causing vision deterioration, often to 20/100 or worse.

The EOG is abnormal in all affected patients and in carriers. This disorder is one of the few in which the EOG is abnormal and the ERG is normal. Carriers can be identified by the presence of an abnormal-appearing EOG in the absence of morphologic abnormalities. The condition is caused by mutations in the *vitelliform macular dystrophy gene (VMD2)*, also called *bestrophin*, on chromosome 11.

Wabbels B, Preising MN, Kretschmann U, Demmler A, Lorenz B. Genotype-phenotype correlation and longitudinal course in ten families with Best vitelliform macular dystrophy. *Graefes Arch Clin Exp Ophthalmol.* 2006;244(11):1453–1466.

Hereditary Vitreoretinopathies

The vitreoretinopathies include a broad range of disease entities. The ones discussed here characteristically present in childhood.

Juvenile Retinoschisis

Juvenile retinoschisis is an X-linked disease caused by mutations in the *RS1* gene, which encodes for the retinal protein, retinoschisin, an adhesion protein that is believed to be essential to the health of Müller cells. The disease mainly affects males. Foveal retinoschisis is present in almost all cases of juvenile retinoschisis. About 50% of patients have peripheral retinoschisis in addition to foveal involvement. The retinoschisis occurs in the nerve fiber layer. The fovea has a star-shaped or spokelike configuration that may resemble cystoid macular edema and become less distinct over time. Vitreous veils or strands

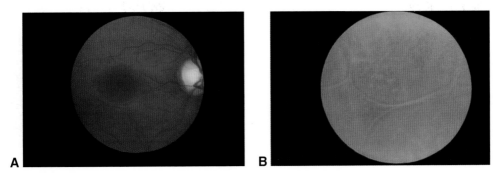

Figure 23-17 Juvenile retinoschisis. **A,** Central (macular) and **(B)** peripheral schisis may be present. Note vitreous veils. *(Part A courtesy of Richard A. Lewis, MD.)*

are common (Fig 23-17), and vitreal syneresis, or liquefaction, is prominent. Visual acuity varies but may gradually deteriorate to the finger-counting range. Complications include vitreous hemorrhages and retinal detachments. The ERG shows a reduction of the scotopic b-wave with preservation of the a-wave; the EOG is normal. Optical coherence tomography scans show schisis spaces in the middle layers of the macula. There has been some success with gene replacement in mouse models.

Sikkink SK, Biswas S, Parry NR, Stanga PE, Trump D. X-linked retinoschisis: un update. *J Med Genet.* 2007;44(4):225–232.

Stickler Syndrome

Stickler syndrome is characterized by flat midface, progressive hearing loss, cleft palate, Pierre Robin sequence, mitral valve prolapse, and progressive arthropathy with spondyloepiphyseal dysplasia. The ophthalmic manifestations are frequent and vision-threatening. The most common is high myopia, with a high incidence of retinal detachment secondary to retinal breaks, lattice degeneration, and proliferative vitreoretinopathy. A hallmark of the syndrome is vitreous liquefaction that results in an optically empty vitreous cavity, except for vitreous veils that may be attached to the retina. Angle anomalies, ectopia lentis, cataracts, ptosis, and strabismus are less frequently associated. The incidence of vitreous loss during cataract surgery is high, as is the rate of subsequent retinal detachments. Retinal folds and breaks should be treated before cataract extraction. The role of prophylactic retinopexy is controversial.

There are several types of Stickler syndrome. Types 1 and 2 present with the classic systemic and ocular features of the disease. Type 3 Stickler syndrome displays only systemic features and no ocular features, and a fourth type displays only ocular features. All 4 forms are autosomal dominant and display different mutations in the genes that encode for collagen.

Although the arthropathy may not be symptomatic initially, children with Stickler syndrome often show radiographic abnormalities of long bones and joints. Early diagnosis may aid in preventing some of the severe complications of the ocular pathology and allow treatment of mild joint involvement.

Familial Exudative Vitreoretinopathy

Familial exudative vitreoretinopathy (FEVR) is now divided into 2 types. Type 1 is autosomal dominant and caused by a mutation on chromosome 11. Type 2 is an X-linked recessive disorder caused by a mutation in the *NDP* gene, the same gene involved in Norrie disease. The two types share similar features: retinal traction, folds, breaks, and detachment secondary to vitreous traction, posterior vitreous detachment, avascular peripheral retina, and thick peripheral intraretinal and subretinal exudates. Family members can show marked variation of severity, from minimal straightening of vessels and peripheral nonperfusion to total retinal detachment. Some patients have bilateral retinal folds. The differential diagnosis includes ROP and Coats disease.

Cryopexy, photocoagulation, retinal detachment surgery, vitrectomy, and cataract surgery have all been used to manage this disorder.

Norrie Disease

Norrie disease is an X-linked recessive disorder caused by a mutation in the gene *(NDP)* encoding for the protein norrin. The condition is characterized by a distinctive retinal appearance: a globular, severely dystrophic retina with pigmentary changes in the avascular periphery. Norrie disease causes congenital blindness and varying degrees of hearing impairment and mental retardation. Affected boys are typically born blind. During the first few days or weeks of life, a yellowish retinal detachment appears bilaterally, followed by a whiter mass behind the clear lens. Over time, the lenses, and later the cornea, opacify; phthisis bulbi may ensue by age 10 years or earlier. Female carriers demonstrate peripheral retinal abnormalities. ROP, X-linked familial exudative vitreoretinopathy, and Coats disease are phenocopies.

Goldmann-Favre Vitreoretinal Dystrophy

Goldmann-Favre vitreoretinal dystrophy consists of vitreous strands and veils as well as foveal and peripheral retinoschisis. The fundus may appear similar to that seen in retinitis pigmentosa, including optic nerve pallor and attenuation of the retinal vessels. The pigmentary disturbance tends to be in a nummular (circular), rather than a bone-spicule, configuration; in some cases, little pigment is seen. Decreased central acuity and night blindness are prominent early findings in the second decade of life, and complicated cataracts subsequently develop. Inheritance is autosomal recessive.

Systemic Diseases and Disorders With Retinal Manifestations

Diabetes Mellitus

Type 1, or *insulin-dependent, diabetes mellitus* was formerly called *juvenile-onset diabetes mellitus.* The prevalence of retinopathy in this condition is directly proportional to the duration of diabetes after puberty. Retinopathy rarely occurs less than 5 years after the onset of diabetes mellitus. Fundus photography or angiography reveals that about 50% of patients have nonproliferative (background) retinopathy after 7 years, although only half of these cases can be recognized by direct ophthalmoscopy. The prevalence of retinopathy increases to approximately 90% in patients who have had type 1 diabetes for 15 years or more. Proliferative diabetic retinopathy is rare in pediatric cases and is not covered in this section. For further discussion, see BCSC Section 12, *Retina and Vitreous.*

A variety of nonproliferative changes may occur in the pediatric age group. These changes are thought to result from obstruction of retinal capillaries and abnormal capillary permeability. Microaneurysms are the first ophthalmoscopic sign; they may be followed by retinal hemorrhages, areas of retinal nonperfusion, cotton-wool spots, hard exudates, intraretinal microvascular abnormalities, and venous dilation. A rapid rise of blood glucose may produce myopia, and sudden reduction of blood glucose can induce hyperopia, because of osmotic changes in the lens and alteration of its refractive status. Several weeks may be required before acuity returns to normal.

True diabetic cataracts are uncommon, occurring most often in patients with poorly controlled disease. Such cataracts resemble a snowstorm that affects the anterior and posterior cortices of young patients. Diabetes mellitus, especially in young children, may be part of the *DIDMOAD syndrome* (*diabetes insipidus, diabetes mellitus, optic atrophy, and deafness*), also known as *Wolfram syndrome.*

Management

The American Academy of Ophthalmology recommends annual ophthalmic examinations beginning 3–5 years after the onset of diabetes mellitus (http://www.aao.org/ppp). The American Diabetes Association recommends the first ophthalmic examination be obtained once the child is 10 years of age or older and has had diabetes for 3–5 years (www.diabetes.org). The American Academy of Pediatrics (AAP) recommends an initial ophthalmic examination 3–5 years after diagnosis if the patient is older than 9 years, with annual follow-up examinations thereafter (www.aap.org). Specifically, the AAP states that children younger than 9 years do not require screening examinations. The reason for this is that the incidence of diabetic retinopathy is negligibly low in this age group.

Lueder GT, Silverstein J; American Academy of Pediatrics Section on Ophthalmology and Section on Endocrinology. Screening for retinopathy in the pediatric patient with type 1 diabetes mellitus. *Pediatrics.* 2005;116(1):270–273.

Leukemia

In leukemia, the most common eye findings are retinal hemorrhages, especially flame-shaped lesions in the nerve fiber layer. They involve the posterior fundus and can have some correlation with other aspects of the disease such as anemia, thrombocytopenia, or coagulation abnormalities. At times, these hemorrhages have white centers. The retinal hemorrhages in leukemia can resemble those associated with intracranial hemorrhages and trauma. Collections of leukocytes have also been found on histopathologic examination. Retinal hemorrhages have been reported as the first manifestation of leukemia. Other forms of retinal involvement include localized perivascular infiltrations, microinfarction, and discrete tumor infiltrations.

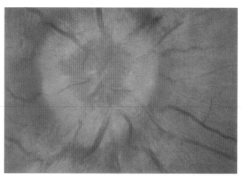

Figure 23-18 Leukemic infiltration of optic nerve.

Optic nerve involvement occurs if the disc is infiltrated by leukemic cells (Fig 23-18). Translucent swelling of the disc obscures the normal landmarks; with florid involvement, only a white mass is visible in the region of the disc. A papilledema-like fundus picture may occur, with loss of central vision. Therefore, a leukemic child with disc edema and loss of central vision should be considered to have this complication. Early optic nerve involvement in leukemia constitutes a medical emergency because permanent loss of central vision is imminent. Generally, such patients should undergo radiation therapy as soon as possible.

Leukemia may also involve the anterior segment and orbit. This topic is discussed in Chapter 26.

Albinism

Albinism is a group of various conditions that involve the melanin system of the skin and eye *(oculocutaneous albinism [OCA])*, or the eye alone *(ocular albinism [OA])* (Table 23-5; see also BCSC Section 12, *Retina and Vitreous*). OCA is a group of 4 autosomal recessive disorders; OA is X-linked (uncommonly autosomal recessive).

The major ophthalmic findings in all types of OCA and OA are iris transillumination from decreased pigmentation, foveal aplasia or hypoplasia, and a characteristic deficit of pigment in the retina, especially peripheral to the posterior pole (Fig 23-19). Nystagmus, light sensitivity, high refractive errors, and reduced central acuity are often present, and visual acuity ranges from 20/25 to 20/200. If a child has significant foveal hypoplasia, nystagmus will begin at 2–3 months of life. The severity of the visual defect tends to be proportional to the degree of nystagmus and pigmentation. An abnormally large number of crossed fibers appear in the optic chiasm of patients and animals with albinism, precluding stereopsis and often inducing strabismus. Asymmetric visually evoked potentials (VEPs) reflect this abnormality. Absence of misrouting on VEP precludes the diagnosis of albinism.

There are 4 known types of OCA: OCA1–OCA4. OCA1 is caused by a mutation in the tyrosinase gene *(TYR)*, and there are 2 subtypes, OCA1A and OCA1B. In OCA1A, tyrosinase is inactive, so the skin and hair are white, and the skin does not tan. In OCA1B, tyrosinase is minimally active; thus, the hair, which is initially white, may darken to blonde, and the skin is slightly more pigmented and may tan. Visual acuity is poorest in this type.

Table 23-5 Albinism

Disease	Ocular Manifestations	Systemic Manifestations	Inheritance
OCA1A (tyrosinase-negative or complete lack of tyrosinase activity)	Iris is thin, pale blue; characteristic pink reflex from the iris occurs because of marked transillumination defect; prominent choroidal vessels with poorly defined fovea; nystagmus; head-nodding; frequently myopic astigmatism and strabismus; vision 20/100–20/200; marked photophobia	White hair throughout life; skin does not tan; increased susceptibility to skin neoplasia (as with all forms of OCA)	Autosomal recessive, band 11q14–21; tyrosinase gene (*TYR*)
OCA1B (reduced activity of tyrosinase)	At birth, complete albinism with blue, translucent irides and albinotic fundal reflex; nystagmus and photophobia	White hair and skin at birth; increasing pigmentation with yellow-red hair and light normal skin that tans	Autosomal recessive; allelic with OCA1A; *TYR* gene
OCA2	Eye color blue, yellow, or brown (age- and race-dependent); pigment cartwheel effect at pupil and limbus; transillumination minimal to absent in dark-skinned adults; moderate to severe nystagmus; photophobia; moderately severe visual defect; 20/80–20/100	Hair and skin color may be white at birth, darkening over time, but patients are typically born with some pigment; increased susceptibility to skin neoplasia; hyperkeratoses and freckling in exposed areas of skin	Autosomal recessive, band 15q11.2–q12; *OCA2* gene (formerly, the *P* gene)
OCA3	Blue to brown irides; transillumination of irides; retinal hypopigmentation; nystagmus; strabismus	Skin and hair red-brown; freckles present; areas of hypopigmentation	Autosomal recessive; *TYRP1* gene
OCA4	Same as OCA2	Same as OCA2	Autosomal recessive; *MATP* gene

(Continued)

Table 23-5 *(continued)*

Disease	Ocular Manifestations	Systemic Manifestations	Inheritance
OA1	In affected men, marked deficiency of pigment in iris and choroid; nystagmus and myopic astigmatism; if darkly pigmented, may be limited to nystagmus, foveal hypoplasia, and tessellated fundus; mosaic pigment pattern in fundi. Carrier females display mild abnormalities.	Normal pigmentation elsewhere; occasional hypopigmented cutaneous macules; patients appear more lightly pigmented than their relatives	X-linked recessive, Xp22.3; *OA1* gene
Chédiak-Higashi syndrome	Partial albinism; diminished uveal and retinal pigmentation with photophobia and nystagmus	Early death from recurrent infections; silver tinge to hair; neutropenia, anemia, thrombocytopenia, hepatosplenomegaly, lymphadenopathy, leukemia	Autosomal recessive, band 1q42-43; *LYST* gene
Hermansky-Pudlak syndrome	Eye color blue-gray to brown (age- and race-dependent); iris normal to cartwheel effect; transillumination present in light-skinned individuals; mild to severe nystagmus and photophobia; slight to moderate decrease in visual acuity; high frequency in Puerto Rico	Platelet bleeding disorder, pulmonary fibrosis; hair color variable, white to dark red-brown; cream-colored skin; melanosis on exposed skin; pigmented nevi and freckles; susceptibility to skin neoplasia; ceroid storage throughout the body	Autosomal recessive, 10q2; *HPS1* gene, others

Adapted from Nelson LB, Calhoun JH, Harley RD, eds. *Pediatric Ophthalmology*. 3rd ed. Philadelphia: Saunders; 1991. Updated from Online Mendelian Inheritance in Man, OMIM. Baltimore: Johns Hopkins University Press; 2009. http://www.ncbi.nlm.nih.gov/omim/. Accessed May 18, 2009.

OCA2 is caused by mutations in the *OCA2* gene, formerly known as the *P* gene, which helps tyrosinase function. In affected persons, the amount of pigment present at birth is minimal and increases over time (see Fig 23-19C). Hair color ranges from blonde to light brown. OCA2 is the most prevalent type worldwide, and there is a high frequency of OCA2 mutant alleles in the African population.

OCA3 is caused by a mutation in the tyrosinase-related protein 1 gene *(TYRP1)*. This type occurs mainly in persons of African descent and has been termed *red OCA* or *Rufous OCA*. Affected individuals have red hair and reddish brown skin. Visual abnormalities are often mild.

OCA4 is caused by mutations in the membrane-associated transporter protein gene *(MATP)*. Persons with OCA4 have the same phenotype as those with OCA2.

Ocular albinism (OA1), also called *Nettleship-Falls albinism*, is usually caused by a mutation in the *OA1* gene on the X chromosome. An autosomal recessive form of OA has been reported. Vision in OA varies from 20/60 to 20/400, with some patients reported to have vision as good as 20/25. Affected individuals appear to have decreased pigment in the eyes but not the skin. The melanocytes are normal in size and number in the eyes and skin, but there are abnormalities in the melanosomes within the melanocytes (giant melanocytes). The systemic nature of the melanosome defect in OA1 suggests that this disorder is actually a type of OCA in which the major manifestations are in the eye.

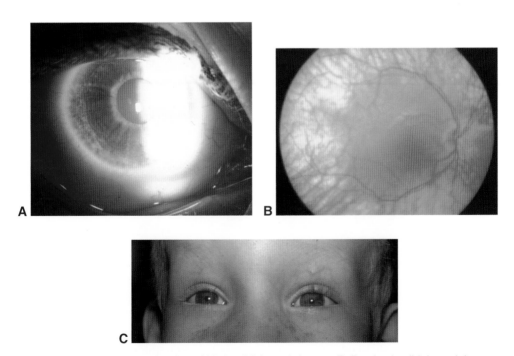

Figure 23-19   **A,** Transillumination of iris in albinism, right eye. **B,** Fundus in albinism, right eye, demonstrating complete lack of pigment and macular agenesis. **C,** Child with oculocutaneous albinism type 2 (OCA2). Note white hair, eyebrows, and lashes, and light-colored irides and freckles. *(Parts A and C courtesy of Edward L. Raab, MD.)*

Albinism can be part of a broader syndrome, such as Hermansky-Pudlak syndrome or Chédiak-Higashi syndrome, both of which are autosomal recessive. *Hermansky-Pudlak syndrome* occurs with higher frequency in Puerto Rico and is characterized by interstitial fibrosis and mild bleeding problems. *Chédiak-Higashi syndrome* is a rare condition characterized by increased susceptibility to bacterial infections. Whenever a patient is diagnosed with albinism, the clinician should inquire about bleeding or bruising tendencies as well as previous infections, as a positive response could indicate one of these syndromes, which have potentially serious consequences.

All patients with OCA are at risk for skin cancer and should be counseled.

Dorey SE, Neveu MM, Burton LC, Sloper JJ, Holder GE. The clinical features of albinism and their correlation with visual evoked potentials. *Br J Ophthalmol.* 2003;87(6):767–772.

Grønskov K, Ek J, Brondum-Nielsen K. Oculocutaneous albinism. *Orphanet J Rare Dis.* 2007;2:43.

Familial Oculorenal Syndromes

Lowe syndrome (the oculocerebrorenal syndrome of Lowe) is an X-linked recessive disorder characterized by a renal tubulopathy (Fanconi-type) that occurs in the first year of life, producing aminoaciduria, metabolic acidosis, proteinuria, and rickets. Affected children are severely hypotonic at birth, and mental retardation is common.

The most common eye defect is congenital bilateral cataract. The lenses are small, thick, and opaque and may demonstrate posterior lenticonus. Congenital glaucoma often develops. Surgery is often difficult, with recurrent cyclitic membranes and recalcitrant glaucoma. Mothers of affected children may have punctate snowflake opacities oriented in a radial fashion within the lens cortex that indicate their carrier status.

Alport syndrome is usually transmitted as an X-linked disorder but can be autosomal recessive or dominant. It is a disorder of basement membranes that produces progressive renal failure, deafness, anterior lenticonus, cataract of the crystalline lens, and fleck retinopathy. Hematuria begins in childhood. Proteinuria and renal casts develop, with hypertension and kidney failure occurring late in the course of the disease.

Senior-Loken syndrome is an autosomal recessive disease characterized by nephronophthisis, renal failure, and a pigmentary retinal degeneration similar to LCA. The ERG is flat.

Neurometabolic Disorders

When neurometabolic disorders, especially some of the lipid storage diseases, are suspected, ophthalmologists are often consulted to determine whether a cherry-red spot is present, because its presence is diagnostic of these disorders. The appearance of a cherry-red spot in the macula is caused by loss of transparency of the perifoveal retina due to edema or deposition of abnormal materials in the retinal ganglion cells. Normally, the fovea, which is very thin and almost devoid of ganglion cells (the site of storage material accumulation in storage disease), appears to be red to brown, depending on the patient's race. With infiltration of the retinal ganglion cells, the surrounding, thicker perifoveal retina becomes white and its color contrasts with that of the fovea, creating the "cherry-red spot." The most common diseases to cause a cherry-red spot are

- GM_1 gangliosidosis
- Tay-Sachs disease (GM_2 gangliosidosis type I)
- Sandhoff disease (GM_2 gangliosidosis type II)
- Niemann-Pick disease
- sialidosis
- Farber lipogranulomatosis
- metachromatic leukodystrophy
- central retinal artery occlusion
- trauma (retinal edema) (See also BCSC Section 12, *Retina and Vitreous.*)

The cherry-red spot will disappear over time as the intumescent ganglion cells die and atrophy. Optic atrophy often results. Therefore, the absence of a spot should not be used to rule out a diagnosis, especially in older children.

Gangliosidoses

GM_1 type I gangliosidosis is an autosomal recessive lysosomal storage disease in which all 3 β-galactosidase isoenzymes (hexosaminidase A, B, and C) are absent. There are 3 forms of this disease: infantile, juvenile, and adult. In the infantile form, a cherry-red spot is present in 50% of patients. Acuity is greatly diminished, and pendular nystagmus is present. Tortuous conjunctival vessels with saccular microaneurysms, optic atrophy, occasional corneal clouding, papilledema, and high myopia may be present. Other features of this disease include hepatosplenomegaly, psychomotor retardation, hypotonia, Hurler-like facial features, kyphosis, and congestive heart failure. Affected children usually die by 1–2 years of age.

GM_2 type I gangliosidosis (Tay-Sachs disease), also an autosomal recessive lysosomal storage disease, is caused by a mutation in the alpha unit of hexosaminidase A. A foveal cherry-red spot occurs in all affected patients by age 6 months, and vision is reduced by age 12–18 months. Nystagmus, optic atrophy, and narrowing of the retinal vessels develop. The disease is characterized by developmental retardation, onset in infancy, followed by paralysis, dementia, and blindness. Patients with Tay-Sachs usually die by 24–30 months of age.

This disease is the most common of the gangliosidoses. It is approximately 100 times more common in infants of Eastern European Jewish (Ashkenazi) descent than in those of non-Jewish descent. Genetic screening and counseling programs in that population have reduced the number of cases of Tay-Sachs disease by 90% in the United States. Other groups, such as French Canadians, can also be affected more often than the general population. The heterozygous condition can be identified so that carriers can be counseled, and the homozygous state can be diagnosed in utero by amniocentesis.

In *GM_2 type II gangliosidosis (Sandhoff disease),* hexosaminidase B beta chain is deficient. The inheritance pattern of this disorder and the ocular and systemic findings are indistinguishable from those of Tay-Sachs disease.

The causative genes for many of the gangliosidoses are known, and carrier detection and treatment strategies are evolving.

Poll-The BT, Maillette de Buy Wenniger-Prick LJ, Barth PG, Duran M. The eye as a window to inborn errors of metabolism. *J Inherit Metab Dis.* 2003;26(2-3):229–244.

HIV/AIDS

The ocular complications of HIV (human immunodeficiency virus) infection and AIDS, including cytomegalovirus retinitis, have been observed only rarely since the advent of highly active antiretroviral therapy (HAART). Such complications typically occur only in children with advanced HIV infection/AIDS and severe immunocompromise. For more information, see BCSC Section 12, *Retina and Vitreous.*

CHAPTER 24

Optic Disc Abnormalities

Developmental Anomalies

Morning Glory Disc Anomaly

Morning glory disc anomaly is caused by either an abnormal closure of the embryonic fissure or abnormal development of the distal optic stalk at its junction with the primitive optic vesicle. Clinically, the anomaly appears as a funnel-shaped excavation of the posterior fundus that incorporates the optic disc. The surrounding retinal pigment epithelium is elevated, with an increased number of blood vessels looping at the edges of the disc (Fig 24-1). A central core of white glial tissue occupies the position of the normal cup. This tissue may have contractile elements, and the optic cup can actually be seen to open and close with some periodicity. Morning glory disc anomaly occurs more frequently in females and is typically unilateral. Visual acuity can range anywhere from 20/20 to no light perception but in general is approximately 20/100 to 20/200. Serous retinal detachments can occur in approximately one-third of affected patients, but the source of the subretinal fluid is unknown. Morning glory disc anomaly has been associated with basal encephalocele in patients with midfacial anomalies. Abnormalities of the carotid circulation, including moyamoya disease (progressive steno-occlusion of the proximal intracranial arteries combined with hypertrophy of collateral vessels at the base of the brain), are associated findings. Therefore, magnetic resonance imaging (MRI) and magnetic resonance angiography of the brain should be obtained in patients with morning glory disc anomaly.

Lenhart PD, Lambert SR, Newman NJ, et al. Intracranial vascular anomalies in patients with morning glory disc anomaly. *Am J Ophthalmol.* 2006;142(4):644–650.

Massaro M, Thorarensen O, Liu GT, Maguire AM, Zimmerman RA, Brodsky MC. Morning glory disc anomaly and moyamoya vessels. *Arch Ophthalmol.* 1998;116(2):253–254.

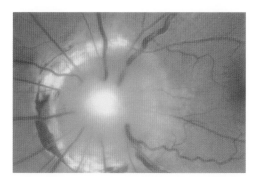

Figure 24-1 Morning glory disc anomaly, left eye.

Coloboma of the Optic Nerve

Coloboma of the optic nerve may be part of a complete chorioretinal coloboma that involves the entire embryonic fissure, or the coloboma may involve only the optic disc. Mild optic disc colobomas resemble deep physiologic cupping and may be confused with glaucomatous damage. More extensive disorders appear as an enlargement of the peripapillary area with a deep central excavation lined by a glistening white tissue, with blood vessels crossing over the edge of this deep cavity (Fig 24-2). The defects usually extend inferonasally and are often associated with retinal coloboma in the periphery. Nonrhegmatogenous or rhegmatogenous retinal detachments may occur. This condition may be unilateral or bilateral and can be very asymmetric. Visual acuity may be mildly or severely decreased and is difficult to predict from the optic disc appearance. Ocular colobomas may also be accompanied by multiple systemic abnormalities (eg, CHARGE association: *c*oloboma, *h*eart, choanal *a*tresia, mental *r*etardation, *g*enitourinary abnormalities, and *e*ar abnormalities; see Chapter 19).

Myelinated (Medullated) Retinal Nerve Fibers

Normal myelination starts at the lateral geniculate ganglion and stops at the lamina cribrosa. Occasionally, some of the fibers in the retina acquire a myelin sheath. Clinically, this appears as a white superficial retinal area whose frayed and feathered edges tend to follow the same orientation as the normal retinal nerve fibers (Fig 24-3). Retinal vessels that pass within the superficial layer of the nerve fibers are obscured. The myelinated fibers may occur as a single spot or as several noncontiguous isolated patches. The most common location is along the disc margin. Vision loss can occur from macular involvement or from unilateral high myopia and amblyopia. In these cases, the macula can also be hypoplastic. Treatment of amblyopia should be attempted but is often unsuccessful. Absolute scotomata correspond to the area of the myelination.

Straatsma BR, Heckenlively JR, Foos RY, Shahinian JK. Myelinated retinal nerve fibers associated with ipsilateral myopia, amblyopia, and strabismus. *Am J Ophthalmol*. 1979;88(3 Pt 1): 506–510.

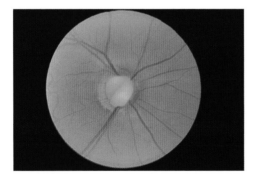

Figure 24-2 Optic nerve coloboma, right eye.

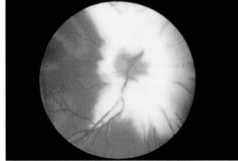

Figure 24-3 Myelinated nerve fibers of optic nerve and retina, right eye.

Tilted Disc Syndrome

In tilted disc syndrome, or *Fuchs coloboma,* the superior pole of the optic disc may appear elevated with posterior displacement of the inferior nasal disc, or the disc can be horizontally tilted, resulting in an oval-appearing optic disc with an obliquely oriented long axis (Fig 24-4). This condition is often accompanied by a scleral crescent located inferiorly or inferonasally, situs inversus (a nasal detour of the temporal retinal vessels as they emerge from the disc before turning back temporally), and posterior ectasia of the inferior nasal fundus. Many affected eyes are myopic.

Because of the fundus abnormality, affected patients have myopic astigmatism. Patients may demonstrate a bitemporal hemianopia, which is typically incomplete and preferentially involves the superior quadrants. The hemianopia can usually be distinguished from a chiasmal lesion because the defect does not respect the vertical midline. Large and small isopters are fairly normal; medium-sized isopters are severely constricted. Appropriate refractive correction often results in elimination of the visual field defect. Tilted discs, myopic astigmatism, bilateral decreased vision, and visual difficulty at night should suggest the possibility of X-linked congenital stationary night blindness (see Chapter 23).

Bergmeister Papilla

To varying extents, the hyaloid artery may not be resorbed before birth. The entire artery may remain as a fine thread or cord extending from the optic disc to the lens and can be associated with *persistent fetal vasculature* (formerly called *persistent hyperplastic primary vitreous*). The hyaloid artery may be patent and contain blood where it was attached to the posterior lens capsule. In mild cases, the attachment to the posterior lens capsule is located inferonasally (Mittendorf dot) and is usually visually insignificant. When all that remains of the hyaloid artery is glial tissue on the disc in association with avascular prepapillary veils and epipapillary membranes, the term *Bergmeister papilla* is used.

Megalopapilla

Megalopapilla features an abnormally large optic disc diameter and is often associated with an increased cup–disc ratio that can be confused with normal-tension glaucoma. Visual acuity is usually normal or slightly decreased, and visual fields may demonstrate

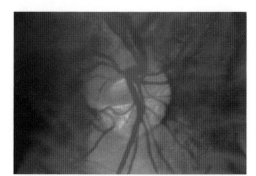

Figure 24-4 Tilted disc syndrome, right eye.

a slightly enlarged blind spot. Rarely, megalopapilla has been associated with optic nerve glioma. The condition can be unilateral or bilateral, and the cause is unknown.

Optic Nerve Hypoplasia

Histologically, optic nerve hypoplasia (ONH) is characterized by a decreased number of optic nerve axons. Clinically, the disc is pale or gray and smaller than normal. This condition can be unilateral or bilateral and is often asymmetric (Fig 24-5). It may be associated with a yellow to white ring around the disc *(double ring sign)*. The outer ring corresponds with the normal junction between the sclera and the lamina cribrosa, and the inner ring corresponds with the abnormal extension of the retina and pigment epithelium over the outer portion of the lamina cribrosa. Because the size of the surrounding ring often corresponds to the normal disc diameter, careful observation is necessary to avoid mistaking the entire hypoplastic disc/ring complex for a normal-sized disc. The vascular pattern is also abnormal and can be associated with too few or too many disc vessels. Retinal vascular tortuosity is common.

Visual acuity ranges from normal to light perception and is related to the integrity of the macular fibers; it often does not correlate with the overall size of the disc. Frequently, visual fields contain localized defects combined with visual field constriction. Children with bilateral ONH often present with congenital sensory nystagmus, and those affected unilaterally often present with sensory strabismus. Because patients with ONH can have strabismus, unilateral vision loss may result from superimposed amblyopia and respond to patching therapy.

Midline central nervous system (CNS) anomalies are associated with bilateral and unilateral ONH. Septo-optic dysplasia *(de Morsier syndrome)* denotes the association of ONH with absence of the septum pellucidum and agenesis of the corpus callosum.

The advent of MRI has expanded the spectrum of CNS anomalies associated with ONH. Patients with ONH may have any combination of absence of the septum pellucidum, agenesis of the corpus callosum, cerebral hemisphere abnormalities, and pituitary gland abnormalities. Cerebral hemisphere abnormalities such as schizencephaly, periventricular leukomalacia, or encephalomalacia occur in approximately 45% of patients with ONH and are associated with neurodevelopmental defects.

MRI shows pituitary gland abnormalities in approximately 15% of patients with ONH. Normally, the posterior pituitary gland appears bright on T1-weighted images. However,

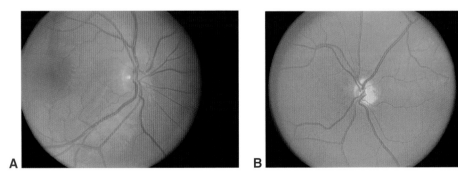

Figure 24-5 Optic nerve hypoplasia. **A,** Normal right optic nerve. **B,** Hypoplastic left optic nerve.

in patients with ONH, this bright spot and/or the pituitary infundibulum may be absent, and an ectopic posterior pituitary bright spot may appear at the upper infundibulum. These abnormalities suggest pituitary hormone deficiency, requiring further endocrinologic workup.

Absence of the septum pellucidum or agenesis of the corpus callosum alone (without cerebral hemisphere or pituitary abnormalities) is not associated with neurodevelopmental defects or endocrinologic dysfunction.

Patients with ONH are at risk for hypothalamic and pituitary dysfunction, such as growth hormone deficiency, hypothyroidism, hyperprolactinemia, panhypopituitarism, and diabetes insipidus. A history of neonatal jaundice suggests hypothyroidism; neonatal hypoglycemia or seizures indicate possible panhypopituitarism. Patients with ONH and diabetes insipidus can have significant problems with thermal regulation and must be monitored carefully during febrile illnesses. Laboratory evaluation of patients with ONH is directed by their clinical appearance and MRI findings. Referral to a pediatric endocrinologist should be considered for patients with either clinical signs of endocrinologic dysfunction or pituitary abnormalities on MRI.

ONH denotes injury to the optic nerve prior to complete development. Thus, ONH can occur from any prenatal or perinatal injury to the optic nerve. Frequently, the etiology is unknown. In patients with associated midline CNS abnormalities (absent septum pellucidum, posterior pituitary ectopia), early gestational injuries to these structures may either directly injure adjacent optic axons or secondarily disrupt axonal migration.

ONH has been associated with maternal ingestion of phenytoin, quinine, and LSD, as well as with fetal alcohol syndrome. Segmental hypoplasia can sometimes occur in children whose mothers have type 1 diabetes mellitus.

Children with *periventricular leukomalacia (PVL)* display an unusual form of ONH. The optic nerves demonstrate a large cup within a normal-sized optic disc. This form of ONH occurs secondary to transsynaptic degeneration of optic axons caused by bilateral lesions in the optic radiations.

Ahmad T, Garcia-Filion P, Borchert M, et al. Endocrinological and auxological abnormalities in young children with optic nerve hypoplasia: a prospective study. *J Pediatr.* 2006;148(1): 78–84.

Brodsky MC, Glasier CM. Optic nerve hypoplasia. Clinical significance of associated central nervous system abnormalities on magnetic resonance imaging. *Arch Ophthalmol.* 1993; 111(1):66–74.

Hoyt WF, Kaplan SL, Grumbach MM, Glaser JS. Septo-optic dysplasia and pituitary dwarfism. *Lancet.* 1970;1(7652):893–894.

Jacobson L, Hellström A, Flodmark O. Large cups in normal-sized optic discs: a variant of optic nerve hypoplasia in children with periventricular leukomalacia. *Arch Ophthalmol.* 1997; 115(10):1263–1269.

Phillips PH, Spear C, Brodsky MC. Magnetic resonance diagnosis of congenital hypopituitarism in children with optic nerve hypoplasia. *J AAPOS.* 2001;5(5):275–280.

Optic Nerve Aplasia

Optic nerve aplasia is rare. There are no optic nerve axons or retinal blood vessels, making the choroidal pattern clearly visible.

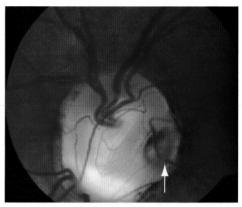

Figure 24-6 Left optic nerve with temporal optic nerve pit *(arrow)* and mild inferonasal disc coloboma. Cilioretinal vessels emanate from the optic nerve pit. *(Courtesy of Paul Phillips, MD.)*

Optic Nerve Pits or Holes

Optic nerve pits (Fig 24-6) are usually unilateral and typically appear in the inferotemporal quadrant or central portion of the disc. A pit may be shallow or very deep, and it is often covered with a gray veil of tissue. Cilioretinal arteries often emerge from pits. Optic nerve pits are associated with serous retinal detachments occurring mainly during the second and third decades of life.

Peripapillary Staphyloma

Peripapillary staphyloma is a posterior bulging of the sclera in which the optic disc occupies the "bottom of the bowl." The disc may be normal, but it is surrounded by stretched choroid, thereby exposing the white sclera encircling the disc. Visual acuity is usually poor.

Brodsky MC. Congenital optic disk anomalies. *Surv Ophthalmol.* 1994;39(2):89–112.

Optic Atrophy

Optic atrophy in children usually results from anterior visual pathway disease (Table 24-1) such as inflammation (optic neuritis), hereditary optic atrophy, perinatal asphyxia, hydrocephalus, and optic nerve tumors. The workup should include neuroimaging in all cases of uncertain cause (negative family history, normal neurologic examination results), because a tumor or hydrocephalus is present in over 40% of these cases.

Dominant Optic Atrophy

Bilateral slow loss of central vision in childhood may be due to dominant optic atrophy. This condition usually begins before the age of 10 years with mild vision loss, ranging from 20/40 to 20/100. Visual fields show central or cecocentral scotomata with normal peripheral isopters. Color vision testing may be diagnostic, revealing a tritan dyschromatopsia. Clinically, the optic disc shows temporal pallor with an area of triangular excavation. Inheritance is autosomal dominant, although family pedigrees may be hard to elicit. Long-term prognosis is good, with visual function rarely reduced to the 20/200 level.

Table 24-1 Causes of Acquired Optic Atrophy in Childhood

Craniopharyngioma
Optic nerve/chiasmal glioma
Hydrocephalus
Postpapilledema
Optic neuritis
Hereditary optic atrophy
Retinal degenerative disease

A rare recessive optic atrophy can occur with severe bilateral vision loss before age 5 years. Nystagmus is present in approximately half of these patients. Funduscopic examination reveals a pale optic disc with vascular attenuation of the type characteristically seen in retinal degeneration. Electroretinogram results are normal, however.

Behr Optic Atrophy

A hereditary disorder, Behr optic atrophy occurs mainly in males, with onset in childhood. This condition is associated with increased deep tendon reflexes, cerebellar ataxia, bladder dysfunction, mental retardation, hypotonia of the extremities, and external ophthalmoplegia.

Leber Hereditary Optic Neuropathy

A maternally inherited (mitochondrial) disease, Leber hereditary optic neuropathy (LHON) is characterized by acute or subacute bilateral loss of central vision, acquired red-green dyschromatopsia, and central or cecocentral scotomata in otherwise healthy patients (usually males) in their second to fourth decade of life. Clinically, this disorder presents with circumpapillary telangiectasia, pseudoedema of the disc, and absence of fluorescein staining. Optic disc pallor develops within a few weeks of onset of visual disturbance. Final visual acuity is rarely better than 20/200. Associated neurologic abnormalities may include paraplegia, dementia, deafness, migraines, vertigo, spasticity, and a cardiac preexcitation arrhythmia (Wolff-Parkinson-White syndrome).

LHON is transmitted by female carriers and involves the mitochondrial DNA (mtDNA). Most cases are associated with point mutations in the mitochondrial genome responsible for complex I (NADH: ubiquinone oxidoreductase). Molecular genetic analysis of mtDNA from leukocytes is currently available, and the finding of a primary mutation is pathognomonic of the disease. No effective treatment exists, although a small percentage of patients will demonstrate spontaneous improvement. Electrocardiogram testing should be considered in order to detect associated cardiac arrhythmias.

Optic Neuritis

Optic neuritis in childhood frequently presents after systemic infections such as measles, mumps, chickenpox, and viral illnesses. It can also be associated with immunizations and bee stings. Vision loss can be severe. Optic neuritis in children, in contrast with that in adults, is more frequently bilateral and associated with disc edema. In over half of affected children, the history suggests CNS involvement including headache, nausea, vomiting, lethargy, or malaise.

The cause of the postinfectious form of viral optic neuritis is unknown. It has been speculated that a presumed autoimmune process, triggered by previous viral infection, may result in a demyelinative injury.

Optic neuritis in children can occur as an isolated neurologic deficit or as a component of more generalized neurologic disease, such as acute disseminated encephalomyelitis, neuromyelitis optica, or multiple sclerosis. The relationship between optic neuritis and the development of multiple sclerosis, which is common in adults, is less clear in children. A small subset of children with optic neuritis develops signs and symptoms consistent with multiple sclerosis. Most of the neurologic deficits are minor, but disability can be severe.

Treatment of optic neuritis in children remains controversial. As vision loss is often bilateral, treatment with intravenous steroids should be considered in order to hasten visual recovery. The Optic Neuritis Treatment Trial did not specifically address the issue of treatment in children. Optic neuritis in the pediatric population is a different clinical entity, so it is difficult to apply the results of this study to children. BCSC Section 5, *Neuro-Ophthalmology*, discusses the treatment of optic neuritis and the relationship between optic neuritis and multiple sclerosis.

Neuroretinitis denotes inflammatory disc edema associated with macular star formation (Fig 24-7). The etiology is most commonly *Bartonella henselae* infection (cat-scratch disease). Other infectious etiologies of neuroretinitis include mumps, *Toxocara*, tuberculosis, and syphilis. Patients with neuroretinitis are not at risk for developing multiple sclerosis. Neuroretinitis is discussed in BCSC Section 5, *Neuro-Ophthalmology*.

Papilledema

Papilledema refers to optic disc edema secondary to elevated intracranial pressure. It is frequently bilateral. Typically, visual acuity, color vision, and pupillary reactions are initially normal. However, visual dysfunction may occur from severe or chronic papilledema.

Increased intracranial pressure in children can be caused by hydrocephalus, mass lesions, meningitis, or pseudotumor cerebri. A full evaluation, including neuroimaging followed by lumbar puncture, is indicated. In infants, increased intracranial pressure results in firmness and distension of the open fontanelles. Significantly elevated pressure is usually accompanied by nausea, vomiting, and headaches. The older child may experience transient visual obscurations. Esotropia and diplopia may result from cranial nerve VI paralysis. The esotropia usually resolves once intracranial pressure is reduced.

Idiopathic Intracranial Hypertension (Pseudotumor Cerebri)

Idiopathic intracranial hypertension (IIH), or *pseudotumor cerebri*, consists of increased intracranial pressure with normal-sized or small ventricles on neuroimaging and normal cerebrospinal fluid content. IIH can occur in children of any age and has been associated with viral infections, drug use (tetracycline, corticosteroids, vitamin A, nalidixic acid,

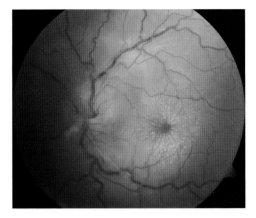

Figure 24-7 Neuroretinitis. Inflammatory optic disc edema with a macular star. *(Courtesy of Paul Phillips, MD.)*

thyroid medications, growth hormone), and cerebral venous sinus thrombosis. *Prepubescent* children with IIH have a lower incidence of obesity compared with adult patients, and the male to female ratio is approximately equal. *Postpubescent* children with IIH have a clinical profile similar to that of adults, with a higher incidence of obesity compared with younger patients and female gender preponderance.

Common presenting symptoms are headache, vision loss, transient visual obscurations, and strabismus observed by the parents. Papilledema may be noted on a routine examination of an asymptomatic child. Ocular examination frequently reveals excellent visual acuity with bilateral papilledema. Unilateral or bilateral cranial nerve VI deficits may be present. The patient should be monitored closely for decreased visual acuity, visual field loss, and worsening headaches. Visual field tests can be difficult to interpret in children but should be obtained, if possible.

Medical treatments include acetazolamide and topiramate (Topamax). Surgical treatment options include optic nerve sheath fenestration and lumbar or ventriculoperitoneal shunts. Optic nerve sheath fenestration and shunting procedures reduce the incidence of vision loss. Shunting procedures are preferred for patients with good visual function and severe headaches that are not responsive to medical management. The visual prognosis is excellent for most patients, although vision loss can occur secondary to chronic papilledema; spontaneous resolution occurs in most cases within 12–18 months.

Rangwala LM, Liu GT. Pediatric idiopathic intracranial hypertension. *Surv Ophthalmol.* 2007; 52(6):597–617.

Pseudopapilledema

Pseudopapilledema refers to any elevated anomaly of the optic disc that resembles papilledema (Table 24-2). Disc anomalies that are frequently confused with papilledema in children include drusen, hyperopia, and prominent glial tissue. Pseudopapilledema can be differentiated from true papilledema by the absence of disc hyperemia, retinal hemorrhages, and exudates and by the lack of any systemic findings that are usually associated

Table 24-2 Conditions Associated With Pediatric Optic Disc Swelling

Papillitis
Optic neuritis (postinfectious)
Toxoplasmosis
Lyme disease
Bartonella infection
Neuroretinitis
Toxocara infection of disc
Leber hereditary optic neuropathy
Papilledema
   Intracranial mass
   Meningitis
   Idiopathic intracranial hypertension
   Dural sinus thrombosis
   Cranial synostosis
   Hydrocephalus
      Chiari malformation
      Aqueductal stenosis
      Dandy-Walker syndrome
      Infection
Hypertension
Astrocytoma of optic disc (tuberous sclerosis)
Optic nerve glioma
Leukemia infiltrate
Pseudopapilledema
   Optic disc drusen
   Hyperopia
   Glial veils

with increased intracranial pressure (Fig 24-8A). Pseudopapilledema is associated with anomalous branching of the large retinal vessels.

Most children with pseudopapilledema do not have other related ophthalmic or systemic abnormalities. However, pseudopapilledema is associated with Down syndrome, Alagille syndrome, and retinitis pigmentosa. Down syndrome is associated with IIH as well; thus, an elevated optic disc in a child with Down syndrome should not be assumed to be benign. If there are clinical symptoms and signs of elevated intracranial pressure (headaches, cranial nerve VI palsy, true papilledema), neuroimaging followed by lumbar puncture should be obtained.

Drusen

Intrapapillary drusen, the most common cause of pseudopapilledema in children, can appear within the first or second decade of life (Fig 24-8B). Drusen are frequently inherited, and examination of the parents is helpful when drusen are suspected in children.

Clinically, the elevated disc does not obscure the retinal arterioles lying anteriorly and often has an irregular border suggesting the presence of drusen beneath the surface. There is no dilation of the papillary network, and retinal hemorrhages and exudates are absent. Peripapillary subretinal hemorrhages and subretinal neovascular membranes rarely occur. When drusen are not buried, they appear as shiny refractile bodies visible on the

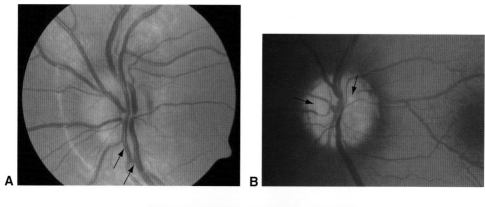

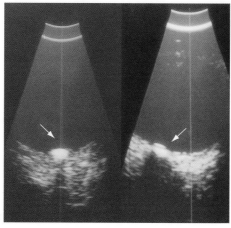

Figure 24-8 **A,** Pseudopapilledema. There is anomalous branching *(arrows)* of the large retinal vessels without disc hyperemia, retinal hemorrhages, or exudates. **B,** Optic nerve head drusen seen as refractile opacities on disc surface *(arrows)*. **C,** Ultrasonographic image of bright spot in nerve *(arrows)* consistent with drusen. *(Parts A and B courtesy of Paul Phillips, MD; part C courtesy of Edward G. Buckley, MD.)*

disc surface, with a gray-yellow translucent appearance. Visual field defects are frequently associated; lower nasal field defects are common. However, concentric narrowing, an arcuate scotoma, and central defects can also occur. These defects can be slowly progressive, and central visual acuity is rarely affected.

Although some patients with drusen can be identified by funduscopic evaluation, occasionally it is difficult to tell for certain that drusen are responsible for the swollen disc appearance. B-scan ultrasonography can be helpful in this situation (Fig 24-8C). This technique permits detection of bright objects in the end of the optic nerve. Computed tomography can also detect these drusen.

Most children with optic disc drusen do not have other related ophthalmic or systemic abnormalities. However, children with pseudoxanthoma elasticum or retinitis pigmentosa have a higher incidence of optic disc drusen compared with the general population.

Auw-Haedrich C, Staubach F, Witschel H. Optic disk drusen. *Surv Ophthalmol.* 2002;47(6): 515–532.

CHAPTER 25

Childhood Nystagmus

The child with nystagmus presents a difficult diagnostic challenge. The primary goal of the ophthalmic evaluation is to determine whether the nystagmus is a sign of a significant neurologic abnormality such as a brain tumor that necessitates immediate intervention, an ocular abnormality that may affect visual development, or a motor defect that is compatible with good visual function. In many children with horizontal nystagmus, the condition occurs because of reduced vision, poor fusion, or both. These ophthalmic causes often can be determined by standard office examination techniques. However, vertical nystagmus and the presence of other neurologic deficits suggest a nonophthalmic etiology that may warrant further neurologic investigation, including neuroimaging. BCSC Section 5, *Neuro-Ophthalmology,* discusses the neurologic implications of nystagmus.

Abadi RV, Bjerre A. Motor and sensory characteristics of infantile nystagmus. *Br J Ophthalmol.* 2002;86(10):1152–1160.

Nomenclature

Nystagmus is an involuntary, rhythmic to-and-fro oscillation of the eyes. In *pendular nystagmus,* the eyes oscillate with equal velocity in each direction. *Jerk nystagmus* denotes a movement of unequal speed; by convention, the fast component defines the direction of the nystagmus—for example, a right jerk nystagmus has a slow movement to the left and a fast movement (jerk) to the right.

The nystagmus movement can be further classified according to the frequency (number of oscillations per unit of time) and the amplitude (the angular distance traveled during the movement). The movements may be horizontal, vertical, rotary, oblique, or circular. Characteristics of the eye movements may change with different gaze direction. A pendular nystagmus can become jerk on extreme gaze.

Certain gaze positions can affect the amplitude and frequency. This is especially true of jerk nystagmus, which typically has a *null point* (the gaze location where the nystagmus is minimal) located in the gaze opposite the fast-phase component *(Alexander's law).* Thus, a right jerk nystagmus becomes much worse on right gaze and improves significantly on left gaze. A patient with a right jerk nystagmus would therefore develop a right head turn and left gaze preference (Fig 25-1).

The National Eye Institute (NEI) has reclassified eye movement abnormalities, including nystagmus. For the discussion of nystagmus in this chapter, we use the traditional, familiar designations. Alternative terminology recommended by the NEI-sponsored Committee for the Classification of Eye Movement Abnormalities and Strabismus (CEMAS) is

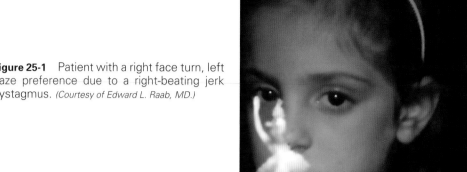

Figure 25-1 Patient with a right face turn, left gaze preference due to a right-beating jerk nystagmus. *(Courtesy of Edward L. Raab, MD.)*

indicated in parentheses. The document produced by the CEMAS committee is available on the NEI website at http://www.nei.nih.gov/news/statements/cemas.pdf.

> Hertle RW; National Eye Institute Sponsored Classification of Eye Movement Abnormalities and Strabismus Working Group. A next step in naming and classification of eye movement disorders and strabismus. *J AAPOS.* 2002;6(4):201–202.

Evaluation

History

Many forms of nystagmus are inherited, either as a direct genetic abnormality or because of an association with other ocular diseases (Table 25-1). A thorough family history is important in the initial evaluation. Questions should be asked about other types of inherited ocular diseases, systemic diseases, or syndromes known to affect visual development. Congenital motor nystagmus may be inherited as an autosomal dominant, recessive, or X-linked trait. Examination of family members with nystagmus can provide valuable prognostic information about the anticipated visual function in affected children.

Events at the time of delivery can significantly affect the developing visual system and, if severe enough, can result in nystagmus. Inquiries as to whether there were problems with labor and delivery, maternal infections, and prematurity can illuminate the cause of nystagmus. In children older than 3 months, parental observations about head tilts, head movements, gaze preference, and viewing distances can aid in diagnosis.

Ocular Examination

The ophthalmic evaluation should concentrate on visual acuity testing, pupillary responses, ocular motility, and funduscopic examination.

Visual acuity testing

The level of visual function can be helpful in determining the cause of nystagmus. Patients with nystagmus and nearly normal visual acuity usually have congenital motor nystagmus,

Table 25-1 Ocular Conditions Associated With Nystagmus

Congenital cataract
Congenital glaucoma
Iridocorneal dysgenesis
Congenital toxoplasmosis
Congenital "macular coloboma"
Bilateral optic nerve hypoplasia/atrophy
Optic nerve coloboma
Retinal coloboma
Foveal hypoplasia
  Aniridia
  Albinism
    Ocular albinism
    Oculocutaneous albinism
Retinal dystrophy
  Leber congenital amaurosis
  Achromatopsia
  Congenital stationary night blindness
Congenital retinoschisis
Retinal dysplasia
Retinoblastoma
Cicatricial retinopathy of prematurity

which is a benign entity. Markedly decreased visual acuity usually implies either retinal or optic nerve abnormalities. Visual acuity should be measured at distance and near as well as under binocular conditions, allowing children to use whatever head position or movement they choose. This last measurement is crucial in establishing the true functional visual performance.

Near visual acuity is usually better than at distance and can indicate the difficulty the child is likely to experience in a school setting. Many children with 20/400 or worse distance acuity can read at the 20/40 to 20/60 level by viewing the material at close range. Glasses or other devices can enable these children to master the school curriculum.

In preverbal children, the *optokinetic nystagmus (OKN)* drum can be used to estimate visual acuity. If vertical rotation of an OKN drum elicits a vertical nystagmus superimposed on the child's underlying nystagmus, the visual function is usually 20/400 or better. Preferential looking also can be used, but the response can be more easily observed with the card held vertically in patients with a horizontal nystagmus.

Pupils
Pupils should be assessed for asymmetry, direct reaction to light, afferent defect, reaction to darkness, and anatomical structure.

Sluggish or absent response to light or an afferent defect indicates anterior visual pathway abnormalities, such as optic nerve or retinal dysfunction. Responses can be normal in mild abnormalities, such as foveal hypoplasia, rod monochromatism, and primary motor nystagmus. The normal response to darkness is the immediate dilation of the pupil. If, instead of dilating, the pupils paradoxically constrict, optic nerve or retinal disease is present (Table 25-2).

Table 25-2 Differential Diagnosis of Paradoxical Pupils

Congenital stationary night blindness
Congenital achromatopsia
Leber congenital amaurosis
Retinitis pigmentosa
Best disease
Albinism
Optic nerve hypoplasia

In addition to pupillary responses, iris structure should be assessed. Defects such as colobomas suggest similar optic nerve or retinal defects. Excess iris transillumination is a hallmark of albinism. Aniridia and albinism are associated with foveal hypoplasia, poor vision, and nystagmus.

Ocular motility

Patients with nystagmus often have strabismus, either as a result of poor vision or as an attempt to damp the nystagmus by converging. Children with manifest latent nystagmus usually fixate with the preferred eye in adduction and turn their heads to look across their noses. They use this maneuver at distance or near to improve visual acuity.

Fundus

Optic nerve or foveal hypoplasia is common in children with nystagmus. Although many of the retinal disorders are associated with visible abnormalities, in some, the fundus appears normal or there are subtle retinal pigmentary changes (Table 25-3). In patients with nystagmus and normal-appearing posterior poles, electrophysiologic testing may be necessary to identify the cause.

Childhood Nystagmus Types

Some authors have described a transient nystagmus occurring in children before 2 months of age and subsiding after about 6 months. In the absence of other causes, the nystagmus was attributed to as-yet immature and unstable motor control.

Good WV, Hou C, Carden SM. Transient, idiopathic nystagmus in infants. *Dev Med Child Neurol.* 2003;45(5):304–307.

Table 25-3 Conditions Associated With Decreased Vision and Minimal Fundus Changes

Leber congenital amaurosis
Rod monochromacy
Blue-cone monochromacy
Congenital stationary night blindness
Ocular albinism
Optic nerve hypoplasia
Hereditary optic atrophy

Congenital Nystagmus (Infantile Nystagmus Syndrome)

Congenital motor nystagmus

Congenital motor nystagmus is a binocular conjugate nystagmus that is usually horizontal and commonly remains so on upgaze and downgaze (uniplanar). Congenital motor nystagmus can be pendular, jerk, circular, or elliptical, and more than 1 type may exist in the same individual. The characteristic waveform of congenital motor jerk nystagmus is a slow phase with an exponential increase in velocity. A null point, or *neutral zone,* may be present; this is a gaze position in which the intensity of oscillations is diminished and the visual acuity improves. If the null point is not in primary position, anomalous head postures may be adopted to damp the nystagmus and provide the best visual acuity. Head bobbing or movement may also be present at first, although this usually decreases with age. Oscillopsia is rare. See Table 25-4.

Congenital motor nystagmus is damped by convergence and therefore is often associated with esotropia. This combination of nystagmus and esotropia has been termed *nystagmus blockage syndrome,* a distinction from those cases in which esotropia and nystagmus happen to coexist. Patients with nystagmus blockage syndrome characteristically present with an esotropia that "eats up prism" on attempted measurement and exhibit an increased jerk nystagmus on attempted lateral gaze.

Purely congenital motor nystagmus is not associated with other central nervous system abnormalities. Visual function can be near normal. Patients develop a preferred gaze position to utilize a null location, thereby increasing foveation time, during which their acquisition of visual information occurs. This head position becomes more obvious as the child reaches school age.

Approximately two-thirds of these patients exhibit a paradoxical inversion of the OKN response. Normally, if a patient with right jerk nystagmus views an OKN drum rotating to the patient's left (eliciting a pursuit left, jerk right response), the right jerk nystagmus will increase. However, patients with congenital motor nystagmus exhibit either a damped right jerk nystagmus or possibly even a left jerk nystagmus. This paradoxical response occurs only in congenital nystagmus.

Stevens DJ, Hertle RW. Relationship between visual acuity and anomalous head posture in patients with congenital nystagmus. *J Pediatr Ophthalmol Strabismus.* 2003;40(5):259–264.

Table 25-4 Characteristics of Congenital Nystagmus

Bilateral
Conjugate
Horizontal
Uniplanar
Worsens with attempted fixation
Improves with convergence
Null point often present with head position
Two-thirds of patients have "inverted" OKN response
Oscillopsia usually not present

Congenital sensory nystagmus

Congenital sensory nystagmus, another form of congenital nystagmus, is secondary to a bilateral, pregeniculate, afferent visual pathway abnormality. Inadequate image formation results in failure of development of the normal fixation reflex. If this is present at birth, the resulting nystagmus begins in the first 3 months of life. Its severity depends on that of the vision loss.

The nystagmus is typically horizontal and uniplanar and has a waveform identical to that of congenital motor nystagmus. Pendular nystagmus is most common and on lateral gaze, the nystagmus may become jerk.

Searching, slow, wandering conjugate eye movements may also be observed. Searching nystagmus, defined as a roving or drifting, typically horizontal, movement of the eyes without fixation, is usually observed in children whose vision is worse than 20/200. Pendular nystagmus occurs when the visual acuity is better than 20/200 in at least 1 eye. Jerk nystagmus is often associated with visual acuity between 20/60 and 20/100.

The associated bilateral, pregeniculate afferent abnormality may be obvious, such as in children with bilateral cataracts or corneal opacities. The ocular abnormality may be more subtle, such as in children with optic nerve hypoplasia or foveal hypoplasia. A child with congenital sensory nystagmus from a retinal dystrophy may have mild vascular attenuation, optic disc pallor, or a completely normal retinal appearance. An electroretinogram may be required for diagnosis. See Table 25-1 for the ocular conditions that can give rise to sensory nystagmus.

> Hamed LM. Congenital nystagmus: in search of simplicity on the other side of complexity. *J AAPOS.* 1999;3(2):67–68.
>
> Hertle RW, Dell'Osso LF. Clinical and ocular motor analysis of congenital nystagmus in infancy. *J AAPOS.* 1999;3(2):70–79.

Periodic alternating nystagmus

Periodic alternating nystagmus (PAN; *central vestibular instability nystagmus*) is an unusual form of congenital motor jerk nystagmus that periodically changes direction. The motion typically starts with a jerk nystagmus in 1 direction that lasts for 60–90 seconds and then slowly begins to damp, until it reaches a period of no nystagmus that lasts from 10 to 20 seconds, followed by nystagmus that jerks in the opposite direction in a repeating process. Some children adopt an alternating head position to take advantage of the changing null position. The cause of congenital PAN is unknown, but this condition has been associated with oculocutaneous albinism.

Latent nystagmus

Latent nystagmus *(fusion maldevelopment nystagmus syndrome)* is a congenital conjugate horizontal jerk nystagmus that is a marker of fusion maldevelopment. Latent nystagmus occurs in children with decreased fusion, which results from either early onset strabismus or decreased vision in 1 or both eyes. When 1 eye is occluded, a jerk nystagmus develops in both eyes, with the fast phase directed toward the uncovered eye. Thus, a left jerk nystagmus of both eyes occurs when the right eye is covered, and a right jerk nystagmus of both eyes occurs when the left eye is covered. This nystagmus is the only form that reverses direction as driven by a change in fixation. Similarly, the null point and corresponding head position reverse with a change in fixation (Fig 25-2). The null point is with the fixating eye in adduction. Therefore, occlusion of the right eye induces a left jerk nystagmus with a null point in right gaze (left head turn). Occlusion of the left eye induces a right jerk nystagmus with a null point in left gaze (right head turn). Asymmetries in amplitude, frequency, and velocity of the nystagmus also can be present, depending on which eye is covered.

Latent nystagmus usually is noted in early childhood, particularly in patients with congenital esotropia and dissociated vertical deviation. The cause is unknown but may be related to the mechanism of vestibular nystagmus, as well as fusion maldevelopment. Because latent nystagmus is induced when an eye is covered, binocular visual acuity is better than monocular, and occlusion must be avoided during monocular tests of vision. Use of polarizing lenses and a polarized chart, blurring of the nontested eye with a +5.00 D sphere, or repositioning of the occluder several inches in front of the eye not being tested can be effective.

Latent nystagmus is damped by fusion and increased with disruption of fusion (such as ocular occlusion). Latent nystagmus may become manifest (manifest latent nystagmus) when both eyes are open but only 1 eye is being used for vision (ie, the other eye is suppressed or amblyopic). Occlusion of the preferred eye results in a change in the direction of the jerk nystagmus. Electronystagmographic evaluation of latent and manifest latent nystagmus reveals a similar waveform with an exponential decrease in velocity of the slow phase—a pattern opposite that of congenital motor nystagmus, which shows an exponential increase in slow-phase velocity (Fig 25-3).

Brodsky MC, Tusa RJ. Latent nystagmus: vestibular nystagmus with a twist. *Arch Ophthalmol.* 2004;122(2):202–209.

Gottlob I. Nystagmus. *Curr Opin Ophthalmol.* 2001;12(5):378–383.

Richards M, Wong A, Foeller P, Bradley D, Tychsen L. Duration of binocular decorrelation predicts the severity of latent (fusion maldevelopment) nystagmus in strabismic macaque monkeys. *Invest Ophthalmol Vis Sci.* 2008;49(5):1872–1878.

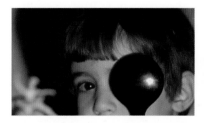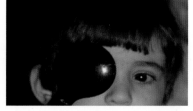

Figure 25-2 Latent nystagmus. There is a right face turn during fixation with the right eye. The head turn reverses during fixation with the left eye. The null point is with the fixating eye in adduction. *(Courtesy of Edward L. Raab, MD.)*

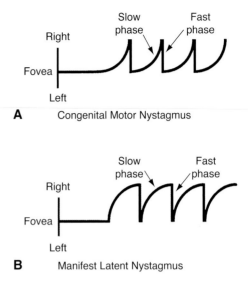

Figure 25-3 Left jerk nystagmus. **A,** Electronystagmographic evaluation of congenital motor nystagmus shows an exponential increase in velocity of the slow phase. **B,** Manifest latent nystagmus shows a waveform with an exponential decrease in velocity of the slow phase.

Acquired Nystagmus

Spasmus nutans

Spasmus nutans *(spasmus nutans syndrome)* is an acquired nystagmus that occurs in children during the first 2 years of life, presenting as a triad of nystagmus, head nodding, and torticollis. The nystagmus generally is bilateral and of small amplitude and high frequency (shimmering); however, it can be monocular, asymmetric, and variable in different gaze positions. It can be horizontal, vertical, or rotary and is occasionally intermittent. The head nodding and torticollis appear to be compensatory movements that reduce the frequency and asymmetry of the nystagmus and therefore maximize vision.

Spasmus nutans occasionally can be familial and has been present in monozygotic twins. It usually disappears by age 3–4 years. It is a benign idiopathic disorder in most cases, but nystagmus characteristic of spasmus nutans has been associated with chiasmal or suprachiasmal tumors and retinal dystrophies such as congenital stationary night blindness in children. Neuroradiologic investigation is warranted if spasmus nutans occurs with evidence of optic nerve dysfunction (optic disc pallor, relative afferent pupillary defect). As subtle optic disc pallor and relative afferent pupillary defects are difficult to detect in children, some investigators believe that neuroimaging is indicated for all children with spasmus nutans, although this view is controversial. Electroretinography should be considered in children with spasmus nutans and clinical signs of a retinal dystrophy such as myopia or paradoxical pupils.

Gottlob I, Wizov SS, Reinecke RD. Spasmus nutans. A long-term follow-up. *Invest Ophthalmol Vis Sci.* 1995;36(13):2768–2771.

Lambert SR, Newman NJ. Retinal disease masquerading as spasmus nutans. *Neurology.* 1993;43(8):1607–1609.

Shaw FS, Kriss A, Russel-Eggitt I, Taylor D, Harris C. Diagnosing children presenting with asymmetric pendular nystagmus. *Dev Med Child Neurol.* 2001;43(9):622–627.

Unsöld R, Ostertag C. Nystagmus in suprasellar tumors: recent advances in diagnosis and therapy. *Strabismus.* 2002;10(2):173–177.

See-saw nystagmus

See-saw nystagmus *(vision loss nystagmus)*, an unusual but dramatic type of nystagmus, has both vertical and torsional components. The name derives from the action of the familiar playground device. If 2 eyes were placed on a see-saw, one at either end, they would "roll down the plank" as the see-saw rose, with the high eye intorting and the low eye extorting. As the direction of the see-saw changed, so would that of the eye movement. Thus, the eyes make alternating movements of elevation and intorsion followed by depression and extorsion.

This type of nystagmus is often associated with a lesion in the rostral midbrain or the suprasellar area. In children, the most likely associated intracranial tumor is a craniopharyngioma. Confrontation visual fields may elicit a bitemporal defect. Neuroradiologic evaluation is necessary. The treatment for see-saw nystagmus is removal of the inciting cause.

Convergence-retraction nystagmus

Convergence-retraction nystagmus *(induced convergence-retraction)* is part of the dorsal midbrain syndrome associated with paralysis of upward gaze, defective convergence, eyelid retraction, and pupillary light–near dissociation. In the pediatric age group, convergence-retraction nystagmus is commonly secondary to congenital aqueductal stenosis or a pinealoma. It is best elicited on attempted upgaze saccades (eg, by asking the patient to track a downwardly rotating OKN drum). Co-contraction of all the horizontal extraocular muscles occurs, and the eyes are pulled into the orbit. In addition, the medial rectus muscles overpower the lateral rectus muscles, causing the eyes to converge on attempted upgaze (hence the term *convergence-retraction*). However, voluntary convergence is minimal. The abnormal eye movements in convergence-retraction nystagmus are actually saccades. Therefore, convergence-retraction nystagmus is not a true nystagmus and is considered a disjunctive saccadic oscillation.

Opsoclonus

Opsoclonus is an extremely rare eye movement disorder that, like convergence-retraction nystagmus, is not a true nystagmus. Rather, it is a bizarre, rapid, and involuntary ocular oscillation. Opsoclonus can be present intermittently and often has a very-high-frequency, low-amplitude movement. The movements are so fast and chaotic that they are not easily confused with other forms of infantile nystagmus.

Common causes of opsoclonus in children are acute postinfectious cerebellar ataxia and epidemic viral encephalitis. Opsoclonus can also be a paraneoplastic manifestation of occult neuroblastoma.

Downbeat nystagmus

Downbeat nystagmus is a jerk nystagmus with the fast component downward. It obeys Alexander's law (see the section Nomenclature, earlier in this chapter) and is maximum in downgaze and down to the left and right. Downbeat nystagmus often has a null position in upgaze. When congenital, this condition is associated with good vision and normal neurologic findings, although a hereditary form of downbeat nystagmus may precede spinocerebellar degeneration.

More commonly, downbeat nystagmus is acquired, secondary to structural abnormalities such as the Arnold-Chiari malformation. In this condition, the cerebellar tonsils herniate through the foramen magnum, compressing the brain stem and resulting in downbeat nystagmus. Decompression of this area often results in complete resolution. Pharmacologic agents such as codeine, lithium, tranquilizers, and anticonvulsants may also cause this condition.

Monocular nystagmus

Monocular nystagmus has been reported to occur in severely amblyopic and blind eyes. The oscillations are pendular, chiefly vertical, slow, small in amplitude, and irregular in frequency.

Dissociated nystagmus

Nystagmus only in the abducting eye (dissociated nystagmus) occurs in several conditions, the most familiar being internuclear ophthalmoplegia. Myasthenia gravis may simulate an internuclear ophthalmoplegia. Surgical weakening of the medial rectus muscle has been reported to cause a nystagmus of the contralateral abducting eye similar to that seen with internuclear ophthalmoplegia but without the slowing of saccades in the adducting eye that occurs in the latter condition.

Differential Diagnosis

Figure 25-4 presents the signs and symptoms of various forms of horizontal nystagmus in children, along with guidelines for testing and systemic associations.

Treatment

Prisms

Prisms can optically improve head positions by shifting the image into the null zone, or they can improve visual acuity by inducing convergence. They can be used as the sole treatment or as a trial to predict surgical success. Fresnel Press-On prisms are useful for this because powers of 10Δ–20Δ are often necessary. However, Fresnel prisms are not transparent and may reduce visual acuity. Ground-in prisms are transparent and may maximize visual acuity for children who require smaller amounts of prism. Surfacing laboratories are able to grind as much as 12Δ into spectacle lenses.

To correct head positions, each prism is mounted with the apex pointing to the direction of the null zone. For example, with a left head turn and a null zone in right gaze, prisms before the right eye should be oriented base-in and prisms before the left eye should be oriented base-out. This shifts the image to the right and decreases the amount of head turn the patient requires to gain the same visual benefit. If this technique improves the head position, strabismus surgery is also likely to be effective. A limitation of prism

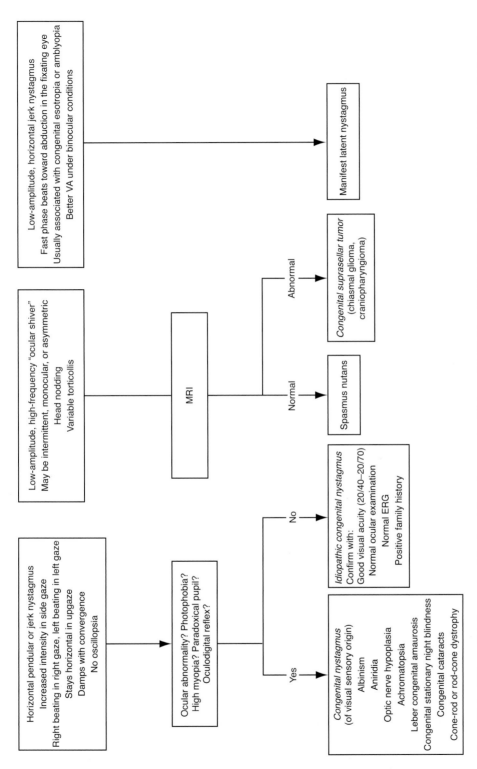

Figure 25-4 Differential diagnosis of horizontal nystagmus in children. *(Modified from Brodsky MC, Baker RS, Hamed LM. Pediatric Neuro-Ophthalmology. New York: Springer-Verlag; 1995:339.)*

treatment is that, unlike surgery, it does not bring the eyes out of the gaze position necessary to achieve the null zone.

Prism spectacles may improve visual acuity by stimulating fusional convergence, which damps the nystagmus. In this situation, base-out prisms are placed in front of both eyes in amounts determined by trial and error.

Nystagmus Surgery

Extraocular muscle surgery for nystagmus is indicated to correct a head turn by shifting the null point closer to the primary position. Surgery can also improve visual acuity by decreasing nystagmus intensity and therefore improving foveation time. The types of surgery typically recommended are a recession-resection procedure performed on both eyes *(Kestenbaum-Anderson)* or a 4-horizontal-muscle recession.

In the Kestenbaum-Anderson procedure, the eyes are surgically rotated toward the direction of the head turn and away from the null zone or preferred position of gaze. Each eye undergoes a recession-resection procedure to move the eyes in the same direction. For example, if a patient with congenital nystagmus has a left face turn and null zone in right gaze, the eyes are surgically rotated to the left by recession of the right lateral and left medial rectus muscles and by resection of the right medial and left lateral rectus muscles. This makes it more difficult for the patient to look into right gaze, thereby damping the nystagmus more toward the primary position (Fig 25-5).

The amount of recession-resection performed in the Kestenbaum-Anderson procedure has been modified through experience. Table 25-5 describes the original operation plus 2 modifications in which the amount of surgery is increased by 40% or 60%. The resulting amounts are rounded off to the nearest 0.5 mm. The total amount of surgery for each eye (as measured in millimeters) is equal in order to rotate each globe an equal amount. For face turns of 30°, the 40% augmented procedure is recommended; for turns of 45°, the 60% augmentation procedure is employed. The augmented procedures may cause restriction of motility, which is usually necessary to achieve a satisfactory result.

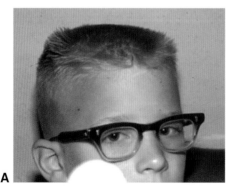
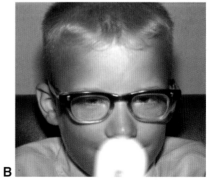

A   B

Figure 25-5 **A,** Congenital motor nystagmus with the null point in right gaze. **B,** Null point shifted by the Kestenbaum-Anderson procedure, eliminating the necessity for a head turn. *(Courtesy of Edward L. Raab, MD.)*

Table 25-5 **Kestenbaum-Anderson Procedure and Modifications**

Procedure	Kestenbaum	40% Augmented	60% Augmented
Recess medial rectus	5.0 mm	7.0 mm	8.0 mm
Resect medial rectus	6.0 mm	8.4 mm	9.6 mm
Recess lateral rectus	7.0 mm	9.8 mm	11.2 mm
Resect lateral rectus	8.0 mm	11.2 mm	12.8 mm
Total surgery	13.0 mm	18.2 mm	20.8 mm
R + R	(5 + 8) = (6 + 7)	(7 + 11.2) = (8.4 + 9.8)	(8 + 12.8) = (9.6 + 11.2)

If vertical torticollis is present with congenital nystagmus, chin-up or chin-down posturing may be ameliorated in some cases by vertical prism (again, apex toward the null zone) or by surgery on the vertical rectus muscles or the oblique muscles. As with horizontal nystagmus, the eyes are rotated away from the null point. Thus, if a chin-up, eyes-down posture is present, the inferior rectus muscles are recessed and the superior rectus muscles are resected. The amount of surgery is usually 5–7 mm of recession and resection of the vertical rectus muscles of each eye.

Recession of all the horizontal rectus muscles to a position posterior to the equator is an alternative to the Kestenbaum-Anderson procedure. It usually requires 8–10 mm of recession of both medial rectus muscles and 10–12 mm of recession of both lateral rectus muscles. This approach may be especially beneficial for improving visual function when the head position is not a problem, but a newly generated deviation is possible. Further, recent studies have found that merely disinserting and reattaching the horizontal rectus muscles, without recession or resection, may be beneficial to damp the nystagmus and improve visual function. Nystagmus surgery in the absence of abnormal head posture is controversial.

Surgery for nystagmus blockage syndrome involves recession of the medial rectus muscles, usually with amounts that are slightly larger than normal. This can be combined with posterior fixation sutures to enhance the effect.

For nystagmus patients with strabismus, the surgery must be performed on the dominant fixating eye; surgery on the nondominant eye is adjusted to account for the strabismus. For example, a patient who is right-eye dominant and has a right head turn and left gaze null zone would undergo a right medial rectus recession and right lateral rectus resection in the amounts indicated in Table 25-5. This procedure could lessen or eliminate a coexisting esotropia and would increase an exotropia. Surgery on the nonpreferred eye is tailored to these possibilities.

Hertle RW, Dell'Osso LF, FitzGibbon EJ, Thompson D, Yang D, Mellow SD. Horizontal rectus tenotomy in patients with congenital nystagmus: results in 10 adults. *Ophthalmology.* 2003;110(11):2097–2105.

Reinecke RD. Costenbader Lecture. Idiopathic infantile nystagmus: diagnosis and treatment. *J AAPOS.* 1997;1(2):67–82.

Roberts EL, Saunders RA, Wilson ME. Surgery for vertical head position in null point nystagmus. *J Pediatr Ophthalmol Strabismus.* 1996;33(4):219–224.

Zubcov AA, Stärk N, Weber A, Wizov SS, Reinecke RD. Improvement of visual acuity after surgery for nystagmus. *Ophthalmology.* 1993;100(10):1488–1497.

Low Vision Rehabilitation

Children with nystagmus often have permanent reduced visual acuity, even after treatment with prisms and surgery. Children with reduced vision require formal low vision assessments and low vision rehabilitation. (For patients whose visual function could be helped or enhanced by vision rehabilitation, the American Academy of Ophthalmology provides the SmartSight website: http://one.aao.org/CE/EducationalContent/Smartsight.aspx.)

CHAPTER **26**

Ocular and Periocular Tumors in Childhood

Ocular and orbital tumors, both benign and malignant, occur relatively frequently in infants and children. Benign masses are much more common than malignant ones. Ocular and orbital tumors can be classified by location and type (Table 26-1). See also BCSC Section 4, *Ophthalmic Pathology and Intraocular Tumors,* and Section 7, *Orbit, Eyelids, and Lacrimal System.*

Shields JA, Shields CL. Pediatric ocular and periocular tumors. *Pediatr Ann.* 2001;30(8): 491–501.

Orbital Tumors

A wide variety of space-occupying lesions can develop in the region of the orbit during childhood. Several of the most important pediatric malignancies show a predilection for orbital involvement. Benign adnexal masses are common and, in many cases, constitute a threat to vision.

Differential Diagnosis

The diagnosis of space-occupying lesions in the orbit is a particular challenge because the clinical manifestations of these lesions are both nonspecific and relatively limited in variety:

- proptosis or other displacement of the globe
- swelling or discoloration of the eyelids
- palpable subcutaneous mass
- ptosis
- strabismus

The problem of differential diagnosis in childhood is compounded by the fact that in young patients, both benign and malignant tumors often enlarge very rapidly, making them difficult to distinguish from one another; from infectious and inflammatory disorders such as orbital cellulitis; and from the effects of trauma, which occurs with high frequency and often without a reliable history. Furthermore, mild to moderate proptosis can be difficult to detect in an uncooperative child with associated eyelid swelling.

Table 26-1 Ocular and Orbital Tumor Classification

I. Orbital lesions
  A. Cystic lesions
    1. Developmental orbital cysts
      a. Choristoma, dermoid, epidermoid
      b. Teratoma
      c. Congenital cystic eye
      d. Colobomatous cyst
    2. Acquired orbital cysts
      a. Cystic vascular lesions
      b. Epithelial appendage cysts
      c. Epithelial implantation cysts
      d. Lacrimal duct cysts
      e. Optic nerve sheath meningocele
      f. Hematic cyst
      g. Aneurysmal bone cyst
      h. Cystic myositis
      i. Parasitic cysts: hydatid, cysticercus cellulosae
      j. Chocolate cyst
      k. Cholesterol granulomatous cyst
    3. Adjacent structure cysts
      a. Mucocele
      b. Mucopyocele
      c. Dacryocele
      d. Cephalocele
      e. Enterogenous cysts
      f. Dentigerous cysts
  B. Vascular lesions
    1. Capillary hemangioma
    2. Cavernous hemangioma
    3. Lymphangioma
    4. Orbital varix
    5. Arteriovenous malformation
    6. Hemangiopericytoma
    7. Malignant hemangioendothelioma
    8. Organizing hematoma (hematic cysts, cholesterol granuloma)
    9. Sturge-Weber syndrome
    10. Klippel-Trénaunay-Weber syndrome
  C. Inflammatory masses
    1. Preseptal and orbital cellulitis
    2. Idiopathic orbital inflammatory syndrome
    3. Other orbital inflammatory syndromes
  D. Histiocytic, hematopoietic, and lymphoproliferative masses
    1. Langerhans cell histiocytosis
      a. Histiocytosis X
      b. Hand-Schüller-Christian disease
      c. Letterer-Siwe disease
    2. Juvenile xanthogranuloma (non–Langerhans cell histiocytosis)
    3. Sinus histiocytosis
    4. Leukemia and granulocytic sarcoma
    5. Lymphoma
  E. Mesodermal tumors
    1. Fibroma
    2. Myofibromatosis
    3. Lipoma

(Continued)

Table 26-1 *(continued)*

    4. Leiomyoma
    5. Fibrous dysplasia
    6. Juvenile ossifying fibroma
    7. Giant cell (reparative) granuloma of bone
    8. Aneurysmal bone cyst
    9. Cartilaginous hamartoma
   10. Sarcoma
       a. Osteogenic sarcoma
       b. Leiomyosarcoma
       c. Fibrosarcoma
       d. Malignant fibrous histiocytoma
       e. Alveolar soft part sarcoma
   11. Rhabdomyosarcoma
 F. Neurogenic tumors
    1. Glioma
    2. Meningioma
    3. Neurofibroma
    4. Schwannoma
    5. Esthesioneuroblastoma
    6. Paraganglioma
    7. Melanotic neuroectodermal tumor of infancy
 G. Lacrimal gland
    1. Pleomorphic adenoma (benign mixed tumor)
    2. Adenocarcinoma (malignant mixed tumor)
 H. Metastatic
    1. Neuroblastoma
    2. Ewing sarcoma
    3. Wilms tumor
    4. Rhabdomyosarcoma (rarely)

II. Eyelid lesions
 A. Chalazion
 B. Hordeolum
 C. Benign epithelial and appendage tumors: syringoma, porosyringoma, myoepithelioma, apocrine hidrocystoma (sudiferous cyst; originating from a blocked excretory duct of Moll's apocrine sweat gland), eccrine hidrocystoma (derived from lid eccrine sweat gland), sebaceous cyst (pilar cyst; retention cyst of the pilosebaceous structure), milia (cystic expansion of the pilosebaceous structure due to obstruction of the orifice), epidermal inclusion cyst, pilomatrixoma (calcifying epithelioma of Malherbe; a solid or cystic mass derived from hair matrix cells), conjunctival inclusion cyst
 D. Papilloma
 E. Molluscum contagiosum
 F. Cutaneous horn
 G. Rhabdomyosarcoma

III. Epibulbar tumors
 A. Papilloma
 B. Limbal dermoid
 C. Choroidal osteoma
 D. Choroidal melanoma
 E. Teratoma
 F. Rhabdomyosarcoma

Nevertheless, typical presentations of the common benign orbital and periorbital masses in infants and children (hemangioma, dermoid cyst) are sufficiently distinctive to permit confident clinical diagnosis in most cases. A malignant process should be suspected when proptosis and eyelid swelling suggestive of cellulitis are not accompanied by warmth of the overlying skin or when periorbital ecchymosis or hematoma develops in the absence of an unequivocal trauma history.

The current widespread availability of high-quality imaging permits orbital masses to be differentiated noninvasively in most cases. For initial diagnostic evaluation of the orbit, computed tomography (CT) has advantages over magnetic resonance imaging (MRI) because of CT's high sensitivity to disturbances of bony architecture, avoidance of interference from the high-MRI signal intensity of orbital fat, and greater ease of use (although sedation is still generally required for young children). Dermoid cysts, teratomas, colobomatous cysts, and encephaloceles have highly distinctive appearances on CT, as do the blood-filled cavities found in acutely deteriorated lymphangiomas. The superior ability of MRI to differentiate various tissue types makes this imaging modality a valuable adjunctive study in many cases, and its lack of radiation is an advantage when repeated imaging is required. In experienced hands, ultrasonography may also provide important diagnostic information about the orbit.

Definitive diagnosis still often requires biopsy. A pediatric oncologist should be consulted when appropriate, and a metastatic workup should be considered before resorting to orbital surgery, because other, more easily accessible sites can sometimes be used as tissue sources.

Pseudoproptosis can result from a mismatch between the volume of the globe and the capacity of the orbit. Examples include the elongation of the eyeball from primary congenital glaucoma or high myopia and the shallowness of the orbit in craniofacial syndromes with midfacial hypoplasia or plagiocephaly.

Gorospe L, Royo A, Berrocal T, Garcia-Raya P, Moreno P, Abelairas J. Imaging of orbital disorders in pediatric patients. *Eur Radiol.* 2003;13(8):2012–2026.

Primary Malignant Neoplasms

Malignant diseases of the orbit include primary tumors arising from orbital tissue elements, secondary growth of solid tumors originating elsewhere in the body (metastasis), and abnormally proliferating cells of the hematopoietic and lymphoreticular systems. A large majority of primary malignant tumors of the orbit in childhood are sarcomas. Tumors of epithelial origin (eg, carcinoma of the lacrimal gland) are extremely rare.

Rhabdomyosarcoma

The most common primary pediatric orbital malignant tumor is rhabdomyosarcoma. The incidence of this disease (which is found in about 5% of orbital biopsies of children and adolescents) exceeds that of all other sarcomas combined. The orbit is the origin of 10% of rhabdomyosarcomas; an additional 25% develop elsewhere in the head and neck, occasionally involving the orbit secondarily. The average age of onset is about 5–7 years, although onset can occur at any age. Rhabdomyosarcoma in infancy is more aggressive and carries a poorer prognosis.

Although ocular rhabdomyosarcoma usually originates in the orbit, it can occasionally arise in the conjunctiva, eyelid, or anterior uveal tract. Patients generally present with proptosis (80%–100%), globe displacement (80%), blepharoptosis (30%–50%), conjunctival and eyelid swelling (60%), palpable mass (25%), and pain (10%) (Fig 26-1). Onset of symptoms and signs is usually rapid. CT or MRI demonstrates an irregular but well-circumscribed mass of uniform density.

A biopsy is required for confirmation of the diagnosis whenever a rhabdomyosarcoma is suspected. Fine-needle aspiration biopsy (FNAB) should not be used to make the primary diagnosis. The most common histopathologic type is embryonal, which shows few cells containing characteristic cross-striations. Second in frequency is the prognostically unfavorable alveolar pattern, showing poorly differentiated tumor cells compartmentalized by orderly connective tissue septa. Botryoid (grapelike), or well-differentiated pleomorphic tumors, are rarely found in the orbit but may originate from conjunctiva. It is now widely accepted that rhabdomyosarcoma arises independently of the muscles and probably develops from undifferentiated mesenchymal cells.

Small encapsulated or otherwise well-localized rhabdomyosarcomas should be totally excised when possible. For larger or more extensive tumors, chemotherapy and radiation are used in conjunction with surgery. Exenteration of the orbit is seldom indicated.

Much of the current information on diagnosis and treatment of rhabdomyosarcoma has been obtained through the collaborative endeavors of the Intergroup Rhabdomyosarcoma Study Group (IRSG). A staging classification of rhabdomyosarcoma is employed by the IRSG. In brief, Group I is defined as localized disease that is completely resected, Group II is microscopic disease remaining after biopsy, Group III is gross disease remaining after biopsy, and Group IV is distant metastasis present at onset. This classification can help the clinician in selecting treatment and in establishing a prognosis. Primary orbital rhabdomyosarcoma has a relatively good prognosis, with patients with alveolar cell type having a 74% 5-year survival and patients with embryonal cell type, a 94% 5-year survival.

After completion of treatment, affected children should have a comprehensive ocular examination every 3–4 months initially, every 4–6 months for several years, and then yearly, with periodic orbital CT or MRI, depending on the clinical findings.

Shields JA, Shields CL. Rhabdomyosarcoma: review for the ophthalmologist. *Surv Ophthalmol.* 2003;48(1):39–57.

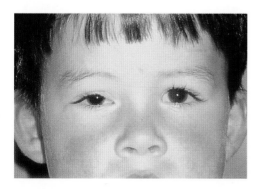

Figure 26-1 Rhabdomyosarcoma in a 4-year-old boy presenting with right upper eyelid ptosis of 3 weeks' duration and a palpable subcutaneous mass.

Other sarcomas

Osteosarcoma, chondrosarcoma, and fibrosarcoma can also develop in the orbit during childhood. The risk of sarcoma increases in children with a history of heritable retinoblastoma, particularly when external-beam radiation treatment has been given.

Metastatic Tumors

The orbit is the most common site of ocular metastasis in children, in contrast to adults, in whom the uvea is the most frequently affected.

Neuroblastoma

One of the most common childhood cancers is neuroblastoma, the most frequent source of orbital metastasis. It usually originates in either the adrenal gland or the sympathetic ganglion chain in the retroperitoneum or mediastinum. Approximately 20% of all patients with neuroblastoma show clinical evidence of orbital involvement, which is sometimes the initial manifestation of the tumor.

Unilateral or bilateral proptosis and eyelid ecchymosis are the classic presentations of metastatic neuroblastoma (Fig 26-2). Patients may also have eyelid swelling, ocular motility disturbances, and ptosis. Other signs and symptoms may include abdominal fullness and pain, venous obstruction and edema, hypertension caused by renal vascular compromise, and bone pain. Incisional biopsy shows small, round blue cells and confirms the diagnosis. Urinalysis for catecholamines is positive in 90%–95% of cases.

The mean age at diagnosis of patients with orbital neuroblastoma metastasis is approximately 2 years. Even with intensive treatment including radiation and chemotherapy, only about 10%–25% of affected patients survive. The prognosis for disseminated neuroblastoma is considerably better in infants under age 1 year than in older children.

Opsoclonus, characterized by rapid, multidirectional saccadic eye movements, is a unique paraneoplastic syndrome that is associated with neuroblastoma and is not related to orbital involvement. It is associated with a good prognosis for survival, although neurologic deficits may persist. Horner syndrome can occur from a *primary* cervical or apical thoracic neuroblastoma that involves the sympathetic chain (Fig 26-3). Horner syndrome does not occur from metastatic neuroblastoma.

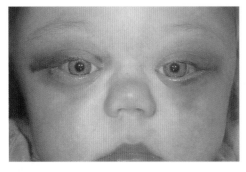 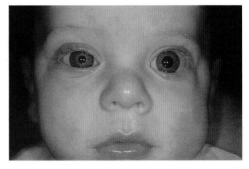

Figure 26-2 Bilateral orbital metastasis of neuroblastoma, presenting with periorbital ecchymosis in a 2-year-old girl.

Figure 26-3 Right Horner syndrome, the presenting sign of localized intrathoracic neuroblastoma in a 6-month-old boy.

Weinstein JL, Katzenstein HM, Cohn SL. Advances in the diagnosis and treatment of neuro-blastoma. *Oncologist.* 2003;8(3):278–292.

Ewing sarcoma

Ewing sarcoma is a tumor that is composed of small round cells and that usually originates in the long bones of the extremities or the axial skeleton. Ewing sarcoma is the second most frequent solid tumor source of orbital metastasis. Contemporary treatment regimens involving surgery, radiation, and chemotherapy permit long-term survival in many cases with disseminated disease.

Leukemia

By far the most common malignant disease of childhood, leukemia is acute in 95% of cases, more often lymphocytic than myelocytic. Although the most common clinical manifestation of leukemia is leukemic retinopathy (discussed later in this chapter; see also Chapter 23), all ocular structures can be affected. Leukemic infiltration of the orbit is relatively uncommon and more characteristic of acute myelogenous leukemia. Orbital involvement may be difficult to distinguish from bacterial or fungal orbital cellulitis. Orbital infiltration can cause proptosis, eyelid swelling, and ecchymosis and may be best managed by radiation therapy. Infiltration of the optic nerve by leukemic cells may cause optic disc edema and loss of vision and requires prompt treatment with low-dose radiation.

Granulocytic sarcoma, or chloroma (in reference to the greenish color of involved tissue), is a localized accumulation of myeloid leukemic cells in the orbit. This lesion may develop several months before leukemia becomes hematologically evident.

Lymphoma

In contrast with adult disease, lymphoma in children very rarely involves the orbit. Burkitt lymphoma, endemic to east Africa and uncommon in North America, is the most likely form to involve the orbit.

Histiocytosis X

Histiocytosis X (Langerhans cell histiocytosis) is the collective term for a group of disorders involving abnormal proliferation of histiocytes, often within bone. More specifically, the cells are of the dendritic type, which are considered to be immune accessory cells or antigen-processing and antigen-presenting cells, as opposed to phagocytic cells. *Eosinophilic granuloma,* the most localized and benign form of histiocytosis, produces bone lesions that involve the orbit, skull, ribs, and long bones in childhood or adolescence. Symptoms may include proptosis, ptosis, and periorbital swelling; localized pain and tenderness are relatively common. Radiography and CT characteristically demonstrate sharply demarcated osteolytic lesions without surrounding sclerosis (Fig 26-4). Treatment consists of observation of isolated asymptomatic lesions, excision of painful and easily accessible lesions, systemic corticosteroid administration, or low-dose radiation; all modalities have a high rate of success.

Hand-Schüller-Christian disease is a more disseminated and aggressive form of histiocytosis X that is likely to produce proptosis from involvement of the bony orbit in childhood. Diabetes insipidus is common. Chemotherapy is often required, but the prognosis is generally good. Children with this condition usually present between 2 and 5 years of age.

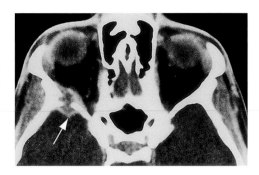

Figure 26-4 Axial CT image showing eosinophilic granuloma with partial destruction of the right posterior lateral orbital wall *(arrow)* in a 15-year-old boy, who presented with retrobulbar pain and mild edema and erythema of the right upper eyelid.

Letterer-Siwe disease is the most severe and malignant variety of histiocytosis X, usually affecting infants younger than 2 years. It is characterized by soft tissue lesions of multiple viscera (liver, spleen) but rarely involves the eye.

Huang F, Arceci R. The histiocytoses of infancy. *Semin Perinatol.* 1999;23(4):319–331.

Benign Tumors

Vascular lesions: hemangiomas

Advances in the biological characterization of vascular lesions have led to a revision of their classification. The current classification of vascular lesions establishes clear clinical, histopathologic, and prognostic differences between hemangiomas and vascular malformations. The older terms *capillary* and *strawberry hemangioma* should be translated into the single term *hemangioma.* In contrast, cavernous hemangiomas, port-wine stains, and lymphangiomas all should be called "malformations." This nomenclature has been incorporated into the medical literature but has not been used consistently in the ophthalmic literature.

Hemangiomas are hamartomatous growths composed of proliferating capillary endothelial cells. They show a characteristic early phase of active growth in early infancy, with a subsequent period of regression and involution.

Hemangiomas can be classified by their depth of skin involvement:

- superficial, arising only on the skin and immediate subjacent skin and having a bright red appearance
- deep, arising only in the deeper subcutaneous tissue and having a bluish hue (Fig 26-5)
- compound/mixed, having components of both

Alternatively, hemangiomas can be classified by type of orbital involvement:

- preseptal, involving the skin and preseptal orbit
- intraorbital, involving the postseptal orbit
- compound/mixed, involving the preseptal and postseptal orbit

Hemangiomas occur in 1%–3% of term newborns and are more common in premature infants and females and after chorionic villus sampling. Most hemangiomas are

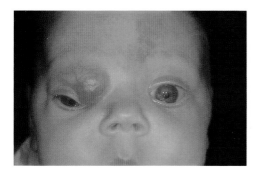

Figure 26-5 Capillary hemangioma in a 2-month-old girl involving the right upper eyelid and orbit with displacement of the globe and induction of 8 D of astigmatic refractive error.

clinically insignificant at birth; they can be inapparent or can appear as an erythematous macule or a telangiectasia. The natural history is rapid proliferation and growth over the first several months of life, rarely lasting beyond 1 year. During this phase, the lesion may ulcerate, hemorrhage, or cause amblyopia by inducing astigmatism or obstructing the visual axis. After the first year of life, the lesion usually begins to regress, although the rate and degree of involution vary. Children and their parents may also suffer psychologically if a marked deformity persists.

Systemic disease associated with hemangiomas   *PHACE(S)* is an acronym for *p*osterior fossa malformations, *h*emangiomas, *a*rterial anomalies, *c*oarctation of the aorta and cardiac defects, *e*ye abnormalities (including increased retinal vascularity, microphthalmia, optic nerve hypoplasia, exophthalmos, choroidal hemangiomas, strabismus, colobomas, cataracts, and glaucoma), and *s*ternal clefting and *s*upraumbilical raphe. The PHACE(S) syndrome should be considered in any infant presenting with a large, segmental, plaque-like facial hemangioma involving 1 or more dermatomes (Fig 26-6).

Kasabach-Merritt syndrome is a thrombocytopenic coagulopathy with a high mortality rate. It is caused by sequestration of platelets within a vascular lesion that is now thought not to be a true hemangioma, but 1 of 2 distinct vascular lesions, either the kaposiform hemangioendothelioma or the tufted angioma.

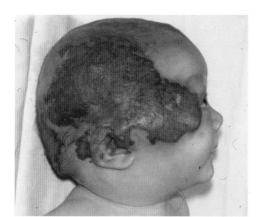

Figure 26-6 Plaque hemangioma in a child with PHACE(S) syndrome. *(Courtesy of Ken K. Nischal, FRCOphth.)*

Diffuse neonatal hemangiomatosis is a potentially lethal condition that occurs in infants, with multiple small cutaneous hemangiomas associated with visceral lesions affecting the liver, gastrointestinal tract, and brain. These hemangiomas are initially asymptomatic but can lead to cardiac failure and death within weeks. Infants with more than 3 cutaneous lesions should be evaluated for visceral lesions.

Maffucci syndrome is a rare genetic disorder affecting both males and females. It is characterized by benign enlargement of cartilage (enchondromas); bone deformities; and dark, irregularly shaped hemangiomas. Approximately 30%–37% of enchondromas develop into a chondrosarcoma. Malignant transformation of vascular lesions is possible but exceedingly rare.

Treatment of hemangiomas If the diagnosis is unclear on clinical grounds, MRI can be useful to distinguish hemangioma from plexiform neurofibroma, lymphatic malformation, and rhabdomyosarcoma, each of which may be associated with rapid growth and proliferation or progressive proptosis. MRI or Doppler ultrasonography may also be helpful in delineating the posterior extent of the tumor if it cannot be determined clinically.

Observation is indicated when hemangiomas are small and there is no risk of amblyopia from either obstruction of the visual axis or induced astigmatism.

Steroids are used during the proliferative phase of the tumor to arrest growth and accelerate involution of the lesion. They can be administered topically, intralesionally, or systemically. Topical clobetasol propionate cream 0.05% may be preferred for small superficial lesions. Intralesional injections of a combination of a long-acting and a short-acting steroid are commonly used for localized periocular hemangiomas (it is essential to use a steroid preparation that is approved for intralesional administration). If the hemangioma is diffuse or extensively involves the posterior orbit, then systemic steroids may be employed, with recommended dosages of prednisone or prednisolone ranging from 2 to 5 mg/kg/day.

Steroids are associated with myriad well-known complications, the risks of which must be weighed against the potential benefits of treatment and discussed with the family. Adrenal suppression and growth retardation can occur with all routes of administration, including topical creams. Intralesional injections carry the risks of bilateral retinal artery embolization, subcutaneous linear fat atrophy, and eyelid depigmentation. It may also be necessary to postpone immunizations for children receiving high doses of steroids. Consultation with a child's primary care provider is recommended.

Interferon alfa-2a, though effective, has been associated with an unacceptably high side-effect profile and is usually reserved for severe, recalcitrant, or life-threatening tumors. Vincristine may be a promising alternative, but it is still under investigation.

A pulsed-dye laser can be used to treat superficial hemangiomas with few complications, but it has little effect on deeper components of the tumor.

Surgical excision of periocular hemangiomas is feasible for some well-localized lesions (Fig 26-7). In other cases, surgery may be used as a reconstructive tool years after medical treatment.

Propranolol has recently been described for the treatment of hemangiomas and appears to be effective.

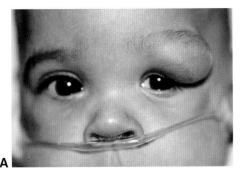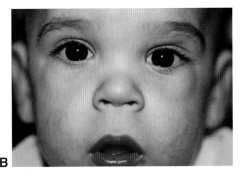

A **B**

Figure 26-7 **A,** Five-month-old boy with well-circumscribed capillary hemangioma in left upper eyelid. Preoperative refraction was –6.00 +8.00 × 40°. **B,** At 6 months postoperative, induced astigmatism has resolved and refraction was –0.25 +0.25 × 80°. *(Courtesy of David A. Plager, MD.)*

Léauté-Labrèze C, Dumas de la Roque E, Hubiche T, Boralevi F, Thambo JB, Taïeb A. Propranolol for severe hemangiomas of infancy. *N Engl J Med.* 2008;358(24):2649–2651.

Vascular lesions: malformations

Vascular malformations are developmental anomalies that can be derived from capillary venous, arterial, or lymphatic vessels. In contrast to hemangiomas, vascular malformations remain relatively static, with growth of the lesion correlating to growth of the child. The age and mode of clinical presentation vary, but, in general, vascular malformations manifest later in life, although cutaneous vascular malformations such as port-wine stains are evident from birth.

Orbital lymphangioma Orbital lymphangioma, a lymphatic malformation, may produce proptosis at birth or, more commonly, in the second or third decade of life. Lymphangioma of the orbit is best managed conservatively. Exacerbations tend to occur during upper respiratory tract infections and may be managed with short-course systemic corticosteroids. Rapid expansion may also be seen in cases of intralesional hemorrhage (Fig 26-8). In these cases, partial resection and drainage may be required to manage acute orbital symptoms and compressive optic neuropathy. Because of the infiltrative character of this malformation, complete removal is considered impossible. Intralesional injection of a sclerosing

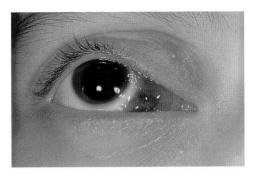

Figure 26-8 Lymphangioma with hemorrhage involving the right orbit, upper eyelid, and conjunctiva in a 15-year-old girl.

agent may hold promise but requires further investigation before it can be recommended for general use.

Orbital venous malformations   Orbital venous malformations, or varices, can be divided into primary and secondary types. The primary type is confined to the orbit and has no association with arteriovenous malformations (AVMs). The secondary orbital varix occurs as a result of an intracranial AVM shunt that causes the orbital veins to dilate. Orbital venous malformations usually become symptomatic after years of progressive congestion and rarely manifest before the second decade of life. Treatment is reserved for highly symptomatic lesions.

Orbital arteriovenous malformations   Arteriovenous malformations isolated to the orbit are extremely rare. Patients with congenital AVM aneurysms of the retina and midbrain, a condition known as *Wyburn-Mason syndrome* (see Chapter 27), may have orbital involvement. AVMs of the bony orbit rarely manifest in childhood but are characterized by pulsatile exophthalmos, chemosis, congested conjunctival vessels, and raised intraocular pressure. AVMs may be treated by embolization, surgical resection, or both.

Capillary malformations   Port-wine stains manifest as a flat red or pink cutaneous lesion that may lighten during the first year but then tends to become darker, thicker, and more nodular over time. *Sturge-Weber syndrome,* or *encephalotrigeminal angiomatosis,* is a capillary malformation of the leptomeninges with or without ocular or facial involvement. The classic manifestations are a port-wine stain of the face that usually follows the distribution of the trigeminal nerve, an intraocular choroidal hemangioma, and seizures. Glaucoma can occur in affected eyes and can be difficult to treat. The development of new lasers has provided additional treatment options for patients with port-wine stains.

Ceisler EJ, Santos L, Blei F. Periocular hemangiomas: what every physician should know. *Pediatr Dermatol.* 2004;21(1):1–9.

Garza G, Fay A, Rubin PAD. Treatment of pediatric vascular lesions of the eyelid and orbit. *Int Ophthalmol Clin.* 2001;41(4):43–55.

Other vascular tumors   Other orbital tumors composed of vascular elements are rare in childhood. *Hemangiopericytoma* is a benign tumor of pericytes that manifests as slow proptosis of the globe and has the potential for malignant transformation.

Tumors of bony origin

During the early years of life, a variety of uncommon benign orbital tumors of bony origin may present with gradually increasing proptosis. Fibrous dysplasia and ossifying fibroma are similar disorders characterized by destruction of normal bone and replacement by fibro-osseous tissue. In both conditions, orbital radiography and CT show varying degrees of lucency and sclerosis.

Fibrous dysplasia has a slow progression that ceases when skeletal maturation is complete. The most serious complication is vision loss caused by optic nerve compression, which may occur acutely. Periodic assessment of vision, pupil function, and optic disc appearance is indicated. Surgical treatment is indicated for functional deterioration or disfigurement.

Histopathologically, *ossifying fibroma* is distinguished by the presence of osteoblasts. Ossifying fibroma tends to be a more locally invasive lesion than is fibrous dysplasia; some authorities recommend early excision.

Brown tumor of bone is an osteoclastic giant cell reaction resulting from hyperparathyroidism. *Aneurysmal bone cyst* is a degenerative process in which normal bone is replaced by cystic cavities containing fibrous tissue, inflammatory cells, and blood, producing a characteristic radiographic appearance.

Tumors of connective tissue origin

Benign orbital tumors originating from connective tissue are rare in childhood. *Juvenile fibromatosis* may present as a mass in the inferior anterior portion of the orbit. These tumors, sometimes called *myofibromas* or *desmoid tumors,* are composed of relatively mature fibroblasts. They tend to recur locally after excision and can be difficult to control, but they do not metastasize.

Tumors of neural origin

Optic pathway glioma is the most important orbital tumor of neural origin in childhood. Optic pathway gliomas are usually low-grade astrocytomas; however, the rate of growth with or without therapeutic intervention is unpredictable. Accordingly, the management of these tumors is controversial and depends largely on their location. Approximately 20% of optic pathway gliomas are associated with neurofibromatosis 1. *Plexiform neurofibroma* nearly always occurs in the context of neurofibromatosis and not infrequently involves the eyelid and orbit. (These tumors are discussed in detail in Chapter 27.) Orbital *meningioma* and *schwannoma* (neurilemoma, neurinoma) are rare before adulthood and also usually appear in patients with neurofibromatosis. Meningioma typically presents with progressive vision loss, mild proptosis, and restriction of ocular motility; most patients are female. Childhood meningiomas tend to be locally aggressive and should be totally excised if possible, unless the involved eye retains good vision.

Steinbok P. Optic pathway tumors in children. *J Chin Med Assoc.* 2003;66(1):4–12.

Ectopic Tissue Masses

The term *choristoma* is applied to growths consisting of normal cells and tissues appearing at an abnormal location. The growths may result from abnormal sequestration of germ layer tissue during embryonic development or from faulty differentiation of pluripotential cells. Masses composed of such ectopic tissue growing in the orbit can also be a consequence of herniation of tissue from adjacent structures.

Cystic lesions

Dermoid cysts are benign developmental choristomas thought to be the most common space-occupying orbital lesions of childhood. These cysts are congenital, arising from primitive dermal elements that have been sequestered in fetal suture lines at the time of closure. The tissue forms a cyst lined with keratinized epithelium and dermal appendages, including hair follicles, sweat glands, and sebaceous glands. Cysts containing squamous epithelium without dermal appendages are called *epidermoid cysts.*

Orbital dermoid cysts presenting in childhood most commonly arise in the supero-nasal and superotemporal quadrants (Fig 26-9) but sometimes extend into the bony suture line. Clinically, the dermoid cyst in children presents as a painless mass that is unattached to overlying skin and is mobile, smooth, and nontender. Episodes of inflammation may occur with small ruptures of the cyst wall and consequent extrusion of cyst contents into the surrounding tissue. Most patients have no visual symptoms. CT can confirm the diagnosis, revealing a well-circumscribed lesion with a low-density lumen and often bony remodeling (Fig 26-10). Deeper orbital lesions may show complete bony defects.

Management of dermoid cysts is surgical. Early excision may avoid the increased risk of traumatic rupture with ambulation. An infrabrow or eyelid crease incision is used, and the cyst is carefully dissected. If possible, rupture of the cyst at the time of surgery is avoided to limit lipogranulomatous inflammation and scarring. If the cyst is entered, the site should be irrigated. Sutural cysts often cannot be removed intact because of their communication into or through bone. To limit the possibility of recurrence, the surgeon must attempt removal of all remaining cyst lining.

Shields JA, Kaden IH, Eagle RC Jr, Shields CL. Orbital dermoid cysts: clinicopathologic correlations, classification, and management. The 1997 Josephine E. Schueler Lecture. *Ophthal Plast Reconstr Surg.* 1997;13(4):265–276.

Teratomas

Choristomatous tumors that contain multiple tissues derived from all 3 germinal layers (ectoderm, mesoderm, and endoderm) are known as *teratomas*. Skin and dermal appendages, neural tissue, muscle, and bone are typically present; endodermal elements such as respiratory and intestinal tract epithelium are less consistently found. Most teratomas are partially cystic, with varying fluid content. Orbital teratomas account for a very small fraction of both orbital tumors and teratomas in general, which usually arise in the gonads or sacrococcygeal region. The clinical presentation of orbital teratomas is particularly dramatic, however, with massive proptosis evident at birth (Fig 26-11). In contrast with teratomas in other locations, which tend to show malignant growth, most orbital lesions are benign. Surgical excision, facilitated by prior aspiration of fluid, can often be accom-

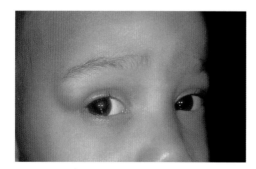

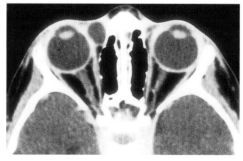

Figure 26-9 Three-year-old girl with periorbital dermoid cyst, right eye, with typical superotemporal location.

Figure 26-10 Axial CT image showing a dermoid cyst of the superonasal anterior orbit, right eye, in a 6-year-old boy.

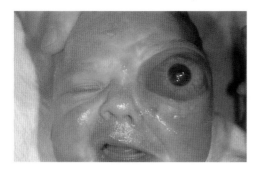

Figure 26-11 Congenital cystic teratoma originating in the left orbit of a 1-day-old girl.

plished without sacrificing the globe. Permanent optic nerve damage from stretching and compression usually results in poor vision in the involved eye.

Ectopic lacrimal gland

A rare choristomatous lesion, ectopic lacrimal gland may present with proptosis in childhood. Cystic enlargement and chronic inflammation sometimes aggravate the problem.

Colobomatous cyst

Also known as *microphthalmos with cyst,* the colobomatous cyst is composed of tissues that originate from the eye wall of a malformed globe with posterior segment coloboma. Most fundus colobomas show some degree of scleral ectasia, resulting from a deficiency of tissue in the region where apposing edges of the embryonic neuroectodermal fissure have failed to fuse properly. In extreme cases, a bulging globular appendage grows to become as large as or larger than the globe itself, which is invariably microphthalmic, sometimes to a marked degree.

Like other colobomatous malformations, microphthalmos with cyst may occur either as an isolated congenital defect or in association with a variety of intracranial or systemic anomalies. Frequently, the other eye shows evidence of coloboma as well. The wall of a colobomatous cyst consists of thin sclera lined by rudimentary tissue of neuroectodermal origin, occasionally incorporating hyperplastic glial tissue accumulations; the cyst contains aqueous fluid with a few suspended cells. The usual location is inferior or posterior to the globe, with which the cyst is always in contact. The cyst interior communicates with the vitreous cavity, sometimes through a channel so small it is undetectable even with high-resolution imaging.

Posteriorly located colobomatous cysts may or may not cause proptosis, depending on the size of the globe and the cyst. Inferiorly located cysts present as a bulging of the lower eyelid or a bluish subconjunctival mass (Fig 26-12). If fundus examination does not make the diagnosis obvious, other possibilities can be excluded by using CT, MRI, or ultrasonography to demonstrate a cystic lesion with the uniform internal density of vitreous attached to the globe. The goal of treatment is to promote normal growth of the orbit, and a variety of methods are used, including aspiration of the cyst, surgical excision of the cyst, and orbital expanders and conformers.

McLean CJ, Ragge NK, Jones RB, Collin JR. The management of orbital cysts associated with congenital microphthalmos and anophthalmos. *Br J Ophthalmol.* 2003;87(7):860–863.

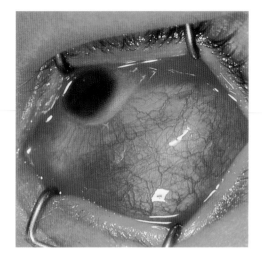

Figure 26-12 Colobomatous cyst (associated with microphthalmos), left eye.

Mucocele

Mucoceles are cystic lesions that originate from the paranasal sinuses and may expand over time, potentially causing destruction of bone and possibly eroding into the orbit or intracranial space. These lesions most commonly arise from the frontal or anterior ethmoidal sinuses, resulting in inferior or medial displacement of the globe. The differential diagnosis includes encephalocele with skull base deformity. Treatment involves reestablishing normal sinus drainage and removing the cyst wall.

Encephalocele or meningocele

Encephaloceles or meningoceles in the orbital region may result from a congenital bony defect that permits herniation of intracranial tissue or may develop after trauma that disrupts the bone and dura mater of the anterior cranial fossa. An intraorbital location leads to proptosis or downward displacement of the globe. Anterior presentation takes the form of a subcutaneous mass that can be misdiagnosed as a dacryocele. However, encephaloceles and meningoceles are typically located above the medial canthal ligament. In contrast, dacryoceles are typically located below the medial canthal ligament. Pulsation of the globe or the mass from the transmission of intracranial pulse pressure is characteristic. Neuroimaging readily confirms the diagnosis of this rare condition.

Childhood Orbital Inflammations

Several noninfectious, nontraumatic disorders that may simulate an orbital mass lesion deserve brief mention. Thyroid eye disease, the most common cause of proptosis in adults, rarely occurs in prepubescent children but occasionally affects adolescents (Fig 26-13). (See also Chapter 11.)

Idiopathic orbital inflammatory disease

Idiopathic orbital inflammatory disease *(orbital pseudotumor)* is an inflammatory cause of proptosis in childhood that differs significantly from the adult form. The typical pediatric presentation is acute and painful, resembling orbital cellulitis more than tumor or thyroid eye disease (Fig 26-14). Bilaterality and episodic recurrence are common, as are associated

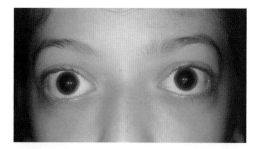

Figure 26-13 Thyroid eye disease with bilateral exophthalmos in a 15-year-old girl.

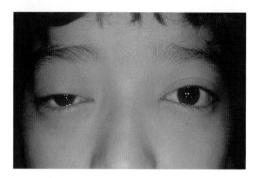

Figure 26-14 Bilateral idiopathic orbital inflammatory disease (orbital pseudotumor) in an 11-year-old boy with a 1-week history of eye pain. Ocular rotation was markedly limited in all directions. CT confirmed proptosis and showed enlargement of all extraocular muscles. Laboratory workup was negative for thyroid disease and rheumatologic disorders. Complete resolution occurred after 1 month of corticosteroid treatment.

systemic manifestations such as headache, nausea and vomiting, and lethargy. Uveitis is common and occasionally constitutes the dominant manifestation. Imaging studies may show increased density of orbital fat, thickening of posterior sclera and the Tenon layer, or enlargement of extraocular muscles. As opposed to orbital cellulitis, sinusitis is typically not present. Treatment with a systemic corticosteroid usually provides prompt and dramatic relief, but recurrent disease is common.

Orbital myositis

Orbital myositis describes idiopathic orbital inflammatory disease that is confined to 1 or more extraocular muscles. The clinical presentation depends on the amount of inflammation. Diplopia, conjunctival chemosis, and orbital pain are common. Symptoms can be subacute for weeks or can progress quite rapidly. Visual function is rarely involved unless massive muscle enlargement is present. CT or MRI findings consist of diffusely enlarged muscles with the enlargement extending all the way to the insertion (unlike with thyroid myopathy, which mainly involves the muscle belly). Corticosteroid treatment usually results in resolution of symptoms, but prolonged treatment (4–6 weeks) is often necessary and recurrence is common.

Eyelid and Epibulbar Lesions

Malignant tumors arising from eyelid skin or conjunctiva (basal cell carcinoma, squamous cell carcinoma, melanoma) are relatively common in adults, but they are extremely rare in childhood. These tumors are discussed elsewhere in the BCSC (see Section 4, *Ophthalmic Pathology and Intraocular Tumors;* Section 7, *Orbit, Eyelids, and Lacrimal System;* and Section 8, *External Disease and Cornea*). Pediatric cases are likely to be associated with underlying systemic disorders that predispose to malignancy, such as basal cell nevus syndrome or xeroderma pigmentosum. In addition, rhabdomyosarcoma may present atypically as an eyelid or conjunctival mass.

Benign lesions of the ocular surface and surrounding skin are common, and these may be classified as originating from epithelium, melanocytes, or vascular tissue.

Papillomas

Papillomas are benign epithelial proliferations that usually appear as sessile masses at the limbus or as pedunculated lesions of the caruncle, fornix, or palpebral conjunctiva. Papillomas may be transparent, pale yellow, or salmon-colored, sometimes speckled with red dots. Papillomas in children usually result from viral infection and are likely to disappear spontaneously. Surgical excision is indicated if there is persistent associated conjunctivitis or keratitis or if new lesions continue to appear. Recurrence following surgical excision is possible. Oral cimetidine can induce papilloma regression.

Conjunctival Epithelial Inclusion Cysts

Usually resulting from surgery or trauma, conjunctival epithelial inclusion cysts are filled with clear fluid. Excision is indicated only if they are a source of bothersome symptoms.

Epibulbar Limbal Dermoid Tumors

Although both are classified as choristomas, dermoid tumors are completely distinct from dermoid cysts. Epibulbar limbal dermoid tumors are evident at birth as whitish dome-shaped masses, straddling the limbus in the inferotemporal quadrant in about three-quarters of cases, with a diameter of about 2–10 mm and a thickness of 1–3 mm. They are composed of keratinizing surface epithelium and have an underlying dermal layer that frequently contains a few hair follicles and a small amount of fatty tissue. Little if any postnatal growth occurs. Apart from their undesirable appearance, epibulbar limbal dermoids may cause ocular irritation and interfere with vision by inducing astigmatism or haziness of adjacent clear cornea.

There is no urgency to remove an epibulbar dermoid tumor unless irritating symptoms or amblyopia persists. The tumor is removed by excising the episcleral portion flush with the plane of surrounding tissue. In general, the surgeon need not remove underlying clear corneal tissue, mobilize surrounding tissue, or apply a patch graft over the resulting surface defect; however, because some lesions may extend into the anterior chamber, tissue should be available in the event that a patch graft is required. Cornea and conjunctiva heal within a few days to several weeks, generally with some scarring and imperfect corneal transparency; nevertheless, the appearance can be improved considerably.

Lipodermoid

A conjunctival lesion, the lipodermoid (*dermolipoma*) is usually located near the temporal fornix and is composed of adipose tissue and dense connective tissue. The overlying conjunctival epithelium is normal, and hair follicles are absent. Lipodermoids may be extensive, sometimes involving orbital tissue, lacrimal gland, and extraocular muscle. Both epibulbar limbal dermoid tumors and conjunctival lipodermoids are frequently associated with Goldenhar syndrome (Fig 26-15). In patients with Goldenhar syndrome, the lesions are accompanied by a variety of other anomalies, including ear deformities (preauricular appendages, aural fistulas, microtia), maxillary or mandibular hypoplasia (hemifacial microsomia), vertebral deformities, colobomas or notching of the eyelid, and Duane syndrome.

Lipodermoids rarely require excision. If surgery is undertaken, the surgeon should attempt to remove only the portion of the lesion visible within the palpebral fissure, disturbing conjunctiva and the Tenon layer as little as possible to minimize scarring. Even with a conservative operative approach, cicatrization may be a problem that requires surgical revision.

Conjunctival Nevi

Conjunctival nevi are relatively common in childhood. The lesions may be flat or elevated. Histopathologically, most of these nevi are compound (nevus cells are found in both epithelium and substantia propria); others are junctional (nevus cells confined to the interface between epithelium and substantia propria). Nevi are typically brown, but approximately one-third are nonpigmented, having a pinkish appearance. The lesions are occasionally noted at birth but more commonly develop during later childhood or adolescence (Fig 26-16).

Malignant melanoma of the conjunctiva and primary acquired melanosis, a premalignant nevoid lesion of adulthood, are extremely rare in childhood.

Congenital Nevocellular Nevi of the Skin

Congenital nevocellular nevi can occur on the eyelids and may cause amblyopia or undergo malignant transformation (Fig 26-17). The risk of malignant transformation increases with the size of the lesion, with large lesions (>20 cm) having a 5%–20% risk of

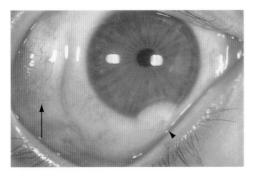

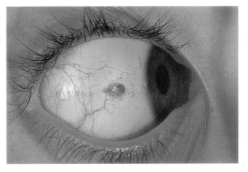

Figure 26-15 Small inferior limbal dermoid *(arrowhead)* and larger lipodermoid *(arrow)* involving the temporal conjunctival fornix, right eye, in a child with Goldenhar syndrome.

Figure 26-16 Pigmented nevus of the bulbar conjunctiva, right eye, recently developed in a 4-year-old girl.

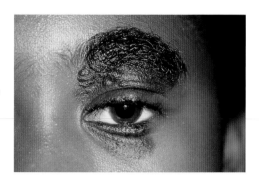

Figure 26-17 Congenital nevocellular nevus of the eyelid, present since birth. *(Courtesy of Amy Hutchinson, MD.)*

malignant transformation. Observation is often recommended for small (<1.5 cm) and medium-sized (1.5–20 cm) lesions.

Ocular Melanocytosis

A congenital pigmentary lesion, ocular melanocytosis *(melanosis oculi)* is characterized by unilateral patchy but extensive slate-gray or bluish discoloration of the sclera (not conjunctiva). Intraocular pigmentation is also increased, which contributes to a higher incidence of glaucoma and increases the risk of malignant melanoma. Some patients, particularly persons of Asian ancestry, may have associated involvement of eyelid and adjacent skin with dermal hyperpigmentation that produces brown, bluish, or black discoloration without thickening or other abnormality *(oculodermal melanocytosis, nevus of Ota)*. Small patches of slate-gray scleral pigmentation, typically bilateral and without clinical significance, are common in black and Asian children. Melanosis of skin and sclera is occasionally associated with Sturge-Weber syndrome and Klippel-Trénaunay-Weber syndrome (Fig 26-18).

> Akor C, Greenberg MF, Pollard ZF, Grossniklaus HE. Conjunctival melanoma in a child. *J Pediatr Ophthalmol Strabismus*. 2004;41(1):56–58.

Inflammatory Conditions

Inflammatory masses of the eyelids and ocular surface are much more common than tumors. *Chalazia* are caused by blockage of the meibomian glands, and *hordeola* arise from

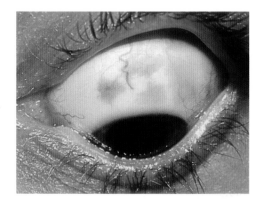

Figure 26-18 Congenital ocular melanocytosis.

blocked eccrine and apocrine glands. Treament of both includes eyelid hygiene and warm compresses, with surgical treatment reserved for large, painful, or chronic lesions. Doxycycline can be used safely in children who are at least 8 years old but should be avoided in younger children. Pyogenic granuloma is a pedunculated, fleshy pink growth of granulation tissue that develops, sometimes rapidly and exuberantly, from the conjunctiva overlying a chalazion or site of trauma.

Phlyctenular keratoconjunctivitis and *ligneous conjunctivitis* are 2 uncommon inflammatory disorders of the conjunctiva that typically occur in young patients and may result in the formation of ocular surface masses. *Nodular episcleritis* occasionally is seen in childhood. Eyelid and epibulbar lesions can develop in juvenile xanthogranuloma, which is discussed later in the chapter. See also BCSC Section 8, *External Disease and Cornea.*

Intraocular Tumors

Iris and Ciliary Body Lesions

Both primary and secondary malignant tumors of the iris are very rare in children. Leukemic infiltration of iris tissue may create a mass lesion, which is one of the less common ocular manifestations of pediatric leukemia. Solid tumors almost never metastasize to the uveal tract in childhood.

A number of relatively common and entirely benign iris lesions may generate concern about the possibility of malignancy in childhood. For pigmented iris nevi and freckles large enough to be noticed by family members or primary care physicians, repeated observation is sometimes required in order to provide reassurance concerning the harmless nature of the lesions. Children with neurofibromatosis 1 occasionally develop melanocytic lesions similar to the common Lisch nodule that are large enough to be considered benign tumors. Nodules of iris-pigmented epithelium at the pupillary margin may be present as an insignificant congenital anomaly or may develop after prolonged use of miotic drops (eg, echothiophate for treatment of strabismus).

Juvenile xanthogranuloma

Juvenile xanthogranuloma is a nonneoplastic histiocytic proliferation that develops in infants younger than 2 years. It is characterized by the presence of Touton giant cells. Skin involvement is typically but not always present in the form of 1 or more small round papules, orange or tan in color. Iris lesions are relatively rare and virtually always unilateral. The fleshy yellow-brown mass may be small and localized or diffusely infiltrative of the entire iris, with resulting heterochromia. Spontaneous bleeding with hyphema is a characteristic clinical presentation. Secondary glaucoma may cause acute pain and photophobia and ultimately significant vision loss (Fig 26-19).

Juvenile xanthogranuloma is a self-limited condition that usually regresses spontaneously by age 5 years, but treatment is indicated for ocular involvement to avoid complications. Topical corticosteroids and pharmacologic agents to lower intraocular pressure, given as necessary, are generally sufficient to control the problem; surgical excision or radiation should be considered if intractable glaucoma is present.

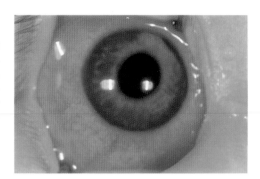

Figure 26-19 Juvenile xanthogranuloma of iris, right eye, in a 1-year-old boy with a 3-day history of redness and light sensitivity. Note small hyphema layered superonasally adjacent to the tan-colored iris lesion. The lesion regressed without further complications over 6 months with topical corticosteroid treatment.

Medulloepithelioma

A medulloepithelioma *(diktyoma)* originates from the nonpigmented epithelium of the ciliary body and most often presents as an iris mass during the first decade of life. Secondary glaucoma, hyphema, and ectopia lentis are less frequent initial manifestations. This rare lesion shows a spectrum of clinical and pathologic characteristics, ranging from benign to malignant. Although metastasis is rare, local invasiveness can lead to death. Teratoid elements are often present. Enucleation is usually required and is curative in a large majority of cases.

Choroidal and Retinal Pigment Epithelial Lesions

A pigmented fundus lesion in a child is usually benign. Flat choroidal nevi are common as an incidental fundus finding in children and need not be viewed as a particular cause for concern. Patients with neurofibromatosis 1 often have flat, tan-colored spots in the choroid.

Congenital hypertrophy of the retinal pigment epithelium (CHRPE) is a sharply demarcated, flat, hyperpigmented lesion that may be isolated or multifocal (Fig 26-20). Such lesions are sometimes grouped, in which case they are also known as *bear tracks*. A specific subgroup of these lesions has been associated with familial adenomatous polyposis (Gardner syndrome). Patients with Gardner syndrome are at very high risk for adenocarcinoma of the colon by 50 years of age. The CHRPE lesions associated with Gardner syndrome have a halo of surrounding depigmentation with a tail of depigmentation that is oriented radially and directed toward the optic nerve. Patients with Gardner syndrome may also have skeletal hamartomas and various other soft tissue tumors. The presence of 4 or more CHRPE lesions not restricted to 1 sector of the fundus or bilateral involvement should raise suspicion of familial polyposis syndrome.

Combined hamartoma of the retina and retinal pigment epithelium is an ill-defined, elevated, variably pigmented tumor that may be juxtapapillary or located in the retinal periphery. In the peripheral location, dragging of the retinal vessels is a prominent feature. Tumors have a variable composition of glial tissue and retinal pigment epithelium. This condition can be associated with neurofibromatosis 2, incontinentia pigmenti, X-linked retinoschisis, and facial hemangiomas.

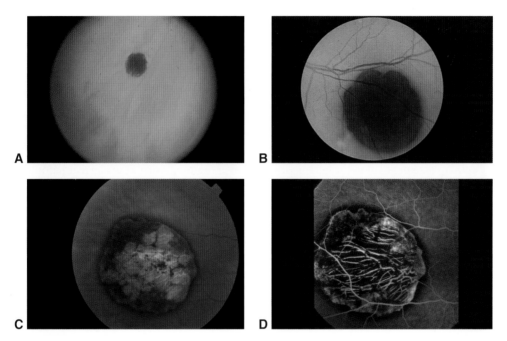

Figure 26-20 Congenital hypertrophy of the RPE (CHRPE). Examples of varying clinical appearances. **A,** Small CHRPE. **B,** Medium-sized CHRPE; note the homogeneous black color and well-defined margins of this nummular lesion. **C, D,** Color fundus photograph and corresponding fluorescein angiogram of a large CHRPE. Note the loss of RPE architecture and highlighted choroidal vasculature. *(Parts A, C, and D courtesy of Timothy G. Murray, MD.)*

Melanocytoma is a darkly pigmented tumor with little or no growth potential that usually involves the optic disc and adjacent retina (Fig 26-21). Malignant melanoma of the choroid is extremely rare in children.

Choroidal osteoma is a benign bony tumor of the uveal tract that may occur in childhood, usually presenting with decreased visual acuity.

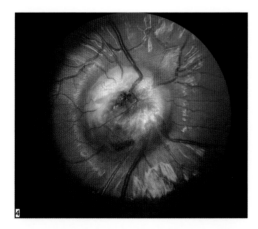

Figure 26-21 Melanocytoma of the optic disc and adjacent retina. *(Courtesy of Scott Lambert, MD.)*

Isolated localized choroidal hemangioma is extremely rare in childhood. Diffuse hemangioma of the choroid associated with Sturge-Weber syndrome is discussed in Chapter 27.

Leukemia

Childhood leukemias can be associated with tumor infiltration of the retina, optic disc, and uvea. Optic disc edema, retinal and choroidal thickening with hemorrhage, and retinal detachment may be observed. Ocular involvement is highly correlated with central nervous system involvement when the cerebrospinal fluid contains abnormal cells. Histopathologically, the choroid is the most frequently affected ocular tissue, but choroidal involvement is usually not apparent clinically. Indirect ophthalmoscopy sometimes reveals mildly pale fundus areas, but choroidal involvement is more accurately detected ultrasonically.

Leukemic infiltrates in the anterior segment may lead to heterochromia iridis; a change in the architecture of the iris; frank iris infiltrates; spontaneous hyphemas; leukemic cells in the anterior chamber; and hypopyon. Keratic precipitates may be seen, and some affected eyes develop glaucoma from tumor cells clogging the trabecular meshwork. Anterior chamber paracentesis for cytologic studies may be diagnostic in cases involving the anterior segment. Topical steroids and local irradiation are effective for anterior segment complications. Leukemic involvement of the iris may be confused with juvenile xanthogranuloma.

Intraocular leukemic infiltrates may respond to systemic chemotherapy and irradiation, but the prognosis is poor.

Retinoblastoma

Retinoblastoma is the most common malignant ocular tumor of childhood and one of the most common pediatric solid tumors, with an incidence of 1:14,000–1:20,000 live births. Retinoblastoma is typically diagnosed during the first year of life in familial and bilateral cases and between ages 1 and 3 in sporadic unilateral cases. Onset later than age 5 is rare but can occur. The most common initial sign is leukocoria (white pupil), which is usually first noticed by the family and described as a glow, glint, or cat's-eye appearance (Fig 26-22A). Approximately 25% of cases present with strabismus (esotropia or exotropia). Less common presentations include vitreous hemorrhage, hyphema, ocular or periocular inflammation, glaucoma, proptosis, and pseudohypopyon. BCSC Section 4, *Ophthalmic Pathology and Intraocular Tumors,* also discusses retinoblastoma.

A retinoblastoma is a neuroblastic tumor, biologically similar to neuroblastoma and medulloblastoma. Diagnosis of retinoblastoma can usually be based on its ophthalmoscopic appearance. Intraocular retinoblastoma can exhibit a variety of growth patterns. With endophytic growth, it appears as a white to cream-colored mass that breaks through the internal limiting membrane (Fig 26-22B). Endophytic retinoblastoma is sometimes associated with vitreous seeding, in which individual cells or fragments of tumor tissue become separated from the main mass, as shown in Figure 26-23A. Vitreous seeds may be few and localized or so extensive that the clinical picture resembles endophthalmitis. Occasionally, malignant cells enter the anterior chamber and form a pseudohypopyon.

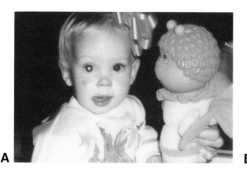
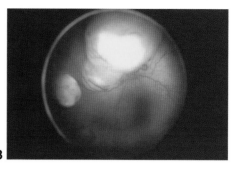

A

B

Figure 26-22 **A,** Leukocoria of the right eye shown in family photograph of a 1-year-old girl with retinoblastoma. **B,** Wide-angle fundus photograph showing multiple retinoblastoma lesions, left eye. *(Courtesy of A. Linn Murphree, MD.)*

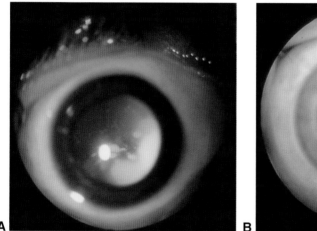
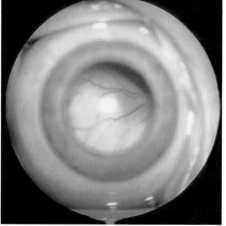

A

B

Figure 26-23 **A,** Endophytic retinoblastoma with vitreous seeding. **B,** Exophytic retinoblastoma with overlying detached retina.

Exophytic tumors are usually yellow-white and occur in the subretinal space so that the overlying retinal vessels are commonly increased in caliber and tortuosity (Fig 26-23B). Exophytic retinoblastoma growth is often associated with subretinal fluid accumulation that can obscure the tumor and closely mimic the appearance of an exudative retinal detachment suggestive of advanced Coats disease. Retinoblastoma cells have the potential to implant on previously uninvolved retinal tissue and grow, thereby creating an impression of multicentricity in an eye with only a single primary tumor.

Large tumors often show signs of both endophytic and exophytic growth. Small retinoblastoma lesions appear as a grayish mass and are frequently confined between the internal and external limiting membranes. A third pattern, diffuse infiltrating growth retinoblastoma, is usually unilateral and nonhereditary. It is found in children older than 5 years. The tumor presents with conjunctival injection, anterior chamber seeds, pseudohypopyon, large clumps of vitreous cells, and retinal infiltration of tumor. Because no distinct tumor mass is present, diagnostic confusion with inflammatory conditions is common.

Spontaneous regression of retinoblastoma is also possible and can be asymptomatic, resulting in the development of a benign retinocytoma, or it can be associated with inflammation and, ultimately, phthisis bulbi. In either case, the genetic implications are the same as for an individual with an active retinoblastoma.

Pretreatment evaluation of a patient with presumed retinoblastoma requires imaging of the head and orbits, which can confirm the diagnosis and can assist in evaluating possible extraocular extension and potential intracranial disease (Fig 26-24). CT may facilitate the diagnosis by demonstrating intraocular calcification. However, MRI and ultrasonography, which avoid the use of radiation, may be preferable to CT, because the risk of secondary tumors is high in many of these patients. Other, more invasive tests are reserved for atypical cases. Aspiration of ocular fluids for diagnostic testing should be performed only under the most unusual circumstances because such procedures can disseminate malignant cells and usually are not necessary.

The retinoblastoma gene *(RB1)* maps to a locus within the q14 band of chromosome 13 and codes for a protein, pRB, that functions as a suppressor of tumor formation. pRB is a nucleoprotein that binds to DNA and controls the cell cycle at the transition from the G_1 phase to the S-phase, thereby inhibiting cellular proliferation. Approximately 60% of retinoblastoma cases arise from somatic nonhereditary mutations of both alleles of *RB1* in a retinal cell. These mutations generally result in unifocal and unilateral tumors. In the other 40% of patients, a mutation in 1 of the 2 alleles of *RB1* either is inherited from an affected parent (10%) or occurs spontaneously in 1 of the gametes. A second somatic mutation occurs in 1 or more retinal cells, resulting in multicentric and usually bilateral tumor formation.

Genetic counseling for the families of retinoblastoma patients is complex and challenging (Table 26-2). Both of the patient's parents and all siblings should also be examined. In about 1% of cases, a parent may be found to have an unsuspected fundus lesion that represents a spontaneously regressed retinoblastoma or retinocytoma.

Genetic testing for retinoblastoma is available but has limitations. Karyotypic studies can identify only large deletions spanning 2 to 5 million base pairs, which account for only 3%–5% of retinoblastoma patients. Other direct and indirect methods can be used to detect smaller mutations; however, indirect methods require the presence of 2 or more affected family members, and the accuracy of these analyses greatly increases with examination of tumor-derived DNA, which is not available if the proband is being treated with

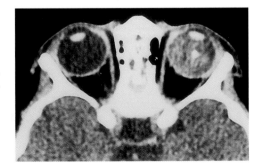

Figure 26-24 Axial CT image showing retinoblastoma filling most of the posterior segment of left eye, with localized calcification.

Table 26-2 Genetic Counseling for Retinoblastoma

If Parent:	Has Bilateral Retinoblastoma	Has Unilateral Retinoblastoma	Is Unaffected
Chance of offspring having retinoblastoma	45% affected → / 55% unaffected →	7%–15% affected → / 85%–93% unaffected →	<1% affected → / 99% unaffected →
Laterality	From affected: 85% bilateral →, 15% unilateral →; unaffected: 0% →	From affected: 85% bilateral →, 15% unilateral →; unaffected: 0% →	From affected: 33% bilateral →, 67% unilateral →; unaffected: 0% →
Focality	85% bilateral → 100% multifocal →; 15% unilateral → 96% multifocal → / 4% unifocal →; 0% →	85% bilateral → 100% multifocal →; 15% unilateral → 96% multifocal → / 4% unifocal →; 0% →	33% bilateral → 100% multifocal →; 67% unilateral → 15% multifocal → / 85% unifocal →; 0% →
Chance of next sibling having retinoblastoma	45%, 45%, 45%, 45%	45%, 45%, 45%, 7%–15%	5%*, <1%*, <1%*, <1%

*If parent is a carrier, then 45%

Table created by David H. Abramson, MD.

methods other than enucleation. Direct methods are time-consuming and costly and fail to find the mutation in up to 20% of cases. Preimplantation genetic testing can be performed, and in vitro fertilization techniques have been used to select embryos that are free from the germinal *RB1* mutation, successfully resulting in the birth of children unaffected by retinoblastoma.

The differential diagnosis of leukocoria is shown in Table 26-3. The most common retinal lesion simulating retinoblastoma is Coats disease. The presence of crystalline material, extensive subretinal fluid, and peripheral vascular abnormalities, combined with absence of calcium, suggests Coats disease. *Astrocytic hamartomas* and *hemangioblastomas* are benign retinal tumors that may simulate the appearance of small retinoblastomas. Both are usually associated with the neurocutaneous syndromes discussed in Chapter 27.

The characteristic histopathologic features of retinoblastoma include Flexner-Wintersteiner rosettes, which are usually present, and fleurettes, which are less common. Both represent limited degrees of retinal cellular differentiation. Homer Wright rosettes are also frequently present but are less specific for retinoblastoma because they are common in other neuroblastic tumors. Calcification of varying extent is usually present.

Classification of retinoblastoma

The Reese-Ellsworth classification (Table 26-4) was originally developed to predict globe salvage after external beam radiotherapy and chemotherapy. Although it is still useful for comparing contemporary treatment modalities to older ones, new classification schemes are emerging, such as the Philadelphia practical classification, and the International Classification of Retinoblastoma. No single new scheme has yet been widely accepted.

> Murphree AL. Intraocular retinoblastoma: the case for a new group classification. *Ophthalmol Clin North Am.* 2005;18(1):41–53.
> Shields CL, Shields JA. Basic understanding of current classification and management of retinoblastoma. *Curr Opin Ophthalmol.* 2006;17(3):228–234.

Management of retinoblastoma

The management of retinoblastoma has changed dramatically over the past decade and continues to evolve. External beam radiotherapy is seldom used as the primary treatment of intraocular retinoblastoma because of its high association with the development of craniofacial deformity and secondary tumors in the field of radiation. When the likelihood of salvaging vision is low, primary enucleation of eyes with advanced unilateral retinoblastoma is still recommended to avoid the side effects of systemic chemotherapy. To prevent extraocular spread of the tumor, the surgeon should avoid unnecessary manipulation of the globe and obtain a long segment of optic nerve.

Primary systemic chemotherapy (chemoreduction) followed by local therapy (consolidation) is now the most commonly used vision-sparing technique (Fig 26-25). Most studies of chemoreduction for retinoblastoma have employed vincristine, carboplatin, and an epipodophyllotoxin, either etoposide or teniposide. Others have added cyclosporine. The choice of agents as well as number and frequency of cycles varies from institution to institution. Chemotherapy is rarely successful when used alone, but in some cases, local therapy (cryotherapy, laser photocoagulation, thermotherapy, or plaque radiotherapy)

Table 26-3 Differential Diagnosis of Leukocoria

Clinical Diagnosis in Suspected Retinoblastoma
Retinoblastoma
Persistent fetal vasculature
Retinopathy of prematurity
Cataract
Coloboma of choroid or optic disc
Uveitis
Larval granulomatosis (toxocariasis)
Congenital retinal fold
Coats disease
Organizing vitreous hemorrhage
Retinal dysplasia
Corneal opacity
Familial exudative vitreoretinopathy (FEVR)
High myopia/anisometropia
Myelinated nerve fibers
Norrie disease
Retinal detachment
Photographic artifact

Table 26-4 Reese-Ellsworth Classification of Retinoblastoma

Group I
  a. Solitary tumor, less than 4 disc diameters in size, at or behind the equator
  b. Multiple tumors, none over 4 disc diameters in size, all at or behind the equator
Group II
  a. Solitary tumor, 4 to 10 disc diameters in size, at or behind the equator
  b. Multiple tumors, 4 to 10 disc diameters in size, behind the equator
Group III
  a. Any lesion anterior to the equator
  b. Solitary tumors larger than 10 disc diameters behind the equator
Group IV
  a. Multiple tumors, some larger than 10 disc diameters
  b. Any lesion extending anterior to the ora serrata
Group V
  a. Massive seeding involving over half the retina
  b. Vitreous seeding

can be used without chemotherapy. Adverse effects of chemoreduction treatment include low blood count, hair loss, hearing loss, renal toxicity, and neurologic and cardiac disturbances. Acute myelogenous leukemia has been reported after a chemoreduction regimen that included etoposide. Local administration of chemotherapy, which has the potential to minimize systemic complications, is being investigated.

Intra-arterial chemotherapy with melphalan via cannulation of the ophthalmic artery is a relatively new treatment modality for intraocular retinoblastoma. The initial description of this treatment modality appears promising as a means of reducing the need for external beam radiotherapy.

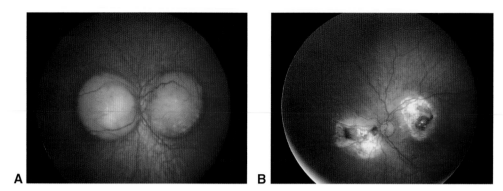

Figure 26-25 **A,** Left eye of infant with bilateral retinoblastoma. Two tumors straddle the optic nerve. **B,** After chemoreduction and laser consolidation, all tumors are nonviable. The child's vision was 20/25 at age 5 years.

Treated retinoblastoma sometimes disappears altogether, but more often it persists as a calcified mass (type 1, or cottage cheese, pattern) or a noncalcified, translucent grayish lesion (type 2, or fish flesh, pattern, which is difficult to distinguish from untreated tumor). Type 3 regression has elements of both types 1 and 2, and type 4 regression is a flat, atrophic scar. A child with treated retinoblastoma must be observed closely, with frequent examinations under anesthesia.

Extraocular retinoblastoma, though uncommon in the United States, is still problematic in developing countries, primarily because of delay in diagnosis. The 4 major types are optic nerve involvement, orbital invasion, central nervous system involvement, and distant metastasis. Treatment of extraocular retinoblastoma includes intensive multimodality chemotherapy, autologous hematopoietic stem cell rescue, and external beam radiation therapy. Exenteration is rarely necessary. Long-term disease-free survival is possible if the central nervous system is not involved; otherwise, the prognosis is usually poor.

Patients with trilateral retinoblastoma have a primitive neuroectodermal tumor of the pineal gland or parasellar region, in addition to retinoblastoma. The risk of trilateral retinoblastoma has been less than 0.5% and 5%–15% in patients with unilateral and bilateral retinoblastoma, respectively. However, the rate of trilateral retinoblastoma appears to be reduced in patients treated with chemoreduction therapy. Serial MRI to monitor for intracranial neoplasms has been recommended by some investigators, but this approach has not been shown to reduce mortality from this condition. Treatment includes systemic and intrathecal chemotherapy and external beam, stereotactic, or gamma knife radiation therapy. Favorable responses have been obtained in some cases, but the prognosis is frequently poor.

Abramson DH, Dunkel IJ, Brodie SE, Kim JW, Gobin YP. A phase I/II study of direct intraarterial (ophthalmic artery) chemotherapy with melphalan for intraocular retinoblastoma initial results. *Ophthalmology.* 2008;115(8):1398–1404.

Duncan JL, Scott IU, Murray TG, Gombos DS, van Quill K, O'Brien JM. Routine neuroimaging in retinoblastoma for the detection of intracranial tumors. *Arch Ophthalmol.* 2001;119(3): 450–452.

Monitoring

Close monitoring of patients with retinoblastoma and their family members is crucial. Even patients with unilateral unifocal tumors have an almost 20% chance of developing retinoblastoma in their fellow eye. This risk is diminished with age and is low after age 24 months. If the retinoblastoma is the hereditary form, the patient and siblings should be examined every 4 months until age 3 or 4 years and then every 6 months until age 6 years.

Nonocular tumors are common in patients with germinal mutations, estimated to occur with an incidence of 1% rate per year of life (eg, 10% prevalence by age 10, 30% by age 30). The incidence is higher for patients treated with external beam radiotherapy before 1 year of age. The most common secondary tumors are osteogenic sarcoma of the skull and long bones, soft tissue sarcomas, cutaneous melanoma, breast cancer, lung cancer, brain tumors, and Hodgkin lymphoma. Patients who develop second, nonocular tumors are at even greater risk for additional malignancies.

Abramson DH, Schefler AC. Update on retinoblastoma. *Retina.* 2004:24(6):828–848.

Ellsworth RM. The practical management of retinoblastoma. *Trans Am Ophthalmol Soc.* 1969; 67:462–534.

Gunduz K, Shields CL. Retinoblastoma update. *Focal Points: Clinical Modules for Ophthalmologists.* San Francisco: American Academy of Ophthalmology; 2005, module 7.

Shields CL, Mashayekhi A, Demirci H, Meadows AT, Shields JA. Practical approach to management of retinoblastoma. *Arch Ophthalmol.* 2004;122(5):729–735.

Shields CL, Meadows AT, Leahey AM, Shields JA. Continuing challenges in the management of retinoblastoma with chemotherapy. *Retina.* 2004;24(6):849–862.

Shields CL, Meadows AT, Shields JA, Carvalho C, Smith AF. Chemoreduction for retinoblastoma may prevent intracranial neuroblastic malignancy (trilateral retinoblastoma). *Arch Ophthalmol.* 2001;119(9):1269–1272.

CHAPTER 27

Phakomatoses

The phakomatoses, or *neurocutaneous syndromes,* are a group of disorders featuring multiple discrete lesions of 1 or a few histologic types that are found in 2 or more organ systems, including the skin and central nervous system (CNS). The lesions are usually hamartomas (abnormal proliferations of tissues normally found in the involved organs). Each syndrome is defined not by the characteristics of the individual lesions but by their multiplicity or association with one another. Eye involvement is frequent and may constitute an important source of morbidity or provide information of critical importance to diagnosis. Four major disorders have traditionally been designated phakomatoses, and all have important eye manifestations:

- neurofibromatosis (von Recklinghausen disease)
- tuberous sclerosis (Bourneville disease)
- angiomatosis of the retina and cerebellum (von Hippel–Lindau disease)
- encephalofacial or encephalotrigeminal angiomatosis (Sturge-Weber syndrome)

Other conditions sometimes classified as phakomatoses include

- ataxia-telangiectasia (Louis-Bar syndrome)
- incontinentia pigmenti (Bloch-Sulzberger syndrome)
- racemose angioma (Wyburn-Mason syndrome)

Table 27-1 describes the features of the phakomatoses.

Korf BR. The phakomatoses. *Clin Dermatol.* 2005;23(1):78–84.

Neurofibromatosis

Patients with neurofibromatosis (NF), or *von Recklinghausen disease,* manifest characteristic lesions composed of melanocytes or neuroglial cells, which are both primarily derivatives of neural crest mesenchyme. Although the melanocytic and glial lesions in NF are often called *hamartomas,* this designation is questionable in that most lesions do not become evident until years after birth and many are histologically indistinguishable from low-grade neoplasms originating in the same tissues.

NF has 2 forms (NF1 and NF2) that are distinguished by differences in genetics, diagnostic criteria, morbidity, and treatment. Both are familial disorders that show autosomal dominant inheritance with very high penetrance (virtually 100% in NF1). However, a large percentage of cases (nearly half in NF1) are sporadic, presumably reflecting the high rate of mutation known to be true for the responsible gene. The genetic locus of NF1

363

Table 27-1 The Phakomatoses

Condition	Description	Associated Ocular Condition	Associated Conditions and Risks	Transmission
Neurofibromatosis (von Recklinghausen disease)	Occasionally congenital, widespread hamartomas of peripheral nerves and tissue of neural crest derivation	Neurofibromas of eyelid and orbit, uveal melanocytic nevi, retinal glial hamartomas, congenital glaucoma, optic nerve glioma, absence of greater wing of sphenoid with pulsating exophthalmos	Similar hamartomas of central nervous system, peripheral and cranial nerves, gastrointestinal tract; malignant transformation possible	Autosomal dominant NF1: band 17q11.2 NF2: band 22q12.2
Tuberous sclerosis (Bourneville disease)	Variable mental deficiency, seizures, and adenoma sebaceum	Angiofibromas of eyelid, skin; glial hamartomas of retina and optic disc	Adenoma sebaceum (angiofibromas), cerebral glial hamartomas	Autosomal dominant, bands 9q34, 16p13.3
von Hippel–Lindau disease (retinal angiomatosis)	Retinal angioma supplied by dilated tortuous arteriole and venule; may be multiple	Retinal exudates, hemorrhages, retinal detachment, glaucoma	Cerebellar capillary hemangiomas, malformation of visceral organs	Autosomal dominant, 3p26–p25
Sturge-Weber syndrome (encephalofacial angiomatosis)	Capillary hamartia (nevus flammeus) of skin, conjunctiva, episclera, and/or uveal tract, and of meninges	Glaucoma (especially with upper eyelid involvement by nevus flammeus)	Diffuse meningeal hemangioma with seizure disorder, hemiplegia or hemianopia, or mental retardation	Sporadic
Ataxia-telangiectasia (Louis-Bar syndrome)	Progressive cerebellar ataxia, ocular and cutaneous telangiectasia, pulmonary infections	Conjunctival telangiectasia, anomalous ocular movements, and nystagmus	Dysarthria, coarse hair and skin, immunologic deficiency, and mental and growth retardation	Autosomal recessive, chromosome 11q22–23
Incontinentia pigmenti (Bloch-Sulzberger syndrome)	Cutaneous; dental, central nervous system, and ocular changes	ROP-like vasculopathy may progress to retinal detachment and retrolental membrane formation	"Splashed paint" hyperpigmented macules, microcephaly, seizures, and mental deficiency	X-linked dominant
Wyburn-Mason syndrome (racemose angioma)	Retinal and midbrain arteriovenous (A-V) communication (aneurysms and angiomas) and facial nevi	A-V communication (racemose angioma) of retina, with vision loss depending on location of A-V communication	A-V aneurysm at midbrain; intracranial calcification	Sporadic

Modified from Isselbacher K, Braunwald E, Wilson JD, eds. *Harrison's Principles of Internal Medicine.* 13th ed. New York: McGraw-Hill; 1994:2207–2210.

is on the long arm of chromosome 17 (17q11.2), and that of NF2 is on the long arm of chromosome 22 (22q12.2). The NF1 gene has been isolated and cloned. It appears to code for the protein *neurofibromin,* which is involved in regulation of cellular proliferation and tumor suppression. NF1 is by far the more common condition, with a prevalence of 1 in 3000–5000.

Neurofibromatosis Type 1

The clinical and pathologic manifestations of NF1 are discussed in the following sections.

Melanocytic lesions

Almost all adults with NF1 have melanocytic lesions involving both the skin and the eye. The most common cutaneous expression, café-au-lait spots, appears clinically as flat, sharply demarcated, uniformly hyperpigmented macules of varying size and shape. At least a few are usually present at birth, but their number and size increase during the first decade of life. Clusters of small café-au-lait spots, or freckling, in the axillary or inguinal regions are particularly characteristic of NF1, occurring in a majority of patients older than age 10.

Many unaffected people have 1 to 3 café-au-lait spots, but greater numbers are rare except in association with NF. In the past, NF was often diagnosed solely on the basis of multiple café-au-lait spots, but it is now recognized that a few persons with this finding never develop other stigmata of the disease and may have offspring with a similarly limited condition, suggesting the existence of a genetic disorder distinct from NF1. Currently, NF1 is diagnosed only when 2 or more criteria from the following group of 7 are met:

- 6 or more café-au-lait spots >5 mm in diameter in prepubescents or >15 mm in diameter in postpubescents
- 2 or more neurofibromas of any type or 1 plexiform neurofibroma
- freckling of axillary, inguinal, or other intertriginous areas
- optic nerve glioma
- 2 or more iris Lisch nodules
- a distinctive osseous lesion, such as sphenoid bone dysplasia or thinning of the long-bone cortex, with or without pseudarthrosis
- a first-degree relative with NF1, according to the above criteria

Neurofibromatosis. Conference Statement. National Institutes of Health Consensus Development Conference. *Arch Neurol.* 1988;45(5):575–578.

Occasionally, eyelid skin or conjunctiva is hyperpigmented in NF1, but melanocytic lesions of the uveal tract are far more common ocular manifestations. In the iris, these lesions take the form of small (usually ≤1 mm), sharply demarcated, dome-shaped excrescences known as *Lisch nodules* (Fig 27-1; see also Chapter 19, Fig 19-3). Clinically, Lisch nodules usually appear to have smooth surfaces and a translucent interior suggesting a gelatinous consistency, but in some people they look solid and wartlike. Color varies but can be described as tan in most cases. In heavily pigmented brown irides, the nodules tend to stand out as lighter nodules against the smooth, dark anterior surface and may be visible

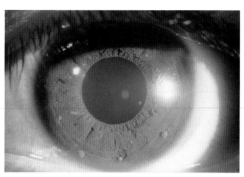

Figure 27-1 Lisch nodules of iris, left eye, in child with type 1 neurofibromatosis. Also see Figure 19-3 (Lisch nodules).

to the unaided eye. When overall iris stromal pigmentation is lighter, Lisch nodules are usually slightly darker than the rest of the iris but can be partly hidden within recesses in the stromal tissue and may be overlooked unless a slit lamp is used. They may be difficult to differentiate from small clumps of normal pigmented tissue, especially when they are few and the patient is less than fully cooperative during the examination. Histopathologically, the lesions consist primarily of uniform spindle-shaped, melanin-containing cells, indistinguishable from those found in iris nevi and low-grade spindle-cell melanomas.

Most Lisch nodules develop during childhood or adolescence. They are seen infrequently before age 3 years, appear in a majority of cases of NF1 between ages 5 and 10 years, and are present in nearly 100% of affected adults. The finding of 2 or more Lisch nodules is a diagnostic criterion for NF1, but an affected adult's eye typically has dozens and occasionally 100 or more (see also Chapter 19).

Choroidal lesions have been reported to occur in one-third to one-half of adults with NF1. These lesions are described as flat with indistinct borders and hyperpigmented in relation to the surrounding fundus but ranging from yellow-white to dark brown. Their number varies from 1 to 20 per eye, with each lesion typically 1 to 2 times the size of the optic disc. Direct histopathologic correlation for this clinical finding is lacking, but it is presumed to represent localized concentration of melanocytes similar to a choroidal nevus.

Neither the vision nor the health of the eye is affected by these lesions, regardless of their extent, except for the association with glaucoma in iris ectropion. People with NF1 are thought to be predisposed to uveal melanoma as well as a number of other malignant neoplasms. However, the prevalence of iris, and especially choroidal, tumors is still quite low.

Glial cell lesions

Nodular neurofibromas   Among lesions of neuroglial origin in NF1, *nodular cutaneous* and *subcutaneous neurofibromas,* or *fibroma molluscum,* are by far the most common. These are soft papulonodules, often pedunculated, with color ranging from that of normal skin to violescent. They typically begin to appear in late childhood and increase in number throughout adolescence and adulthood; nearly all adults with NF1 have at least a few. In some cases, hundreds of these lesions are present, causing considerable disfigurement.

Plexiform neurofibromas   Of much greater clinical significance than nodular neurofibromas are the less common plexiform neurofibromas, which occur in approximately 30%

of patients with NF1. These neurofibromas are very rarely seen in other contexts. The lesions appear clinically as extensive subcutaneous swellings with indistinct margins. Hyperpigmentation or hypertrichosis of the overlying skin is common, as is hypertrophy of underlying soft tissue and bone (regional gigantism). The consistency of plexiform neurofibromas is typically soft and not easily distinguished from that of normal tissue; the oft-repeated statement that they feel like a "bag of worms" applies in only a minority of cases.

Plexiform neurofibromas develop earlier than nodular lesions, frequently becoming evident in infancy or childhood. These neurofibromas often show considerable enlargement over time, resulting in severe disfigurement and functional impairment. Rarely, the lesions undergo malignant degeneration, producing a neurofibrosarcoma capable of widespread metastasis.

Approximately 10% of plexiform neurofibromas involve the face, commonly the upper eyelid and orbit. At onset, the involved upper eyelid is thicker than normal and usually appears mildly ptotic (Fig 27-2). Its inner surface may override the lower eyelid margin and lashes when the eye is closed. Characteristically, the greater involvement of the upper eyelid's temporal portion gives the eyelid margin an S-shaped configuration and an overall appearance of an eyelid that is too big for the eye. The lesion undergoes considerable and sometimes massive growth during childhood and adolescence, although extension across the facial midline is rare. Complete ptosis may eventually result from the increasing bulk and weight of the upper eyelid. Irritation of the upper palpebral conjunctiva caused by rubbing against the lower lashes can create significant discomfort. Glaucoma in the ipsilateral eye is found in as many as half of cases.

Complete excision of a plexiform neurofibroma involving the eyelid is generally not possible. Treatment is directed toward the relief of specific symptoms and is likely to be partially successful at best. Distorted and chronically inflamed conjunctiva sometimes requires resection. Surgical debulking and frontalis suspension procedures can reduce ptosis sufficiently to permit binocular vision, but the condition is usually progressive.

Optic glioma This low-grade pilocytic astrocytoma involves the optic nerve, chiasm, or both (optic glioma) and is among the most characteristic and potentially serious complications of NF1. Symptomatic optic gliomas (ie, tumors producing significant vision loss,

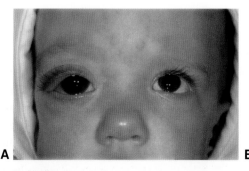
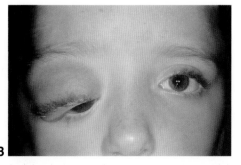

A **B**

Figure 27-2 Plexiform neurofibroma involving the right upper eyelid, associated with ipsilateral buphthalmos, in girl with NF1. **A,** Age 8 months. **B,** Age 8 years.

proptosis, or other complications) occur in 1%–5% of individuals with NF1. When CT or MRI is performed prospectively on unselected NF1 patients, abnormalities of the optic nerve (often bilateral) or chiasm, indicating the presence of glioma, are found in approximately 15% of cases.

Typically, the entire orbital portion of an involved optic nerve shows cylindrical or fusiform enlargement (Fig 27-3). A relatively narrow central core usually differs from surrounding tissue because of the characteristic growth pattern of optic nerve glioma in NF1: most cellular proliferation occurs in the perineural intradural space (arachnoidal gliomatosis) associated with production of abundant mucinous material that gives this tissue the signal characteristics of water. This core shows higher density in CT; with MRI, the core shows higher density on T1-weighted images and lower density on T2-weighted images.

Exaggerated sinuousness or kinking of the optic nerve often occurs, creating an appearance of discontinuity or localized constriction on axial images. These appearances distinguish optic glioma from the principal differential diagnostic alternative, optic nerve sheath meningioma, which also occurs with increased frequency in NF. However, optic nerve sheath meningioma occurs much less commonly than optic glioma and rarely in childhood.

Gliomas involving the intracranial optic nerve or chiasm in NF1 produce enlargement of these structures on both CT and MRI and, frequently, abnormal signal intensity on MRI, which is now the preferred means of diagnosis. Associated contiguous involvement of the orbital portion of 1 or both optic nerves usually occurs, and extension into the optic tracts and posterior visual pathways is often evident, especially on MRI. Intraocular extension has also been reported.

Optic gliomas that become symptomatic in patients with NF1 nearly always do so before age 10 years, often apparently following a brief period of rapid enlargement. Even

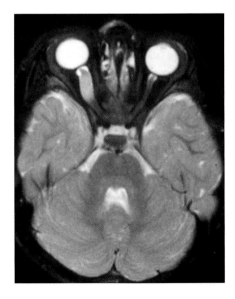

Figure 27-3 Axial MRI of a right optic nerve glioma in a child with NF1. *(Courtesy of Ken K. Nischal, FRCOphth.)*

without treatment, some gliomas then appear to enter a phase of stability or much slower growth, and spontaneous improvement has been documented in a few cases.

Tumors confined to the optic nerve at the time of clinical presentation infrequently extend into the chiasm subsequently and only rarely develop extradural extension or distant metastasis. New chemotherapy regimens may be effective in halting growing masses, and radiation therapy can be useful, especially in cases of sudden vision loss or rapid growth. However, there are clinicians who believe that the efficacy of chemotherapy is difficult to evaluate, even in large studies, because of the widely variable natural history of this disease. Surgical treatment remains controversial. Some authorities recommend complete excision through a transfrontal approach that preserves the globe but sacrifices any remaining vision on the involved side, but it has not been demonstrated that this approach improves the prognosis for sight in the other eye. Subtotal orbital excision for relief of disfiguring proptosis can also be considered.

In addition to bilateral vision loss, tumors primarily involving the chiasm may produce significant morbidity, including hydrocephalus and hypothalamic dysfunction leading to precocious puberty or hypopituitarism. Glioma of the chiasm carries a reported mortality rate of 50% or higher. In the past, most deaths occurred within months of diagnosis, but recent series show longer survival, reflecting earlier detection and improved management of complications, in addition to more effective treatment of the tumor itself with chemotherapy. Radiation therapy, which is used after a failure of chemotherapy treatment, appears to retard or reverse progression in many cases, but it is not firmly established that this therapy can substantially reduce the ultimate rate of tumor-related blindness and death, which may occur as late as 20 years after presentation.

Other neuroglial abnormalities   Abnormal proliferation of peripheral neuroglial or other neural crest–derived cells may occur in relation to deeper tissues and visceral organs as well as skin (spinal and gastrointestinal neurofibromas, pheochromocytoma). Prominence of corneal nerves, thought to represent glial hypertrophy, may be noted on slit-lamp examination in as many as 20% of cases. A frequent histopathologic finding in the choroid is the presence of so-called ovoid bodies, onionlike formations that appear to consist of hyperplastic Schwann cells surrounding peripheral nerve axons. Rarely, a localized neurofibroma develops within the orbit in association with NF. Retinal hamartomas indistinguishable from those seen in tuberous sclerosis have also been found in patients with NF1.

Other manifestations

NF1 is associated with an increased, but still generally low, incidence of a number of conditions that cannot be explained by abnormal proliferation of neural crest–derived cells. These conditions include a variety of benign tumors that may involve skin or eye (juvenile xanthogranuloma, capillary hemangioma) and several forms of malignancy (leukemia, rhabdomyosarcoma, pheochromocytoma, Wilms tumor). Also relatively common are bony defects such as scoliosis, pseudarthrosis of the tibia, and hypoplasia of the sphenoid bone, which may result in ocular pulsation. Sphenoid dysplasia may be progressive and may be associated with neurofibromas in the ipsilateral superficial temporal fossa as well as in deep orbit. Neuroimaging should be obtained in any patient with ocular pulsations, neurofibromas in this area, or other reasons for clinical suspicion. A number of ill-defined abnormalities of the CNS (macrocephaly, aqueductal stenosis, seizures, and usually minor intellectual deficits) are also seen with increased frequency in patients with NF1.

The most significant ophthalmic disorder in this category is glaucoma, which is usually unilateral. In most cases, glaucoma is associated with ipsilateral plexiform neurofibroma of the upper eyelid or with the iris abnormality known as *congenital iris ectropion* (see discussion in Chapter 19). Buphthalmos, or enlargement of the cornea and the globe as a whole, is seen if intraocular pressure (IOP) is elevated during the first 2 years of life. In some cases, excessive growth of the eyeball may also be a manifestation of regional hypertrophy, at least in part. Corneal edema and high myopia can result from high pressure in early or later childhood.

The pathogenesis of glaucoma in NF1 is unknown. Abnormal trabecular meshwork development in some patients can lead to early-onset childhood or congenital glaucoma. In other patients, synechial closure of the angle may result from neurofibromatous tissue posterior to the iris or neurofibromatous infiltration of the angle directly. Medical management of the glaucoma can be attempted but frequently fails. A variety of surgical procedures have been employed with moderate success; achievement of adequate pressure control often requires several operations. Contributing to the poor prognosis are frequently associated, significant orbital and optic nerve abnormalities, as well as refractory amblyopia (anisometropic or deprivation).

A child or adult who appears to have any one of the abnormalities typically associated with NF1 should undergo an eye examination that includes the following:

- assessment of vision (acuity and color discrimination)
- pupillary light reaction, including careful scrutiny for relative afferent defect
- slit-lamp examination with particular attention to the iris
- ophthalmoscopy to identify disc pallor or edema and choroidal lesions
- measurement of IOP, when indicated by other findings

The discovery of Lisch nodules has been used to confirm the presence of NF1 in a patient with café-au-lait spots, and the absence of such nodules in an adult patient has been said to virtually rule out the diagnosis. However, the use of iris changes as a diagnostic marker for NF1 has been questioned by some practitioners. Iris changes in patients with known NF1 may be more diverse than the classic descriptions of Lisch nodules, and interobserver reliability for the diagnosis of NF1 based on iris findings can be inconsistent.

Although the role of routine screening with MRI remains controversial, abnormalities of vision, pupil function, or optic disc appearance indicate a need for neuroimaging studies to look for optic glioma. Screening neuroimaging in preverbal children, in whom vision and visual fields cannot be accurately assessed, should be considered. However, some clinicians do not recommend routine neuroimaging in children, even if preverbal, unless there are other abnormalities (eg, apparent decreased vision, relative afferent pupillary defect). An appropriate interval for periodic ophthalmic reassessment in childhood is 1–2 years unless a significant abnormality requires closer observation. New onset of significant eye involvement is less likely in adults, but blood pressure should be regularly monitored because of the risk of pheochromocytoma.

Jacquemin C, Bosley TM, Liu D, Svedberg H, Buhaliqa A. Reassessment of sphenoid dysplasia associated with neurofibromatosis type 1. *Am J Neuroradiol.* 2002;23(4):644–648.

Listernick R, Ferner RE, Liu GT, Gutmann DH. Optic pathway gliomas in neurofibromatosis-1: controversies and recommendations. *Ann Neurol.* 2007;61(3):189–198.

Trovó-Marqui AB, Goloni-Bertollo EM, Teixeira MF, Tajara EH. Presence of the R1748X mutation in the NF1 gene in a Brazilian patient with ectropion uveae. *Ophthalmic Res.* 2004;36(6):349–352.

Neurofibromatosis Type 2

NF2 is less common than NF1 by a factor of at least 10. NF2 is diagnosed by the presence of bilateral acoustic neuromas (eighth nerve tumors) or by a first-degree relative with NF2 and presence of a unilateral acoustic neuroma, neurofibroma, meningioma, schwannoma, glioma, or early-onset posterior subcapsular cataract.

Patients with NF2 typically present in their teens to early adulthood with symptoms related to the eighth nerve tumor(s), including decreased hearing or tinnitus. Ocular findings may predate the onset of symptoms. Therefore, the alert ophthalmologist may be able to help diagnose the potential for CNS tumors before they become symptomatic. The most characteristic eye finding in NF2 is lens opacity, especially posterior subcapsular cataract or wedge cortical cataracts. Other, less common findings are retinal hamartoma and combined hamartomas of the retina and retinal pigment epithelium (RPE). Lisch nodules of the iris can occur in NF2, but are not expected.

Kaiser-Kupfer MI, Freidlin V, Datiles MB, et al. The association of posterior capsular lens opacities with bilateral acoustic neuromas in patients with neurofibromatosis type 2. *Arch Ophthalmol.* 1989;107(4):541–544.

Tuberous Sclerosis

Tuberous sclerosis (TS), or *Bourneville disease,* is a familial disorder associated with a variety of abnormalities involving the skin, eye, CNS, and other organs. Estimates of the prevalence of TS range from as high as 1:6000 to 1:100,000 or lower. Two distinct genes giving rise to TS have been identified: *TSC1* at band 9q34 and *TSC2* at band 16p13.3, whose proteins, *hamartin* and *tuberin* respectively, are tumor growth suppressors. Transmission as an autosomal dominant trait has been documented in numerous pedigrees, but new mutations account for as many as 80% of cases.

The 3 classic findings, known as the Vogt triad, are mental retardation, seizures, and facial angiofibromas, although all 3 are present in only about 30% of patients with TS. The disease is characterized by benign tumor growth in multiple organs, predominantly the skin, brain, heart, kidney, and eye. Primary features of this disorder, any one of which is sufficient to diagnose TS, are

- facial angiofibroma
- ungual fibromas (multiple)
- cortical tuber
- subependymal nodule (giant cell astrocytoma)

- multiple subependymal nodules protruding into the ventricle
- multiple retinal astrocytomas

Several distinct skin lesions are characteristic of TS (Fig 27-4). The earliest cutaneous sign to appear is the white spot, or hypopigmented macule, which is present in almost all cases at birth or in infancy. These lesions are sharply demarcated, with a shape that often resembles an ash leaf, and are thus called "ash leaf spots." Ultraviolet light from a Wood's lamp increases the visibility of white spots in light-skinned people. Histopathologically, these spots have decreased melanin but normal numbers of melanocytes.

Facial angiofibromas, often called *adenoma sebaceum,* begin to appear in childhood and increase progressively in number; they are present in three-quarters of adolescents and adults with TS. These lesions are often mistaken for common acne. Subungual and periungual fibromas are also common after puberty; gingival fibromas may occur as well. A thickened plaque of skin known as a shagreen patch, or collagenoma, occurs in approximately one-quarter of cases, typically in the lumbosacral area. Plaques involving the forehead that sometimes extend into the eyelids may be present at birth.

Seizures occur in 80% of patients with TS and may be difficult to control. Severe mental retardation is present in 50% of patients, but intelligence is often normal. Characteristic findings in neuroimaging studies include nodular periventricular or basal ganglion calcifications (representing benign astrocytomas) and tuberous malformations of the cortex (Fig 27-5). Malignant astrocytomas occur infrequently. Obstruction of the foramen of Munro by tumor may produce hydrocephalus, and cardiac tumors (rhabdomyomas) can lead to early death or severe disability. Lesions of bone and kidney are common but usually produce no significant disturbance of function.

Hypopigmented lesions analogous to white spots of the skin are occasionally seen in the iris or choroid, but the most frequent and characteristic ocular manifestation of TS is the retinal phakoma (Fig 27-6). Pathologically, this growth arises from the innermost layer of the retina and is composed of nerve fibers and relatively undifferentiated cells that appear to be of glial origin; the growth is frequently called an *astrocytic hamartoma.* Phakomas can develop anywhere in the fundus but are usually found near the posterior pole, involving the retina, the optic disc, or both. They vary in size from about half to twice the diameter of the disc. Vision is rarely affected significantly.

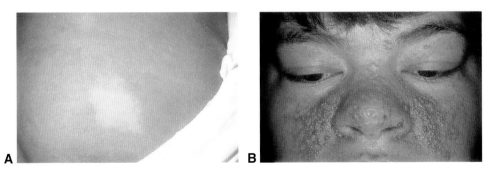

A **B**

Figure 27-4 Cutaneous lesions of tuberous sclerosis. **A,** Hypopigmented macule. **B,** Adenoma sebaceum of the face.

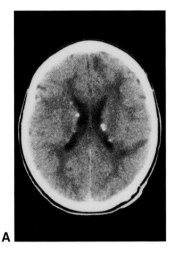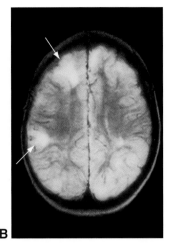

A   B

Figure 27-5 Brain lesions of tuberous sclerosis. **A,** Axial CT image showing small periventricular calcifications in the basal ganglia bilaterally. **B,** Axial T2-weighted MRI showing 2 tuberous malformations *(arrows)* of the right hemisphere cortex.

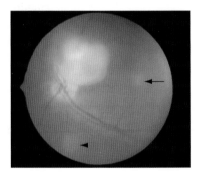

Figure 27-6 Fundus lesions of tuberous sclerosis, left eye. In addition to the large phakoma partially overlying the optic disc, a small hypopigmented lesion *(arrow)* appears in the temporal macula, and a barely visible second phakoma *(arrowhead)* partially obscures a retinal blood vessel near the edge of the photograph, directly below the disc. The lesions of tuberous sclerosis can vary considerably in their opaqueness and visibility.

Retinal phakomas usually have 1 of 2 distinct appearances, although intermediate forms can occur. The first type is typically found in very young children and is relatively flat with a smooth surface, indistinct margins, and gray-white color. These lesions are translucent to a degree that at times makes them difficult to detect ophthalmoscopically. The examiner can most easily locate them by tracing retinal vessels from the disc peripherally and scrutinizing points at which a vessel is partially obscured by overlying tissue. Domelike elevations can then be perceived with the binocular indirect ophthalmoscope by carefully observing the surface light reflection while shifting viewing direction slightly. The second type of phakoma is sharply demarcated and more elevated than the first type, with an irregular surface that has been compared to a mulberry or a cluster of tapioca grains or fish eggs. These lesions are opaque, glistening, and yellow-white as a result of calcification. They are found relatively more often in older patients and on or adjacent to the optic disc. The term *giant drusen* has been applied to disc involvement by a mulberry phakoma because of its resemblance to the common but unrelated condition known as *drusen* (or *hyaline bodies*) of the optic nerve head.

The reported frequency of phakomas in persons with TS varies greatly, but data from series suggest that they are present in one-third to more than one-half of cases. One to several may be found in a single eye, and the rate of bilateral involvement is about 40%. There is no evidence that the number of lesions increases with age, although individual tumors have been documented to grow over time. Phakomas are not pathognomonic of TS; they occur occasionally in association with neurofibromatosis and in the eyes of unaffected persons.

Alcorn DM. Ocular oncology. *Ophthalmol Clin North Am.* 1999;12:2.

von Hippel–Lindau Disease

von Hippel–Lindau (VHL) disease, or *retinal angiomatosis,* is an autosomal dominantly inherited disorder of incomplete penetrance manifesting both benign and malignant tumors of many organ systems. It is the result of a mutation of a tumor suppressor gene located on 3p26–p25. The prevalence of VHL is approximately 1 in 36,000 births. Its most common abnormalities are vascular tumors *(hemangioblastomas)* of the retina and CNS, most often the cerebellum. These tumors have only limited proliferative capacity, but exudation across thin vessel walls in the lesions leads to the formation of fluid accumulations that may attain considerable size and compromise vital structures. Cysts and tumors occur frequently in numerous other organs, including the kidneys *(renal cell carcinoma),* pancreas, liver, epididymis, and adrenal glands *(pheochromocytoma).* Despite its well-accepted classification as a neurocutaneous syndrome, VHL disease rarely has significant cutaneous manifestations, although café-au-lait spots and port-wine stains *(nevus flammeus)* are seen occasionally. Mental deficiency is not a feature of the disease. Associated malignant tumors make it a potentially fatal disease.

Pedigree studies suggest that ocular involvement occurs in most cases of VHL disease. (Identical eye disease without familial transmission or systemic involvement is 3 to 4 times more common than the complete syndrome.) The retinal lesions originally described by von Hippel usually become visible ophthalmoscopically between ages 10 and 35 years, with an average age of onset of 25 years, about a decade before the peak clinical incidence of cerebellar disease. Tumors are multiple in the same eye in about one-third of cases and bilateral in as many as one-half of cases. Tumors typically occur in the peripheral fundus, but lesions adjacent to the optic disc have also been described.

The incipient retinal lesion appears as a minor, nonspecific vascular anomaly or a small reddish dot in the fundus that gradually enlarges into a flat or slightly elevated grayish disc. The lesion ultimately acquires the fully developed appearance of a pink globular mass 1 to 3 or more disc diameters in size. The hallmark of the mature tumor is a pair of markedly dilated vessels (artery and vein) running between the lesion and the optic disc, indicating significant arteriovenous shunting (Fig 27-7). Recent observations suggest that characteristic paired or twin retinal vessels of normal caliber may be present before the tumor becomes visible.

Histopathologically, retinal angiomas consist of relatively well-formed capillaries; however, fluorescein angiography shows these vessels to be leaky. Transudation of fluid

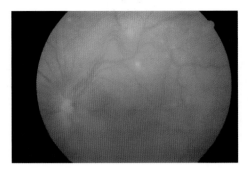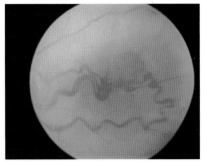

Figure 27-7   von Hippel–Lindau disease (retinal angiomatosis), left eye.

into the subretinal space causes lipid accumulation, retinal detachment, and consequent loss of vision in many involved eyes. Secondary degenerative changes, including cataract and glaucoma, often occur in blind eyes with long-standing retinal detachment; ultimately, enucleation may become necessary.

Retinal angiomas can be effectively treated with cryotherapy or laser photocoagulation in two-thirds or more of cases, particularly when the lesions are still small. Multiple treatment sessions may be necessary to achieve complete success. Early diagnosis increases the likelihood of successful treatment, yet the ocular lesions of VHL are asymptomatic prior to retinal detachment. Therefore, children known to be at risk for the disease should undergo periodic ophthalmologic evaluation beginning at about age 5 years.

Systemically, early tumor diagnosis can significantly reduce morbidity and mortality. The Cambridge screening protocol recommends that patients with VHL undergo annual complete physical examination and dilated eye examinations, renal ultrasonography, and 24-hour urine collection for vanillylmandelic acids. These patients should undergo neuroimaging every 3 years to age 40 and every 5 years thereafter. At-risk relatives should also undergo thorough annual screening for the disorder. Molecular genetic testing has been suggested for patients with early-onset cerebellar hemangioblastoma (<30 years old), early-onset retinal angioma, or familial clear cell renal carcinoma.

Chang JH, Spraul CW, Lynn ML, Drack A, Grossniklaus HE. The two-stage mutation model in retinal hemangioblastoma. *Ophthalmic Genet.* 1998;19(3):123–130.

Sturge-Weber Syndrome

Sturge-Weber syndrome (SWS), or *encephalofacial angiomatosis,* consists of a facial cutaneous angioma (port-wine stain) with an ipsilateral leptomeningeal vascular malformation that typically results in the following:

- cerebral calcification
- seizures, which may show a jacksonian pattern, progressing from focal to grand mal
- focal neurologic deficits (hemianopia, hemiparesis)
- a highly variable degree of mental deficiency (with normal intelligence in some affected persons)

SWS is unique among the 4 major neurocutaneous syndromes in that it is not a genetically transmitted disorder. However, lesions are always present at birth. The distribution of cutaneous and cerebral involvement suggests a disturbance very early in embryonic development (4–8 weeks' gestation), when primitive facial structures overlie the future occipital lobes of the developing brain. The prevalence of SWS is not reliably known.

Calcium deposits characteristic of SWS form after birth in brain parenchyma, usually involving the occipital lobe and varying portions of the parietal, temporal, and occasionally frontal lobes. Curvilinear densities, paralleling cerebral convolutions to produce the so-called railroad track sign, can be demonstrated by means of CT earlier and more consistently than by conventional radiographs, but these densities are often not detectable before age 2 years. MRI is less sensitive than CT for identifying calcification but may provide better delineation of other abnormalities associated with the angiomatous malformation that can confirm the diagnosis in very young children (Fig 27-8). These abnormalities include cerebral volume reduction, abnormal signal intensity in cortex and white matter, prominent deep venous system, and enlarged choroid plexus.

The Sturge-Weber skin lesion, which can be quite disfiguring, consists of dilated and excessively numerous but well-formed capillaries in the dermis. The lesion usually involves the forehead and upper eyelid on the same side as the cerebral vascular malformation, with varying extension to the ipsilateral lower eyelid and maxillary and mandibular regions (Fig 27-9). The sharply demarcated area of the port-wine nevus occasionally does not conform to the distribution of the trigeminal divisions, and involvement of the contralateral face, the scalp, and the trunk and extremities is common. (The designation *Klippel-Trénaunay-Weber syndrome* is sometimes applied to cases with extensive lesions of the extremities, although this syndrome may not be a true phakomatosis.) Hypertrophy of soft tissue and bone underlying the angioma is common in childhood, and thickening of the involved skin (sometimes with a nodular pattern) may develop later in life. Treatment of affected skin with a pulsed-dye laser has been shown to markedly reduce vascularity, considerably improving appearance without causing significant damage to dermal tissue.

It is noteworthy that not all children who have a port-wine stain necessarily have SWS.

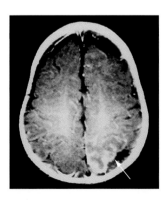

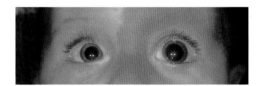

Figure 27-8 Axial gadolinium-enhanced T1-weighted MRI shows vascular malformation with underlying cortical atrophy *(arrow)* in the left occipital lobe of a 4-month-old girl with Sturge-Weber syndrome.

Figure 27-9 Facial port-wine nevus involving the left eyelids, associated with ipsilateral buphthalmos in an infant girl with Sturge-Weber syndrome.

Ocular Involvement

Any portion of the ocular circulation may be anomalous in SWS when the skin lesion involves the eyelids. Increased conjunctival vascularity commonly produces a pinkish discoloration. Frequently, an abnormal plexus of episcleral vessels appears, although it may be hidden by the overlying tissue of the Tenon layer. The retina sometimes shows tortuous vessels and arteriovenous communications.

The choroid is the site of the most significant, purely vascular anomaly of the eye associated with SWS. In a majority of cases of SWS with ocular involvement, increased numbers of well-formed choroidal vessels give the fundus a uniform bright red or red-orange color that has been compared to tomato catsup (Fig 27-10). Typically, the region of the posterior pole is involved; in some cases, there is gradual transition to a normal vascular pattern in the periphery, whereas in others the entire fundus seems to be affected. Choroidal angiomatosis usually remains asymptomatic in childhood. During adolescence or adulthood, however, the choroid sometimes becomes markedly thickened. Degeneration or detachment of the overlying retina with severe vision loss may follow, but the frequency of this progression is not established. No treatment is known to effectively prevent or reverse such deterioration, although scattered application of laser photocoagulation, which has proven useful in the management of circumscribed choroidal angiomas not associated with SWS, may help.

Glaucoma is the most common and serious ocular complication, reported to occur in up to approximately 70% of patients. The cause of elevated IOP is uncertain but is likely secondary to elevated episcleral venous pressure, hyperemia of the ciliary body with hypersecretion of aqueous, or developmental anomaly of the anterior chamber angle. Involvement of the upper-eyelid skin seems to increase the likelihood of glaucoma. Onset of glaucoma can be at birth or later in childhood. If IOP is elevated during early infancy, enlargement of the cornea can occur.

Management

When SWS is first documented or suspected, a complete ophthalmic evaluation is essential, including measurement of IOP. Sedation or general anesthesia may be necessary for uncooperative children. Examination should be repeated periodically throughout

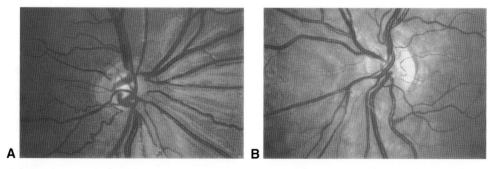

A   **B**

Figure 27-10   Fundus appearance in an adolescent boy with Sturge-Weber syndrome. **A,** Right eye. Note glaucomatous disc cupping and deeper red color of surrounding choroid, compared with normal fellow eye. **B,** Left eye.

childhood even if no ocular abnormality is initially detected. SWS glaucoma is difficult to treat, and there is no universally accepted treatment scheme. Initial therapy with topical drops can be effective, especially when onset occurs later. Surgery is indicated in early-onset cases and when medical treatment is inadequate. Adequate long-term pressure control can frequently be achieved, although multiple operations are typically necessary. Aqueous shunts, or setons, have shown promise in the management of otherwise intractable glaucoma in patients with SWS (see BCSC Section 10, *Glaucoma*). A particular risk of glaucoma surgery in SWS is massive intraoperative or postoperative exudation or hemorrhage from anomalous choroidal vessels, caused by rapid ocular decompression. Special care must be taken with implanted drainage devices to prevent excessive early postoperative hypotony. Choroidal or subretinal fluid accumulation after surgery may be dramatic, but spontaneous resorption usually occurs within 1–2 weeks. Angle surgery in the form of goniotomy and trabeculotomy has been used successfully in some SWS patients.

Thomas-Sohl KA, Vaslow DF, Maria BL. Sturge-Weber syndrome: a review. *Pediatr Neurol.* 2004;30(5):303–310.

Ataxia-Telangiectasia

Ataxia-telangiectasia (AT), or *Louis-Bar syndrome,* is an autosomal recessive disorder that primarily involves the CNS (particularly the cerebellum), the ocular surface, the skin, and the immune system. Though rare (prevalence is about 1:40,000), AT is thought to be the most common cause of progressive ataxia in early childhood. Truncal ataxia is usually noted during the second year of life, with subsequent development of dysarthria, dystonia, and choreoathetosis. Progressive deterioration of motor function leads to serious disability by age 10 years. Intellectual impairment, if present, is usually mild.

Recognition of ocular features is often the key to diagnosis of AT. Ocular motor abnormalities are found in many patients with AT and are frequently among the earliest manifestations. Characteristically, the ability to initiate saccades with preservation of vestibulo-ocular movements is poor, very similar to congenital ocular motor apraxia. Head thrusts are used to compensate for saccades. Strabismus and nystagmus may also be present.

Telangiectasia of the conjunctiva develops between the ages of 3 and 5 years. In one study, 91% of AT patients had conjunctival telangiectasia. Involvement is initially interpalpebral but away from the limbus, eventually becoming generalized (Fig 27-11). Similar, though less obvious, vessel changes can appear in the skin of the eyelids and other sun-exposed areas. A variety of skin changes that suggest accelerated aging are common in older children and adults with AT.

Individuals with AT show greatly increased sensitivity to the tissue-damaging side effects of therapeutic radiation and many chemotherapeutic agents. Defective T-cell function in patients with AT is usually associated with hypoplasia of the thymus and decreased levels of circulating immunoglobulin. Recurrent respiratory tract infections are a serious problem, frequently causing death in adolescence or young adulthood even with optimal antimicrobial and supportive treatment. The increased susceptibility to various

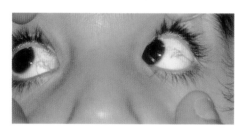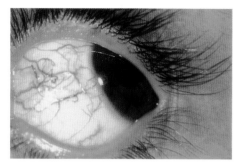

Figure 27-11 Abnormally dilated and tortuous interpalpebral conjunctival vessels in a child with ataxia-telangiectasia, seen only in the interpalpebral fissure.

malignancies, particularly lymphomas and leukemias, contributes to early mortality in one-third to one-half of cases.

The causative gene in AT is called *ATM* (ataxia-telangiectasia mutated gene) and is found on chromosome 11q22.3. The protein of ATM is involved in the repair of DNA and the regulation of tumor suppressor genes, including *BRCA1*. A new rapid test from peripheral blood can diagnose AT accurately. AT heterozygosity is present in an estimated 1%–3% of the population. Although gene carriers are generally healthy and cannot be identified except in the context of a known AT pedigree, they are at significantly increased risk for common forms of malignancy and show greater-than-normal sensitivity to radiation. In women heterozygous for the AT gene, breast cancer is about 7 times more frequent than in noncarriers and may account for nearly 10% of all cases in the United States.

Butch AW, Chun HH, Nahas SA, Gatti RA. Immunoassay to measure ataxia-telangiectasia mutated protein in cellular lysates. *Clin Chem.* 2004;50(12):2302–2308.

Farr AK, Shalev B, Crawford TO, Lederman HM, Winkelstein JA, Repka MX. Ocular manifestations of ataxia-telangiectasia. *Am J Ophthalmol.* 2002;134(6):891–896.

Incontinentia Pigmenti

Incontinentia pigmenti (IP), or *Bloch-Sulzberger syndrome,* involves the skin, brain, and eyes and shows the unusual inheritance pattern of X-linked dominance with a presumed lethal effect on the hemizygous male fetus. Nearly all affected persons are female, with mother-to-daughter transmission in familial cases. IP results from a mutation of the *NEMO (NF-kB essential modulator)* gene located on band Xq28. BCSC Section 2, *Fundamentals and Principles of Ophthalmology,* details this inheritance pattern in the chapters on genetics.

The cutaneous manifestations of IP are distinctive. The skin usually appears normal at birth, but erythema and bullae develop during the first few days of life, usually on the extremities, and persist for weeks to months (Fig 27-12A). A second distinct phase characterized by verrucous changes begins at about 2 months of age, subsiding after a few more months. Finally, clusters of small hyperpigmented macules in a characteristic "splashed paint" distribution make their appearance, most prominently on the trunk (Fig 27-12B).

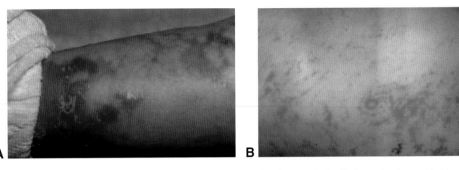

Figure 27-12 Pigmented skin lesions of incontinentia pigmenti. **A,** Bullous lesions. **B,** Hyper-pigmented macules. *(Courtesy of Edward L. Raab, MD.)*

Histopathologically, the early vesicular lesions show local accumulation of unusually large macrophages and eosinophils, accompanied by peripheral blood eosinophilia. In the lesions of the pigmentary stage, which persist for years before gradually fading, free melanin granules are found abnormally scattered in the dermis. Though present in all cases, skin involvement varies considerably in extent, occasionally being so limited that it is completely overlooked at 1 or more of its stages.

About one-third of patients with IP have CNS problems that may include microcephaly, hydrocephalus, seizures, and varying degrees of mental deficiency. Dental abnormalities (missing and malformed teeth) are found in roughly two-thirds of cases. Other, less common findings include scoliosis, skull deformities, cleft palate, and dwarfism.

Ocular involvement occurs in at least one-quarter to one-third of cases, typically in the form of a proliferative retinal vasculopathy that closely resembles retinopathy of prematurity. At birth, the only detectable abnormality may be incomplete peripheral retinal vascularization. Abnormal arteriovenous connections, microvascular abnormalities, and neovascular membranes develop at or near the junction of the vascular and avascular retina (Fig 27-13). Rapid progression sometimes leads to total retinal detachment and retrolental membrane formation (pseudoglioma) within the first few months of life. Other affected eyes show gradual deterioration over a period of several years; still others have proliferative lesions of limited extent that may persist for decades. Microphthalmos,

Figure 27-13 Vascular abnormalities of the temporal retina, right eye, in a 2-year-old child with incontinentia pigmenti. Note avascularity peripheral to the circumferential white vasoproliferative lesion, which showed profuse leakage on fluorescein angioscopy.

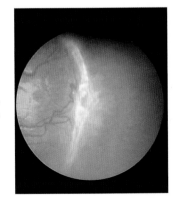

cataract, glaucoma, optic atrophy, strabismus, and nystagmus occur occasionally, representing secondary consequences of end-stage retinopathy in most if not all cases.

The retinopathy of IP has been managed by photocoagulation or cryotherapy in a small number of cases, with varying degrees of reported success. Treatment is usually applied primarily to the avascular peripheral retina, as in the currently preferred approach to management of retinopathy of prematurity.

Catalano RA. Incontinentia pigmenti. *Am J Ophthalmol.* 1990;110(6):696–700.

Wyburn-Mason Syndrome

Wyburn-Mason syndrome, or *racemose angioma,* is a nonhereditary arteriovenous malformation of the eye and brain, typically involving the optic disc or retina and the midbrain. Skin lesions are present in a minority of cases. The complete syndrome is considerably less common than an isolated occurrence of similar ocular or intracranial disease.

Seizures, mental changes, hemiparesis, and papilledema may result from the CNS lesions, which are frequently a source of hemorrhage, unlike the hemangioma of SWS.

Ocular manifestations are unilateral and congenital but may progress somewhat during childhood. The typical lesion consists of markedly dilated and tortuous vessels that shunt blood flow directly from arteries to veins; these vessels do not leak fluid (Fig 27-14). Vision ranges from normal to markedly reduced in the involved eye, and intraocular hemorrhage and secondary neovascular glaucoma are possible complications. No treatment is indicated for primary lesions.

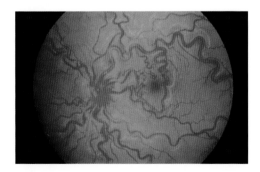

Figure 27-14 Racemose angioma of the retina, left eye.

CHAPTER **28**

Craniofacial Malformations

Craniosynostosis

Craniosynostosis is the premature closure of 1 or more cranial sutures during the embryonic period or early childhood. Cranial sutures are present throughout the skull, which is divided into 2 parts, the *calvarium* and the *skull base,* via an imaginary line drawn from the supraorbital rims to the base of the occiput (Fig 28-1).

Bony growth of the skull occurs in osteoblastic centers located at the suture sites. Bone is laid down parallel and perpendicular to the direction of the suture. Premature suture closure prevents perpendicular growth but allows parallel growth. This pattern is termed *Virchow's law* and leads to clinically recognizable cranial bone deformations, all of which carry specific nomenclature (Fig 28-2). The following are important terms associated with craniosynostosis.

Plagiocephaly   The term *plagiocephaly* literally means "oblique head." Most often it is the consequence of a unilateral coronal suture synostosis. On the synostotic side, the forehead and supraorbital rim are retruded (depressed), the interpalpebral fissure is wider, and the orbit is often higher than on the nonsynostotic side. Because of brain growth and necessary cranial vault expansion, the nonsynostotic side will display protrusion or bulging of the forehead, lower supraorbital rim, narrower interpalpebral fissure, and often a lower orbital position (Fig 28-3).

Oxy-, turri-, acrocephaly   These terms all mean "tower head." The condition occurs most often with multiple suture closures, such as both coronals, the sagittal, and possibly the lambdoidals.

Brachycephaly   "Short head"; specifically refers to growth in the anterior-posterior axis. Brachycephaly is often the result of bilateral closure of the coronal sutures. The forehead is most often wide and flat.

Scaphocephaly   "Boat head." Scaphocephaly usually results from premature closure of the sagittal suture; the skull is thus long in the anterior-posterior axis and narrow bitemporally.

Dolichocephaly   "Long head"; the skull shape is much like that in scaphocephaly.

Kleeblattschädel   "Cloverleaf skull"; the skull shape is trilobar. Kleeblattschädel is typically the result of synostosis of the coronal, lambdoidal, and sagittal sutures.

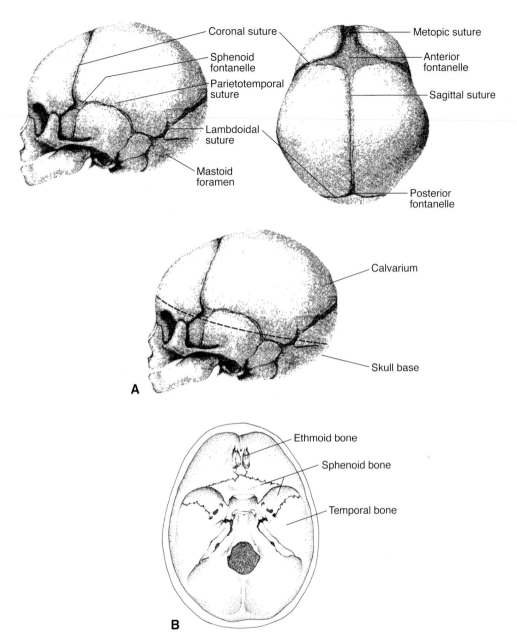

Figure 28-1 **A,** Normal sutures and fontanelles of the fetal skull. **B,** Adult cranial base, complete with sutures. *(Illustration by C.H. Wooley.)*

Hypertelorism, orbital   Excessive distance between the medial orbital walls. This diagnosis is made not clinically but rather radiographically.

Hypertelorism, ocular   Excessive interpupillary distance when compared to standard nomograms; it implies orbital hypertelorism.

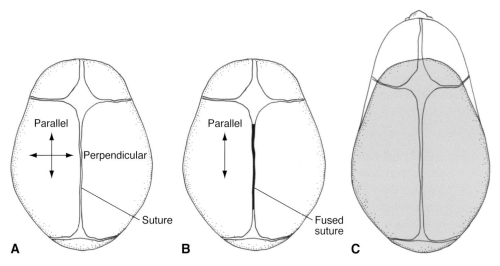

Figure 28-2 **A,** Normal sutures. Bone growth occurs at the suture, laid down parallel and perpendicular to the direction of the suture. **B,** Virchow's law. Prematurely fused sutures allow bone growth only in the parallel direction; perpendicular growth is inhibited. **C,** An example of Virchow's law. Closure of the sagittal suture produces scaphocephaly (boatlike skull) when compared to the normal skull (shaded area). *(Illustration by C.H. Wooley.)*

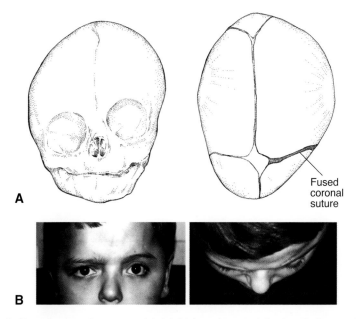

Figure 28-3 **A,** Fused coronal suture, with inhibition of perpendicular skull growth. **B,** Patient with left coronal synostosis. Note retruded left forehead, elevated brow, and wider interpalpebral fissure, with compensatory protrusion of the right forehead, lower brow, and narrowed interpalpebral fissure. *(Part A illustration by C.H. Wooley; part B courtesy of Jane Edmond, MD.)*

Telecanthus Increased distance between the medial canthi. This may be secondary to hypertelorism, but it can be a primary soft tissue abnormality.

Calvarial suture fusion affects cranial shape and orbital development. Skull base suture fusion affects facial and orbital development. In contrast to calvarial suture fusion, which causes different cranial deformations, skull base suture fusion causes just 1 constellation of abnormalities, midface hypoplasia (Fig 28-4), specifically consisting of the following:

- maxillary hypoplasia
- beak-shaped nose
- hypertelorism
- shallow orbits with proptosis and lagophthalmos
- high-arched palate with dental malocclusion
- relative mandibular prognathism (prominent-appearing jaw is due to retruded maxilla)

Not all skull deformities are secondary to synostosis of a suture. Deformational plagiocephaly is a skull deformation secondary to intrauterine constraint (eg, oligohydramnios) and is characterized by ipsilateral occipital flattening with contralateral forehead flattening. The skull takes on a trapezoidal shape when viewed from above. The ear is displaced anteriorly on the side of the flattened occiput.

Etiology of Craniosynostosis

Early suture fusion can occur sporadically as an isolated abnormality (eg, sagittal suture synostosis and most cases of unilateral coronal suture synostosis), or it can be associated with other abnormalities and part of a genetic syndrome. Craniosynostosis syndromes are usually autosomal dominant conditions, and many of these syndromes have associated

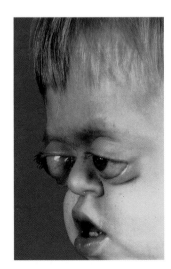

Figure 28-4 Note the manifestations of skull base suture fusion—namely, severe midface retrusion, shallow orbits, proptosis, beak-shaped nose—in this child with Crouzon syndrome. *(Reproduced by permission from Miller MT. Ocular abnormalities in craniofacial malformations. Int Ophthalmol Clin. 1984;24(1):148.)*

limb abnormalities. The most frequent craniosynostosis syndromes are Apert, Crouzon, Pfeiffer, and Saethre-Chotzen.

Many of the craniosynostosis syndromes have overlapping features, making accurate diagnosis based on clinical findings difficult. Advances in gene discovery have revealed that many of these syndromes are caused by mutations in the fibroblast growth factor receptor *(FGFR)* genes 1, 2, and 3 and the *TWIST* gene. These mutations result in increased calvarial cell differentiation and bone matrix formation. Mutations are found in approximately 50% of craniosynostosis syndrome patients.

Craniosynostosis Syndromes

Common systemic features of the craniosynostosis syndromes include fusion of multiple calvarial sutures and skull base sutures. Syndactyly and brachydactyly, ranging in severity, are also hallmarks of these syndromes—with one notable exception, Crouzon syndrome.

Crouzon Syndrome

Crouzon syndrome is the most common autosomal dominant craniosynostosis syndrome. Over 30 mutations cause the Crouzon phenotype, all occurring on the *FGFR2* gene on chromosome 10.

Calvarial bone synostosis often includes both coronal sutures, resulting in a broad, retruded forehead; brachycephaly; and tower skull. The skull base sutures are also involved, leading to varying degrees of midface retrusion. There is often marked variability of the skull and facial features, with milder cases escaping diagnosis through multiple generations. Hypertelorism and proptosis, with inferior scleral show (lower eyelid below limbus with scleral baring), are the most frequent features of Crouzon syndrome (Fig 28-5). Intelligence is usually normal. Findings are usually limited to the head. There are no obvious hand or foot abnormalities, such as those encountered in Apert and other

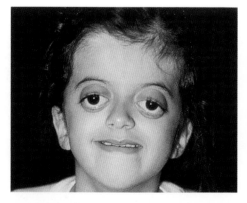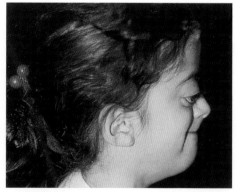

Figure 28-5 Crouzon syndrome. This patient evidences turribrachycephaly with forehead retrusion, proptosis, inferior scleral show, and a small, beaklike nose. Also visible is the emerging midface hypoplasia. *(Reproduced with permission from Katowitz JA, ed. Pediatric Oculoplastic Surgery. New York: Springer; 2002:fig 31-23.)*

craniosynostosis syndromes, which can greatly aid the clinician in the diagnosis of Crouzon. Hydrocephalus is common.

Apert Syndrome

Patients with Apert syndrome usually have multiple fused calvarial sutures, most often both coronal sutures, and skull base suture fusion. Although the skull shape and facial features of these patients may resemble those of patients with Crouzon syndrome, the former display an often extreme amount of syndactyly, causing all the digits (hands and feet) to be completely fused. Apert syndrome is likely to be associated with internal organ malformations (cardiovascular and genitourinary) and mental deficiency. Hydrocephalus is less common. The condition is autosomal dominant. Two mutations, both on the *FGFR2* gene on chromosome 10, account for most patients who carry this diagnosis (Fig 28-6).

Patients with *Pfeiffer syndrome* have craniofacial abnormalities similar to those of Apert syndrome patients, often with more severe craniosynostosis, resulting in a cloverleaf skull. In Pfeiffer syndrome, the syndactyly is much less severe, and patients have characteristic short, broad thumbs and toes. This syndrome is autosomal dominant and secondary to mutations on *FGFR* genes 1 or 2.

Saethre-Chotzen Syndrome

In general, the features of Saethre-Chotzen syndrome are much milder than those of other craniosynostosis syndromes; this syndrome is therefore often underdiagnosed. Early suture fusion is not a constant feature but, when present, typically involves 1 coronal suture (plagiocephaly), inducing an asymmetric face, a characteristic cited as a classic feature of Saethre-Chotzen syndrome. Other common features are ptosis, low hairline, and ear abnormalities. The hands and feet display slightly shortened digits (brachydactyly) and mild syndactyly. Intelligence is usually normal. The condition is autosomal dominant. Mutations in the *TWIST* gene on chromosome 7 cause the Saethre-Chotzen phenotype (Fig 28-7).

Ocular Complications

Proptosis

Proptosis (or exorbitism) in craniosynostosis results from the reduced volume of the bony orbit that usually occurs in syndromes with coronal and/or skull base suture fusion. The severity of the proptosis in these patients is not uniform and frequently increases with age because of the impaired growth of the bony orbit.

Corneal Exposure

Because the eyelids may not close completely over the proptotic globes, corneal exposure may occur secondary to inadequate blink and/or nocturnal lagophthalmos, with possible development of exposure keratitis. Exposure keratitis, in the short term, leads to punctate epithelial erosions, epithelial defects, and possible infectious keratitis. If exposure keratitis is not prevented or treated, scarring of the cornea will ensue and result in vision loss.

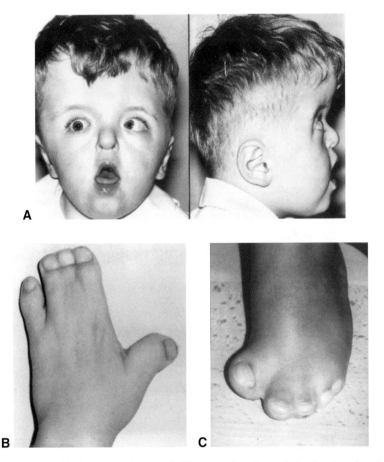

Figure 28-6 Patient with Apert syndrome. **A,** Note turribrachycephaly, forehead and superior orbital rim retrusion, maxillary hypoplasia, beaklike nose with depression of nasal bridge, and trapezoid-shaped mouth (common in infancy in Apert syndrome). **B,** Extreme syndactyly of the digits; the thumb is spared but is broad and deviated. When all digits are fused, it is termed *mitten deformity.* **C,** Syndactyly of the toes analogous to that of the hands. *(Reproduced by permission from Cohen MM Jr, Maclean R. Craniosynostosis: Diagnosis, Evaluation, and Management. 2nd ed. New York: Oxford University Press; 2000:figs 24-18, 24-46A, 24-51B.)*

Aggressive lubrication is necessary to prevent corneal drying. Tarsorraphies can decrease the exposure. Surgically expanding the orbital volume, thereby eliminating the proptosis, is the treatment when the proptosis and exposure are severe and lubrication and tarsorraphies fail.

Globe Luxation

Patients with extremely shallow orbits may suffer globe luxation when their eyelids are manipulated or when there is increased pressure in the orbits, such as occurs with a Valsalva maneuver. The globe is luxated forward, with the eyelids closing behind the equator of the globe. The condition is very painful and can cause corneal exposure; it may also possibly compromise the blood supply to the globe, which is a medical emergency.

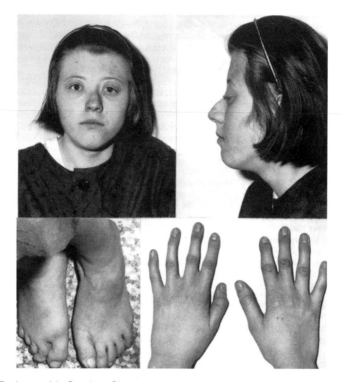

Figure 28-7 Patient with Saethre-Chotzen syndrome. Note the facial asymmetry, flat fore-head, low-set hairline, mild left ptosis, classic lateral deviation of the great toes, shortened toes, and partial syndactyly of fingers 2 and 3. *(Reproduced by permission from Cohen MM Jr, Maclean R. Craniosynostosis: Diagnosis, Evaluation, and Management. 2nd ed. New York: Oxford University Press; 2000:fig 28-4.)*

Physicians and patients (or their caregivers) should quickly replace the globe behind the eyelids. The best technique for doing this is to place a finger and thumb over the conjunctiva within the interpalpebral fissure and exert gentle but firm pressure to reposition the globe; this technique does not damage the cornea. For recurrent luxation, the short-term solution is tarsorraphy; the long-term solution is orbital volume expansion.

Vision Loss

Patients with craniofacial syndromes commonly suffer vision loss owing to a variety of causes: corneal scarring from exposure, uncorrected refractive errors, amblyopia, and optic nerve compromise. Most cases of vision loss can be prevented.

Amblyopia

Amblyopia is common in patients with craniofacial syndromes and is secondary to high uncorrected refractive errors, anisometropia, and strabismus, all of which occur more frequently in these patients.

Strabismus

Patients with craniosynostosis show a variety of horizontal deviations in primary position; exotropia is the most frequent. The most consistent finding, however, is a marked

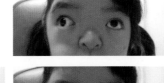

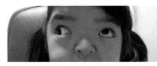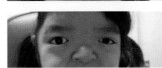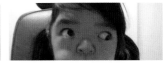

Figure 28-8 Patient with Apert syndrome. Note the good alignment in primary position with marked elevation of adducted eyes (inferior oblique overaction) and exotropia in upgaze (V pattern). *(Courtesy of John Simon, MD.)*

V pattern. This V pattern is often accompanied by a marked apparent overaction (pseudo-overaction) of the inferior oblique muscles, especially when 1 or both coronal sutures are synostosed, as occurs in unicoronal synostosis and Apert and Crouzon syndromes (Fig 28-8). The apparent inferior oblique overaction on the side of the coronal suture fusion may be due to the following: orbital and secondary globe extorsion, which causes the medial rectus to be offset superiorly, converting it into an elevator when the eye is in adduction; superior oblique trochlear retrusion (because of superior orbital rim retrusion), which induces superior oblique underaction and secondary true inferior oblique overaction; anomalous extraocular muscle insertions or agenesis (occurs more frequently in craniofacial patients); and/or orbital pulley abnormalities.

Optic Nerve Abnormalities

Because the synostosed cranial vault is unable to expand as the brain grows, the intracranial contents become crowded, elevating intracranial pressure (ICP). Papilledema can occur because of elevated ICP, and chronic papilledema can eventually lead to optic atrophy and vision loss. Hydrocephalus is another cause of elevated ICP and occurs in up to 40% of patients with Apert, Crouzon, and especially Pfeiffer syndromes. The severe midface retrusion that these conditions produce may cause breathing problems and sleep apnea. Idiopathic intracranial hypertension secondary to sleep apnea can also cause elevated ICP and papilledema. Optic atrophy may also occur with or without antecedent papilledema. Children with elevated ICP may not complain of a headache. Therefore, young patients with multiple fused sutures should be examined yearly or biyearly.

Optic nerve edema and/or atrophy can also occur secondary to optic nerve foramina synostosis, where the bony canal stenoses. This is rare but has been described in patients with craniofacial syndromes.

Ocular Adnexa Abnormalities

Patients with craniosynostosis syndromes display more adnexal abnormalities than do patients with isolated suture fusion. Common abnormalities include orbital hypertelorism, telecanthus, abnormal slant of the palpebral fissures secondary to superior displacement of the medial canthi, ptosis, and nasolacrimal apparatus abnormalities such as duct obstruction and punctal anomalies. Epiphora is a common finding in these patients and may be secondary to nasolacrimal apparatus abnormalities that produce obstruction;

poor blink secondary to proptosis; obliquity of the palpebral fissures; or ocular irritation from corneal exposure.

Management

In recent decades, there have been major advances in reconstructive surgery for severe craniofacial malformation. This surgery is frequently extensive and involves en bloc movement of the facial structures. The status of the visual system should be documented preoperatively, with attention to vision, the eyelids and orbit, and the motility examination. Postoperatively, the function of the visual system should be reevaluated and appropriate treatment instituted.

In many centers, a specialized craniofacial team—comprising facial plastic surgeons, neurosurgeons, ophthalmologists, and oral surgeons—collaborates to determine the timing of the reconstructive surgery by prioritizing the child's multiple problems. Common surgical procedures include frontoorbital advancement; Le Fort II, or midface advancement; orbital hypertelorism repair; and a variety of jaw procedures. The first 2 procedures involve manipulation of the orbits and expansion of orbital volume.

In addition, reconstructive surgery that involves moving the orbits may significantly change the degree or type of strabismus, thereby modifying the indicated form of strabismus surgery. Another consideration is that improved binocular function may not be attainable in these patients because of their unusual and incomitant form of ocular muscle imbalance. Thus, early strabismus surgery may offer no particular advantage, and deferring treatment until craniofacial surgery is completed may be appropriate.

Gorlin RJ, Cohen MM, Hennekam RCM. *Syndromes of the Head and Neck.* 4th ed. New York: Oxford University Press; 2001.

Katowitz J, ed. *Pediatric Oculoplastic Surgery.* New York: Springer-Verlag; 2002.

Nonsynostotic Craniofacial Conditions

Many craniofacial syndromes do not involve synostosis. A few of particular importance to the ophthalmologist are discussed in the following sections.

Branchial Arch Syndromes

Branchial arch syndromes are caused by disruptions in the embryonic development of the first 2 branchial arches, which are responsible for the formation of the maxillary and mandibular bones, the ear, and facial musculature. The best known of these syndromes are *oculoauriculovertebral (OAV) spectrum,* which includes hemifacial microsomia and Goldenhar syndrome, and *Treacher Collins syndrome.*

Oculoauriculovertebral spectrum

There has been no firm agreement about the nomenclature involved with this condition, but most believe that hemifacial microsomia (HFM) is the forme fruste of the OAV spectrum. Hemifacial microsomia affects aural, oral, and mandibular growth. Patients with

HFM may display, on the involved side, decreased jaw and cheek growth, ear abnormalities such as microtia or anotia (small or absent external ear), pretragal skin tags, deafness, and facial weakness (cranial nerve VII courses through the middle ear). Macrostomia can also occur. Hemifacial microsomia is usually unilateral but may be bilateral.

Patients with the OAV spectrum may have characteristic vertebral abnormalities such as hemivertebrae and vertebral hypoplasia. They may also have neurologic, cardiovascular, and genitourinary abnormalities. Most cases are sporadic, but there are rare familial cases.

Goldenhar syndrome   Goldenhar syndrome is a more severe presentation of the OAV spectrum. Patients with Goldenhar syndrome have HFM (unilateral or bilateral) in addition to characteristic ophthalmic abnormalities. Most cases are sporadic.

Epibulbar and limbal dermoids are the ocular hallmarks of Goldenhar syndrome. Epibulbar dermoids (also termed *lipodermoids*) usually occur in the inferotemporal quadrant, covered by conjunctiva and often hidden by the lateral upper and lower eyelids. Limbal dermoids are reported more frequently than lipodermoids and can be bilateral (in approximately 25% of cases). They occasionally impinge on the visual axis but more commonly interfere with visual acuity by causing astigmatism; they can also cause anisometropic amblyopia. Eyelid colobomas may occur. Other abnormalities include microphthalmia, cataract, and iris abnormalities (Fig 28-9). Duane syndrome is more common in patients with Goldenhar syndrome than in the general population.

Treacher Collins syndrome

Abnormal growth and development of the first and second branchial arch in Treacher Collins syndrome (mandibulofacial dysostosis) give rise to underdevelopment and even agenesis of the zygoma and malar eminences bilaterally. The cheeks and lateral orbital rims are depressed and the palpebral fissures slant downward because of lateral canthal

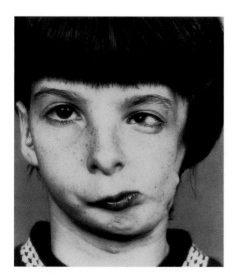

Figure 28-9 Hemifacial microsomia, Goldenhar variant. Patient has facial asymmetry, a hypoplastic left ear (microtia), an ear tag near the right ear, limbal lipodermoid in the left eye, and esotropia. Patient also has a left Duane syndrome.

dystopia. Pseudocolobomas (and, uncommonly, true colobomas) are found in the outer third of the lower eyelids. Meibomian glands may be absent. The cilia of the lower eyelid may be absent, medial to the pseudocoloboma. The ears are malformed and hearing loss is common. The mandible is typically hypoplastic, leading to micrognathia. Macrostomia is common. Intelligence is normal. The syndrome is inherited in an autosomal dominant fashion and displays variable expression (Fig 28-10). Most patients with this syndrome have a mutation in the *TCOF1* gene.

Pierre Robin Sequence

The Pierre Robin sequence (also *anomaly, deformity*) is characterized by respiratory problems, micrognathia, glossoptosis, and cleft palate. These abnormalities occur in a variety of syndromes, and the Pierre Robin sequence is a frequent finding in Stickler syndrome. Associated ocular anomalies include retinal detachment, microphthalmos, congenital glaucoma, cataracts, and high myopia.

Fetal Alcohol Syndrome

Fetal alcohol syndrome is an example of a craniofacial condition caused by in utero exposure to a teratogen, in this case ethanol. Alcohol and other teratogens can produce a wide range of effects on the developing fetus, depending on consumption or dose, timing of intake, genetic background, and other factors. A pattern of malformations has been observed in children born to women with a history of heavy alcohol use during pregnancy. *Fetal alcohol syndrome,* the term applied to this pattern, is characterized by prenatal and postnatal growth retardation, central nervous system abnormalities, and a wide spectrum of malformations, the most typical of these being craniofacial (Fig 28-11). Other facial features include a thin vermilion border of the upper lip. Mental retardation, ranging from mild to severe, occurs often in children with this syndrome.

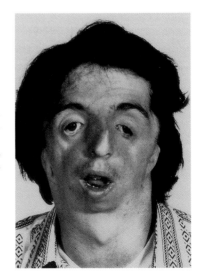

Figure 28-10 Mandibulofacial dysostosis (or Treacher Collins syndrome). Note downward slant of palpebral fissure, low-set abnormal ears, notch or curving of the inferotemporal eyelid margin, and maxillary and mandibular hypoplasia. *(Reproduced by permission from Peyman GA, Sanders DR, Goldberg MF. Principles and Practice of Ophthalmology. Philadelphia: Saunders; 1980:2411.)*

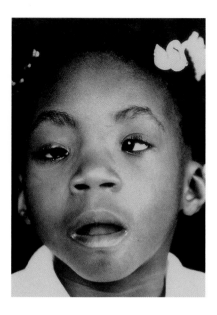

Figure 28-11 Fetal alcohol syndrome. Asymmetric ptosis; telecanthus; strabismus; long, flat philtrum; anteverted nostrils. This child also had Peters anomaly of the left cornea and myopia of the right eye. See also BCSC Section 2, Fig 4-17. *(Reproduced by permission from Miller MT, Israel J, Cuttone J. Fetal alcohol syndrome.* J Pediatr Ophthalmol Strabismus. *1981;18(4):6–15.)*

The classic ocular characteristics of fetal alcohol syndrome are short palpebral fissures, telecanthus, epicanthus, ptosis, microphthalmos, and strabismus, namely esotropia. Anterior segment dysgenesis, optic nerve hypoplasia, and high refractive errors have also been reported. Half of children with this syndrome, which is underdiagnosed, will suffer some form of visual impairment.

CHAPTER 29

Ocular Findings in Inborn Errors of Metabolism

In a 1985 survey of McKusick's *Mendelian Inheritance in Man,* the eye was involved in at least 25% of approximately 3000 diseases noted, making it the fourth most common system affected by genetic disease. More than 200 loci for genetic ocular disease have been mapped. For additional discussion of genetic disorders, see also BCSC Section 2, *Fundamentals and Principles of Ophthalmology.*

Hereditary eye disorders may be isolated and confined to the eyes or may be part of a larger disorder in which the eye abnormalities are associated with single-organ or multiple-organ system disease. Some of these genetic multisystem diseases are nonmetabolic disorders, while others are caused by inborn errors of metabolism. The latter are characterized by the genetic absence, either physical or functional, of 1 or more enzymes. There are several ways in which this enzyme deficiency can cause eye abnormalities: direct toxicity of abnormal metabolic products; accumulation of abnormal (or normal) metabolites; errors of synthetic pathways; or deficient production of energy. Inborn errors of metabolism are generally inherited as recessive disorders, either autosomal or X-linked, rarely as autosomal dominant or mitochondrial disorders. Germline mutations (genetic errors of the gametes only) may also occur. Carriers of inborn errors of metabolism possess half the normal quantity of an enzyme, as would be expected in persons with 1 normal gene and 1 defective one. This usually results in adequate metabolic function but subnormal serum levels. Measurement of enzyme levels in fetal cells obtained through amniocentesis may allow prenatal detection of many of these metabolic conditions. The causative genes are known for many of these disorders, allowing preconception or prenatal testing in some cases.

The age of onset of eye abnormalities in inborn errors of metabolism is variable, with some abnormalities present at birth and others occurring in early childhood. Knowledge of these ocular manifestations is critical for proper diagnosis and treatment, as the ophthalmologist may be called to help confirm a diagnosis, or the pediatric patient with this disorder may initially present to the ophthalmologist. Many of these disorders now have treatments that are more effective if instituted early. Consultation with a geneticist is warranted for any patient with ocular findings suggestive of an inborn error of metabolism.

Inborn errors of metabolism can be categorized according to the processes and biochemical pathways affected by enzyme deficiencies (specific disorders are listed in parentheses):

- carbohydrate synthesis (galactosemia)
- amino acid metabolism (homocystinuria)
- organic acid metabolism (methylmalonic aciduria)
- mitochondrial metabolism (Kearns-Sayre syndrome)
- urea cycle (ornithine transcarbamylase deficiency)
- peroxisome function (adrenoleukodystrophy, Zellweger disease)
- steroid pathway (Smith-Lemli-Opitz syndrome)
- lipid storage (Tay-Sachs, Gaucher disease)
- transport (cystinosis)
- lysosomal storage (mucopolysaccharidoses, cystinosis, neuronal ceroid-lipofuscinosis)
- metal metabolism (Wilson disease)

These disorders can also be categorized by the ocular structure that is affected. Metabolic diseases cloud the cornea via accumulation of a pathway product. If the product is produced in the cornea, the clouding may be found throughout the cornea. If the level of the product is elevated in the blood, then the peripheral cornea alone may be involved. Diseases that affect the cornea include the mucopolysaccharidoses (MPS; types I H, I S, IV, VI, and VII) (Fig 29-1), cystinosis, and Wilson disease. Cystinosis causes crystalline-like deposits throughout the cornea and symptoms of photophobia. Wilson disease may present with a peripheral brown Kayser-Fleischer ring.

In many multisystem diseases, cataracts occur (eg, as a feature of Smith-Lemli-Opitz syndrome and all the galactosemias). In galactokinase deficiency, cataracts may be the sole manifestation of the disease. Lens dislocation occurs in homocystinuria.

Over 400 known inherited diseases involve the retina. Retinitis pigmentosa (RP) is one of the most common of these. RP may occur as a primary defect in the photoreceptors or as a secondary event from sensitivity of the photoreceptors of the pigment epithelium to a generalized metabolic defect. Retinal degeneration is found in peroxisomal disorders (Zellweger disease, Refsum disease), lysosomal disorders (neuronal ceroid-lipofuscinosis), and mitochondrial disorders (Kearns-Sayre).

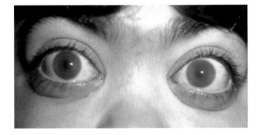

Figure 29-1 Mucopolysaccharidosis I H (Hurler). *(Courtesy of Edward L. Raab, MD.)*

Table 29-1 summarizes the common ophthalmic manifestations of the major inborn errors of metabolism that affect the eye. For patients suspected to have these disorders, evaluation should include

- complete ocular and family history
- examination of other family members for additional evidence or findings that confirm the carrier state
- complete ocular examination focusing on the expected findings
- appropriately directed laboratory testing

Kamboj M. Clinical approach to the diagnoses of inborn errors of metabolism. *Pediatr Clin North Am.* 2008;55(5):1113–1127.

Poll-The BT, Maillette de Buy Wenniger-Prick LJ, Barth PG, Duran M. The eye as a window to inborn errors of metabolism. *J Inherit Metab Dis.* 2003;26(2-3):229–244.

Treatment

Many previously untreatable metabolic disorders now have treatment options, either through clinical trials or by established standards of care. Often, the earlier a patient is referred to a geneticist, the better the chance of a beneficial effect from such treatments. These treatments include enzyme replacement therapy (eg, MPS I, Fabry), bone marrow or umbilical cord blood stem cell transplant (mucopolysaccharidoses and leukodystrophies), and dietary changes (eg, homocystinuria, Refsum disease, tyrosinemia, gyrate atrophy, galactosemia). Gene therapy is promising but is still on the horizon.

Examples of treatable metabolic disorders with ocular findings are homocystinuria and cystinosis. Classic homocystinuria is caused by cystathionine β-synthase deficiency, which is usually detected shortly after birth if neonatal screening measures are employed. Milder forms may be diagnosed later in life. Dietary restriction of methionine and supplementation of folate, pyridoxine (vitamin B6), vitamin B12, and/or betaine (N,N,N-trimethylglycine) can markedly reduce plasma homocysteine levels and prevent progression of disease in homocystinuria. Most untreated patients with classic homocystinuria will develop mental retardation and ectopia lentis; thrombotic events will likely occur in 50% before 30 years of age. The risk of these sequelae is greatly decreased by metabolic control.

In patients with cystinosis, systemic cysteamine can ameliorate renal disease, and topical cysteamine eyedrops can prevent or reverse painful crystalline keratopathy.

Patients and families can also be reassured that much research is ongoing. In vitro studies of cells from albino mice have been successful in repairing the tyrosinase gene, allowing previously amelanotic cells to produce melanin, and preliminary in vivo animal results look promising. Nonsteroidal anti-inflammatory agents have been shown to slow progression of disease in the Sandhoff disease mouse, whereas tamoxifen and vitamin E are beneficial in the mouse model of Niemann-Pick C. Gene therapy in Fabry mice using lentivirus vectors and in MPS I mice using adeno-associated virus vector has shown positive results. Transplantation of genetically modified bone marrow cells directly into the brains of MPS VII mice corrects the brain pathology, and using an adeno-associated

Table 29-1 Ocular Findings in Mucopolysaccharidoses, Mucolipidoses, Lipidoses, Gangliosidoses, and Miscellaneous Disorders

Disease	Enzyme Deficiency	Corneal Clouding	Motility Disorders	Cherry-Red Spot	RPE Degeneration	Optic Atrophy	Other	Inheritance
Mucopolysaccharidoses								
MPS I H, I S Hurler (2528)* Scheie	α-iduronidase	+++	-	-	+++	+	glaucoma papilledema	AR
MPS II Hunter (30990)	iduronate sulfatase	-	-	-	++	+	-	XR
MPS III Sanfilippo (25290)	A: heparan N-sulfatase B: N-acetyl-α-D-glucosaminidase	-	-	-	++	rare	late blindness	AR
MPS IV Morquio (25300)	A: N-acetyl-galactosamine-6-sulfatase B: β-galactosidase	++	-	-	rare	rare	-	AR
MPS VI Maroteaux-Lamy (25320)	arylsulfatase B	++	-	-	-	+	papilledema glaucoma	AR
MPS VII Sly (25322)	β-glucuronidase	+	-	-	-	-	-	AR
Mucolipidoses								
Type I (25240) sialidosis (type 2) cherry-red spot myoclonus syndrome	neuraminidase	-	+	+	+	-	hearing loss	AR
Type II I-cell disease (25250)	multiple lysosomal enzymes	++	-	-	-	-	Hurler-like	AR
Type III pseudo-Hurler polydystrophy (25260)	multiple lysosomal enzymes	+++	-	-	-	-	Hurler-like puffy eyelids (25260)	AR
Type IV (25265)	partial ganglioside sialidase	+++	-	-	++	+	photophobia	AR
Lipidoses								
Niemann-Pick disease (25720)	sphingomyelinase	+	nystagmus	+	-	+	eventual vision loss	AR
Fabry disease (30150)	α-galactosidase A	whorl-like	-	-	-	-	angiokeratoma, spokelike cataract, aneurysmal conjunctival vessels	XR
Gaucher disease (Type I 23080) (Type II 23090) (Type III 23100)	glucocerebrosidase	-	paralytic strabismus, looped saccades	-	+	-	pinguecula, conjunctival pigmentation	AR
Metachromatic leukodystrophy (25010)	arylsulfatase A	-	nystagmus	+	-	+	blindness, decreased pupil reaction	AR
Krabbe disease (24520)	galactocerebrosidase	-	nystagmus	rare	-	+	cortical blindness	AR
Fucosidosis (23000)	α-L-fucosidase	-	-	-	+	-	Hurler-like features, angiokeratoma, tortuous conjunctival vessels	AR

Gangliosidoses

Disease	Enzyme Deficiency	Conjunct. Tortuosity	Corneal Clouding	Motility Disorders	Cherry-Red Spot	RPE Degeneration	Optic Atrophy	High Myopia	Blindness	Inheritance
Generalized (GM₁) gangliosidosis										
(1) Type I (23050)	β-galactosidase A, B, and C	+	±	ET, nystagmus	50% of patients	–	+	+	+	AR
(2) Type II (23060) Derry disease juvenile GM₁	β-galactosidase B and C	–	–	ET, nystagmus	–	+	±	–	late	AR
(3) Type III (23065) adult GM₁	β-galactosidase (partial)	±	rare	–	–	–	–	–	–	AR
GM₂ gangliosidosis										
(1) Type I (27280) Tay-Sachs disease	hexosaminidase A	–	–	nystagmus, ophthalmoplegia	+	–	+	–	+	AR
(2) Type II (26880) Sandhoff disease	hexosaminidase A and B	–	rare	ET	+	–	±	–	+	AR
(3) Type III (23065) juvenile GM₂ Bernheimer-Seitelberger disease	hexosaminidase A (partial)	–	–	–	–	+	+	–	late	AR

Disease	Enzyme Deficiency	Corneal Clouding	Motility Disorders	Cherry-Red Spot	RPE Degeneration	Optic Atrophy	Other	Inheritance
Miscellaneous Disorders								
Galactosialidosis	β-galactosidase neuraminidase	+	–	+	–	+	dwarfism, seizures, coarse facies	AR
Ceroid-lipofuscinosis (20420)								
Hagberg-Santavuori disease	PPT-1	–	+	Macular	+	+	blindness	AR
Jansky-Bielschowsky disease	PPT-1	–	+	bull's	+	+	blindness	AR
Spielmeyer-Vogt disease	unknown	–	+	eye	+	+	blindness	AR
Kufs disease	unknown	–	–	–	–	–		AR
Cystinosis (21980)	unknown	crystals	–	–	++	–	conjunctival crystals, renal problems	AR
Galactosemia (23040)	gal-1-PO₄ uridyl transferase	–	–	–	–	–	cataracts if not treated	AR
Mannosidosis (24850)	α-mannosidase	++	–	–	–	pallor, blurred margin	Hurler-like, spokelike cataract	AR
Homocystinuria (23620)	cystathionine β-synthase	–	–	–	+	–	dislocated lens, cataract	AR
Refsum disease (26650)	phytanic acid α-hydrolase	–	–	–	++	–	cataract, night blindness	AR

*These code numbers refer to the system developed by Victor McKusick (McKusick VA, Francomano CA, Antonarakis SE. *Mendelian Inheritance in Man: Catalogs of Autosomal Dominant, Autosomal Recessive, and X-Linked Phenotypes.* 10th ed. Baltimore: The Johns Hopkins University Press; 1992). Plus (+) and minus (–) signs indicate the relative likelihood of occurrence of ocular findings in these systemic disorders.

virus vector, researchers have performed gene therapy intravitreally with improved retinal function. A clinical trial of gene therapy in the brains of children with late infantile neuronal ceroid-lipofuscinosis is ongoing. The ophthalmologist should have a high suspicion for these devastating disorders in order to direct patients to the best treatment options as early as possible.

Online Mendelian Inheritance in Man, OMIM. Baltimore, MD: Johns Hopkins University Press; 2009. http://www.ncbi.nlm.nih.gov/omim/.

CHAPTER **30**

Ocular Trauma in Childhood

Trauma is one of the most important causes of ocular morbidity in childhood. Only strabismus ranks higher in frequency among reasons for pediatric eye surgery, and only amblyopia is responsible for more early monocular vision loss. Children 11–15 years old have a particularly high incidence of severe eye injury compared with other age groups. Injured boys outnumber girls by a factor of 3 or 4 to 1.

Most ocular trauma in younger children occurs during casual play with other children. Older children and adolescents are most likely to be injured while participating in sports. A majority of serious childhood eye injuries could thus, in principle, be prevented by appropriate adult supervision and by regular use of protective eyewear for sports. Fireworks and BB guns are among the less frequent causes of pediatric ocular trauma, but they are likely to cause severe injuries.

The management of eye trauma in very young patients requires several special considerations. First, the difficulty of evaluation and treatment is often considerably increased by inadequate cooperation. Even school-aged children, stressed by the recent injury, may strenuously resist any approach to the eye. Overcoming the child's opposition by force risks exacerbating the damage caused by penetrating wounds or blunt impact. In a child older than 3 years, a forceful approach may make it exceedingly difficult to establish the rapport needed for subsequent treatment. Instilling topical anesthetic and giving the child a chance to calm down in quiet surroundings can facilitate examination in cases likely to involve minor injury. When preliminary assessment indicates that prompt surgical treatment may be necessary, it is appropriate to defer detailed physical examination of the eye until the patient is in the operating room and under general anesthesia.

A second issue in the care of children with eye trauma is the potential for the injury or its treatment to lead to vision loss from amblyopia. In children younger than 5 years, visual deprivation amblyopia associated with traumatic cataract or other media opacity may be more likely to cause severe long-term reduction of acuity than the original physical damage. Minimizing the interval between the injury and restoration of optimal media clarity and optics, including adequate aphakic refractive correction, must be a high priority. Monocular occlusion following injury should be kept to a minimum as well; the expected benefit from an occlusive dressing must be weighed against the risk of disturbing binocular function or inducing amblyopia in a very young child.

American Academy of Pediatrics, Committee on Sports Medicine and Fitness; American Academy of Ophthalmology, Eye Health and Public Information Task Force. Protective eyewear for young athletes. *Ophthalmology.* 2004;111(3):600–603.

Child Abuse

Although most eye injuries in childhood are accidental or innocently caused by other children, a significant portion results from physical abuse by adults. Child abuse is a pervasive problem in our society, with an estimated 2 million victims per year in the United States. Abusive behavior in a parent or other caregiver usually reflects temporary loss of control during a period of anger or stress rather than premeditated cruelty. Lack of knowledge of the proper way to care for or discipline a child is also a frequent contributing factor. In the relatively rare *Munchausen syndrome by proxy,* the child is physically harmed by a psychopathic parent to create signs of illness in an effort to manipulate medical care providers.

A reliable history is often difficult to obtain when child abuse has occurred. Suspicion should be aroused when repeated accounts of the circumstances of injury or histories obtained from different individuals are inconsistent or when the events described seem to conflict with the extent of injuries (eg, bruises on multiple aspects of the head after a fall) or with the child's developmental level (eg, a 2-month-old rolling off a bed or a 6-month-old climbing out of a high chair).

Any physician who suspects that child abuse might have occurred is required by law in every US state and Canadian province to report the incident to a designated governmental agency. Once this obligation has been discharged, the ophthalmologist is probably best advised to leave full investigation of the situation to appropriate specialists or authorities.

The presenting sign of child abuse involves the eye in approximately 5% of cases, and ocular manifestations are detected in the course of evaluating many others. Blunt trauma inflicted with fingers, fists, or implements such as belts or straps is the usual mechanism of nonaccidental injury to the ocular adnexa or anterior segment. Periorbital ecchymosis, subconjunctival hemorrhage, and hyphema should raise suspicion of recent abuse if the explanation provided is less than completely plausible. Cataract and lens dislocation may be signs of repeated injury or trauma inflicted more remotely in the past. A majority of rhegmatogenous retinal detachments that occur in childhood have a traumatic origin; abuse should be suspected when such a finding is encountered in a child without a history of injury or an apparent predisposing factor such as high myopia.

Shaking Injury

A unique complex of ocular, intracranial, and sometimes other injuries occurs in infants who have been abused by violent shaking. Because the essential features of what is now generally known as *shaken baby syndrome* were identified in the early 1970s, it has become widely recognized as one of the most important manifestations of child abuse.

Victims of shaking injury are always younger than 3 years and usually younger than 12 months. When a reliable history is available, it typically involves a parent or other caregiver who shook an inconsolably crying baby in anger or frustration. Often, however, the only information provided is that the child's mental status deteriorated or that seizures or respiratory difficulty developed; or the involved caregiver may relate that an episode of relatively minor trauma occurred, such as a fall from a bed. Even without a supporting history, the diagnosis of shaken baby syndrome can still be made with confidence on the basis of characteristic clinical findings. It must be kept in mind, however, that answers to important questions concerning the timing and circumstances of injury and the identity of the perpetrator frequently cannot be inferred from medical evidence alone.

Intracranial injury in shaken infants almost always includes subdural hematoma, typically bilateral over the cerebral convexities or in the interhemispheric fissure. Evidence of subarachnoid bleeding is also often apparent. Although initial scans may be normal in many cases, cerebral parenchymal damage is manifest on neuroimaging, acutely as edema, ischemia, or contusion and in later stages as atrophy. These findings are thought to result from repetitive abrupt deceleration of the child's head as it whiplashes back and forth during the shaking episode. Some authorities, citing the frequency with which shaken baby syndrome victims also show evidence of having received blows to the head, think that impact is an essential component. Displacement of the brain in relation to the skull and dura mater ruptures bridging vessels, and compression against the cranial bones produces further damage. The infant's head is particularly vulnerable to such effects because of its relatively large mass in relation to the body and poor stabilization by neck muscles.

Ocular involvement

The most common ocular manifestation of shaking injury, present in a large majority of cases, is retinal hemorrhage. Preretinal, nerve fiber layer, deep retinal, or subretinal localization may be seen. Hemorrhages tend to be concentrated in or near the macular region, but sometimes are so extensive that they occupy nearly the entire fundus (Fig 30-1). Vitreous hemorrhage may also develop, usually as a secondary phenomenon resulting from migration of blood that was initially intraretinal. Occasionally, the vitreous becomes almost completely opacified by dispersed hemorrhage within a few days of injury. Retinal hemorrhages in shaken infants resolve over a period ranging from 1 or 2 weeks to several months. Vitrectomy should be considered if amblyopia is likely secondary to persistent vitreous hemorrhage.

Some eyes of shaken infants show evidence of retinal tissue disruption in addition to hemorrhage. Full-thickness perimacular folds in the neurosensory retina, typically with circumferential orientation around the macula that creates a craterlike appearance, are highly characteristic. Splitting of the retina (traumatic retinoschisis), either deep to

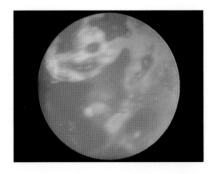

Figure 30-1 Extensive retinal hemorrhages in a 2-month-old infant suspected to have been violently shaken.

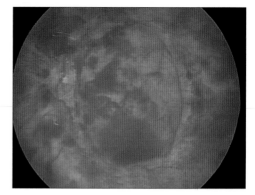

Figure 30-2 Traumatic retinoschisis. *(Courtesy of Ken K. Nischal, FRCOphth.)*

the nerve fiber layer or superficial (involving only the internal limiting membrane), may create partially blood-filled cavities of considerable extent, also usually in the macular region (Fig 30-2). Full-thickness retinal breaks and detachment are rare. Retinal folds usually flatten out within a few weeks of injury, but schisis cavities can persist indefinitely.

A striking feature of shaken baby syndrome is the typical lack of external evidence of trauma. The ocular adnexa and anterior segment appear entirely normal. Occasionally, the trunk or extremities show bruises representing the imprint of the perpetrator's hands. In a minority of cases, broken ribs or characteristic metaphyseal fractures of the long bones result from forces generated during shaking. It must be kept in mind, however, that many shaken babies are also victims of other forms of abuse. In particular, signs of impact to the head must be carefully sought.

When extensive retinal hemorrhage accompanied by perimacular folds and schisis cavities is found in association with intracranial hemorrhage or other evidence of trauma to the brain in an infant, shaking injury can usually be diagnosed with confidence regardless of other circumstances. Extensive retinal hemorrhage without other ocular findings strongly suggests that intracranial injury has been caused by shaking, but alternative possibilities such as a coagulation disorder must be considered as well. Although severe accidental head trauma (eg, sustained in a fall from a second-story level or a motor vehicle collision) is infrequently accompanied by retinal hemorrhage, which is virtually never extensive, it has been hypothesized that severe, fatal, acute head crush injury may rarely cause a significant hemorrhagic retinopathy with perimacular folds. Retinal hemorrhage is rare and has never been documented to be extensive following cardiopulmonary resuscitation by trained personnel. Spontaneous subarachnoid hemorrhage occurs rarely in young children and may be associated with some degree of intraocular bleeding. Retinal hemorrhages resulting from the birth trauma of vaginal delivery are common in newborns, but seldom persist beyond age 1 month. Though much less frequent, retinal hemorrhages may also be noted after cesarean delivery.

Emerson MV, Pieramici DJ, Stoessel KM, Berreen JP, Gariano RF. Incidence and rate of disappearance of retinal hemorrhage in newborns. *Ophthalmology*. 2001;108(1):36–39.

Levin AV. Retinal hemorrhages of crush head injury: learning from outliers. *Arch Ophthalmol*. 2006;124(12):1773–1774.

Lueder GT, Turner JW, Paschall R. Perimacular retinal folds simulating nonaccidental injury in an infant. *Arch Ophthalmol.* 2006;124(12):1782–1783.

Prognosis

In one large study, 29% of children with shaken baby syndrome died of their injuries. Poor visual and pupillary response were correlated with a higher risk of mortality. Survivors often suffered permanent impairment ranging from severe retardation and quadriparesis to mild learning disability and motor disturbances. Vision loss from traumatic retinoschisis, optic nerve damage, or cortical injury occurred in 20% of patients, but nearly complete recovery of vision was common. Dense vitreous hemorrhage, usually associated with deep traumatic retinoschisis, carried a poor prognosis for both vision and life.

McCabe CF, Donahue SP. Prognostic indicators for vision and mortality in shaken baby syndrome. *Arch Ophthalmol.* 2000;118(3):373–377.

Morad Y, Kim YM, Armstrong DC, Huyer D, Mian M, Levin AV. Correlation between retinal abnormalities and intracranial abnormalities in the shaken baby syndrome. *Am J Ophthalmol.* 2002;134(3):354–359.

Pierre-Kahn V, Roche O, Dureau P, et al. Ophthalmologic findings in suspected child abuse victims with subdural hematomas. *Ophthalmology.* 2003;110(9):1718–1723.

Superficial Injury

Corneal abrasion is one of the most common ocular injuries occurring in children, as it is in older people. Use of a pressure patch to keep the eyelids closed so that an abrasion will heal faster in a preschool child has been questioned by some practitioners. Obtaining and maintaining the desired effect can be difficult in this age group. Even without patching, moderately large traumatic corneal epithelial defects usually heal within 1–2 days in young children. However, patching does reduce blinking and rubbing of the eye, possibly diminishing the discomfort from the abrasion and accelerating healing. Use of topical cycloplegic drops and antibiotic ointment may also help reduce discomfort and risk of infection, respectively.

Cigarette burns of the cornea are the most common thermal injuries to the ocular surface in childhood. Usually, these occur in the age range of 2–4 years and are accidental, not manifestations of abuse. These burns result from the toddler's running into a cigarette held at eye level by an adult. Despite the alarming initial white appearance of coagulated corneal epithelium, cigarette burns typically heal rapidly and without scarring. Treatment is the same as for mechanical abrasions.

Chemical burns in childhood are generally caused by organic solvents or soaps found in household cleaning agents. Even burns involving almost total loss of corneal epithelium are likely to heal in a week or less with or without patching. Acid and alkali burns in children, as in adults, can be much more serious. The initial and most important step in management of all chemical injuries is immediate copious irrigation and meticulous removal of any particulate matter from the conjunctival fornices. See also BCSC Section 8, *External Disease and Cornea.*

Corneal foreign bodies in children can sometimes be dislodged with a forceful stream of irrigating solution from a small bottle; sharp instruments can thus be avoided.

If mechanical removal proves necessary, use of a slit lamp in the office or microscope in either a minor treatment room or operating room is required.

Penetrating Injury

Unless an adult has witnessed a traumatic incident, the history cannot be relied on to exclude the possibility of penetrating injury to the globe. The anterior segment and fundus must be thoroughly inspected in suspicious circumstances, with general anesthesia used if necessary. An area of subconjunctival hemorrhage or chemosis or a small break in the skin of the eyelid may be the only surface manifestation of scleral perforation by a sharp-pointed object, such as a pencil or scissors blade (Fig 30-3). Distortion of the pupil may be the most evident sign of a small corneal or limbal perforation. Computed tomography (CT) of the orbits should be considered if there is any reason to suspect an intraocular or deeply situated foreign body.

Corneoscleral lacerations in children are repaired according to the same principles as for adults. Corneal wounds heal relatively rapidly in very young patients, however, and sutures should be removed correspondingly earlier.

Fibrin clots often form quickly in the anterior chamber of a child's eye after a penetrating injury to the cornea, and these can simulate the appearance of fluffy cataractous

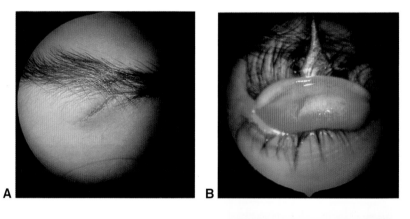

A   B

Figure 30-3 A, Small skin entry wound created by a thrown dart, right brow region, in a 7-year-old boy. **B,** Conjunctival exit wound indicates complete perforation of the eyelid. **C,** Extensive injury to the anterior segment of the same eye.

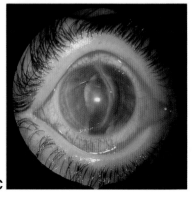

C

lens cortex to a remarkable degree. To avoid unnecessarily rendering the eye aphakic (and thereby compromising visual rehabilitation), the clinician should not perform lens removal in the course of primary wound repair unless absolutely certain that the anterior capsule has been ruptured. Even if lens cortex is exposed, postponing cataract surgery for 1–2 weeks until severe posttraumatic inflammation has quieted down may result in a smoother postoperative recovery and reduced risk of complications, without significantly worsening the visual prognosis. See also BCSC Section 11, *Lens and Cataract.*

Small conjunctival lacerations are often self-sealing. Full-thickness eyelid lacerations should be repaired meticulously, especially those involving a canaliculus, and sedation or general anesthesia may be required, even in older children. Otherwise, working near the eyes with sharp instruments and draping the face to create a sterile field are likely to frighten the patient and add to the difficulty of the repair. Clearly superficial wounds can be repaired in the emergency room. Use of an absorbable suture is an acceptable alternative if the physician wishes to avoid the need for removal of nonabsorbable sutures.

Blunt Injury

Hyphema

The management of hyphema in infants and children requires special considerations. As with all forms of pediatric trauma, the precise occurrence that led to intraocular bleeding may be difficult to determine. The possibility of abuse must be considered, as must the possibility of nontraumatic etiology: retinoblastoma, juvenile xanthogranuloma of the iris, and bleeding diathesis resulting from leukemia or other blood dyscrasia are relatively rare but important causes of spontaneous hyphema during the early years of life. Ultrasonography or CT should be performed to rule out intraocular tumor in suspicious cases if the iris and fundus cannot be adequately seen, and a complete blood count should be performed routinely, with coagulation studies, if a bleeding disorder is suspected.

Intraocular pressure (IOP), an important parameter for therapeutic decision-making with traumatic hyphema, is often difficult to monitor in the pediatric patient. The risks of inaccurate measurements and of further traumatizing the injured eye may outweigh the potential value of obtaining results in uncooperative children. With small amounts of blood pooling in the anterior chamber, concern about pressure tends to be greatest in patients with sickle cell trait or disease (Fig 30-4). Such patients may develop sickling in the anterior chamber, elevating IOP and retarding resorption of blood, or in the retinal circulation, causing vascular occlusion. A sickle preparation *("sickle cell prep"),* followed by *hemoglobin electrophoresis* for those with a positive screen in order to distinguish sickle cell trait from disease, is required for all African-American children with traumatic hyphema.

It was once common practice to hospitalize all patients with hyphema and place them on bed rest with bilateral patching of the eyes. Such extreme restriction has never been shown to improve prognosis, however, and is likely to be unproductive in children. On the other hand, some decrease in normal childhood running, jumping, and rough play is both reasonable and appropriate, as is placing a protective metal shield over the affected eye. Hospitalization during the first 5 days after injury, when risk of rebleeding is greatest,

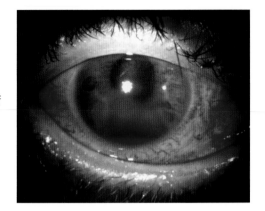

Figure 30-4 Small hyphema; note layering of blood inferiorly. *(Courtesy of Edward L. Raab, MD.)*

remains justifiable and is one way to ensure the opportunity for daily follow-up evaluation, especially when parental cooperation is questionable. Outpatient management with close follow-up is an acceptable alternative if the child's caregiver is compliant.

Medical management of hyphema remains controversial in children as in adults. Many ophthalmologists routinely use cycloplegic and corticosteroid drops to facilitate fundus examination, improve comfort, and reduce the risk of inflammatory complications and possibly of rebleeding as well. The value of these topical agents is unproven, however, and some clinicians prefer to use them selectively for control of pain or obvious inflammation or avoid them altogether to minimize manipulation of the eye. Pressure-lowering medication is appropriate for eyes known or strongly suspected to be hypertensive. Aspirin-containing compounds should be scrupulously avoided because of their antiplatelet action.

Oral administration of an antifibrinolytic agent (ε-aminocaproic acid, 50 mg/kg every 4 hours to a maximum of 30 g daily; or tranexamic acid, 25 mg/kg every 8 hours to a maximum of 4.5 g daily, for 5 days) has been shown to reduce the incidence of rebleeding in traumatic hyphema. However, one study found an insignificant decrease in the incidence of rebleeding among patients treated with tranexamic acid; gastric upset and hypotension may be significant adverse effects of oral ε-aminocaproic acid. Recently, topical aminocaproic acid was demonstrated to be an effective alternative. It is important to note that IOP may become transiently elevated after these antifibrinolytic agents are discontinued. Oral prednisolone has also been advocated in a dosage of 0.75 mg/kg/day in 2 divided doses (to a maximum of 40 mg/day in children). None of these treatments is universally accepted.

Surgical evacuation of hyphema is usually performed in adults when early corneal blood staining is detected or when significant IOP elevation has persisted for 5–7 days. The difficulty of detecting early blood staining in a child and the risk that corneal staining may cause severe deprivation amblyopia, coupled with the problems of accurately measuring IOP, justify earlier surgical intervention whenever a total hyphema persists for 4–5 days. Even earlier surgery may be necessary if elevated pressures occur in a patient with sickle cell trait or disease. Various operative techniques have been employed; none has been shown to offer particular advantages in childhood.

Late glaucoma is a potential complication of traumatic hyphema in children, as in adults, and may present with no symptoms. Gonioscopy can be performed after the eye has healed and the child can cooperate. Routine annual follow-up should be continued in children who are found to have an angle recession. It is important to remember that children with hyphemas may also have other significant injuries, including damage to the lens, retina, or optic nerve.

Pieramici DJ, Goldberg MF, Melia M, et al. A phase III, multicenter, randomized, placebo-controlled clinical trial of topical aminocaproic acid (Caprogel) in the management of traumatic hyphema. *Ophthalmology.* 2003;110(11):2106–2112.

Walton W, Von Hagen S, Grigorian R, Zarbin M. Management of traumatic hyphema. *Surv Ophthalmol.* 2002;47(4):297–334.

Orbital Fractures

Children, like adults, may sustain isolated fractures of orbital bone after blunt impact in the region of the eye. Careful examination of the eye is important to rule out associated ocular damage. CT should be performed to evaluate the fracture and possible associated injuries. The involvement of other specialties, including otolaryngology and neurosurgery, may be helpful in some cases. If there is severe enophthalmos or if the eye movements are extremely compromised, consideration should be given to primary repair of orbital fractures during the first 2 weeks following injury. In many cases, however, the motility will recover or strabismus surgery can be considered after several months if it proves necessary.

Though rare in older patients, orbital roof fractures are common in early childhood (<10 years). Isolated roof fractures typically result from impact to the brow region in a fall, often from a height of only a few feet. The principal external manifestation is hematoma in the upper eyelid (Fig 30-5). Orbital floor fractures are more common in older children because of increased ossification with age.

For further discussion of diagnosis and management of orbital trauma, see Chapter 10 and BCSC Section 7, *Orbit, Eyelids, and Lacrimal System.*

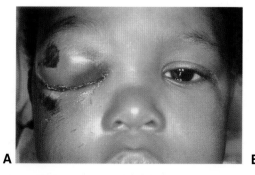
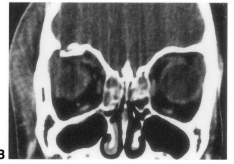

Figure 30-5 Orbital roof fracture in infant who fell with frontal impact. **A,** Marked right upper eyelid swelling from hematoma originating in the superior orbit adjacent to a linear fracture. **B,** Coronal CT image showing a bone fragment displaced into the right orbit.

CHAPTER 31

Decreased Vision in Infants and Children

When an infant has not developed good visual attention or ability to fixate and follow objects by 3–4 months of age, several causes must be considered. Many of these causes are covered elsewhere in this volume, in the chapters on cataracts, glaucoma, retinal disorders, and malformations. Some ocular abnormalities are relatively easily diagnosed by standard ophthalmic examinations. Others, however, are subtle and difficult to detect.

Normal Visual Development

Visual development is a highly complex maturation process. Structural changes occur in both the eye and the central nervous system. Laboratory and clinical research has shown that normal vision develops as a result of both genetic coding and experience in a normal visual environment.

Vision in the infant usually is assessed qualitatively by clinical appraisal as well as by psychophysical tests such as *optokinetic nystagmus (OKN)* responses, or *visually evoked cortical potential (VECP*; also abbreviated *VEP* or *VER* for *visually evoked potential* or *response*), and preferential looking techniques. A blink reflex to bright light should be present several days after birth. The pupillary light reflex is usually present after 31 weeks' gestation, but it can be difficult to evaluate because of miosis in the newborn.

At about 6 weeks of age, the normal baby should be able to make and maintain eye contact with other humans and react with facial expressions. Infants 2–3 months old should be interested in bright objects. Premature infants can be expected to reach these landmarks later, depending on their degree of prematurity.

Disconjugate eye movements, skew deviation, and *sunsetting* (tonic downward deviation of both eyes) may be noted in normal infants, but these should not persist after 4 months of age. Signs of actual poor visual development include wandering eye movements, lack of response to familiar faces and objects, and nystagmus. Staring at bright lights and forceful rubbing of the eyes in an otherwise visually disinterested infant *(oculodigital reflex)* are other signs of poor visual development and suggest an ocular cause for the deficiency.

Weinacht S, Kind C, Mönting JS, Gottlob I. Visual development in preterm and full-term infants: a prospective masked study. *Invest Ophthalmol Vis Sci.* 1999;40(2):346–353.

Approach to the Infant With Decreased Vision

A careful history, beginning with a review of vision problems in the family, is essential. If the patient is male, the possibility of an X-linked disorder should be explored. If a sibling has a similar condition not present in previous generations, an autosomal recessive disease is suggested.

Details of the pregnancy should be reviewed: important factors include maternal infection, radiation exposure, drugs, or trauma. Perinatal problems including prematurity, intrauterine growth retardation, fetal distress, bradycardia, meconium staining, and oxygen deprivation are important. The clinician also should inquire about the presence of systemic abnormalities or delayed developmental milestones.

Examination of the infant must include special attention to visual fixation, crispness and equality of pupillary light responses, ocular alignment and motility, and the presence of nystagmus or roving eye movements. A detailed fundus examination and cycloplegic refraction are necessary.

Pupillary responses are sluggish with anterior visual pathway disease such as retinal dystrophies, optic nerve hypoplasia or atrophy, optic nerve coloboma, and morning glory disc anomaly. Paradoxical pupils (pupillary constriction in response to darkness) are most commonly associated with retinal dystrophies but can also occur with optic neuropathies. Pupillary responses are normal in infants with cortical visual impairment.

Congenital sensory nystagmus is characterized as a rhythmic, horizontal, uniplanar, pendular or jerk nystagmus. The jerk component is often right-beating in right gaze and left-beating in left gaze. Congenital nystagmus in children may be an indicator of bilateral pregeniculate visual dysfunction. Although the word *congenital* is used in the name of this entity, the nystagmus usually begins at 2–3 months of age, not at birth. Chapter 25 discusses nystagmus in detail.

Visual deficits in 1 or both eyes can cause abnormal ocular alignment. Esotropic or exotropic deviation can occur.

When an infant presents with poor vision, the workup is predicated on localization of the visual dysfunction. It is useful to classify disorders causing vision loss in infants into those that cause primarily pregeniculate visual dysfunction and those that cause retrogeniculate visual dysfunction (so-called cortical visual impairment). Although this is a useful clinical paradigm, it should be recognized that some disorders affect both the pregeniculate pathway and the retrogeniculate pathway.

Pregeniculate Visual Loss

Congenital sensory nystagmus can be a clinical indicator of bilateral pregeniculate visual loss. Strabismus can occur with unilateral pregeniculate visual loss. The etiology is often apparent on ophthalmic examination. Apparent causes include anterior segment abnormalities, corneal opacities (Peters anomaly, sclerocornea), cataracts, and congenital glaucoma.

Optic nerve hypoplasia is the most common congenital optic disc anomaly resulting in pregeniculate visual loss in infants. Typically, unilateral cases present with sensory strabismus, and bilateral cases present with nystagmus. Endocrinologic evaluation is required in order to detect associated hypopituitarism. Magnetic resonance imaging of the brain should be considered in order to detect associated central nervous system anomalies.

Morning glory disc anomaly, optic disc coloboma, and optic disc staphyloma are other congenital optic disc anomalies that may cause pregeniculate vision loss in infants. They are readily detected on clinical examination. Congenital disc anomalies are discussed in Chapter 24.

Pregeniculate visual loss in infants may also be caused by optic nerve atrophy. Etiologies include hydrocephalus, brain tumors, trauma, hypoxic-ischemic injury, metabolic storage diseases, and inherited genetic optic neuropathies such as Behr optic atrophy. Optic atrophy may be an isolated defect or a facet of a diffuse neurologic or systemic disease. Neuroimaging is generally required. Further systemic and neurologic evaluation depends on associated clinical findings. Optic nerve disorders are discussed in Chapter 24.

Infants with poor vision, nystagmus, and no obvious abnormality on ophthalmic examination may have a retinal disorder. Retinal dystrophies, including Leber congenital amaurosis, achromatopsia, blue-cone monochromatism, and congenital stationary night blindness, cause pregeniculate visual loss. In an infant with a retinal dystrophy, retinal pigment epithelial changes are often absent. Subtle retinal vessel attenuation and optic disc pallor may be present, although the retina may appear completely normal. Clinical signs that suggest a retinal dystrophy include photophobia, nyctalopia, high refractive error (either hyperopic or myopic), paradoxical pupils, and the oculodigital sign (the infant habitually presses on the eye with a finger or fist in an effort to induce entoptic stimulation of the retina).

Electroretinography (ERG) can aid in the diagnosis of these retinal disorders, and some investigators advocate ERG testing for all infants with visual inattentiveness and normal ocular structures. Other researchers think that, in infants, ERG should be reserved only for patients thought to have Leber congenital amaurosis. Obtaining quality ERGs in infants is difficult, and the examiner must be aware of the normal developmental variations that show up in these electrophysiologic tests in the first year of life. Serial testing may be important before definitive diagnostic and prognostic information is provided.

Poor vision and nystagmus in infants may result from *foveal hypoplasia,* another cause of pregeniculate visual loss. Albinism and aniridia are associated conditions. Therefore, infants with nystagmus should be evaluated for the presence of iris transillumination defects, foveal hypoplasia, and fundus hypopigmentation. These findings would indicate albinism. Retinal disorders are discussed in Chapter 23.

Retrogeniculate Visual Loss, or Cortical Visual Impairment

Cortical visual impairment denotes vision loss from pathology posterior to the lateral geniculate nucleus (the retrogeniculate visual pathways). The pathology may involve the optic radiations (which are subcortical), as well as the occipital cortex. Hence, the terms *cerebral visual impairment* and *retrogeniculate visual loss* describe this entity more precisely. However, *cortical visual impairment* is entrenched in the literature and will be used in this discussion.

Cortical visual impairment is the most frequent cause of childhood visual impairment in developed countries. Etiologies may be congenital or acquired. Prenatal and perinatal causes include periventricular leukomalacia (a prominent cause of visual impairment in children born prematurely), intrauterine infection (see Chapter 16), cerebral dysgenesis, asphyxia, intracranial hemorrhage, hydrocephalus, and infection. Acquired causes include trauma and child abuse (see Chapter 30), shunt malfunction, meningitis, and encephalitis.

Infants with cortical visual impairment demonstrate varying degrees of visual attentiveness. Both the family and the ophthalmologist may be uncertain as to whether the baby can see. Examination reveals normal ocular structures, normal pupillary responses, and searching eye movements. Rhythmic nystagmus movements are typically not present. Descending optic atrophy (from transsynaptic degeneration) may coexist. In preterm infants, optic disc cupping resembling glaucomatous cupping can occur from transsynaptic degeneration, most commonly secondary to periventricular leukomalacia.

The ERG results appear normal; the VEP results may be normal or subnormal. Neuroimaging may be normal or reveal changes such as atrophy and porencephaly in the occipital (striate or parastriate) cortex, damage to the optic radiations, or periventricular leukomalacia. Children with normal neuroimaging studies may have a more favorable prognosis.

Depending on the etiology, cortical visual impairment may be transient or permanent and can be an isolated finding or associated with multiple neurologic deficits.

Brodsky MC, Fray KJ, Glasier CM. Perinatal cortical and subcortical visual loss: mechanisms of injury and associated ophthalmologic signs. *Ophthalmology.* 2002;109(1):85–94.

Good WV. Development of a quantitative method to measure vision in children with chronic cortical visual impairment. *Trans Am Ophthalmol Soc.* 2001;99:253–269.

Delayed Visual Maturation

Sometimes, when eye examination results are totally normal but fixation is poor, the problem is merely delayed maturation of the visual system. In such children, neurologic examination results may be normal except for poor visual attention. Some patients, however, have evidence of other neurologic impairment. The problem is especially common in children with other developmental disabilities.

If the infant's visual behavior does not begin to progress toward normal within a few months, further investigation is warranted. Visually evoked cortical potentials recorded very early in life may initially be abnormal; this determination is more valid as the child approaches 12 months of age. Such testing can be omitted when the infant's visual behavior is clearly progressing toward normal.

Low Vision Rehabilitation

Low vision rehabilitation comprises the treatment of visually impaired patients who have exhausted medical and surgical options. Unfortunately, low vision rehabilitation is often neglected in children. However, children with visual impairment require formal low vision assessments that will provide rehabilitative treatment options, including correction of refractive errors, magnification for reading, bifocal glasses, telescopic magnification devices for viewing distance targets, prisms, and a variety of selective transmission lenses aimed at reduction of glare and photostress. See also Chapter 9, Vision Rehabilitation, in BCSC Section 3, *Clinical Optics.*

For patients whose visual function could be helped or enhanced by vision rehabilitation, the American Academy of Ophthalmology provides the SmartSight website: http://one.aao.org/CE/EducationalContent/Smartsight.aspx. See also Table 31-1, which lists resources for further information.

> Hutcheson KA, Drack AV. Diagnosis and management of the infant who does not see. *Focal Points: Clinical Modules for Ophthalmologists.* San Francisco: American Academy of Ophthalmology; 1998, module 12.
>
> Markowitz SN. Principles of modern low vision rehabilitation. *Can J Ophthalmol.* 2006:41(3): 289–312.
>
> Preferred Practice Patterns Committee, Vision Rehabilitation Panel. *Vision rehabilitation for adults.* San Francisco: American Academy of Ophthalmology; 2007. Available online at http://one.aao.org/CE/PracticeGuidelines/PPP.aspx.

Table 31-1 Sources of Information on Low Vision

American Foundation for the Blind, 11 Penn Plaza, Ste 300, New York, NY 10001; (212) 502-7600 or (800) 232-5463; www.afb.org. For the publication *Reach Out and Teach: Meeting the Training Needs of Parents of Visually and Multiply Handicapped Young Children* by KA Ferrell, PhD (AFB, 1985), call (800) 232-3044.

American Printing House for the Blind (APH), 1839 Frankfort Avenue, PO Box 6085, Louisville, KY 40206-0085; (502) 895-2405 or (800) 223-1839; www.aph.org. Large-print and braille books, tapes, talking computer software, and low vision aids.

Family Support America, 205 W. Randolph St, Ste 2222, Chicago, IL 60606; (312) 338-0900; www.familysupportamerica.org. Identifies parent support groups all over the country.

Lighthouse for the Blind, Lighthouse Center for Education, Information, and Resource Service: (800) 829-0500. Independent organizations in every state; check local directories for listings.

National Association for the Visually Handicapped (NAVH), 22 West 21st St, 6th floor, New York, NY 10010, (212) 889-3141; www.navh.org. Large-print textbooks, library material on request. Sources of information and guidance on resources for the visually handicapped.

National Association of Parents of Children With Visual Impairments (NAPVI), PO Box 317, Watertown, MA 02471; (800) 562-6265; www.spedex.com/napvi. Some areas have a state organization as well; NAPVI can direct the parent.

National Dissemination Center for Children With Disabilities (NICHCY), 1825 Connecticut Ave NW, Ste 700, Washington, DC 20009; (800) 695-0285.

National Library Service for the Blind and Physically Handicapped (NLS), Library of Congress, 1291 Taylor St NW, Washington, DC 20011; (202) 707-5100 or (800) 424-8567. Books and magazines in braille and audio.

National Organization for Albinism and Hypopigmentation (NOAH), PO Box 959, East Hampstead, NH 03826-0959; (800) 473-2310; www.albinism.org.

Prevent Blindness America, 211 West Wacker Drive, Ste 1700, Chicago, IL 60606; (800) 331-2020; www.preventblindness.org.

Recording for the Blind & Dyslexic, 20 Roszel Road, Princeton, NJ 08540; (866) 732-3585 (866-RFBD-585); www.rfbd.org.

Retinoblastoma Support News (newsletter for families of children with retinoblastoma) and *Parent to Parent* (newsletter for families of blind or visually impaired or multihandicapped children). Published by Institute for Families, PO Box 54700, mail stop 111, Los Angeles, CA 90054-0700; (323) 669-4649; www.instituteforfamilies.org.

(Continued)

Table 31-1 *(continued)*

National Toll-Free Numbers
  American Council of the Blind (800) 424-8666
  Better Hearing Institute (800) 327-9355 (800-EAR-WELL)
  Epilepsy Information Line (800) 332-1000 [(800) EFA-1000]
  Cystic Fibrosis Foundation (800) 344-4823
  National Down Syndrome Society (800) 221-4602
  National Easter Seal Society (800) 221-6827
  National Health Information Center (800) 336-4797
  Spina Bifida (800) 621-3141
  United Cerebral Palsy Association (800) 872-5827
  National Fragile X Foundation (800) 688-8765
  American Kidney Fund (800) 638-8299
  The Arc of the United States (formerly Association for Retarded Citizens) (800) 433-5255
  Sickle Cell Association (800) 421-8453
  Retina International (formerly International Retinitis Pigmentosa Association) (800) 344-4877

Sources of Large-Print Publications
  New York Times Large-Print Weekly, 229 West 43rd Street, New York, NY 10036; (800) 631-2580
  Library for the Blind and Physically Handicapped, Free Library of Philadelphia, 919 Walnut St,
    Philadelphia, PA 19107-5289; (800) 222-1754
  Reader's Digest Large Print, PO Box 8177, Red Oak, IA 51591-1177; (800) 807-2780

Basic Texts

Pediatric Ophthalmology and Strabismus

Brodsky MC, Baker RS, Hamed LM. *Pediatric Neuro-Ophthalmology.* New York: Springer-Verlag; 1995.

Buckley EG, Freedman S, Shields MB. *Atlas of Ophthalmic Surgery, Vol III: Strabismus and Glaucoma.* St Louis: Mosby-Year Book; 1995.

Cibis GW, Tongue AC, Stass-Isern ML. *Decision Making in Pediatric Ophthalmology.* St Louis: Mosby-Year Book; 1993.

Del Monte MA, Archer SM. *Atlas of Pediatric Ophthalmology and Strabismus Surgery.* New York: Churchill Livingstone; 1993.

Helveston EM. *Surgical Management of Strabismus: An Atlas of Strabismus Surgery.* 4th ed. St Louis: Mosby-Year Book; 1993.

Helveston EM, Ellis FD. *Pediatric Ophthalmology Practice.* 2nd ed. St Louis: Mosby; 1984.

Isenberg SJ, ed. *The Eye in Infancy.* 2nd ed. St Louis: Mosby-Year Book; 1994.

Jones KL. *Smith's Recognizable Patterns of Human Malformation.* 6th ed. Philadelphia: Elsevier Saunders; 2005.

Katowitz JA, ed. *Pediatric Oculoplastic Surgery.* New York: Springer; 2002.

Leigh RJ, Zee DS. *The Neurology of Eye Movements.* 4th ed. New York: Oxford; 2006.

Miller NR, Newman NJ, Biousse V, Kerrison JB, eds. *Walsh and Hoyt's Clinical Neuro-Ophthalmology.* 6th ed. Philadelphia: Lippincott Williams & Wilkins; 2005.

Nelson LB, Olitsky SE, eds. *Harley's Pediatric Ophthalmology.* 5th ed. Philadelphia: Lippincott Williams & Wilkins; 2005.

Parks MM. *Atlas of Strabismus Surgery.* Philadelphia: Harper & Row; 1983.

Parks MM. *Ocular Motility and Strabismus.* Hagerstown: Harper & Row; 1975.

Plager DA, Parks MM, von Noorden GK. *Strabismus Surgery: Basic and Advanced Strategies.* Ophthalmology Monograph 17. New York: Oxford University Press; 2004.

Renie WA, ed. *Goldberg's Genetic and Metabolic Eye Disease.* 2nd ed. Boston: Little, Brown & Co; 1986.

Rosenbaum AL, Santiago AP, eds. *Clinical Strabismus Management: Principles and Surgical Techniques.* Philadelphia: Saunders; 1999.

Scott WE, D'Agostino DD, Lennarson LW, eds. *Orthoptics and Ocular Examination Techniques.* Baltimore: Williams & Wilkins; 1983.

Spencer WH, ed. *Ophthalmic Pathology: An Atlas and Textbook.* 4th ed. Philadelphia: Saunders; 1996.

Tasman W, Jaeger EA, eds. *Duane's Clinical Ophthalmology.* Philadelphia: Lippincott Williams & Wilkins; 2007.

Traboulsi EI. *A Compendium of Inherited Disorders and the Eye.* New York: Oxford University Press; 2006.

von Noorden GK. *Atlas of Strabismus.* 4th ed. St Louis: Mosby; 1983.

von Noorden GK, Campos EC. *Binocular Vision and Ocular Motility: Theory and Management of Strabismus.* 6th ed. St Louis: Mosby; 2002.

von Noorden GK, Helveston EM. *Strabismus: A Decision Making Approach.* St Louis: Mosby; 1994.

Wilson ME, Saunders RA, Trivedi RH, eds. *Pediatric Ophthalmology.* Berlin: Springer; 2009.

Wright KW, ed. *Color Atlas of Strabismus Surgery: Strategies and Techniques.* 3rd ed. New York: Springer; 2007.

Wright KW, Spiegel PH, eds. *Pediatric Ophthalmology and Strabismus.* 2nd ed. New York: Springer; 2003.

Related Academy Materials

Focal Points: Clinical Modules for Ophthalmologists

Coats DK. Adult strabismus (Module 12, 2009).

Curnyn KM, Longest C. Why do kids do that? (Module 6, 2006).

Gunduz K, Shields CL. Retinoblastoma update (Module 7, 2005).

Hertle RW, Kowal LM, Yeates KO. The ophthalmologist and learning disabilities (Module 2, 2005).

Mets MB, Noffke AS. Ocular infections of the external eye and cornea in children (Module 2, 2002).

Meyer DR. Congenital ptosis (Module 2, 2001).

Pelton RW, Klapper SR. Preseptal and orbital cellulitis (Module 11, 2008).

Robb RM. Nasolacrimal duct obstruction in children (Module 8, 2004).

Suh DW. Acquired esotropia in children and adults (excluding pediatric accommodative esotropia) (Module 10, 2003).

Trigler L. Managing accommodative esotropia patients and their parents (Module 5, 2008).

Wallace DK. Retinopathy of prematurity (Module 12, 2008).

Wygnanski-Jaffe T, Levin AV. Introductory genetics for the ophthalmologist (Module 5, 2005).

Print Publications

Arnold AC, ed. *Basic Principles of Ophthalmic Surgery* (2006).

Dunn JP, Langer PD, eds. *Basic Techniques of Ophthalmic Surgery* (2009).

Parke DW II, ed. *The Profession of Ophthalmology: Practice Management, Ethics, and Advocacy* (2005).

Plager DA, ed. *Strabismus Surgery: Basic and Advanced Strategies.* Written by Buckley EG, Plager DA, Repka MX, Wilson ME, with contributions by Parks MM, von Noorden GK. American Academy of Ophthalmology Monograph Series No. 17. New York: Oxford University Press; 2004.

Rockwood EJ, ed. *ProVision: Preferred Responses in Ophthalmology.* Series 4. Self-Assessment Program, 2-vol set (2007).

Wilson FM II, Blomquist PH, eds. *Practical Ophthalmology: A Manual for Beginning Residents.* 6th ed. (2009).

Preferred Practice Patterns

Preferred Practice Patterns are available at http://one.aao.org/CE/PracticeGuidelines/PPP.aspx.

Preferred Practice Patterns Committee, Pediatric Ophthalmology Panel. *Amblyopia* (2007).
Preferred Practice Patterns Committee, Pediatric Ophthalmology Panel. *Esotropia and Exotropia* (2007).
Preferred Practice Patterns Committee, Pediatric Ophthalmology Panel. *Pediatric Eye Evaluations* (2007).

Ophthalmic Technology Assessments

Ophthalmic Technology Assessments are available at http://one.aao.org/CE/Practice Guidelines/Ophthalmic.aspx. Assessments are published in the Academy's journal, *Ophthalmology*. Individual reprints may be ordered at http://www.aao.org/store.

Ophthalmic Technology Assessment Committee. *Strabismus Surgery for Adults* (2003).

Policy Statement

Learning Disabilities, Dyslexia, and Vision. A Joint Statement of the American Academy of Pediatrics, American Association for Pediatric Ophthalmology and Strabismus, American Association of Certified Orthoptists, and American Academy of Ophthalmology, 2009. Available at www.aao.org.

CDs/DVDs

Basic and Clinical Science Course (Sections 1–13) (DVD-ROM; 2009).
Clinical Skills DVD Series. *Strabismus Evaluation and Surgery* (DVD-ROM; reviewed for currency 2007).
Demer JL, Lambert SR, Tychsen L. *LEO Clinical Update Course on Pediatric Ophthalmology and Strabismus* (CD-ROM; 2008).
Johns KJ, ed. Understanding and Preventing Amblyopia. In: *Eye Care Skills: Presentations for Physicians and Other Health Care Professionals, Version 3.0* (CD-ROM; 2009).

Online Materials

Preferred Practice Patterns and Ophthalmic Technology Assessments are available at http://one.aao.org/CE/PracticeGuidelines/default.aspx.

Basic and Clinical Science Course (Sections 1–13); http://one.aao.org/CE/Educational Products/BCSC.aspx

Clinical Education and Ethics Courses; http://one.aao.org/CE/EducationalContent/Courses.aspx

Clinical Education Cases; http://one.aao.org/CE/EducationalContent/Cases.aspx

Focal Points modules; http://one.aao.org/CE/EducationalProducts/FocalPoints.aspx

Hebson CB, Murchison AP, Grossniklaus HE. Toddler With Ecchymosis and Eyelid Edema. Academy Grand Rounds (May 2009); http://one.aao.org/CE/EducationalContent/Cases.aspx

MOC Exam Study Kit, Compass Version 2.0 (2008); http://one.aao.org/CE/EducationalContent/CompassExam.aspx

MOC Exam Study Kit, Version 2.0 (2007); http://one.aao.org/CE/MOC/default.aspx

Plager DA, Carter BC. Surgical Management of Pediatric Cataracts (October 2009); http://one.aao.org/CE/EducationalContent/Courses.aspx

Reddy AK, Marx D, Edmond JC. Unilateral Proptosis in a 3-Year-Old Boy. Academy Grand Rounds (December 2008); http://one.aao.org/CE/EducationalContent/Cases.aspx

Rockwood EJ, ed. *ProVision: Preferred Responses in Ophthalmology.* Series 4. Self-Assessment Program, 2-vol set (2007); http://one.aao.org/CE/EducationalProducts/Provision.aspx

To order any of these materials, please order online at www.aao.org/store, or call the Academy's Customer Service toll-free number, 866-561-8558, in the U.S. If outside the U.S., call 415-561-8540 between 8:00 AM and 5:00 PM PST.

Credit Reporting Form

Basic and Clinical Science Course, 2010–2011
Section 6

The American Academy of Ophthalmology is accredited by the Accreditation Council for Continuing Medical Education to provide continuing medical education for physicians.

The American Academy of Ophthalmology designates this educational activity for a maximum of 15 *AMA PRA Category 1 Credits*™. Physicians should only claim credit commensurate with the extent of their participation in the activity.

If you wish to claim continuing medical education credit for your study of this Section, you may claim your credit online or fill in the required forms and mail or fax them to the Academy.

To use the forms:

1. Complete the study questions and mark your answers on the Section Completion Form.
2. Complete the Section Evaluation.
3. Fill in and sign the statement below.
4. Return this page and the required forms by mail or fax to the CME Registrar (see below).

To claim credit online:

1. Log on to the Academy website (www.aao.org/cme).
2. Select Review/Claim CME.
3. Follow the instructions.

Important: These completed forms or the online claim must be received at the Academy by June 2013.

I hereby certify that I have spent _____ (up to 15) hours of study on the curriculum of this Section and that I have completed the study questions.

Signature: _____

Date

Name: _____

Address: _____

City and State: _____   Zip: _____

Telephone: (_____) _____   Academy Member ID# _____

area code

Please return completed forms to: **Or you may fax them to: 415-561-8575**
American Academy of Ophthalmology
P.O. Box 7424
San Francisco, CA 94120-7424
Attn: CME Registrar, Customer Service

2010–2011
Section Completion Form

Basic and Clinical Science Course

Answer Sheet for Section 6

Question	Answer	Question	Answer	Question	Answer
1	a b c d	18	a b c d	35	a b c d
2	a b c d	19	a b c d	36	a b c d
3	a b c d	20	a b c d	37	a b c d
4	a b c d	21	a b c d	38	a b c d
5	a b c d	22	a b c d	39	a b c d
6	a b c d	23	a b c d	40	a b c d
7	a b c d	24	a b c d	41	a b c d
8	a b c d	25	a b c d	42	a b c d
9	a b c d	26	a b c d	43	a b c d
10	a b c d	27	a b c d	44	a b c d
11	a b c d	28	a b c d	45	a b c d
12	a b c d	29	a b c d	46	a b c d
13	a b c d	30	a b c d	47	a b c d
14	a b c d	31	a b c d	48	a b c d
15	a b c d	32	a b c d	49	a b c d
16	a b c d	33	a b c d	50	a b c d
17	a b c d	34	a b c d		

Section Evaluation

Please complete this CME questionnaire.

1. To what degree will you use knowledge from BCSC Section 6 in your practice?

   ☐ Regularly

   ☐ Sometimes

   ☐ Rarely

2. Please review the stated objectives for BCSC Section 6. How effective was the material at meeting those objectives?

   ☐ All objectives were met.

   ☐ Most objectives were met.

   ☐ Some objectives were met.

   ☐ Few or no objectives were met.

3. To what degree is BCSC Section 6 likely to have a positive impact on health outcomes of your patients?

   ☐ Extremely likely

   ☐ Highly likely

   ☐ Somewhat likely

   ☐ Not at all likely

4. After you review the stated objectives for BCSC Section 6, please let us know of any additional knowledge, skills, or information useful to your practice that were acquired but were not included in the objectives.

5. Was BCSC Section 6 free of commercial bias?

   ☐ Yes

   ☐ No

6. If you selected "No" in the previous question, please comment.

7. Please tell us what might improve the applicability of BCSC to your practice.

Study Questions

Although a concerted effort has been made to avoid ambiguity and redundancy in these questions, the authors recognize that differences of opinion may occur regarding the "best" answer. The discussions are provided to demonstrate the rationale used to derive the answer. They may also be helpful in confirming that your approach to the problem was correct or, if necessary, in fixing the principle in your memory. The Section 6 faculty would like to thank the Self-Assessment Committee for working with them to provide these study questions and discussions.

1. Congenital nasolacrimal duct obstruction is most commonly caused by an obstruction of
    a. the upper canaliculus
    b. the valve of Hasner
    c. the lower punctum
    d. the valve of Rosenmüller

2. What is the most appropriate surgical management for a patient with unilateral superior oblique paralysis where excyclotorsion is the primary problem?
    a. superior oblique tenotomy
    b. superior rectus recession
    c. fadenoperation
    d. Harada-Ito procedure

3. A 23-year-old man is diagnosed with A-pattern exotropia. Testing of versions is most likely to reveal
    a. superior oblique overaction
    b. inferior oblique overaction
    c. superior rectus overaction
    d. inferior rectus overaction

4. A patient is found to have A-pattern exotropia with a compensatory head posture. The most likely head posture is
    a. chin-up
    b. chin-down
    c. right head tilt
    d. right face turn

5. Which of the following clinical features will most likely help differentiate Duane syndrome from a sixth nerve paralysis?
    a. limited adduction of the affected eye
    b. incomitant esodeviation
    c. anomalous head posture
    d. limited abduction of the affected eye

6. A 34-year-old patient undergoes strabismus surgery under general anesthesia. During the procedure, he develops tachycardia, a rise in body temperature, and muscular rigidity. The next step should be to do what?

   a. Cool skin with ice and administer benzodiazepine.

   b. Cool skin with ice and administer intravenous beta-blocker.

   c. Discontinue anesthetic agents, hyperventilate with oxygen, and administer dantrolene.

   d. Release tension on extraocular muscles and administer atropine.

7. Four weeks after bilateral medial rectus recession surgery, a patient presents with a new 15 prism-diopter (Δ) exotropia. On examination, there is limited adduction of the right eye. The most likely diagnosis is

   a. anterior segment ischemia

   b. adherence syndrome

   c. conjunctival scarring

   d. slipped muscle

8. A 10-month-old patient with a history of strabismus surgery for congenital esotropia presents with a history of a right eye that has begun to spontaneously drift upward several times a day. The most likely diagnosis is

   a. superior oblique paralysis

   b. orbital fat adherence syndrome

   c. consecutive hypertropia

   d. dissociated vertical deviation

9. A patient with thyroid eye disease complains of gradually worsening vision in the left eye. Best-corrected acuity in the left eye is 1 line worse than at the last visit, and there is a 6Δ exophoria at near. What is the most appropriate initial workup?

   a. Evaluate pupillary function and color vision.

   b. Prescribe increased lubrication.

   c. Prescribe a trial of Fresnel prisms on glasses.

   d. Obtain an orbital computerized axial tomography (CT) scan.

10. Pertinent clinical features used to confirm the diagnosis of a dacryocele in a 2-week-old infant include which of the following?

    a. the presence of a bluish swelling just below and nasal to the medial canthus

    b. the presence of a bluish swelling just below and temporal to the medial canthus

    c. the presence of a bluish swelling just above and temporal to the medial canthus

    d. the presence of a bluish swelling just above and nasal to the medial canthus

11. The crowding phenomenon in visual acuity testing describes which one of the following?

    a. need for siblings to leave the examination room to avoid distracting the patient

    b. increase in performance when reading a single optotype compared to a full line

    c. decrease in performance after repeated testing

    d. optimal distance to hold Teller acuity cards to avoid approaching the patient too closely

12. Which form of bilaterally symmetric refractive error at a level of 3.5 diopters would place a child at the greatest risk for isometric amblyopia?

    a. myopia

    b. hyperopia

    c. astigmatism

    d. no risk of isometric amblyopia

13. Which of the following is the most appropriate test for quantifying torsion during a pre-operative strabismus evaluation?

    a. red-glass test

    b. double Maddox rod test

    c. Hess screen test

    d. afterimage test

14. Which method of clinical measurement of the accommodative convergence to accommodation ratio (AC/A) employs the distance and near deviations and their relationship?

    a. near point of accommodation

    b. near point of convergence

    c. gradient method

    d. heterophoria method

15. A 3-year-old African-American girl presents with a recently acquired esotropia of 40Δ. Cyclopentolate refraction is +3.50 OU. With this prescription, she has a residual esotropia of 12Δ. The next step in management should be

    a. redoing cycloplegic refraction

    b. surgery for the entire angle of deviation

    c. contact lenses

    d. decreasing the hyperopic correction of the spectacles

16. A patient undergoes bilateral lateral rectus recession for intermittent exotropia. The patient should be told that a stable postoperative result will be known in what period of time?

    a. immediately after surgery

    b. 48–72 hours after surgery

    c. 6–8 weeks after surgery

    d. 4–6 months after surgery

17. Which of the following types of exodeviations is the most common?

    a. pseudoexotropia

    b. congenital exotropia

    c. Duane syndrome type 2

    d. intermittent exotropia

18. Which of the following is the most appropriate description of the cornea after birth?

    a. It flattens, reaching adult power by the age of 12 years.

    b. It has a diameter of approximately 8 mm.

    c. It changes most in the first 5 years, reaching adult diameter by age 8 years.

    d. It is cloudy at birth, because of edema and endothelial immaturity.

19. Which of the following findings is most likely considered to be normal in a 1-month-old infant on eye examination?

    a. 20/30 vision with preferential viewing techniques

    b. episodes of large-angle esotropia

    c. normal horizontal and vertical movements

    d. higher intraocular pressure than adults

20. One of the risk factors for developing inferior oblique muscle overaction is

    a. sensory esotropia

    b. craniosynostoses

    c. superior oblique muscle overaction

    d. Duane syndrome

21. A 2-week-old infant is suspected of having persistent fetal vasculature (PFV). On anterior segment examination, what findings would support this diagnosis?

    a. congenital bilateral cataracts

    b. normal axial lengths

    c. iris hypoplasia

    d. anteriorly displaced ciliary processes

22. In patients with aniridia, careful screening must be performed to rule out the following systemic disease:

    a. retinoblastoma

    b. Wilms tumor

    c. rhabdomyosarcoma

    d. pheochromocytoma

23. Wilms tumor is most often associated with which of the following types of aniridia?

    a. autosomal dominant

    b. autosomal recessive

    c. sporadic

    d. X-linked recessive

24. A 12-year-old boy presents to the emergency department with severe bilateral ocular pain, redness, and photophobia resulting from a chemical burn 15 minutes ago. The most appropriate initial management is

    a. copious irrigation with saline solution

    b. application of mild antibiotic ointment

    c. neutralization of the pH

    d. topical N-acetyl cysteine followed by pressure patching

25. Intraocular inflammation associated with juvenile idiopathic arthritis (JIA) is usually of what type?

    a. anterior and nongranulomatous

    b. multifocal choroiditis

    c. acute retinal necrosis

    d. vitritis

26. The most common mode of inheritance of neurofibromatosis type 1 (NF1) is

    a. autosomal recessive

    b. X-linked recessive

    c. mitochondrial

    d. autosomal dominant

27. The presence of a plexiform neurofibroma of the upper eyelid in a child with NF1 mandates serial examinations for which of the following conditions?

    a. cataract

    b. amblyopia

    c. strabismus

    d. optic atrophy

28. A 12-year-old African-American patient is diagnosed with a 5-mm traumatic hyphema OD. Intraocular pressure (IOP) is 22 mm Hg OD and 12 mm Hg OS. The following laboratory test is indicated:

    a. HLA-B27 testing

    b. ANA titer testing

    c. sickle cell testing

    d. beta-thalassemia testing

29. An 11-month-old girl presents for evaluation and is found to have epiblepharon. The child is playful and asymptomatic, and there is no evidence of corneal involvement. What would be the best initial treatment for this child's condition?

    a. observation

    b. artificial tear eyedrops every 4 hours

    c. surgery to remove a strip of skin and orbicularis muscle from beneath the lid margin

    d. Quickert suture repair

30. When consulting with the parents of a child with decreased visual acuity from corneal tears in Descemet's membrane, what statement is most correct?

    a. Correction of the refractive error and amblyopia therapy are usually successful in treating this condition.

    b. Early small-graft penetrating keratoplasty is indicated when Haab striae are seen.

    c. Topical hypertonic saline does not appear to be helpful.

    d. It is important to observe the contralateral eye for the development of Haab striae.

31. During the initial examination of a 5-year-old child, you note the presence of asymptomatic tears in Descemet's membrane in the child's left eye. Horizontal corneal diameter is equal and normal in both eyes. What is the most likely cause of the findings on examination?

    a. acute hydrops

    b. forceps birth injury

    c. nonincidental trauma

    d. congenital glaucoma

32. Which of the following is the most likely risk factor for uveitis in patients with juvenile idiopathic arthritis?

    a. arthritis onset after age 2 years

    b. more than 4 joints involved at onset

    c. female gender

    d. absence of ANA positivity

33. Pseudoptosis may be associated with which of the following conditions of the affected eye?

    a. hypotropia

    b. heterochromia

    c. Duane syndrome

    d. Kawasaki syndrome

34. What is the most appropriate type of surgical needle for scleral reattachment during resectioning of an extraocular muscle?

    a. cutting

    b. reverse cutting

    c. tapered at the point

    d. spatulated

35. A needle perforating the sclera during strabismus surgery can result in various clinical manifestations. The most common outcome is

    a. vitreous hemorrhage

    b. chorioretinal scar

    c. retinal detachment

    d. endophthalmitis

36. The positions of gaze in which 1 extraocular muscle is the prime mover of each eye are called the

    a. secondary positions

    b. midline positions

    c. diagnostic positions

    d. cardinal positions

37. A patient is diagnosed with inferior oblique muscle overaction. Findings on testing of versions would be

    a. overelevation of the affected eye in adduction

    b. overelevation of the affected eye in abduction

    c. overelevation of the affected eye in adduction and abduction

    d. overelevation of the affected eye in primary position

38. Individuals at greater risk for developing anomalous retinal correspondence include which one of the following?

    a. a 7-year-old boy with a history of congenital esotropia

    b. a 12-year-old girl with a 3-week history of decreased vision in her right eye

    c. a 15-year-old boy with a 1-week history of esotropia

    d. a 7-year-old girl with a history of exophoria

39. Which one of the following is a pertinent clinical feature of monofixation syndrome?

    a. esotropia of $>10\Delta$ with simultaneous prism and cover testing

    b. evidence of central fusion without peripheral sensory fusion

    c. evidence of peripheral sensory fusion without central fusion

    d. evidence of peripheral sensory fusion without motor fusion

40. Botulinum toxin injection is most effective in treating which of the following forms of strabismus?

    a. dissociated vertical deviation

    b. small-angle esotropia

    c. chronic thyroid eye disease

    d. A-pattern exotropia

41. Botulinum toxin is an effective treatment for which of the following disorders?

    a. ptosis

    b. phthisis

    c. dry eye

    d. essential blepharospasm

42. Which systemic medication is the most appropriate treatment for an infant with ophthalmia neonatorum secondary to *Chlamydia trachomatis?*

    a. erythromycin

    b. doxycycline

    c. ofloxacin

    d. azithromycin

43. An 11-year-old patient presents with red, itchy eyes. On examination, gray, jellylike limbal nodules with vascular cores are seen. This is suggestive of what diagnosis?

    a. phlyctenular keratoconjunctivitis

    b. atopic keratoconjunctivitis

    c. vernal keratoconjunctivitis

    d. superior limbic keratoconjunctivitis

44. The majority of congenital glaucoma cases are inherited based on the following pattern:

    a. autosomal dominant

    b. sporadic

    c. X-linked recessive

    d. autosomal recessive

45. The mechanism of glaucoma in Sturge-Weber syndrome is

    a. increased episcleral venous pressure

    b. angle-closure glaucoma

    c. neovascular glaucoma

    d. pupillary block glaucoma

46. A 1-month-old baby is diagnosed with unilateral anterior polar cataract that is approximately 1.5 mm in diameter. The most appropriate initial management is

    a. close observation

    b. lensectomy

    c. lensectomy with intraocular lens implant

    d. chronic dilation

47. A newborn infant with nystagmus is diagnosed with aniridia. Optic nerve examination is most likely to reveal

    a. coloboma

    b. pallor

    c. hypoplasia

    d. swelling

48. A 12-year-old boy is diagnosed with well-controlled intermittent exotropia. Stereopsis testing is most likely to reveal

    a. monofixation syndrome

    b. no stereopsis because of temporal hemiretinal suppression

    c. no stereopsis because of diplopia

    d. excellent stereopsis

49. Pseudopapilledema is most frequently seen in conjunction with which of the following findings after complete ophthalmologic examination?

    a. hyperopia

    b. myopia

    c. esotropia

    d. exotropia

50. An infant is diagnosed with cortical visual impairment. The most likely finding on pupillary examination is

    a. paradoxical pupillary response

    b. bilateral sluggishly reactive pupils

    c. unilateral relative afferent pupillary defect

    d. normal pupillary examination

Answers

1. **b.** Nasolacrimal duct obstruction most typically occurs at the most distal portion of the lacrimal duct, because of incomplete canalization, at or about full-term gestation (40 weeks), of what was a solid structure in the fetus. This occurs at the valve of Hasner. The canaliculi and puncta and the valve of Rosenmüller, which is in the region of the junction of the canaliculi, are more proximal and more likely to have canalized normally.

2. **d.** Whether unilateral or bilateral, the Harada-Ito procedure is the preferred surgical approach when the main subjective symptoms are those of torsional imbalance. In this operation, the anterior fibers of the distal portion of the superior oblique tendon are advanced toward the lateral rectus muscle, creating a tightening effect that compensates for the extorsion caused by the paralysis. Weakening an already paralytic superior oblique muscle would contribute to further torsional misalignment. Neither a superior rectus recession nor a fadenoperation (posterior fixation) would compensate by assisting intorsion.

3. **a.** The superior oblique muscles are accessory abductors, especially inferiorly. Alignment that is relatively more divergent or less convergent in downgaze compared to upgaze defines an A pattern. The inferior oblique muscles are abductors in the superior gaze position, and this action tends to generate a V pattern. The vertical rectus muscles are accessory adductors in their respective fields of action but are considered to play a minor role in the etiology of A and V patterns.

4. **b.** Since A and V patterns are variations of a primary position horizontal misalignment, there is no reason for a compensatory head position unless it allows single binocular vision. For a patient with A-pattern exotropia, single binocular vision, if achievable, is attained only with the eyes directed upward; hence, a chin-down head position is most likely. Head tilting or viewing in lateral gaze does not achieve this result.

5. **a.** Slight limitation of adduction is present in several cases of type 1 Duane syndrome if looked for carefully. Abduction deficiency is a feature of Duane syndrome types 1 and 3, as well as of sixth cranial nerve paralysis; in type 3 Duane syndrome, the limited adduction is also obvious. An anomalous head posture is common in all of these entities.

6. **c.** These signs are highly indicative of malignant hyperthermia. Cooling procedures do not take priority in time. Releasing tension on muscles is a measure against induced *bradycardia*, not tachycardia, and the latter is aggravated by atropine.

7. **d.** Limited adduction in this case is evidence that the medial rectus has reattached too far posteriorly to be effective as an adductor of the eye. Anterior segment ischemia does not typically limit rotation and would not be expected after operation on just one extraocular muscle. Adherence syndrome causing restriction would arise from adherence created on the opposite aspect of the globe, and the lateral rectus was not included in the procedure. Conjunctival scarring over the medial rectus muscle would, if anything, limit abduction.

8. **d.** Dissociated vertical deviation is a frequent accompaniment, concurrently or consecutively, to infantile (congenital) esotropia. The condition is usually bilateral unless 1 eye has deeply reduced vision. Superior oblique muscle paralysis with fixation by the uninvolved eye, and orbital fat adherence syndrome with fixation by the involved eye, could cause a similar picture, but the deviation would tend to be constant rather than intermittent, and these disorders and consecutive hypertropia are not expected with the frequency of dissociated deviation.

9. **a.** More so than exposure or the consequences for ocular motility, optic nerve compression is a serious complication of thyroid eye disease. Direct clinical evidence of optic nerve function compromise, as indicated by pupillary and color vision abnormalities, is more sensitive than an imaging study.

10. **a.** The lacrimal sac lies just nasal to and mostly below the medial canthus. A dacryocele presents at that location. Swelling more laterally in the lower eyelid does not suggest involvement of lacrimal structures. Swelling above the medial canthus raises the suspicion of herniation of intracranial contents (eg, encephalocele) through crevices in the cranial bones.

11. **b.** The crowding phenomenon can cause letters or symbols of a given size to become more difficult to recognize if they are closely surrounded by similar forms. It may reveal that the measured "linear" acuity of an amblyopic eye actually is several lines below that measured with isolated letters. For this reason, for the detection of amblyopia, it is best that isolated letters or pictures not be used to test visual acuity, if possible.

12. **c.** Children with moderate degrees of myopia will see clearly at near and would not be at risk to develop bilateral amblyopia. Children with moderate levels of hyperopia are capable of accommodating to provide themselves with clear vision at distance and at near. Significant levels of astigmatism can lead to isometric amblyopia.

13. **b.** The double Maddox rod test measures torsion. The red-glass test and the afterimage test can be used to determine the direction of the deviation. The Hess screen test is used to measure the magnitude of strabismus in different fields of gaze.

14. **d.** The heterophoria method calculates the AC/A ratio based on the deviation that is present at distance and near fixation. The gradient method uses the change in deviation produced by a change in the stimulus to accommodate at a given fixation distance. The near point of convergence and accommodation do not measure the AC/A ratio.

15. **a.** Some patients do not achieve adequate cycloplegia following instillation of drops. This is more likely to occur in patients with darker-colored eyes. In addition, larger degrees of hyperopia can sometimes be discovered once a patient has been wearing spectacles. Repeating the cycloplegic refraction may uncover more hyperopia, which can be corrected. If surgery is needed, the amount of surgery would target the esotropia with the glasses in place (nonaccommodative portion). Contact lenses would not provide any additional correction of the esotropia, and decreasing the hyperopic correction would make the crossing worse.

16. **c.** Most patients who eventually demonstrate a good result following bilateral lateral rectus recession for exotropia show a small to moderate initial overcorrection shortly after surgery. This overcorrection should be seen immediately after surgery and may persist for several days or weeks. Therefore, evaluation during this period would not allow the surgeon to properly assess the potential stability of the result. The initial overcorrection is generally gone a few weeks after surgery. Examining the patient 6–8 weeks after surgery would give the best evaluation of the success of the surgery.

17. **d.** Intermittent exotropia is the most common exodeviation. Congenital (infantile) exotropia and type 2 Duane syndrome are uncommon entities. Pseudoexotropia is the result of certain facial features or a structural abnormality of the retina and is not a true strabismus disorder.

18. **a.** The average corneal diameter at birth is 9.5–10.5 mm. The cornea reaches adult size by the age of 12 years, but most of the growth occurs in the first year of life—not the first 5 years. The cloudiness present at birth is due to the thickness of the cornea, not edema per se.

19. **b.** In a 1-month-old infant, episodes of strabismus are normal; preferential viewing reveals vision is 20/400; and horizontal movements are normal, but vertical movements are not normal until age 6 months. As stated in the text, intraocular pressure is not higher but lower.

20. **b.** Orbital size and shape variations in craniosynostoses predispose these patients to inferior oblique muscle overactions. The vertical misalignment in sensory esotropia is more likely to be a unilateral dissociated deviation. The superior oblique muscle dysfunction associated with overactive inferior oblique muscles is underaction. The upshoot in Duane syndrome is related to co-contraction of the horizontal rectus muscles, not to an abnormality of the inferior oblique muscle.

21. **d.** Anteriorly displaced ciliary processes are classic for PFV. Cataracts can occur but are not specific for PFV. The axial length is short in PFV. Iris hypoplasia is not a usual finding.

22. **b.** Patients with aniridia are at risk for developing Wilms tumor. Genetic testing can help determine whether periodic surveillance is needed.

23. **c.** Patients with sporadic aniridia are at highest risk for developing Wilms tumor. However, cases of Wilms tumor have been reported in patients with familial aniridia.

24. **a.** The most important initial treatment for a chemical injury of the eye is copious irrigation and meticulous removal of any particulate matter from the conjunctival fornices.

25. **a.** The intraocular inflammation associated with juvenile idiopathic arthritis (previously known as *juvenile rheumatoid arthritis*) is usually bilateral and nongranulomatous, with fine to medium-sized keratic precipitates. However, a minority of patients, especially African Americans, may have granulomatous precipitates. Inflammation of the posterior segment, resulting in a vitritis or retinal inflammation, is rare.

26. **d.** Neurofibromatosis type 1 shows autosomal dominant inheritance. However, almost 50% of cases are sporadic, presumably reflecting the high rate of mutation of the responsible gene.

27. **b.** As in other cases of ptosis, amblyopia may result from occlusion of the pupil or the development of anisometropia. Unlike congenital ptosis, the ptosis resulting from a plexiform neurofibroma may be progressive.

28. **c.** Sickle cell testing must be performed in all African-American hyphema patients. Sickle cell trait or disease may result in an elevated intraocular pressure even in the presence of a small hyphema.

29. **a.** Although epiblepharon may produce an in-turning of the eyelashes, there is often minimal or no irritation of the cornea. If no significant fluorescein staining of the cornea is detected, then only observation is required. The epiblepharon will usually spontaneously resolve with time and seldom requires surgical treatment.

30. **a.** Breaks in Descemet's membrane may be due to forceps injury at birth. Anisometropic astigmatism may result from this injury and produce amblyopia. Early treatment with optical correction of the anisometropia, sometimes also combined with patching of the normal eye, can improve the amblyopia. Keratoplasty usually is not considered as an initial treatment. The contralateral eye is not at increased risk for poor vision.

31. **b.** A normal and symmetrical corneal diameter suggests a forceps injury rather than congenital glaucoma. It is important to obtain a thorough history in order to establish the diagnosis. Acute hydrops is often symptomatic. This type of injury is too localized to suggest nonaccidental trauma.

32. **c.** The most likely risk factor for uveitis in patients with juvenile idiopathic arthritis is female gender. Oligoarthritis is defined as a persistent arthritis lasting more than 6 weeks and affecting 4 or fewer joints during the first 6 months of the disease.

33. **a.** The upper eyelid "follows" the eye in upgaze and downgaze; that is, the eyelid moves in the same direction as the eye. Therefore, the upper eyelid of a hypotropic eye will be lower than that of the fellow eye, producing the false appearance of ptosis. However, note that in the case of monocular elevation deficiency (double elevator palsy), the hypotropic eye may be associated with a true ptosis, pseudoptosis, or both.

34. **d.** The spatulated needle has the thinnest profile and is less likely to cut into or cut out of the sclera.

35. **b.** Small peripheral chorioretinal scars without surrounding retinal detachment are fairly common after surgery for strabismus. Retinal detachments (especially in children) and endophthalmitis are rare even in cases with known scleral perforation.

36. **d.** By having the patient move the eyes to the 6 cardinal positions, the clinician can isolate and evaluate the ability of each of the 6 extraocular muscles to move the eye.

37. **a.** Upward movement of the adducted eye is thought to be accomplished principally by the inferior oblique muscle, although this is somewhat debatable. The superior rectus is the principal elevator when the eye is abducted. The eye is elevated in primary position only in extremely severe cases.

38. **a.** In the development of anomalous retinal correspondence (ARC), the normal sensory development is replaced only gradually and not always completely. The more long-standing the deviation, the more deeply rooted the ARC may become. The period during which ARC may develop probably extends through the first decade of life.

39. **c.** Peripheral fusion without central fusion is the essential feature of this syndrome. There may be a small-angle strabismus (usually <8Δ; usually esotropia), which is noted on simultaneous prism and cover testing, but this is not an invariable feature of the syndrome. Most, but not all, cases will show a latent heterophoria, found on alternate cover testing, in excess of the manifest microtropia.

40. **b.** Botulinum toxin chemodenervation may be a useful treatment for small-angle horizontal strabismus. It is not effective in patients with chronic restrictive strabismus, vertical deviations, or pattern strabismus.

41. **d.** Botulinum toxin is very effective in the treatment of essential blepharospasm, although repeated injections are usually necessary. Adverse effects of treatment include ptosis and dry eyes. Botulinum may also be used to temporarily induce ptosis to promote healing in patients with corneal surface disease, but it is not a long-term treatment for this problem.

42. **a.** Infants who acquire chlamydial disease at birth may present with papillary conjunctivitis during the first week of life. Although the eye infection is usually self-limited, *Chlamydia* may cause pneumonia or gastrointestinal tract infections in neonates. Therefore, systemic treatment with oral erythromycin is indicated.

43. **c.** Vernal keratoconjunctivitis usually presents in older children with symptoms of photophobia and marked itching. A thick, ropy discharge may be present. In limbal vernal keratoconjunctivitis, patients develop gelatinous nodules at the limbus with white centers (Horner-Trantas dots).

44. **b.** Primary congenital glaucoma usually occurs sporadically, but it may be inherited as an autosomal recessive trait. Specific genetic mutations have been identified in some patients.

45. **a.** Patients with Sturge-Weber syndrome have vascular abnormalities that may involve the episcleral vessels. The mechanism of glaucoma is thought to be secondary to increased episcleral venous pressure. The presence of port-wine stains on the eyelids is associated with glaucoma.

46. **a.** Anterior polar cataracts are typically small (<3 mm) white opacities located centrally in the anterior lens capsule. They are not progressive and are not large enough to interfere with vision. However, there is an increased incidence of anisometropia in patients with anterior polar cataracts; refractions should therefore be monitored in these patients.

47. **c.** Of the choices presented, optic nerve hypoplasia is the most likely finding, though only in some patients. Pallor or swelling of the optic nerve should initiate further investigation, as it would in patients with these findings but without aniridia.

48. **d.** Patients with well-controlled intermittent exotropia generally have excellent stereopsis. When the deviation is manifest, they may experience diplopia. If the tropic phase occurs frequently, a young patient may develop suppression and not have diplopia. Later in the course of the disorder, a deviation that is manifest frequently may lead to a decrease in binocular function and some loss of stereopsis.

49. **a.** Structurally full optic discs resembling papilledema are commonly seen in hyperopic patients. Optic discs in myopic patients do not show this appearance. Neither misalignment of the eyes is associated with this finding.

50. **d.** Visual decrease solely from cortical abnormalities does not involve the pupillary pathways.

Index

(*f* = figure; *t* = table)

A-pattern deviations, 107–112, 109*f*
  definition of, 107
  esotropia, 107–112, 109*f*
    treatment of, 112
  exotropia, 107–112, 109*f*
    treatment of, 112
  in inferior oblique muscle paralysis, 122*t*
  pulley system pathology and, 23, 109–110, 110*f*
  surgical treatment of, 110–111, 111*f*, 112
AAO. *See* American Academy of Ophthalmology
AAP. *See* American Academy of Pediatrics
ABC/ABCR transporters. *See* ATP binding cassette
    (ABC/ABCR) transporters
Abducens nerve palsy. *See* Sixth nerve (abducens)
    paralysis
Abduction, 33
  extraocular muscles in
    inferior oblique, 15, 29, 29*t*, 32, 34*f*
    lateral rectus, 13, 17*t*, 29, 29*t*
    superior oblique, 15, 17*t*, 29, 29*t*, 32, 33*f*
  in Möbius syndrome, 140, 140*f*
  nystagmus and (dissociated nystagmus), 326
  in sixth nerve paralysis, 134, 134*f*
Aberrant nerve regeneration
  cranial nerve III (oculomotor), 132
  cranial nerve IV (trochlear nerve), in superior
    oblique myokymia, 142
Abrasions, corneal, 407
Abscesses, subperiosteal, in orbital cellulitis, 195, 196, 196*f*
Abuse, child, ocular trauma and, 404–407, 405*f*, 406*f*
AC. *See* Accommodative convergence
AC/A ratio. *See* Accommodative convergence/
    accommodation ratio
Accommodation
  development of, 170
  near reflex and, 37, 81
Accommodative convergence, 37. *See also*
    Accommodative convergence/accommodation ratio
  assessment of, 81
  in refractive accommodative esotropia, 93
Accommodative convergence/accommodation ratio, 37
  assessment of, 81–82
  high, 94–95
    in intermittent exotropia, 100–101
    management of, 82, 94–95
Accommodative esotropia, 93–95
  high accommodative convergence/accommodative
    (nonrefractive), 94–95
    management of, 82, 94–95
  infantile esotropia and, 91
  partially accommodative, 95
  refractive, 93
Acetazolamide, for glaucoma, 243
Achromatopsia, 291
  incomplete, 291

Acid, ocular injuries caused by, 407
Aciduria, methylmalonic, 398
Acoustic neuromas/neurofibromas, in
    neurofibromatosis type 2, 371
Acquired esotropia, nonaccommodative, 90*t*, 95–98
  basic, 95–96
Acquired strabismus, 11
ACR. *See* American College of Rheumatology
Acrocephaly, 383
Acrylic, for intraocular lenses, 259
Active force generation, 83
Active pulley hypothesis, 23
Acuity. *See* Visual acuity
Aculeiform cataract, 247*t*
Adalimumab, for uveitis, 278
Adduction, 33
  elevation deficiency in (double elevator palsy),
    123–124, 123*f*
  extraocular muscles in
    inferior rectus, 14, 17*t*, 29, 29*t*, 31, 32*f*
    medial rectus, 13, 17*t*, 29, 29*t*
    superior rectus, 14, 17*t*, 29, 29*t*, 31, 31*f*
  in Möbius syndrome, 140, 140*f*
  overdepression in, 115
  overelevation in, 114
Adenoma sebaceum, in tuberous sclerosis, 372, 372*f*
Adenomatous polyposis, familial (Gardner syndrome),
    retinal manifestations of, 352
Adenoviruses/adenoviral infection, 190–191
  epidemic keratoconjunctivitis, 191
  pharyngoconjunctival fever, 191
Adherence syndrome, after strabismus surgery, 158
Adie tonic pupil, 229
Adipose tissue, in orbit, 19, 20*f*
Adjustable sutures, 148–149
Adnexa. *See* Ocular adnexa
Adrenergic agents, for glaucoma, 243
Adrenoleukodystrophy, 398
Adult gangliosidosis (GM_1 gangliosidosis type III), 401*t*
Advancing (extraocular muscle insertion), 147
Afterimage test, in sensory adaptation testing, 58, 58*f*
Age/aging
  eye dimensions and, 167–168, 167*f*, 167*t*, 168*f*
  Lisch nodule prevalence and, 225
  refractive status affected by, 169, 169*f*
Agenesis, 171
Agonist muscles, 33
Ahmed implant, for glaucoma, 241
Aicardi syndrome, 292, 292*f*
AKC. *See* Atopic keratoconjunctivitis
Alagille syndrome, posterior embryotoxon in, 212
Albinism, 298–302, 299–300*t*, 301*f*
  in Chédiak-Higashi syndrome, 300*t*, 302
  in Hermansky-Pudlak syndrome, 300*t*, 302
  iris transillumination in, 231, 298, 301*f*

ocular, 298, 300*t*, 301
  X-linked (Nettleship-Falls), 298, 300*t*, 301
oculocutaneous, 298–301, 299*t*
tyrosinase activity and, 298, 299*t*
Alcohol (ethanol), maternal use/abuse of,
  malformations associated with, 394–395, 395*f*
Alexander's law, 317, 325
Alignment, ocular
  decreased vision and, 414
  tests of, 74–80
  unsatisfactory, after strabismus surgery, 155
Alkalis (alkaline solutions), ocular injuries caused by, 407
Alkylating agents, for uveitis, 278
Allen pictures, for visual acuity testing, 72*t*, 73
Allergic conjunctivitis, 198, 198*t*, 199*t*
Allergic reactions/allergies, 197–200
  atopic keratoconjunctivitis, 200
  conjunctivitis, 198, 198*t*, 199*t*
  to cycloplegics, 88
  drugs for, 198, 198*t*, 199*t*
  to suture materials, in strabismus surgery, 156, 157*f*
  vernal keratoconjunctivitis, 198–200, 199*f*
Allergic shiners, 198
Alpha (α)-interferon, for hemangiomas, 340
Alphagan. *See* Brimonidine
Alport syndrome, 302
Alternate cover test (prism and cover test), 74–75, 76*f*
  for intermittent exotropia evaluation, 100
Alternating fixation, 11
Alternating heterotropia, 74
Alternating nystagmus, periodic, 322
Alternating suppression, 51
Alveolar rhabdomyosarcoma, 335
Amaurosis, Leber congenital, 289–291, 290*f*
Amblyopia, 61–69
  abnormal visual experiences and, 46–48, 47*f*, 61–62
  ametropic, 64
  anisometropic, 63
    visual development affected by, 47–48, 61–62
  classification of, 62–64, 63*f*
  compliance with therapy and, 66–67, 68
  corneal transplantation and, 219
  in craniofacial syndromes, 390
  diagnosis of, 64–65, 65*f*
  history/presenting complaint in, 71
  iatrogenic, 67–68
  in infantile esotropia, 90
  meridional, 64
  in monofixation syndrome, 59
  occlusion, 64, 67–68
    eye trauma and, 403
  "organic," 64
  recurrence of, 69
  refractive errors and, 63, 64. *See also* Ametropic
    amblyopia; Anisometropic amblyopia
  in retinopathy of prematurity, 287
  screening for, 61
  stimulus deprivation, 64
    eye trauma and, 403
    visual development affected by, 46–47, 47*f*, 61–62

strabismic, 62–63, 63*f*
  visual development and, 48–49, 48*f*, 61–62
treatment of, 65–69
  cataract surgery and, 65–66, 255, 259
  complications of, 67–69
  occlusion/optical degradation and, 66–67
  refractive correction and, 66
  unresponsiveness to therapy and, 68–69
Amblyoscope testing, 58–59, 59*f*, 78, 80
American Academy of Ophthalmology
  on eye examination in diabetes, 297
  on fundus examination in premature infant, 285,
    286*t*
  on vision rehabilitation in nystagmus, 330
American Academy of Pediatrics
  on eye examination in diabetes, 297
  on eye examination in juvenile idiopathic (chronic/
    rheumatoid) arthritis, 270, 271*t*
  on fundus examination in premature infant, 285, 286*t*
American Association for Pediatric Ophthalmology and
  Strabismus, on fundus examination in premature
  infant, 285, 286*t*
American College of Rheumatology (ACR), chronic
  childhood arthritis nomenclature and, 267–268,
  269*t*
American Council of the Blind, 418*t*
American Foundation for the Blind, 417*t*
American Kidney Fund, 418*t*
American Printing House for the Blind, 417*t*
Ametropic amblyopia, 64
Aminocaproic acid/ε-aminocaproic acid, for hyphema,
  410
Amniocentesis, trauma from, corneal opacities and, 219
Amplitude, fusional, 41, 41*t*
ANA. *See* Antinuclear antibodies
Anesthesia (anesthetics)
  for extraocular muscle surgery, 160–162
  general, for extraocular muscle surgery, 161
  local (topical/regional)
    for extraocular muscle surgery, 160–161
    for foreign-body removal, 5
  malignant hyperthermia caused by, 161–162
  retrobulbar
    for extraocular muscle surgery, 160–161
    strabismus after, 143
Aneurysmal bone cyst, orbital involvement and, 343
Aneurysms, retinal, in diabetic retinopathy, 297
Angiofibromas, facial, in tuberous sclerosis, 372, 372*f*
Angiomas (angiomatosis)
  choroidal, 377, 377*f*
  racemose (Wyburn-Mason syndrome), 342, 364*t*,
    381, 381*f*
  retinal. *See* Retinal angiomatosis
Angle closure/angle-closure glaucoma
  with iris bombé, 239–240
    topiramate causing, 239
  persistent fetal vasculature (persistent hyperplastic
    primary vitreous) and, 280
Angle kappa, 77, 78*f*
  in retinopathy of prematurity, 287, 287*f*

Aniridia, 223–224, 224*f*
  cataract and, 251*f*
  glaucoma and (iris-induced angle closure), 238
  nystagmus and, 223
  Wilms tumor and, 224
Anisocoria, 229–230
  Adie tonic pupil and, 229
  in Horner syndrome, 230
  physiologic (simple/essential), 229
Anisometropic amblyopia, 63
  visual development affected by, 47–48, 61–62
Ankyloblepharon, 176, 176*f*
  filiforme adnatum, 176, 176*f*
Ankylosing spondylitis, juvenile, 271
Anomalous retinal correspondence, 39, 51*f*, 52–53, 53*f*
  harmonious, 55
  testing in, 52, 53–59
  unharmonious, 55
Antagonist muscles, 34
Anterior capsule, management of in cataract surgery,
  255, 256*f*
Anterior chamber, development of, 169–170
Anterior chamber angle, 236, 237*f*
Anterior chamber cleavage syndrome. *See* Anterior
  segment, dysgenesis of
Anterior ciliary arteries, 16–18
  anterior segment ischemia after strabismus surgery
    and, 158–159
Anterior megalophthalmos, 211
Anterior polar cataract (APC), 247, 247*t*, 248*f*, 250*t*
Anterior segment
  disorders of, 211–221
  dysgenesis of (anterior chamber cleavage syndrome),
    212–214, 213*f*
    glaucoma and, 238
  examination of
    in glaucoma, 236–237, 237*f*
    in penetrating trauma, 408, 408*f*
  ischemia of, after strabismus surgery, 158–159, 158*f*
  leukemic infiltration of, 354
Anterior segment developmental anomalies (ASDA).
  See Anterior segment, dysgenesis of
Anterior uveitis, 267, 267–272, 270*f*, 271*t*. *See also*
  Uveitis
  differential diagnosis of, 268*t*
  HLA association and, 269, 271
  in juvenile idiopathic (chronic/rheumatoid) arthritis,
    268–271, 270*f*, 271*t*
  laboratory tests for, 277*t*
  masquerade syndromes and, 276*t*
  sarcoidosis and, 271
  treatment of, 276–278
  tubulointerstitial nephritis and, 271–272
Anteriorization (extraocular muscle) and recession,
  148*t*
Antiacetylcholine receptor antibodies, in myasthenia
  gravis, 138
Antiangiogenic agents, for retinopathy of prematurity,
  281
Anti-elevation syndrome, 115, 153

Antifibrinolytic agents, for hyphema, 410
Antiglaucoma agents, 242–243
Antihistamines, for ocular allergies, 198, 198*t*, 199*t*
Antimetabolites, for uveitis, 277
Anti-MuSK protein antibodies, in myasthenia gravis,
  138
Antinuclear antibodies, in juvenile idiopathic (chronic/
  rheumatoid) arthritis, 269
APC. *See* Anterior polar cataract
Apert syndrome, 388, 389*f*, 391*f*
APH. *See* American Printing House for the Blind
Aphakia
  after cataract surgery, lensectomy technique and,
    255–256, 257*f*
  congenital, 260
  contact lenses for correction of, 259
  intraocular lenses for correction of, 258–259
  spectacle lenses for correction of, 258, 259
Aphakic glaucoma, 239–240
  cataract surgery and, 239, 260
Aphakic spectacles, 258, 259
Applanation tonometer/tonometry, 236
Apraclonidine
  for glaucoma, 243
  Horner syndrome diagnosis and, 230
Apraxia, ocular motor, 141–142
Aqueous drainage devices/shunts. *See* Glaucoma
  drainage devices
Arachnodactyly, in Marfan syndrome, 263
Arachnoidal gliomatosis, 368
ARC. *See* Anomalous retinal correspondence
Arc of contact, 28
Arteries, extraocular muscles supplied by, 16–18
  surgery and, 25
Arteriohepatic dysplasia (Alagille syndrome), posterior
  embryotoxon in, 212
Arteriovenous malformations, orbital, 342
Arthritis
  juvenile. *See* Juvenile idiopathic (chronic/rheumatoid)
    arthritis
  psoriatic, 269*t*, 270–271
Artificial tears, for Stevens-Johnson syndrome, 201
ASDA (anterior segment developmental anomalies). *See*
  Anterior segment, dysgenesis of
Ash-leaf spot (hypopigmented macule), in tuberous
  sclerosis, 372, 372*f*
Association (genetic), 171
Asthenopia
  corrective treatment of intermittent exotropia and,
    102
  strabismus surgery and, 145
Astigmatism
  amblyopia and, 63, 64, 178
  ptosis and, 178
Astrocytoma (astrocytic hamartoma)
  pilocytic. *See* Optic nerve (optic pathway/chiasm)
    glioma
  retinoblastoma differentiated from, 358
  in tuberous sclerosis, 372
AT. *See* Ataxia-telangiectasia

Ataxia-telangiectasia (Louis-Bar syndrome), 364t, 378–379, 379f
  ATM mutation in, 379
ATM gene, in ataxia telangiectasia, 379
Atopic keratoconjunctivitis, 200
ATP binding cassette (ABC/ABCR) transporters, in Stargardt disease, 293
Atropine
  for amblyopia, 67
  for cycloplegia/cycloplegic refraction, 5, 88, 88t
  side effects of, 88
Autoantibodies, in juvenile idiopathic (chronic/rheumatoid) arthritis, 269
Axenfeld anomaly/syndrome, 213. See also Axenfeld-Rieger syndrome
Axenfeld-Rieger syndrome, 213–214, 213f
  glaucoma associated with, 213, 214, 238
  posterior embryotoxon in, 212, 212f, 213
  pseudopolycoria in, 231, 231f
Axes
  of eye, 11–12
  of Fick, 27, 27f
  visual, 12, 14f, 39
    accommodative convergence and, 37
    muscle action/gaze position and, 30
Axial length, 167–168, 167f, 167t
  congenital glaucoma and, 238
Azathioprine, for uveitis, 277
Azopt. See Brinzolamide

Background diabetic retinopathy. See Diabetic retinopathy, nonproliferative
Bacteria, conjunctivitis caused by
  in children, 189–190, 190f
  in neonates, 187–188, 187f
Baerveldt implant, for glaucoma, 241
Bagolini glasses, in sensory adaptation testing, 56–57, 56f
Balloon dacryoplasty, for congenital nasolacrimal duct obstruction, 209, 209f
Band keratopathy
  in juvenile idiopathic (chronic/rheumatoid) arthritis, 270, 270f
  surgery for, 278
Bartonella henselae (Rochalimaea spp/bartonellosis), cat-scratch disease caused by, 190
  neuroretinitis and, 312
Base-out prism test, in sensory adaptation testing, 57–58, 57f
Basic (acquired) esotropia, 95–96
Bear tracks (grouped pigmentation of retina), 352
Behr optic atrophy, 311
Bell phenomenon, in ptosis evaluation, 179
Bergmeister papilla, 307
Bernheimer-Seitelberger disease (GM₂ gangliosidosis type III), 401t
Best disease (vitelliform macular dystrophy), 293–294, 294f
Bestrophin, mutations in, 294
Beta (β)-blockers, for glaucoma, 242

Beta (β)-hemolytic group A streptococci (Streptococcus pyogenes), orbital cellulitis caused by, 195
Betagan. See Levobunolol
Betaine, for homocystinuria, 399
Betaxolol, for glaucoma, 242
Betimol. See Timolol
Betoptic. See Betaxolol
Better Hearing Institute, 418t
Bielschowsky head-tilt test, 85–86, 85f
  in superior oblique muscle paralysis, 119
Bifixation, in monofixation syndrome, 57–58, 60
Bifocal lenses
  for consecutive esotropia, 103
  for high accommodative convergence/accommodative esotropia, 94, 95
Bilateral acoustic neuroma, in neurofibromatosis type 2, 363, 371
Bimatoprost, for glaucoma, 242–243
Binocular cells, in visual processing, 43f, 44
Binocular eye movements, 34–37. See also specific type
  conjugate (versions), 34, 35, 36f. See also specific type
    assessment of, 81
  disconjugate (vergences), 34, 35–37. See also specific type and Vergences
    assessment of, 86–87
    in infants, 413
Binocular vision
  abnormalities of, 49–50, 50f. See also specific type
    abnormal visual experience and, 46–49, 47f, 48f
    assessment of, 86–87
  physiology of, 39–42, 40f, 41t
  single
    Panum's area of, 40, 40f, 49
    testing field of, 83, 84f
Birth trauma
  corneal opacities and, 216t, 217
  nystagmus caused by, 318
Birth weight, retinopathy and, 281. See also Retinopathy, of prematurity
Blau syndrome (familial juvenile systemic granulomatosis), 274–275
Blepharitis, infectious, 193–194
Blepharophimosis/blepharophimosis syndrome, 178, 179f
Blepharoptosis. See Ptosis
Blepharospasm
  botulinum toxin for, 163–164
  in primary congenital glaucoma, 234
Blindness
  in bright light (day blindness/hemeralopia), in achromatopsia, 291
  in glaucoma, 243
  in inborn errors of metabolism, 401t
  in Norrie disease, 296
  in retinopathy of prematurity, 287
Blinking (blink reflex), in newborn, 413
Bloch-Sulzberger syndrome (incontinentia pigmenti), 364t, 379–381, 380f
Blowout fractures, of orbital floor, 124–126, 125f, 411
  vertical deviations and, 124–126, 125f

Blue-cone monochromacy, 291
Blunt trauma, 409–411, 410*f*, 411*f*
    abuse and, 404
    orbital fractures and, 124, 411, 411*f*
Bone
    brown tumor of, orbital involvement and, 343
    eosinophilic granuloma of, 337, 338*f*
Bone cyst, aneurysmal, orbital involvement and, 343
Bony tumors, of orbit, 342–343
Botryoid rhabdomyosarcoma, 335
Botulinum toxin, type A
    for blepharospasm, 163–164
    complications of use of, 164
    for consecutive esotropia, 103
    indications/techniques/results of, 163–164
    for infantile esotropia, 92
    pharmacology and mechanism of action of, 163
    for residual exotropia, 103
    for sixth nerve paralysis, 134–135
    for strabismus, 163–164
    strabismus caused by, 143
Bourneville disease (tuberous sclerosis), 364*t*, 371–374,
    372*f*, 373*f*
Bowman probe, 208
Brachycephaly, 383
Brachydactyly, in Saethre-Chotzen syndrome, 388, 390*f*
Brain lesions
    in Sturge-Weber syndrome, 376, 376*f*
    in tuberous sclerosis, 372, 373*f*
Branchial arch syndromes, 392–394
Brimonidine, 243
Brinzolamide, 242
Brodmann area 17 (striate cortex), 42
    development of, 44, 45*f*
        abnormal visual experience affecting, 46–49, 47*f*,
        48*f*
Brodmann area 18, 42
Brodmann area 19, 42
Brown syndrome, 122*t*, 130–132, 131*f*
    iatrogenic, tucking procedure causing, 120
    inferior oblique muscle paralysis compared with,
        122*f*, 122*t*
    surgery for, 131–132
Brown tumor of bone, orbital involvement and, 343
Brückner test, for strabismus and amblyopia, 77
Brushfield spots, 227
Bulbar (limbal) vernal keratoconjunctivitis, 199–200
Buphthalmos (megaloglobus)
    in glaucoma, 238
    in neurofibromatosis, 370
Burkitt lymphoma, of orbit, 337
Burns, accidental cigarette burns, 407

Café-au-lait spots
    in neurofibromatosis, 365
    in von Hippel–Lindau disease, 374
CAIs. *See* Carbonic anhydrase inhibitors
Calvarium, 383, 384*f*
    suture fusion and, 386
Canaliculi, lacrimal, atresia/stenosis of, 203

Canthal index, Farcas, 173
Capillary hemangioma. *See* Hemangiomas
Capillary malformations, orbital, 342
Capsulectomy/vitrectomy, for cataract
    lensectomy with intraocular lens implantation and,
        258
    lensectomy without intraocular lens implantation
        and, 256, 257*f*
Capsulorrhexis, 255, 256*f*
Carbonic anhydrase inhibitors, for glaucoma, 242, 243
Cardiff Acuity Test, 73
Cardinal positions of gaze, 28, 28*f*, 80
    extraocular muscle action and, 30–32, 30*f*, 31*f*, 32*f*,
        33*f*, 34*f*
    yoke muscles and, 28*f*, 35, 80
Carrier (genetic), inborn errors of metabolism and, 397
Carteolol, for glaucoma, 242
Cat-scratch disease
    neuroretinitis and, 312
    Parinaud oculoglandular syndrome and, 190
Cataract, 245–260
    abuse and, 404
    age at onset and, 245–246
    amblyopia and, 64, 65–66
    anterior polar, 247, 247*t*, 248*f*, 250*t*
    bilateral, 246*t*
    cerulean, 247*t*
    congenital and infantile, 245
        amblyopia and, 64, 65–66, 246
        hereditary factors in, 247*t*
    in cytomegalic inclusion disease, 184
    diabetic, 247*t*, 297
    etiology of, 245, 246*t*
    evaluation of, 250–251, 253*f*, 254*t*
    hereditary factors in, 246, 247*t*
    in herpes simplex infection, 185
    history in, 251
    lamellar (zonular), 247*f*, 247*t*, 248, 248*f*, 250*t*
    laterality and, 246, 246*t*
    in Lowe syndrome, 247*t*, 302
    metabolic, 253–254, 253*f*, 254*t*, 398
    morphologic types of, 246–250, 246*t*, 248*f*, 249*f*, 251*f*
    in neurofibromatosis type 2, 371
    nuclear, 247–248, 248*f*, 250*t*
    ocular examination and, 252–253
    persistent fetal vasculature (persistent hyperplastic
        primary vitreous) and, 250, 250*t*, 252*f*, 279, 280
    polar, 247, 247*t*, 248*f*, 250*t*
    posterior lenticonus/lentiglobus and, 249, 249*f*, 250*t*
    posterior polar, 247*t*
    removal of. *See* Cataract surgery
    rubella, 183
    starfish, 251*f*
    steroid-induced, uveitis treatment and, 276
    subcapsular, posterior, 249, 250*t*
    surgery for, 254–260, 256*f*, 257*f*. *See also* Cataract
        surgery
    systemic implications of, 245, 246*t*, 253–254, 253*f*,
        254*t*
    traumatic, 251*f*

unilateral, 246t
visual function and, 252
workup for, 253–254, 253f, 254t
zonular (lamellar), 247f, 247t, 248, 248f, 250t
Cataract surgery, 254–260, 256f, 257f
amblyopia and, 65–66, 255, 259
aphakia correction and, 259
complications of, 260
glaucoma after, 239, 260
indications for, 254–255
intraocular lens implantation and, 257–258, 258–259
outcomes of, 260
after penetrating trauma, 409
in persistent fetal vasculature, 280
postoperative care and, 259–260
uveitis and, 278
Cavernous sinus thrombosis, orbital cellulitis and, 196
CCT. See Central corneal thickness of
Cellulitis
orbital, 195–197, 196f
fungal (mucormycosis), 197, 197f
after strabismus surgery, 156, 156f
preseptal, 194–195
after strabismus surgery, 156
CEMAS. See Committee for the Classification of Eye
Movement Abnormalities and Strabismus
Center of rotation, 27, 27f
Central corneal thickness, glaucoma and, 236
Central (pupillary) cysts, 227
Central fusion, 41
Central fusional disruption (horror fusionis), 49–50,
104–105
Central nervous system anomalies, midline, optic nerve
hypoplasia and, 308, 309
Central posterior keratoconus (posterior corneal
depression), 215
Central suppression, 50
Central vestibular instability nystagmus (periodic
alternating nystagmus), 322
Central vision loss, in leukemia, 298
CEP290 gene, in Leber congenital amaurosis, 290
Cerebellar hemangioblastoma, with retinal angiomatosis
(von Hippel–Lindau disease), 364t, 374–375, 375f
Cerebral visual impairment, 415–416
Ceroid-lipofuscinosis, 398, 401t
Cerulean cataract, 247t
Chalazion, 350–351
CHARGE association, 171, 306
CHED. See Congenital hereditary endothelial dystrophy
Chédiak-Higashi syndrome, 300t, 302
Chemical conjunctivitis, in neonates, 188
Chemical injury (burns), 407
Chemodenervation, for strabismus and blepharospasm,
163–164
Chemotherapy/chemoreduction, for retinoblastoma,
358–359, 360f
Cherry-red spot, 302–303
in gangliosidoses, 303, 401t
in inborn errors of metabolism, 400–401t
myoclonus and, 400t

Cherry-red spot myoclonus syndrome, 400t
Chiasm (optic), gliomas involving, in
neurofibromatosis, 367–369
Chickenpox. See Varicella
Children
abuse of
cataract and, 404
gonococcal conjunctivitis and, 189
ocular trauma and, 404–407, 405f, 406f
cataract surgery in, 254–260, 256f, 257f. See also
Cataract surgery
corneal transplantation in, 219
decreased/low vision in, 413–417, 417–418t
examination of, 3–5
preparation for, 3, 4f
rapport and, 3–5
eye development in, 167–171, 167f, 167t, 168f, 169f
abnormalities of, 171. See also specific type and
Congenital anomalies
intraocular lens implantation in, 257–258, 258–259
nystagmus in, 288–289, 289t, 317–330, 319t. See also
Nystagmus
ocular infection in, 181–197
ocular trauma in, 403–411
abuse and, 404–407, 405f, 406f
Chlamydia/Chlamydia trachomatis, conjunctivitis in
neonates caused by, 187–188
Chlorambucil, for uveitis, 278
Chloroma (granulocytic sarcoma), 337
Cholinesterase/acetylcholinesterase inhibitors, for
high accommodative convergence/accommodative
esotropia, 94, 95
Chondrosarcoma, of orbit, 336
Choriomeningitis, lymphocytic, 186
Chorioretinitis, in syphilis, 185
Choristomas, of orbit, 343
Choroid
dark, in Stargardt disease, 293
hemangiomas of, 354, 377, 377f
in leukemia, 354
in neurofibromatosis, 352, 366
nevus of, 352
osteoma of, 353
in Sturge-Weber syndrome, 377, 377f
tumors of, 352–355
Chronic progressive external ophthalmoplegia (CPEO),
137, 139t
CHRPE. See Congenital hypertrophy of retinal pigment
epithelium
CHSD. See Congenital hereditary stromal dystrophy
Cigarette burns of cornea, 407
Cigarette smoking, thyroid disease and, 135
Ciliary arteries, anterior, 16–18
anterior segment ischemia after strabismus surgery
and, 158–159
Ciliary body, neoplastic disorders of, 351–352
Clobetasol, for hemangiomas, 340
Clostridium botulinum, toxin derived from, 163
CMV. See Cytomegaloviruses
CNGA3 gene, in achromatopsia, 291

CNGB3 gene, in achromatopsia, 291
Coats disease, 287–288, 288*f*
   retinoblastoma differentiated from, 358
Cocaine, Horner syndrome diagnosis and, 230
Cogan twitch, 137
Collagenoma, in tuberous sclerosis, 372
Colobomas
   eyelid, 175, 176*f*
     in mandibulofacial dysostosis (Treacher Collins
      syndrome), 394
   Fuchs (tilted disc syndrome), 307, 307*f*
   in Goldenhar syndrome, 175, 393
   iris, 224–225, 225*f*
   lens, 260–261, 261*f*
   optic nerve/optic disc, 306, 306*f*, 415
Colobomatous cyst (microphthalmos with cyst), 345, 346*f*
Color vision defects
   achromatopsia, 291
   blue-cone monochromacy, 291
   in dominant optic atrophy, 310
Combined hamartoma, of retina and retinal pigment
   epithelium, 352
Comitance, spread of, in superior oblique muscle
   paralysis, 120
Comitant (concomitant) deviations, 10
   vertical, 113
     surgery for, 152
Committee for the Classification of Eye Movement
   Abnormalities and Strabismus, 317–318
Compliance with therapy, for amblyopia, 66–67, 68
Compound nevi, of conjunctiva, 349
Computed tomography (CT scan)
   in orbital tumor diagnosis, 334
   in retinoblastoma, 356, 356*f*
   in Sturge-Weber syndrome, 376
Concomitant deviations. *See* Comitant (concomitant)
   deviations
Cone–rod dystrophies/degenerations, Stargardt disease
   differentiated from, 293
Confusion (visual), 49, 50*f*
Congenital anomalies, 171. *See also specific type*
   of cornea, 211–216
   craniofacial malformations, 383–395
   of eyelid, 175–180
   glaucoma associated with, 238
Congenital aphakia, 260
Congenital bilateral mydriasis, 229
Congenital cataract, 245. *See also specific type and*
   Cataract, congenital and infantile
Congenital esotropia. *See* Infantile (congenital)
   esotropia
Congenital fibrosis syndrome, 127, 138–140
Congenital glaucoma (primary congenital glaucoma),
   233–238, 234*f*, 235*t*, 236*f*, 237*f*. *See also* Glaucoma
   corneal opacities and, 218, 234, 235*t*
   genetics of, 233
Congenital hereditary endothelial dystrophy, 216*t*, 217
Congenital hereditary stromal dystrophy, 216*t*, 219
Congenital hypertrophy of retinal pigment epithelium
   (CHRPE), 352, 353*f*

Congenital infection syndrome/TORCHES, 181
Congenital iris ectropion syndrome, 231
   glaucoma in neurofibromatosis and, 370
Congenital lacrimal fistula, 204
Congenital miosis (microcoria), 223, 228–229
Congenital mydriasis, 229
Congenital nevocellular nevi of skin, 349–350, 350*f*
Congenital night blindness, stationary, 291–292
Congenital nystagmus, 288–289, 289*t*, 321–323, 321*t*,
   323*f*, 324*f*
   latent (fusion maldevelopment), 322–323, 323*f*, 324*f*
     dissociated vertical deviation and, 116, 117, 323
   motor, 321
   periodic alternating, 322
   sensory, 322, 414
Congenital ocular motor apraxia, 141
Congenital rubella syndrome, 183–184, 183*f*
Congenital strabismus, 11
Congenital syphilis, 185–186, 221
Congenital tarsal kink, 176–177
Congenital tilted disc syndrome (Fuchs coloboma), 307,
   307*f*
Conjugate eye movements (versions), 34, 35, 36*f*. *See
   also specific type*
   assessment of, 81
   development of, 170
Conjunctiva
   cysts of, 348
     after strabismus surgery, 157, 157*f*
   hemorrhage of, in child abuse, 404
   laceration of, 409
   nevus of, 349, 349*f*
   scarring of, after strabismus surgery, 157, 157*f*
   telangiectasia of, in ataxia-telangiectasia, 378, 379*f*
Conjunctival inclusion cysts, 348
   after strabismus surgery, 157, 157*f*
Conjunctivitis, 188–193, 189*t*
   adenoviruses causing, 190–191
   allergic, seasonal, 198, 198*t*, 199*t*
   bacterial
     in children, 189–190, 190*f*
     in neonates, 187–188, 187*f*
   blepharitis and, 193–194
   chemical, 188
   chlamydial, 187–188
   gonococcal
     in children, 189
     in neonates, 187, 187*f*
   Haemophilus causing, 189
   herpes simplex virus causing
     in children, 191–192, 192*f*
     in neonates, 185, 188
   herpes zoster causing, 192–193, 193*f*
   in infants, 186–188, 187*f. See also* Ophthalmia
     neonatorum
   infectious, 188–193, 189*t*
   in infectious mononucleosis, 193
   ligneous, 351
   meningococcal, 189
   in molluscum contagiosum, 193, 194*f*

in neonates, 186–188, 187f. *See also* Ophthalmia neonatorum
in Parinaud oculoglandular syndrome, 189–190, 190f
in pharyngoconjunctival fever, 191
preseptal cellulitis caused by, 195
seasonal allergic, 198, 198t, 199t
in Stevens-Johnson syndrome, 201, 201f
after strabismus surgery, 156
streptococcal, 189
in trachoma, 190
trachoma-inclusion, in neonates, 187
varicella-zoster virus causing, 192–193, 193f
vernal, 198–200, 199f
viral, 190–193
Connective tissue tumors, of orbit, 343
Consecutive (surgical) esodeviation, 97–98
management of, 103
Consecutive exotropia, 105
Constant exotropia, 103–104
Contact, arc of, 28
Contact lenses, for aphakia, 259
Continuous-tear curvilinear capsulorrhexis, 255, 256f
Contour interaction (crowding phenomenon), 62, 65, 65f
Contour interaction (crowding) bars, for amblyopia evaluation, 65, 65f, 73
Contour stereopsis tests, 87
Convergence, 35
    accommodative, 37
        assessment of, 81
        in refractive accommodative esotropia, 93
    assessment of, 81–82
    development of, 170
    fusional, 37, 41, 41t, 82
    near point of, 81
    near reflex and, 37, 81
    proximal (instrument), 37
    tonic, 36
    voluntary, 37
Convergence insufficiency, 106
    intermittent exotropia and, 101
Convergence paralysis, exotropia and, 106
Convergence-retraction nystagmus (induced convergence-retraction), 325
Convergence tone, 36
Convergent strabismus, 9
Copper, corneal deposition of, 221
Coppock-like cataract, 247
Corectopia, 230
Cornea
    abrasions of, 407
    congenital/developmental anomalies of, 211–216
        central, 214–216, 215f
        peripheral, 212–214, 213f
        of size and shape, 211–212, 212f
    curvature of, 167t, 168, 168f
    development of, 167t, 168, 168f
    diameter of, 167f, 168
        abnormalities of, 211–212, 212f
        glaucoma and, 234, 234f

disorders of, 211–221
    metabolic disorders and, 400–401t
edema of, in glaucoma, 234, 235t
enlargement of
    in glaucoma, 234, 234f, 235t
    in neurofibromatosis, 370
examination of, in glaucoma, 235, 236f
exposure of, in craniosynostosis-induced proptosis, 388–389
foreign body in, 407–408
lacerations of, 408
opacification of, 216–219, 216t, 218f
perforation of, 408
posterior depression of (central posterior keratoconus), 215
shape of, disorders of, 211–212, 212f
size of, disorders of, 211–212
systemic diseases affecting, 220–221, 220f
thickness/rigidity of, glaucoma and, 236
transplantation of, 219
Corneal dystrophies. *See* Endothelial dystrophies; Stromal corneal dystrophies
Corneal light reflex
    eyelid margin distance to (margin-reflex distance), in ptosis, 179
    tests of, 76–78, 77f, 78f
Corneal ulcers
    corneal opacities and, 219
    in vernal keratoconjunctivitis, 200
Corneoscleral laceration, repair of, 408
Correspondence. *See* Retinal correspondence
Cortex, occipital/visual. *See* Occipital (primary visual/calcarine/striate) cortex
Cortical visual impairment, 415–416
Corticosteroids (steroids)
    after cataract surgery, 259
    for hemangiomas, 340
    for hyphema, 410
    for ocular allergies/inflammation, 198, 199t
    for Stevens-Johnson syndrome, 201
    for toxocariasis, 274
    for uveitis, 276–277
Cosopt, for glaucoma, 242
Cottage cheese pattern, in treated retinoblastoma, 360
Cover tests, 74–76, 75f, 76f
    ARC testing and, 53
    for intermittent exotropia evaluation, 100
Cover-uncover test, 74, 75f
CPEO. *See* Chronic progressive external ophthalmoplegia
Cranial dysinnervation disorders, congenital, 127, 139
Cranial nerve III (oculomotor nerve)
    aberrant regeneration of, 132
    extraocular muscles innervated by, 13
Cranial nerve IV (trochlear nerve)
    aberrant regeneration of, superior oblique myokymia and, 142
    extraocular muscles innervated by, 13
Cranial nerve VI (abducens nerve), extraocular muscles innervated by, 13

Cranial nerves, ocular motor, 13
  extraocular muscle surgery and, 24
Cranial sutures
  normal, 384*f*, 385*f*
  premature closure of in craniosynostosis, 383, 385*f*
Craniofacial malformations, 383–395. *See also specific type*
  Apert syndrome, 388, 389*f*, 391*f*
  branchial arch syndromes, 392–394
  craniosynostosis, 383–387, 385*f*, 386*f*
  craniosynostosis syndromes, 387–388, 387*f*, 389*f*, 390*f*
  Crouzon syndrome, 387–388, 387*f*
  in fetal alcohol syndrome, 394–395, 395*f*
  Goldenhar syndrome, 393, 393*f*
  infantile exotropia and, 104
  management of, 392
  mandibulofacial dysostosis, 393–394, 394*f*
  nonsynostotic, 392–395, 393*f*, 394*f*, 395*f*
  ocular complications of, 388–392, 391*f*
  oculoauriculovertebral (OAV) spectrum, 392–393
  Pfeiffer syndrome, 388
  Pierre Robin sequence (anomaly/deformity), 394
  Saethre-Chotzen syndrome, 388, 390*f*
  Treacher Collins syndrome, 393–394, 394*f*
  V-pattern deviations associated with, 110
Craniopharyngiomas, nystagmus caused by, 325
Craniosynostosis, 383–387, 385*f*, 386*f*
  etiology of, 386–387
  ocular complications of, 388–392, 391*f*
  pulley system pathology and, 23
  syndromes associated with, 386–387, 387–388, 387*f*, 389*f*, 390*f*
CRB1 gene, in Leber congenital amaurosis, 290
Credé (silver nitrate) prophylaxis, 188
  chemical conjunctivitis caused by, 188
Cross-fixation, in infantile esotropia, 90
Crossed diplopia, 54, 54*f*
Crouzon syndrome, 387–388, 387*f*
Crowding (contour interaction) bars, for amblyopia evaluation, 65, 65*f*, 73
Crowding phenomenon (contour interaction), 62, 65, 65*f*
CRYO-ROP (Cryotherapy for Retinopathy of Prematurity) study, 282, 283, 285–286, 286*f*
Cryotherapy
  for retinal angiomas/hemangiomas, 375
  for retinopathy of prematurity, 285–286, 286*f*
Cryotherapy for Retinopathy of Prematurity (CRYO-ROP) Study, 282, 283, 285–286, 286*f*
Cryptophthalmos, 175, 175*f*
CSM method, for visual acuity assessment, 72
CSNB. *See* Congenital night blindness, stationary
Cup–disc ratio
  in glaucoma evaluation, 237
  in megalopapilla, 307
Cupping of optic disc
  glaucomatous, 235*t*, 237, 237*f*
  in megalopapilla, 307
Curvature, corneal, 167*t*, 168, 168*f*

Cyclic esotropia, 96
Cycloablation/cyclophotocoagulation, for glaucoma, 241, 241*f*
  endoscopic, 241, 242*f*
Cyclocryotherapy, for glaucoma, 241
Cyclodeviations, double Maddox rod test for evaluation of, 79, 79*f*
Cyclopentolate, for cycloplegia/cycloplegic refraction, 87–88, 88*t*
  in premature infant, 285
Cyclophosphamide, for uveitis, 278
Cyclophotocoagulation. *See* Cycloablation/cyclophotocoagulation
Cycloplegia/cycloplegics
  for amblyopia, 67
  for hyphema, 410
  refraction with. *See* Cycloplegic refraction
  side effects of, 88
Cycloplegic refraction, 87–88, 88*t*
  instilling eyedrops for, 5
Cyclosporine/cyclosporine A, for uveitis, 277–278
Cyclovertical muscle palsies, 3-step test in, 83–86, 85*f*
Cyclovertical strabismus, surgery planning and, 146
CYP1B1 gene, in glaucoma, 233
Cystathionine β-synthase, abnormality of in homocystinuria, 263, 399
Cysteamine, for cystinosis, 220, 399
Cystic Fibrosis Foundation, 418*t*
Cystinosis, 220, 398, 399, 401*t*
  corneal changes in, 220, 220*f*, 401*t*
Cytomegalic inclusion disease, 184–185, 184*f*

Daclizumab, for uveitis, 278
Dacryocele/dacryocystocele, 204–205, 204*f*, 205*f*
Dacryocystitis, dacryocele progressing to, 205
Dacryocystorhinostomy, for congenital nasolacrimal duct obstruction, 210
Dacryoplasty, balloon, for congenital nasolacrimal duct obstruction, 209, 209*f*
Dark choroid, in Stargardt disease, 293
Day blindness (hemeralopia), in achromatopsia, 291
de Morsier syndrome (septo-optic dysplasia), 308
Decreased vision. *See* Low vision; Visual loss/impairment
Degradation, optical, for amblyopia, 67
Delivery (birth), difficult
  corneal opacities and, 216*t*, 217
  nystagmus and, 318
Dellen, after strabismus surgery, 158, 158*f*
Denervation
  with botulinum toxin, 163–164
  and extirpation, 148*t*
Deorsumduction/deorsumversion. *See* Depression of eye
Depression of eye (downgaze), 33, 35
  disorders of in blowout fractures, 125
  extraocular muscles controlling
    inferior rectus, 14, 17*t*, 29*t*
    superior oblique, 15, 17*t*, 29, 29*t*, 31, 33*f*
  3-step test in evaluation of, 83–86, 85*f*

Deprivation amblyopia, 64
  eye trauma and, 403
  visual development affected by, 46–47, 47f, 61–62
Depth perception
  stereoacuity testing of, 87
  stereopsis differentiated from, 42
Dermoids (dermoid cysts/tumors)
  corneal, 218, 218f
    infantile opacities and, 216t, 218, 218f
  epibulbar, 348
  Goldenhar syndrome and, 218, 349f, 393, 393f
  limbal, 218, 218f, 348
    Goldenhar syndrome and, 218, 349f, 393, 393f
  orbital, 343–344, 344f
Dermolipomas (lipodermoids), 348–349, 349f
  Goldenhar syndrome and, 349, 349f, 393, 393f
Derry disease (GM$_1$ gangliosidosis type II), 401t
Descemet's membrane/layer, injuries to, corneal
  opacities and, 216t, 217
Desmoid tumors, of orbit, 343
Deviations. See also specific type and Esodeviations;
  Exodeviations; Horizontal deviations; Strabismus;
  Vertical deviations
  comitant (concomitant), 10
    vertical, 113
      surgery for, 152
  extraocular muscle field of action and, 29
  incomitant (noncomitant), 10
    esodeviations, 90t, 98
    strabismus surgery planning and, 146
    vertical, 113
      strabismus surgery planning and, 146
  primary, 35
  secondary, 35
  skew
    in infants, 413
    inferior oblique muscle paralysis as form of, 121
  strabismic amblyopia and, 62
  strabismus classification and, 11
  terminology in description of, 9–11
Dextrocycloversion, 35
Dextroversion (right gaze), 35
DHD. See Dissociated horizontal deviation
Diabetes mellitus type 1 (insulin-dependent/juvenile-
  onset), 296–297
Diabetic retinopathy, 296–297
  nonproliferative (background), 297
Diagnostic positions of gaze, 80, 80f
Diamox. See Acetazolamide
DIDMOAD syndrome, 297
Diffuse neonatal hemangiomatosis, 340
Diktyoma (medulloepithelioma), 32
Diode laser, for cycloablation/cyclophotocoagulation, in
  glaucoma, 241
Dipivefrin, for glaucoma, 243
Diplopia, 39, 40, 40f, 49–50
  crossed, 54, 54f
  heteronymous, 54, 54f
  homonymous, 54, 54f
  Panum's area and, 40, 40f, 49

paradoxical, 52, 53f
  after strabismus surgery, 155
  testing for (red-glass test), 53–55, 54f
  third nerve paralysis/aberrant regeneration causing, 132
    surgery and, 133
  in thyroid eye disease, 135, 139t
  uncrossed, 54, 54t
Disconjugate eye movements (vergences), 34, 35–37. See
  also specific type
  assessment of, 86–87
  fusional, 41, 41t
  in infants, 413
  supranuclear control systems in, 37
Dislocated lens, 261–265, 261f, 262f, 262t, 264f. See also
  Ectopia lentis
  abuse and, 404
Dissimilar image tests, 78–79, 79f
Dissimilar target tests, 79–80
Dissociated horizontal deviation, 105–106, 105f, 117
Dissociated nystagmus, 326
Dissociated vertical deviation, 105, 105f, 116–118, 117f
  surgery for, 117, 153
Distance-near incomitance, strabismus surgery
  planning and, 146
Distance visual acuity, testing, 71–73, 72t
  nystagmus and, 73, 319
Distichiasis, 177, 177f
Divergence, 35
  fusional, 37, 41t, 82
    in refractive accommodative esotropia, 93
Divergence excess exotropia, 101
Divergence insufficiency/paralysis esodeviation, 97
Divergent strabismus, 9
DNA, mitochondrial, Leber hereditary optic neuropathy
  and, 311
Dolichocephaly, 383
Dominant optic atrophy, 310–311
Dorsal light reflex, dissociated vertical deviation and,
  116
Dorsal midbrain syndrome, nystagmus in, 325
Dorzolamide, for glaucoma, 242
Double elevator palsy (monocular elevation deficiency),
  123–124, 123f
Double Maddox rod testing, 79, 79f
  in superior oblique muscle paralysis, 118
Double-ring sign, in optic nerve hypoplasia, 308
Double vision. See Diplopia
Down syndrome
  Brushfield spots in, 227
  pseudopapilledema in, 314
Downbeat nystagmus, 325–326
Downgaze. See Depression of eye
Doxycycline, for chalazia and hordeola, 351
Drusen, 314–315, 315f
  giant, in tuberous sclerosis, 373
  optic disc/nerve, papilledema/pseudopapilledema
    and, 314–315, 315f
Duane/Duane retraction syndrome, 127–130, 128f
  esotropic, 128, 128f, 129
  exotropic, 105, 128, 128f, 129

Goldenhar syndrome and, 127, 393
  sixth nerve paralysis differentiated from, 134
Ductions, 33–34
  forced. *See* Forced ductions
DVD. *See* Dissociated vertical deviation
Dysautonomia, familial (Riley-Day syndrome), 221
Dyscoria, 223
Dysplasia, of bony orbit, 342
Dysraphia, 171
Dystopia canthorum, 175, 175*f*
Dystrophies
  corneal. *See* Endothelial dystrophies; Stromal corneal
    dystrophies
  vitreoretinal, Goldmann-Favre, 296

E-game, for visual acuity testing, 72*t*, 73
Early-onset (childhood) nystagmus, 288–289, 289*t*,
    317–330, 319*t*. *See also* Nystagmus
Early Treatment for Retinopathy of Prematurity
    (ETROP) study, 281, 283–285, 286
Eccentric fixation, 53, 63
  ARC testing and, 53
Ecchymoses, periorbital
  in child abuse, 404
  in neuroblastoma, 336, 336*f*
Echothiophate
  for glaucoma, 243
  for high accommodative convergence/
    accommodative esotropia, 94
ECP. *See* Endoscopic cyclophotocoagulation
Ectopia lentis, 261
  et pupillae, 229, 230, 262, 262*f*
  in homocystinuria, 263, 264*f*
  in Marfan syndrome, 263
  simple, 262
  in sulfite oxidase deficiency, 264
  treatment of, 264–265
  in Weill-Marchesani syndrome, 264
Ectopic lacrimal gland, 345
Ectopic tissue masses, orbital, 343–346
Ectropion
  congenital, 176
    iris, 231
      glaucoma in neurofibromatosis and, 370
  uveae, 231
Edrophonium, in myasthenia gravis diagnosis, 138,
    138*f*, 139*t*
Ehlers-Danlos syndrome, keratoglobus in, 211
Eighth nerve tumors, in neurofibromatosis type 2, 371
Electromyography, 32
  in myasthenia gravis, 138
Electronystagmography, in latent/latent manifest (fusion
    maldevelopment) nystagmus, 323, 324*f*
Electrophoresis, hemoglobin, in sickling disorders, 409
Electroretinogram
  in achromatopsia, 291
  in congenital stationary night blindness, 291
  in Leber congenital amaurosis, 290
  in low vision evaluation, 415
  in X-linked retinoschisis, 295

Elevated intraocular pressure
  in glaucoma, 234, 235, 236, 243–244
  in hyphema, 409, 410
Elevation of eye (upgaze), 33, 35
  in Brown syndrome, 130, 131, 131*f*
  disorders of, in blowout fractures, 125
  extraocular muscles controlling
    inferior oblique, 15, 17*t*, 29, 29*t*, 32, 34*f*
    superior rectus, 14, 17*t*, 29*t*, 31, 31*f*
    3-step test in evaluation of, 83–86, 85*f*
  in inferior oblique muscle paralysis, 122
  monocular deficiency of (double elevator palsy),
    123–124, 123*f*
Embryonal rhabdomyosarcoma, 335
Embryotoxon, posterior, 212, 212*f*
  in Axenfeld-Rieger syndrome, 212, 212*f*, 213
Emmetropization, 169
Empirical horopter, 39–40, 40*f*
Encephaloceles, of orbit, 346
Encephalofacial/encephalotrigeminal angiomatosis
    (Sturge-Weber syndrome), 342, 364*t*, 375–378, 376*f*,
    377*f*
  glaucoma associated with, 238, 377, 378
  port-wine stain in, 238, 342, 375, 376, 376*f*
Enchondromas, in Maffucci syndrome, 340
Endophthalmitis, postoperative, after strabismus
    surgery, 156
Endoscopic cyclophotocoagulation, for glaucoma, 241,
    242*f*
Endothelial dystrophies, congenital hereditary,
    216*t*, 217
Enophthalmos, in blowout fractures, 126
Enthesitis, in juvenile idiopathic (chronic/rheumatoid)
    arthritis, 269*t*, 271
Entropion, congenital, 176
Enucleation, for retinoblastoma, 358
Enzyme defects, disorders associated with, 397, 398,
    400–401*t*
  management of, 399–402
Eosinophilic granuloma of bone, orbital, 337, 338*f*
Epiblepharon, 176
Epibulbar tumors, 333*t*, 347–351
  dermoids, 348
    Goldenhar syndrome and, 218, 349*f*, 393, 393*f*
Epicanthus, 177–178, 178*f*
  inversus, 177
    in blepharophimosis syndrome, 178, 179*f*
  palpebralis, 177, 178*f*
  supraciliaris, 177
  tarsalis, 177, 178*f*
Epidemic keratoconjunctivitis, 191
  preseptal cellulitis caused by, 195
Epidermoid cysts, of orbit, 343
Epilepsy Information Line, 418*t*
Epinephrine, for glaucoma, 243
Epiphora. *See* Tearing/epiphora
Episcleritis, nodular, 351
Epithelial inclusion cysts, conjunctival, 348
  after strabismus surgery, 157, 157*f*
Epstein-Barr virus infection, 193

Erythema multiforme, major (Stevens-Johnson syndrome), 200–201, 201f
Erythromycin
    for chlamydial conjunctivitis in neonates, 188
    for ophthalmia neonatorum prophylaxis, 188
Eso- (prefix), 9
Esodeviations, 89–98, 90t. *See also specific type and Esotropia*
    divergence insufficiency/paralysis, 97
    incomitant, 90t, 98
    medial rectus muscle restriction causing, 98
    negative angle kappa and, 77, 78f
    sensory deprivation, 96–97
    sixth nerve (abducens) paralysis causing, 98
    strabismic amblyopia and, 62
    surgery for, 150–151, 150t
Esophoria, 89
Esotropia, 89
    A-pattern, 107–112, 109f
        treatment of, 112
    accommodative, 90t, 93–95
    acute, 96
    basic (acquired), 95–96
    cyclic, 96
    divergence insufficiency/paralysis, 97
    in Duane syndrome, 128, 128f, 129
    exotropia following surgery for (consecutive exotropia), 105
    false appearance of (pseudoesotropia), 89, 90t
    with high myopia, 141
    incomitant, 90t, 98
    infantile (congenital), 89–92, 90t, 91f
    intermittent, 89
    management of, 103
    medial rectus muscle restriction causing, 98
    in Möbius syndrome, 140
    nonaccommodative acquired, 90t, 95–98
    with nystagmus, 90t, 92, 321
    red-glass (diplopia) testing and, 54
    sensory deprivation, 96–97
    sixth nerve (abducens) paralysis causing, 98, 134, 134f
    spasm of near synkinetic reflex and, 97
    surgical (consecutive), 97–98
        management of, 103
    V-pattern, 107–112, 108f
        treatment of, 112
Etanercept, for uveitis, 278
ETROP (Early Treatment for Retinopathy of Prematurity) study, 281, 283–285, 286
EULAR. *See* European League of Associations of Rheumatology
European League of Associations of Rheumatology (EULAR), chronic childhood arthritis nomenclature and, 267–268, 269t
Euryblepharon, 177
Ewing sarcoma, of orbit, 337
Examination, ophthalmic, 3–5
    for glaucoma, 234–238, 236f, 237f
    for nystagmus, 318–320, 320t

for retinopathy of prematurity, 285, 286t
for Sturge-Weber syndrome, 377–378
Excyclo- (prefix), 10
Excycloduction. *See* Extorsion
Excyclotorsion, in superior oblique muscle paralysis, 119
Excyclovergence, 35–36
Exo (prefix), 9
Exodeviations, 99–106. *See also specific type and Exotropia*
    esodeviation following surgery for (surgical/consecutive esodeviation), 97–98
        management of, 103
    overcorrection in, value of, 103, 151
    positive angle kappa and, 77, 78f
    surgery for, 150–151, 150t
Exophoria, 99
Exorbitism, 173. *See also* Proptosis
Exotropia
    A-pattern, 107–112, 109f
        treatment of, 112
    consecutive, 105
    constant, 103–105
    convergence insufficiency and, 101, 106
    convergence paralysis and, 106
    in craniosynostosis, 390–391, 391f
    dissociated horizontal deviation and, 105–106, 105f
    in Duane syndrome, 105, 128, 128f, 129
    false appearance of (pseudoexotropia), 99
        in retinopathy of prematurity, 287, 287f
    infantile, 104, 104f
    intermittent, 99–103
    neuromuscular abnormalities causing, 105
    red-glass (diplopia) testing and, 54
    residual, management of, 103
    sensory, 104–105
    V-pattern, 107–112, 108f
        treatment of, 112
Exposure keratitis/keratopathy, in craniosynostosis-induced proptosis, 388–389
External-beam radiation, for retinoblastoma, 358
Extirpation and denervation, 148t
Extorsion (excycloduction), 10, 33
    extraocular muscles in
        inferior oblique, 15, 17t, 29t, 32, 34f
        inferior rectus, 14, 17t, 29, 29t, 31, 32f
Extorsional strabismus, 10
Extraocular muscle surgery, 145–162. *See also specific type or disorder*
    for A-pattern deviations, 110–111, 111f, 112
    acuity considerations and, 145–146
    adjustable sutures used in, 148–149
    anatomical considerations and, 23f, 24–25
    anesthesia for, 160–162
    complications of, 154–160
    for constant exotropia, 103
    cyclovertical strabismus and, 146–147
    for dissociated vertical deviation, 117, 153
    for Duane syndrome, 129

esodeviation after, 97–98
  management of, 103
for esodeviations and exodeviations, 150–151, 150*t*
exotropia after, 105
guidelines for, 149–154, 150*t*
for high accommodative convergence/
    accommodative esotropia, 94
for hypo- and hypertropia, 152–153
incisions for, 154
incomitance and, 146
indications for, 145
for infantile esotropia, 91–92
infections after, 156, 156*f*
for inferior oblique muscle paralysis, 122
for intermittent exotropia, 101–102, 102–103
for monocular elevation deficiency (double elevator
    palsy), 124
monocular recession-resection procedures, 150–151,
    150*t*
for nystagmus, 328–329, 328*f*, 329*t*
oblique muscle procedures and, 148*t*, 151–152
for partially accommodative esotropia, 95
planning, 145–147
posterior fixation in, 148*t*, 149
prior surgery and, 147
pull-over (stay) sutures used in, 149
rectus muscle procedures and, 152–154
for refractive accommodative esotropia, 93
for residual exotropia, 103
for sensory deprivation esodeviation, 96–97
for sixth nerve paralysis, 135
strengthening procedures in, 147–148, 152
for superior oblique muscle paralysis, 120–121
for superior oblique myokymia, 142–143
symmetric, 150, 150*t*
techniques for, 147–149, 148*t*
for third nerve (oculomotor) paralysis, 132–134
in thyroid eye disease, 135–136
transposition procedures in, 149, 153
for V-pattern deviations, 110–111, 111*f*, 112
weakening procedures in, 147, 148*t*, 151–152
Extraocular muscles, 13–25, 14*f*, 16*f*, 17*t*. *See also*
    specific muscle and Ocular motility
  actions of, 13–16, 17*t*, 28–32, 29*t*, 30*f*, 31*f*, 32*f*
    field of, 29
    gaze position and, 30–32, 30*f*, 31*f*, 32*f*, 33*f*, 34*f*
    primary/secondary/tertiary, 13, 28–29, 29*t*
  anatomy of, 13–25, 14*f*, 16*f*, 17*t*
    growth/development and, 170
    surgery and, 23*f*, 24–25
  approaches to in surgery, 154
  arc of contact of, 28
  blood supply/arterial system of, 16–18
    surgery and, 25
  development of, 170
  fascial relationships of, 19–24, 20*f*
  fiber types in, 18–19
  field of action of, 29
  innervation of, 13–16, 17*t*
    surgery and, 24
insertions of, 13–16, 17*t*
  advancing, as strengthening procedure, 147–148
lost, during surgery, 24, 159–160
  esodeviations and, 97–98
orbital relationships of, 19–24, 20*f*
origins of, 13–16, 17*t*
paralysis/paresis of
  in myasthenia gravis, 137, 139*t*
  3-step test in evaluation of, 83–86, 85*f*
physiology of, growth/development and, 170
slipped, surgery and, 24, 160, 160*f*
  esodeviations and, 97–98
structure of, 18–19
venous system of, 18
Exudative vitreoretinopathy, familial, 296
Eye
  axes of, 11–12
  axial length of, 167–168, 167*f*, 167*t*
    in congenital glaucoma, 238
  color of, age affecting, 169
  congenital anomalies of, 171. *See also specific type and*
      Congenital anomalies
    glaucoma associated with, 238
  depression of (downgaze). *See* Depression of eye
  development of, 167–171, 167*f*, 167*t*, 168*f*, 169*f*
    abnormalities of, 171. *See also specific type and*
        Congenital anomalies
  dimensions of, 167–168, 167*f*, 167*t*, 168*f*
  elevation of (upgaze). *See* Elevation of eye
  phthisical (phthisis bulbi), retinoblastoma regression
      and, 356
Eye movements, 32–37. *See also specific type*
  assessment of, 81–83
    convergence and, 81–82
    fusional vergence and, 82–83
    motor tests in, 83
    ocular rotations and, 81
    prism adaptation test in, 86
    3-step test in, 83–86, 85*f*
  binocular, 34–37
    conjugate (versions), 34, 35, 36*f*
      assessment of, 81
    disconjugate (vergences), 34, 35–37. *See also*
        Vergences
      assessment of, 86–87
      in infants, 413
  cortical/supranuclear pathways in control of, 37
  disorders of
    in ataxia-telangiectasia, 378
    history/presenting complaint in, 71
    in inborn errors of metabolism, 400–401*t*
    nystagmus/spontaneous, 320. *See also* Nystagmus
  growth/development and, 170
  monocular (ductions), 33–34
  motor units and, 32–33
Eyedrops (topical medications)
  administration of, 5
  for allergic eye disease, 198, 199*t*
  for glaucoma, 242–243
Eyeglasses. *See* Spectacle lenses (spectacles)

Eyelashes, accessory (distichiasis), 177
Eyelid droop. *See* Ptosis
Eyelid hygiene, for chalazia and hordeola, 351
Eyelids
  coloboma of, 175, 176*f*
    in Goldenhar syndrome, 175, 393
    in mandibulofacial dysostosis (Treacher Collins syndrome), 394
  congenital anomalies of, 175–180
  drooping. *See* Ptosis
  ectropion of, 176
  edema of
    in orbital cellulitis, 195, 196*f*
    in preseptal cellulitis, 194
  entropion of, 176
  fusion of (ankyloblepharon), 176, 176*f*
  infection/inflammation of, 350–351
  lacerations of, repair of, 409
  margin of, distance from corneal reflex and, in ptosis, 179
  in molluscum contagiosum, 193, 194*f*
  plexiform neurofibroma involving, 367, 367*f*
  strabismus surgery affecting position of, 159, 159*f*
  in Sturge-Weber syndrome, 376, 376*f*
  surgery/reconstruction of, for ptosis repair, 179
  tumors of, 333*t*, 347–351

Fabry disease, 399, 400*t*
  cataract and, 247*t*
Facial angiofibromas, in tuberous sclerosis, 372, 372*f*
Facultative suppression, 51
Fadenoperation (posterior fixation suture), 148*t*
  for dissociated vertical deviation, 153
False passage, probing of nasolacrimal duct obstruction and, 208
Familial adenomatous polyposis (Gardner syndrome), retinal manifestations of, 352
Familial dysautonomia (Riley-Day syndrome), 221
Familial exudative vitreoretinopathy, 296
Familial glaucoma iridogoniodysplasia, 213. *See also* Axenfeld-Rieger syndrome
Familial iridoplegia (congenital mydriasis), 229
Familial juvenile systemic granulomatosis (Blau syndrome), 274–275
Familial oculorenal syndromes, 302
Family history/familial factors. *See also under Genetic*
  in cataract, 253–254, 253*f*, 254*t*
  in nystagmus, 318, 319*t*
Family Support America, 417*t*
Fanconi syndrome, 220
Farcas canthal index, 173
Fascia bulbi. *See* Tenon capsule
Fascia lata, autogenous and banked, for frontalis suspension, 179
Fast twitch fibers, 18–19
Fat, orbital, 19, 20*f*
Fetal alcohol syndrome, craniofacial malformations and, 394–395, 395*f*
Fetal vasculature, persistent. *See* Persistent fetal vasculature
FEVR. *See* Familial exudative vitreoretinopathy

FGFR genes, 387
  in Apert syndrome, 388
  in Crouzon syndrome, 387
  in Pfeiffer syndrome, 388
Fibrillin defects, in Marfan syndrome, 263
Fibrin clots, after penetrating trauma, 408–409
Fibroblast growth factor receptor *(FGFR)* genes, 387
  in Apert syndrome, 388
  in Crouzon syndrome, 387
  in Pfeiffer syndrome, 388
Fibroma
  molluscum, 366
  ossifying, of orbit, 343
  in tuberous sclerosis, 372
Fibromatosis, juvenile, of orbit, 343
Fibroplasia, retrolental. *See* Retinopathy, of prematurity
Fibrosarcoma, of orbit, 336
Fibrosis, congenital, 138–140
Fibrous dysplasia, of orbit, 342
Fick, axes of, 27, 27*f*
Field of action, 29
Fine-needle aspiration biopsy (FNAB), of orbit, in rhabdomyosarcoma diagnosis, 335
Fish flesh pattern, in treated retinoblastoma, 360
Fissures, palpebral, 169
  congenital widening of (euryblepharon), 177
  slanting of, 178
    A- and V-pattern deviations and, 110, 110*f*
    in Treacher Collins syndrome, 178, 393–394, 394*f*
  surgery affecting, 24–25
  vertical height of, in ptosis, 179
Fistulas, lacrimal gland, congenital, 204
Fixation (visual)
  alternating, 11
  cataract and, 252
  distance acuity assessment and, 72, 72*t*
  eccentric, 53, 63
    ARC testing and, 53
  monocular, 11
  recruitment during, 33
  strabismus classification and, 11
Fixation duress, for orbital floor fracture, 126
FKHL7 gene. *See FOXC1 (FKHL7)* gene
Flame hemorrhages, in leukemia, 297
Fleurettes, in retinoblastoma, 358
Flexner-Wintersteiner rosettes, in retinoblastoma, 358
Fluorescein, for congenital nasolacrimal duct obstruction evaluation, 206
FNAB. *See* Fine-needle aspiration biopsy
Folate, supplementary, for homocystinuria management, 399
Foldable intraocular lenses, 257, 259
Forced ductions, 83
  in Brown syndrome, 122*t*, 130
  in sixth nerve paralysis, 134
  in thyroid eye disease, 135, 139*t*
Forceps injury, during delivery, corneal opacities and, 216*t*, 217

Foreign bodies, intraocular
anesthesia for removal of, 5
corneal, 407–408
uveitis differentiated from, 276t
Foreign-body granuloma, after strabismus surgery, 156, 156f
Fornix incision, for extraocular muscle surgery, 154
4Δ base-out prism test, in sensory adaptation testing, 57–58, 57f
Fourth nerve (trochlear) palsy, superior oblique muscle paralysis and, 118–121, 119f
Fovea
development of, 44–45
hypoplasia of, 292, 320, 415
Foveal retinoschisis, 294
FOXC1 (FKHL7) gene, in Axenfeld-Rieger syndrome, 214, 233
Fraser syndrome, 175
Freckle, iris, 351
Fresnel prisms
for consecutive esotropia, 103
for esotropia in sixth nerve paralysis, 98
for nystagmus, 326
Frontalis suspension, for ptosis correction, 179
Fuchs coloboma (tilted disc syndrome), 307, 307f
Fucosidosis, 400t
Fundus
albipunctatus, 292
evaluation of
in nystagmus, 320, 320t
in penetrating trauma, 408, 408f
in premature infants, 285, 286t
flavimaculatus (Stargardt disease/juvenile macular degeneration), 292–293, 293f
salt-and-pepper
in rubella, 183, 183f
in syphilis, 185
Fungal orbital infection, 197, 197f
Fusion, 41–42, 41t
peripheral, in monofixation syndrome, 60
strabismus classification and, 10
tenacious proximal, in intermittent exotropia, 100–101
Fusion maldevelopment nystagmus syndrome (latent nystagmus), 322–323, 323f, 324f
dissociated vertical deviation and, 116, 117, 323
Fusional amplitudes, 41, 41t
Fusional convergence, 37, 41, 41t, 82
Fusional divergence, 37, 41t, 82
in refractive accommodative esotropia, 93
Fusional vergence, 41, 41t, 82–83
assessment of, 82

Galactokinase deficiency, 398
Galactosemia, 398, 401t
Galactosialidoses, 401t
β-Galactosidase enzyme deficiency, in gangliosidoses, 303, 401t
Ganglion cells, retinal
development/differentiation of, 44
K system originating in, 44

M system originating in (parasol), 42, 43f
P system originating in (midget), 43, 43f
Gangliosidoses, 303–304, 401t
Gardner syndrome (familial adenomatous polyposis), retinal manifestations of, 352
Gaucher disease, 398, 400t
Gaze, positions of, 27–28, 80
assessment of, 80, 80f
cardinal, 28, 28f, 80
extraocular muscle action and, 30–32, 30f, 31f, 32f, 33f, 34f
yoke muscles and, 28f, 35, 80
diagnostic, 80, 80f
extraocular muscle action affected by, 30–32, 30f, 31f, 32f, 33f, 34f
midline, 80
nystagmus affected by, 317
primary, 13, 27, 80, 80f
secondary, 27
strabismus and, 80, 80f
tertiary, 28
variation of deviation with, 10
Gene therapy
for inborn errors of metabolism, 399–402
for Leber congenital amaurosis, 290
General anesthesia, for extraocular muscle surgery, 161
Generalized gangliosidosis (GM₁ gangliosidosis type I), 303, 401t
Genetic/hereditary factors. See also Inborn errors of metabolism
in cataract, 246, 247t
eye involvement and, 397
in glaucoma, 233
in retinoblastoma, 356–357, 357f
Genetic testing/counseling
in Leber congenital amaurosis, 290
in retinoblastoma, 356–357, 357f
Geniculate body/nucleus/ganglion, lateral, 42
development of, 44
abnormal visual experience affecting, 46
German measles. See Rubella
Gestational age, retinopathy and, 281. See also Retinopathy, of prematurity
Giant cells, Touton, in juvenile xanthogranuloma, 351
Giant drusen, in tuberous sclerosis, 373
Gigantism, regional, 367
Glasses. See Spectacle lenses (spectacles)
Glaucoma, 216t, 233–244
aniridia and, 238
anomalies associated with, 238
aphakic, 239–240
cataract surgery and, 239, 260
Axenfeld-Rieger syndrome and, 213, 214, 238
cataract surgery associated with, 239, 260
clinical features of, 234–238, 234f, 235t, 236f, 237f
corneal opacities and, 218, 234, 235t
corticosteroid-induced, uveitis treatment and, 276
diagnosis/differential diagnosis of, 235–238, 235t, 236f, 237f
examination in, 234–238, 236f, 237f
follow-up care and, 243–244

genetic/hereditary factors in, 233
in Leber congenital amaurosis, 290
juvenile open-angle, 234
lens-induced, 239
in leukemia, 354
in Lowe syndrome, 239, 302
medical therapy for, 242–243
natural history of, 238
in neurofibromatosis, 238, 367, 370
pathophysiology of, 234
persistent fetal vasculature (persistent hyperplastic
    primary vitreous and), 250, 280
Peters anomaly and, 238
primary
    congenital/infantile, 233–238, 234f, 235t, 236f, 237f
    juvenile, 234
prognosis for, 243–244
pseudophakic, 239
secondary, 238–240
    mechanical, 239
in Sturge-Weber syndrome, 238, 377, 378
surgery for, 240–242, 240f, 242f
    uveitis and, 278
systemic disease and, 238–239
tearing/epiphora in, 203, 234, 235t
traumatic hyphema and, 411
treatment of, 240–243, 240f, 242f
Glaucoma drainage devices
    strabismus and, 143
    in Sturge-Weber syndrome, 378
Glaucoma genes, 233
Glaucoma surgery, 240–242, 240f, 242f
GLC1A gene, in glaucoma, 233
GLC3B gene, in glaucoma, 233
GLC3C gene, in glaucoma, 233
Glial cell lesions, in neurofibromatosis, 366–367, 367f,
    368f
Gliomas, optic nerve/pathway/chiasm, 343, 367–369,
    368f
    in neurofibromatosis, 343, 367–369, 368f
    orbital involvement in, 343
Gliomatosis, arachnoidal, 368
Global layer, of extraocular muscle, 18
Globe displacement, in craniosynostosis, 389–390
GM₁ gangliosidosis type I (generalized), 303, 401t
GM₁ gangliosidosis type II (Derry disease), 401t
GM₁ gangliosidosis type III (adult), 401t
GM₂ gangliosidosis type I (Tay-Sachs disease), 303, 398,
    401t
GM₂ gangliosidosis type II (Sandhoff disease), 303, 401t
GM₂ gangliosidosis type III (Bernheimer-Seitelberger
    disease), 401t
GNAT2 gene, in achromatopsia, 291
Goldenhar syndrome, 393, 393f
    colobomas and, 175, 393
    dermoids/dermolipomas and, 218, 349, 349f, 393,
        393f
    Duane syndrome and, 127, 393
Goldmann applanation tonometry, 236
Goldmann-Favre vitreoretinal dystrophy, 296

Goldmann perimetry, in strabismus/amblyopia
    evaluation, 83
Gonioscopy, in glaucoma, 236–237, 237f
Goniotomy, for glaucoma, 240, 240f
    uveitic glaucoma and, 278
Gonococcus (Neisseria gonorrhoeae/gonorrhea),
    conjunctivitis caused by
    in children, 189
    in neonates, 187, 187f
Gradient method, for accommodative convergence/
    accommodation ratio measurement, 81
Granulocytic sarcoma (chloroma), 337
Granulomas
    eosinophilic, orbital, 337, 338f
    foreign-body, after strabismus surgery, 156, 156f
    pyogenic, 351
    in toxocariasis, 273, 273f
Granulomatosis, familial juvenile systemic (Blau
    syndrome), 274–275
Grating acuity, in strabismic amblyopia, 62
Graves eye disease/ophthalmopathy. See Thyroid eye
    disease
Group A β-hemolytic streptococci (Streptococcus
    pyogenes), orbital cellulitis caused by, 195
Grouped pigmentation of retina (bear tracks), 352
GUCY2D gene, in Leber congenital amaurosis, 290

H₁-receptor blockers, for ocular allergy, 198, 199t
Haab striae, 234, 235, 236f
Haemophilus/Haemophilus influenzae
    conjunctivitis caused by, 189
    preseptal cellulitis caused by, 195
Hagberg-Santavuori disease, 401t
Hamartomas
    astrocytic (astrocytomas)
        pilocytic. See Optic nerve (optic pathway/chiasm)
            glioma
        retinoblastoma differentiated from, 358
        in tuberous sclerosis, 372
    combined, of retina and retinal pigment epithelium,
        352
    in neurofibromatosis, 363
    in phakomatoses, 363
Hand-Schüller-Christian disease, orbital involvement
    in, 337
"Hang-back" recession, 147
    for dissociated vertical deviation, 153
Harada-Ito procedure, 121, 148
Harmonious anomalous retinal correspondence, 55
Head-tilt test, Bielschowsky, 85–86, 85f
    in superior oblique muscle paralysis, 119
"Heavy eye syndrome," 23
Hemangioblastomas
    cerebellar, with retinal angiomatosis (von Hippel–
        Lindau disease), 364t, 374–375, 375f
    retinal, 374
        retinoblastoma differentiated from, 358
Hemangiomas (hemangiomatosis)
    of choroid, 354, 377, 377f
    classification of, 339, 339f

definition of, 338
diffuse neonatal, 340
of orbit, 338–341, 339f
systemic disease associated with, 339–340, 339f
Hemangiopericytoma, of orbit, 342
Hemeralopia (day blindness), in achromatopsia, 291
Hemifacial microsomia, 392–393, 393f
Hemoglobin electrophoresis, in sickling disorders, 409
Hemorrhages. See also Hyphema
flame, in leukemia, 297
intracranial, in shaking injury, 404
retinal
in leukemia, 297
in shaking injury, 405, 405f, 406
salmon patch, syphilitic keratitis and, 221
subconjunctival, in child abuse, 404
vitreous, in shaking injury, 405, 407
Hepatolenticular degeneration (Wilson disease),
220–221, 398
cataracts associated with, 247t
Hereditary dystrophies
endothelial, 216t, 217
macular, 292–294
stromal, 216t, 219
vitreoretinal, 294–296
Hereditary optic neuropathy, Leber, 311
Hering's law of motor correspondence, 35, 36f
Hermansky-Pudlak syndrome, 300t, 302
Herpes simplex virus, 185
conjunctivitis caused by
in children, 191–192, 192f
in neonates, 185, 188
keratitis caused by, in newborn, 185
type 1, 185, 191
type 2, 185, 191–192
Herpes zoster, conjunctivitis and, 192–193, 193f
Hess screen test, 80
in superior oblique muscle paralysis, 119
Heterochromia (heterochromia iridis), 227–228, 228f,
228t
in leukemia, 354
Heteronymous diplopia, 54, 54f
Heterophoria method, for accommodative convergence/
accommodation ratio measurement, 81–82
Heterophorias/phorias, 9, 10
cover tests in assessment of, 74–76, 75f
strabismus classification and, 10
Heterotopy, of rectus pulleys, 23
Heterotropias/tropias, 9, 10
A- and V-pattern deviations and, 110
alternating, 74
cover tests in assessment of, 74–76, 75f
strabismic amblyopia and, 62
Hexosaminidase, deficiency of, in gangliosidoses, 303
High accommodative convergence/accommodation
ratio
accommodative (nonrefractive) esotropia and,
94–95
management of, 82, 94–95
intermittent exotropia and, 100–101

High (pathologic/degenerative) myopia
esotropia and, 141
in inborn errors of metabolism, 401t
Hirschberg test, 76–77, 77f
Histiocytosis X (Langerhans cell histiocytosis), orbital
involvement in, 332t, 337–338, 338f
History
in amblyopia, 71
in cataract, 251
in child abuse, 404
decreased vision and, 414
family. See also under Genetic
in cataract, 253–254, 253f, 254t
in nystagmus, 318, 319t
in nystagmus, 318, 319t
in strabismus, 71
HIV infection/AIDS, ocular infection/manifestations
and, 304
cytomegalovirus retinitis, 184
HLA. See Human leukocyte antigens
Holes, optic nerve, 310, 310f
Homatropine
for amblyopia, 67
for cycloplegia/cycloplegic refraction, 88, 88t
Homer Wright rosettes, in retinoblastoma, 358
Homocystinuria, 263–264, 398, 401t
ectopia lentis in, 263, 264f
treatment of, 399
Homonymous diplopia, 54, 54f
Hordeolum, 350–351
Horizontal deviations, 11
A-pattern and V-pattern, 107–112, 108f, 109f. See also
A-pattern deviations; V-pattern deviations
in craniosynostosis, 390–391, 391f
dissociated, 105–106, 105f, 117
in internuclear ophthalmoplegia, 141
strabismus surgery planning and, 146
Horizontal incomitance, strabismus surgery planning
and, 146
Horizontal rectus muscles, 13, 14f. See also Lateral
rectus muscles; Medial rectus muscles
A-pattern deviations associated with dysfunction of,
107–108
action of, 13, 28, 29t
gaze position and, 30, 30f
anatomy of, 13, 14f
surgery of
for A- and V-pattern deviations, 110, 111, 111f, 112
for nystagmus, 328, 329
for third nerve (oculomotor) paralysis, 133
V-pattern deviations associated with dysfunction of,
107–108
Horner syndrome, 230
in neuroblastoma, 230, 336, 336f
Horner-Trantas dots, in vernal keratoconjunctivitis, 200
Horopter, empirical, 39–40, 40f
Horror fusionis (central fusional disruption), 49–50,
104–105
HOTV test, 72t, 73
HPS1 gene, in Hermansky-Pudlak syndrome, 300t

HSV. *See* Herpes simplex virus
Human leukocyte antigens (HLA), in juvenile idiopathic (chronic/rheumatoid) arthritis, 269
Hunter syndrome, 400*t*
Hurler syndrome, 398*f*, 400*t*
  corneal opacities and, 217
Hutchinson triad, 185
Hyaloid artery/system, persistence/remnants of, 250, 252*f*, 279, 307. *See also* Persistent fetal vasculature
Hyper- (prefix), 10
Hyperopia, 169, 169*f*
  amblyopia and, 63, 64
  diabetic retinopathy and, 297
  high accommodative convergence/accommodative esotropia and, 94, 95
  intermittent exotropia and, 102
  refractive accommodative esotropia and, 93
Hyperplasia, 171
Hypersensitivity reactions
  to cycloplegics, 88
  ocular allergy and, 197–198
Hypertelorism, 173, 384
Hyperthermia, malignant, 161–162
Hypertropia, 113
  vertical rectus muscle surgery for, 152–153
Hyphema, 409–411, 410*f*
  abuse and, 404
  sickle cell disease and, 409
Hypo- (prefix), 10
Hypoesthesia, in infraorbital nerve distribution, in blowout fractures, 125
Hypoparathyroidism, cataracts associated with, 247*t*
Hypopigmented macule (ash-leaf spot), in tuberous sclerosis, 372, 372*f*
Hypoplasia, 171. *See also specific structure affected*
Hypotelorism, 173
Hypotony, cycloplegics causing, 88
Hypotropia, 113
  in monocular elevation deficiency (double elevator palsy), 123, 123*f*
  vertical rectus muscle surgery for, 152–153

I-cell disease, 400*t*
Iatrogenic amblyopia, 67–68
ICROP (International Classification of ROP), 282, 282*t*, 283*f*, 284*f*, 285*t*
Idiopathic intracranial hypertension (pseudotumor cerebri), 312–313
Idiopathic orbital inflammatory disease (orbital pseudotumor), 272, 346–347, 347*f*
IGF-I. *See* Insulin-like growth factor I
IIH. *See* Idiopathic intracranial hypertension
ILAR. *See* International League of Associations of Rheumatology
Illiterate E chart (E-game), for visual acuity testing, 72*t*, 73
Immunocompromised host, cytomegalovirus retinitis in, 184
Immunotherapy/immunosuppression, for uveitis, 277, 278

Implant surgery, for glaucoma, 241
Inborn errors of metabolism, 397–402, 400–401*t*
  enzyme defect in, 397, 398, 400–401*t*
  inheritance of, 397, 400–401*t*
  ocular findings in, 397–398, 398*f*, 400–401*t*
  treatment of, 399–402
Incisions, for extraocular muscle surgery, 154
Inclusion conjunctivitis, trachoma (TRIC), 187
Inclusion cysts, epithelial, conjunctival, 348
  after strabismus surgery, 157, 157*f*
Incomitant (noncomitant) deviations, 10
  esodeviations, 90*t*, 98
  strabismus surgery planning and, 146
  vertical, 113
    strabismus surgery planning and, 146
Incomplete achromatopsia, 291
Incontinentia pigmenti (Bloch-Sulzberger syndrome), 364*t*, 379–381, 380*f*
Incyclo- (prefix), 10
Incycloduction. *See* Intorsion
Incyclovergence, 35
Induced tropia test, 72–73
Infantile (congenital) esotropia, 89–92, 90*t*, 91*f*
Infantile exotropia, 104, 104*f*
Infantile glaucoma, 216*t*, 233–238, 234*f*, 235*t*, 236*f*, 237*f*. *See also* Glaucoma
  corneal opacities and, 218, 234, 235*t*
  genetics of, 233
Infantile nystagmus syndrome, 288–289, 289*t*, 321–323, 321*t*, 323*f*, 324*f*. *See also* Congenital nystagmus
Infantile strabismus, 11
Infants
  corneal transplantation in, 219
  decreased/low vision in, 413–417, 417–418*t*
  intraocular lens use in, 255, 258
  ocular infections in, 181–186. *See also specific type*
    conjunctivitis, 186–188, 187*f*. *See also* Ophthalmia neonatorum
  screening eye examinations in, 250–251
  shaking injury and, 404–407, 405*f*, 406*f*
  visually evoked cortical potentials in, 72*t*, 171, 413
Infection (ocular), 181–197
  conjunctivitis, 188–193, 189*t*
  intrauterine and perinatal, 181–186
  ophthalmia neonatorum, 186–188, 187*f*
  orbital and adnexal, 194–197, 196*f*
  after strabismus surgery, 156
Infectious mononucleosis, ocular involvement in, 193
Inferior oblique muscles, 14–15, 14*f*, 16*f*, 17*t*, 18*f*
  action of, 15, 17*t*, 29, 29*t*
    gaze position and, 32, 34*f*
    3-step test in evaluation of, 83–86, 85*f*
  anatomy of, 14–15, 14*f*, 16*f*, 17*t*, 18*f*
    surgery and, 24
  field of action of, 29
  overaction of, 113–115, 114*f*
    in infantile esotropia, 92
    V-pattern deviations associated with, 107, 108*f*
    vertical deviations caused by, 113, 113–115, 114*f*

paralysis of, 121–122, 122f, 122t
pulley system of, 22, 22f, 23
surgery of, 151–152, 152
    for dissociated vertical deviation, 117, 153
    for infantile esotropia, 92
    for superior oblique muscle paralysis, 120–121
    for V-pattern deviations, 110, 112
    for vertical deviations, 114–115
Inferior orbital vein, 18
Inferior rectus muscles, 14, 14f, 16f, 17t, 18f
    action of, 14, 17t, 29t
        gaze position and, 31, 32f
        3-step test in evaluation of, 83–86, 85f
    anatomy of, 14, 14f, 16f, 17t, 18f
        surgery and, 24
    injury of in orbital floor fractures, 125, 126
    surgery of
        for dissociated vertical deviation, 153
        eyelid position changes after, 159, 159f
        for monocular elevation deficiency (double
            elevator palsy), 124
        for nystagmus, 329
        for orbital floor fracture, 126
        for superior oblique muscle paralysis, 120, 121
        for V-pattern deviation, 111
Inferior turbinate, infracture of, for congenital
    nasolacrimal duct obstruction, 208–209
Inflammation (ocular), 350–351
    orbital, 272, 346–347, 347f
Infliximab, for uveitis, 278
Infracture of turbinates, for congenital nasolacrimal
    duct obstruction, 208–209
Infraduction. See Depression of eye
Infraorbital artery, extraocular muscles supplied
    by, 16
Infraorbital nerve, hypoesthesia in distribution of, in
    blowout fractures, 125
Instrument (proximal) convergence, 37
Insulin-dependent diabetes mellitus. See Diabetes
    mellitus type 1
Insulin-like growth factor I, in retinopathy of
    prematurity, 281
Interferon α, for hemangiomas, 340
Intergroup Rhabdomyosarcoma Study Group, 335
Intermediate uveitis, 267, 272, 273f. See also Uveitis
    differential diagnosis of, 268t
    laboratory tests for, 277t
Intermittent tropias, 10
    esotropia, 89
    exotropia, 99–103
Intermuscular septum, 22
    surgery and, 24
International Classification of Retinoblastoma, 358
International Classification of ROP (ICROP), 282, 282t,
    283f, 284f, 285t
International League of Associations of Rheumatology
    (ILAR), chronic childhood arthritis nomenclature
    and, 268, 269t
Internuclear ophthalmoplegia, 141
Interocular distance, abnormal, 173–175, 175f

Intorsion (incycloduction), 10, 29, 33
    extraocular muscles in
        superior oblique, 15, 17t, 29t, 31, 33f
        superior rectus, 14, 17t, 29, 29t, 31, 31f
Intorsional strabismus, 10
Intracranial hemorrhage, in shaking injury, 405
Intracranial hypertension (increased intracranial
        pressure)
    in craniosynostosis, optic nerve abnormalities and, 391
    idiopathic (pseudotumor cerebri), 312–313
    optic disc edema in. See Papilledema
Intraocular lenses (IOLs), 257–258, 258–259
    foldable, 257, 259
    secondary, 259
    visual outcomes and, 260
Intraocular pressure
    drugs for lowering. See Antiglaucoma agents
    in glaucoma, 234, 235, 236, 243–244
    measurement of, 236
    normal range for, 170, 236
    traumatic hyphema and, 409, 410
Intraocular tumors, 351–361
    choroidal and retinal pigment epithelial lesions,
        352–354, 353f
    iris and ciliary body lesions, 351–352, 352f
    leukemic infiltrates, 354
    retinoblastoma, 354–361. See also Retinoblastoma
Intrauterine ocular infection, 181–186. See also specific
        type
Intubation, lacrimal, for congenital lacrimal duct
    obstruction, 209–210
IO. See Inferior oblique muscles
IOLs. See Intraocular lenses
Iopidine. See Apraclonidine
IP. See Incontinentia pigmenti
IR. See Inferior rectus muscles
Iridodonesis, in dislocated lens, 261
Iridogoniodysgenesis anomaly and syndrome, 213, 213f.
        See also Axenfeld-Rieger syndrome
Iridogoniodysplasia, familial glaucoma, 213. See also
        Axenfeld-Rieger syndrome
Iridoplegia, familial (congenital mydriasis), 229
Iris
    abnormalities of, 223–231
        anisocoria and, 229–230
        nystagmus and, 223, 320
    absence of (aniridia), 223–224, 224f
        cataract and, 251f
        glaucoma and (iris-induced angle closure), 238
        nystagmus and, 223, 320
        Wilms tumor and, 224
    in Axenfeld-Rieger syndrome, 213, 214
    coloboma of, 224–225, 225f
    color of, in infants, 169
    cysts of
        primary, 226–227, 226f
        secondary, 227
    dyscoria and, 223
    ectropion of, 231
        glaucoma in neurofibromatosis and, 370

evaluation of, in glaucoma, 237
heterochromia of (heterochromia iridis), 227–228,
    228f, 228t
    in leukemia, 354
hypoplasia of, 213, 214. See also Axenfeld-Rieger
    syndrome
juvenile xanthogranuloma affecting, 226, 351, 352f
in leukemia, 351, 354
neoplastic disorders of, 351–352, 352f
nodules of. See Iris nodules
persistent pupillary membranes and, 228, 229f
pigment epithelium of. See Iris pigment epithelium
pigmentation of, development of, 169
posterior synechiae and, 231
pupillary abnormalities and, 228–231, 231f
stroma of, cysts of, 227
transillumination of, 231
    in albinism, 231, 298, 301f
Iris bombé, glaucoma and, 239–240
Iris freckle, 351
Iris hypoplasia, 213, 214. See also Axenfeld-Rieger
    syndrome
Iris mamillations, 226, 226f
Iris nevus, 351
Iris nodules, 225–226, 225f, 226f. See also Lisch nodules
    in neurofibromatosis, 225, 225f, 365–366, 366f
Iris pigment epithelium, cysts of, 226, 226f
    at pupillary border (central/pupillary cysts), 227
IRSG. See Intergroup Rhabdomyosarcoma Study Group

Jansky-Bielschowsky disease, 401t
Jaw-winking, Marcus Gunn, 180
Jerk nystagmus, 317, 318f, 321, 322–323, 324f, 325. See
    also Nystagmus
JIA. See Juvenile idiopathic (chronic/rheumatoid)
    arthritis
Junctional nevus, of conjunctiva, 349
Juvenile ankylosing spondylitis, 271
Juvenile chronic arthritis. See Juvenile idiopathic
    (chronic/rheumatoid) arthritis
Juvenile fibromatosis, of orbit, 343
Juvenile glaucoma, 234
Juvenile idiopathic (chronic/rheumatoid) arthritis,
    267–271, 269t, 271t
    criteria for, 267–268, 269t
    eye examination schedule for children with, 270, 271t
    nomenclature for, 267–268, 269t
    pauciarticular (oligoarticular/oligoarthritis), 269,
      269t
    polyarticular (polyarthritis), 269, 269t
    uveitis in, 268–271, 270f, 271t
Juvenile macular degeneration (Stargardt disease/
    fundus flavimaculatus), 292–293, 293f
Juvenile-onset diabetes mellitus. See Diabetes mellitus
    type 1
Juvenile-onset vitelliform macular dystrophy. See Best
    disease
Juvenile retinoschisis, 294–295, 295f
Juvenile rheumatoid arthritis. See Juvenile idiopathic
    (chronic/rheumatoid) arthritis

Juvenile systemic granulomatosis, familial (Blau
    syndrome), 274–275
Juvenile xanthogranuloma, 226, 351, 352f
    glaucoma associated with, 351
    of iris, 226, 351, 352f
    uveitis differentiated from, 276t

K system (koniocellular system), 42, 44
    development of, 44
Kasabach-Merritt syndrome, 339
Kawasaki disease (mucocutaneous lymph node
    syndrome), 201–202
Kayser-Fleischer ring, 221
Kearns-Sayre syndrome, 398
Keratitis
    exposure, in craniosynostosis-induced proptosis,
      388–389
    herpes simplex, 185
    interstitial, syphilitic, 186, 221
Keratoconjunctivitis
    atopic, 200
    epidemic, 191
      preseptal cellulitis caused by, 195
    phlyctenular, 351
    vernal, 198–200, 199f
Keratoconus, 212
    central posterior (posterior corneal depression),
      215
Keratoglobus, 211
Keratometry, values for, 168, 168f
Keratopathy
    band
      in juvenile idiopathic (chronic/rheumatoid)
        arthritis, 270, 270f
      surgery for, 278
    exposure, in craniosynostosis-induced proptosis,
      388–389
Keratoplasty, for corneal opacities, 219
Kestenbaum-Anderson procedure, 328–329, 329t
Kleeblattschädel, 383
Klippel-Trénaunay-Weber syndrome, 376
Knapp procedure
    inverse, for orbital floor fracture, 126
    for monocular elevation deficiency (double elevator
      palsy), 124
Koniocellular (K) system, 42, 44
    development of, 44
Krabbe disease, 400t
Krimsky test, 77, 77f
    in infantile exotropia, 104f
Kufs disease, 401t

Labyrinthine reflex system, 37
Lacerations
    conjunctival, 409
    corneoscleral, repair of, 408
    eyelid, repair of, 409
Lacrimal artery, extraocular muscles supplied
    by, 16
Lacrimal canaliculi. See Canaliculi

Lacrimal drainage system, 203–210. *See also* Nasolacrimal duct
  developmental abnormalities of, 203–204
Lacrimal gland fistulas, congenital, 204
Lacrimal glands
  ectopic, 345
  tumors of, 333*t*
Lacrimal intubation, for congenital lacrimal duct obstruction, 209–210
Lacrimal probing
  for congenital dacryocele, 205
  for congenital nasolacrimal duct obstruction, 207, 207–208, 208*f*
Lacrimal puncta. *See* Puncta
Lacrimal sac massage
  for congenital dacryocele, 205, 205*f*
  for congenital nasolacrimal duct obstruction, 206
Lacrimal system, intubation of, for congenital lacrimal duct obstruction, 209–210
Lamellar (zonular) cataracts, 247*f*, 247*t*, 248, 248*f*, 250*t*
  pulverulent, 247*t*
Lancaster red-green test, 80
Lang stereopsis tests, 87
Langerhans cell histiocytosis (histiocytosis X), orbital involvement in, 332*t*, 337–338, 338*f*
Large-print publications, sources of, 418*t*
Larva migrans, visceral, 273
Laser therapy (laser surgery)
  for glaucoma, 241
  for hemangiomas, 340
  for retinal angioma, 375
  for retinopathy of prematurity, 286
Latanoprost, for glaucoma, 242–243
Latent/manifest latent (fusion maldevelopment) nystagmus, 322–323, 323*f*, 324*f*
  dissociated vertical deviation and, 116, 117, 323
Lateral geniculate body/nucleus, 42
  development of, 44
    abnormal visual experience affecting, 46
Lateral incomitance, strabismus surgery planning and, 146
Lateral muscular branch of ophthalmic artery, extraocular muscles supplied by, 16
Lateral rectus muscles, 13, 14*f*, 16*f*, 17*t*, 18*f*
  A-pattern deviations associated with dysfunction of, 107–108
  action of, 13, 17*t*, 29, 29*t*
    gaze position and, 30, 30*f*
  anatomy of, 13, 14*f*, 16*f*, 17*t*, 18*f*
  field of action of, 29
  paralysis of, incomitant esotropia and, 98
  surgery of
    for A- and V-pattern deviations, 111, 111*f*
    for consecutive esotropia, 103
    for constant exotropia, 103
    for Duane syndrome, 129
    for intermittent exotropia, 102–103
    for monocular elevation deficiency (double elevator palsy), 124
    for nystagmus, 328, 329, 329*t*

  for sixth nerve paralysis, 135
  for third nerve (oculomotor) paralysis, 133
  V-pattern deviations associated with dysfunction of, 107–108
Law of motor correspondence, Hering's, 35, 36*f*
Law of reciprocal innervation, Sherrington's, 34
LCA. *See* Leber congenital amaurosis
LCMV. *See* Lymphocytic choriomeningitis virus
LEA symbols, for visual acuity testing, 73
Leber congenital amaurosis, 289–291, 290*f*
Leber hereditary optic neuropathy, 311
Leflunomide, for uveitis, 277
Left gaze (levoversion), 35
Lens (crystalline), 168, 168*f*
  absence of, 260. *See also* Aphakia
  colobomas of, 260–261, 261*f*
  development/embryology of, 168, 168*f*
    congenital anomalies and abnormalities and, 260–261, 261*f*
  dislocated, 261–265, 261*f*, 262*f*, 262*t*, 264*f*. *See also* Ectopia lentis
    abuse and, 404
  disorders of, 245–265
  ectopic. *See* Ectopia lentis
  in homocystinuria, 263, 264*f*
  luxed/luxated, 261, 261*f*. *See also* Ectopia lentis
  in Marfan syndrome, 263
  spherophakic, 260, 260*f*
  subluxed/subluxated, 261, 262*f*. *See also* Ectopia lentis
  in sulfite oxidase deficiency, 264
  in Weill-Marchesani syndrome, 264
Lens-induced glaucoma, 239
Lensectomy
  with intraocular lens, 257–258
  without intraocular lens, 255–256, 257*f*
  for rubella, 183
  for subluxed lenses, 265
Lenses, spectacle. *See* Spectacle lenses
Lenticonus, posterior/lentiglobus, 249, 249*f*, 250*t*
Letterer-Siwe disease/syndrome, orbital involvement in, 338
Leukemia, ocular involvement in, 297–298, 298*f*
  choroid, 354
  iris, 351, 354
  optic disc/optic nerve, 298, 298*f*, 354
  orbit, 337
  retina, 297
  uveitis differentiated from, 276*t*
Leukocoria, in retinoblastoma, 354, 355*f*
  differential diagnosis and, 358, 359*t*
Leukodystrophy, metachromatic, 400*t*
Leukomalacia, periventricular, 309
Levator aponeurosis repair, for ptosis correction, 179
Levator muscle (levator palpebrae superioris), 13, 15–16, 16*f*, 17*t*
  anatomy of, 15–16, 16*f*, 17*t*
  function of, evaluation of in ptosis, 179
  in myasthenia gravis, 137, 139*t*
Levobunolol, for glaucoma, 242
Levocycloversion, 35

Levoversion (left gaze), 35
LGB. *See* Lateral geniculate body/nucleus
LHON. *See* Leber hereditary optic neuropathy
Library for the Blind and Physically Handicapped, 418*t*
Lid-twitch sign, Cogan, 137
Light
  corneal reflex to, in ocular alignment testing, 76–78, 77*f*, 78*f*
  pupillary response to. *See* Pupillary light reflex
Light reflex tests, corneal, 76–78, 77*f*, 78*f*
LIGHT-ROP study, 281
Light toxicity, retinopathy of prematurity and, 281
Lighthouse for the Blind, 417*t*
Ligneous conjunctivitis, 351
Limbal dermoids, 218, 218*f*, 348
  Goldenhar syndrome and, 218, 349*f*, 393, 393*f*
Limbal incision, for extraocular muscle surgery, 154
Limbal (bulbar) vernal keratoconjunctivitis, 199–200
Lipidoses, 400*t*
Lipodermoids (dermolipomas), 348–349, 349*f*
  Goldenhar syndrome and, 349, 349*f*, 393, 393*f*
Lipofuscinosis, neuronal-ceroid, 398, 401*t*
Lisch nodules, 225, 225*f*, 365–366, 366*f*
  in neurofibromatosis, 225, 225*f*, 365–366, 366*f*, 370
Listing's equatorial plane, 27, 27*f*
Lockwood ligament, 22, 23*f*
LogMAR, 73
Longitudinal fasciculus, medial, internuclear ophthalmoplegia caused by lesions of, 141
Lost muscle, surgery and, 24, 159–160
  esodeviations and, 97–98
Louis-Bar syndrome (ataxia-telangiectasia), 364*t*, 378–379, 379*f*
  ATM mutation in, 379
Low birth weight, retinopathy and, 281. *See also* Retinopathy, of prematurity
Low vision, 413–417, 417–418*t*. *See also* Blindness; Visual loss/impairment
  achromatopsia and, 291
  albinism and, 298
  approach to infant with, 414–416
  cataracts and, 252
  craniosynostosis and, 390
  delayed visual maturation and, 416
  in glaucoma, 233, 243
  Leber congenital amaurosis and, 289
  management of, 416–417
  nystagmus and, 330
  optic atrophy and, 310, 415
  optic nerve hypoplasia and, 414–415
  pregeniculate visual loss and, 414–415
  retrogeniculate visual loss/cortical visual impairment and, 415–416
  sources of information on, 417–418*t*
Lowe syndrome (oculocerebrorenal syndrome), 302
  cataract and, 247*t*, 302
  glaucoma and, 239, 302
LPS (levator palpebrae superioris). *See* Levator muscle
LR. *See* Lateral rectus muscles

Lubricants
  for craniosynostosis-induced corneal exposure, 389
  for Stevens-Johnson syndrome, 201
Lumigan. *See* Bimatoprost
Luxed/luxated globe, in craniosynostosis, 389–390
Luxed/luxated lens, 261, 261*f*. *See also* Ectopia lentis
Lymphangiomas, orbital, 341–342, 341*f*
Lymphocytic choriomeningitis virus (LCMV), 186
Lymphomas
  Burkitt, 337
  orbital, 337
Lysosomal storage disorders, 398
  GM_1 gangliosidosis type I and, 303
LYST gene, in Chédiak-Higashi syndrome, 300*t*

M cells (magnocellular neurons/system), 42–43, 43*f*
  development of, 42, 43*f*, 44
    abnormal visual experience affecting, 46
Macula, development of, 170
Macular degeneration, juvenile (Stargardt disease/ fundus flavimaculatus), 292–293, 293*f*
Macular dystrophies, hereditary, 292–294. *See also specific type*
Macular star, inflammatory disc edema with (neuroretinitis), 312, 313*f*
Macular translocation procedures, strabismus and, 143
Macule, hypopigmented (ash-leaf spot), in tuberous sclerosis, 372, 372*f*
Maddox rod/Maddox rod testing, 78
  double, 79, 79*f*
    in superior oblique muscle paralysis, 118
Maffucci syndrome, 340
Magnetic resonance imaging (MRI)
  in neurofibromatosis screening, 370
  in orbital evaluation
    hemangioma diagnosis and, 340
    tumor diagnosis and, 334
  in retinoblastoma, 356
  in Sturge-Weber syndrome, 376, 376*f*
Magnocellular neurons (M cells/system), 42–43, 43*f*
  development of, 42, 43*f*, 44
    abnormal visual experience affecting, 46
Major amblyoscope testing, 58–59, 59*f*, 78, 80
Malformation, 171
Malignant hyperthermia, 161–162
Malpositioning, of rectus pulleys, 23
Mamillations, iris, 226, 226*f*
Mandibulofacial dysostosis (Treacher Collins syndrome), 393–394, 394*f*
Manifest latent nystagmus, 323, 324*f*
Manifest strabismus, 9
  cover tests in assessment of, 74
Mannosidosis, 401*t*
  cataracts in, 247*t*
Marcus Gunn jaw-winking syndrome, 180
Marfan syndrome, 263
  ectopia lentis and, 263
Margin–reflex distance, in ptosis, 179
Marginal myotomy, 148*t*
Maroteaux-Lamy syndrome, 400*t*

Masked bilateral superior oblique muscle paralysis, 120
Masquerade syndromes, uveitis and, 275, 276t
Mast-cell stabilizers, for ocular allergy, 198, 199t
Maternal alcohol use, malformations associated with, 394–395, 395f
Maternal infection transmission, 181–186. *See also specific infection*
MATP gene, in OCA4 (albinism), 299t, 301
Maxillary osteomyelitis, 197
Mechanical glaucomas, secondary, 239
Medial longitudinal fasciculus, internuclear ophthalmoplegia caused by lesions of, 141
Medial muscular branch, of ophthalmic artery, extraocular muscles supplied by, 16
Medial rectus muscles, 13, 14f, 16f, 17f, 18f
   A-pattern deviations associated with dysfunction of, 107–108
   action of, 13, 17t, 29, 29t
      gaze position and, 30, 30f
   anatomy of, 13, 14f, 16f, 17f, 18f
   field of action of, 29
   laceration of during pterygium removal/sinus surgery, 143
   restriction of, incomitant esotropia and, 98
   surgery of, 150, 150t
      for A- and V-pattern deviations, 111, 111f
      for consecutive esotropia, 103
      for constant exotropia, 103
      for convergence insufficiency, 106
      for Duane syndrome, 129
      for infantile esotropia, 92
      lost/slipped muscle and, 159–160, 160f
      for monocular elevation deficiency (double elevator palsy), 124
      for nystagmus, 328, 329, 329t
      for sixth nerve paralysis, 135
   V-pattern deviations associated with dysfunction of, 107–108
Medullated (myelinated) retinal nerve fibers, 306, 306f
Medulloepithelioma (diktyoma), 352
Megalocornea, 211
Megaloglobus (buphthalmos)
   in glaucoma, 238
   in neurofibromatosis, 370
Megalopapilla, 307–308
Megalophthalmos, anterior, 211
Meibomian glands, chalazion caused by obstruction of, 350
Melanocytic tumors, in neurofibromatosis, 355–356, 366f
Melanocytoma, 353, 353f
Melanocytosis
   ocular (melanosis oculi), 350, 350f
   oculodermal (nevus of Ota), 350
Melanomas
   choroidal/uveal, 353
      uveitis differentiated from, 276t
   conjunctival, 349
Melanosis oculi (ocular melanocytosis), 350, 350f
Melphalan, for retinoblastoma, 359

Membrane-associated transporter protein *(MATP)* gene, in OCA4 (albinism), 299t, 301
Meningiomas
   optic nerve, optic glioma differentiated from, 368
   orbital, 343
Meningoceles, orbital, 346
Meningococcus *(Neisseria meningitidis),* conjunctivitis caused by, 189
Meridional amblyopia, 64
Mesectodermal dysgenesis. *See* Anterior segment, dysgenesis of
Mesenchymal dysgenesis. *See* Anterior segment, dysgenesis of
Metabolic disorders. *See also specific type and* Inborn errors of metabolism
   cataracts and, 253–254, 253f, 254t, 398
   corneal changes and, 398, 400–401t
   retinal manifestations of, 302–303, 398, 400–401t
Metachromatic leukodystrophy, 400t
Metastatic eye disease, of orbit, 333t, 336–338, 336f, 338f
Methazolamide, for glaucoma, 243
Methionine, in homocystinuria, dietary restriction in management of, 399
Methotrexate, for uveitis, 277
Methylmalonic aciduria, 398
Metipranolol, for glaucoma, 242
MH. *See* Malignant hyperthermia
Microaneurysms, retinal, in diabetes, 297
Microcoria (congenital miosis), 223, 228–229
Microcornea, 212, 212f
Microphthalmia (microphthalmos)
   in congenital cytomegalovirus infection, 184
   in congenital rubella, 183
   with cyst (colobomatous cyst), 345, 346f
   with linear skin defects, 216
Microsomia, hemifacial, 392–393, 393f
Microspherophakia, in Weill-Marchesani syndrome, 264
Midface hypoplasia, 386, 386f
Midget retinal ganglion cells, 43, 43f
Midline positions of gaze, 80
Miosis/miotic agents
   congenital (microcoria), 223, 228–229
   for consecutive esotropia, 103
   for glaucoma, 243
Mitochondrial DNA, Leber hereditary optic neuropathy and, 311
Mitomycin/mitomycin C, in trabeculectomy, 241
Mitten deformity, 389f
Mittendorf dot, 307
MLF. *See* Medial longitudinal fasciculus
MLS. *See* Microphthalmia (microphthalmos), with linear skin defects
Möbius syndrome/sequence, 140–141, 140f
Moebius syndrome. *See* Möbius syndrome/sequence
Molluscum contagiosum, 193, 194f
Molteno implant, for glaucoma, 241
Molybdenum cofactor deficiency. *See* Sulfite oxidase deficiency

Monochromatism/monochromacy
blue-cone, 291
rod, 291
Monocular cells, in visual processing, 43*f*, 44
Monocular cover-uncover test, 74, 75*f*
Monocular elevation deficiency (double elevator palsy),
123–124, 123*f*
Monocular eye movements (ductions), 33–34
forced. *See* Forced ductions
Monocular fixation, 11
Monocular nystagmus of childhood, 326
Monocular recession-resection procedures, 150–151,
150*t*
Monofixation syndrome, 59–60
Bagolini glasses in evaluation of, 56*f*, 57
4Δ base-out prism test in evaluation of, 57–58, 57*f*
simultaneous prism and cover test in evaluation of,
75–76
Worth 4-dot test in evaluation of, 55
Mononucleosis, infectious, ocular involvement in, 193
Moraxella, conjunctivitis caused by, 189
Morning glory disc anomaly, 305, 305*f*, 415
Morquio syndrome, 400*t*
corneal opacities and, 217
Motor apraxia, ocular, 141–142
Motor correspondence, Hering's law of, 35, 36*f*
Motor fusion, 41, 41*t*
Motor nystagmus, congenital, 321
Motor physiology, 27–37
basic principles and terms related to, 27–32
eye movements and, 32–37
strabismus and, 27–37
Motor tests, in strabismus/amblyopia evaluation, 83
Motor units, 32–33
Moyamoya disease, morning glory disc anomaly in, 305
MPSs. *See* Mucopolysaccharidoses
MPS I H. *See* Hurler syndrome
MPS I S. *See* Scheie syndrome
MPS II. *See* Hunter syndrome
MPS III. *See* Sanfilippo syndrome
MPS IV. *See* Morquio syndrome
MPS VI. *See* Maroteaux-Lamy syndrome
MPS VII. *See* Sly syndrome
MR. *See* Medial rectus muscles
MRD. *See* Margin–reflex distance
mtDNA. *See* Mitochondrial DNA
Mucoceles
nasal, 204–205, 205
orbital invasion by, 346
Mucocutaneous lymph node syndrome (Kawasaki
disease), 201–202
Mucolipidoses, 400*t*
corneal opacities and, 216*t*, 217, 400*t*
Mucopolysaccharidoses, 398, 400*t*
corneal opacities and, 216*t*, 217, 400*t*
Mucor (mucormycosis), orbit involved in, 197, 197*f*
Multiple sclerosis
optic nerve involvement and, 312
uveitis in, differential diagnosis and, 276*t*
Munchausen syndrome by proxy, ocular trauma and, 404

Muscle capsule, of rectus muscles, 19–20
surgery and, 24
Muscle cone, 19, 20*f*
Myasthenia gravis, 137–138, 138*f*, 139*t*
strabismus in, 137–138, 138*f*, 139*t*
Myasthenia Gravis Foundation of America, Inc, 137
Mycophenolate mofetil, for uveitis, 277
Mydriasis/mydriatics, congenital, 229
Myectomy, 148*t*
Myelinated (medullated) retinal nerve fibers, 306, 306*f*
MYOC gene. *See* TIGR/myocilin (*TIGR/MYOC*) gene
Myoclonus, cherry-red spot in, 400*t*
Myofibromas, of orbit, 343
Myokymia, superior oblique, 142–143
Myopathies, extraocular, in thyroid eye disease, 135
Myopia, 169
age of onset and, 169
amblyopia and, 63, 64, 69
diabetic retinopathy and, 297
in inborn errors of metabolism, 401*t*
intermittent exotropia and, 102
retinopathy of prematurity and, 286
in Stickler syndrome, 295
Myositis, orbital, 347
Myotomy, 148*t*
marginal, 148*t*
Myotonic dystrophy, cataracts in, 247*t*

Naproxen, for uveitis, 277
NAPVI. *See* National Association of Parents of Children
With Visual Impairments
Nasal mucoceles, congenital, 204–205, 205
Nasolacrimal duct
congenital obstruction of, 169, 205–210, 206*f*
balloon dacryoplasty for, 209, 209*f*
differential diagnosis of, 206
intubation for, 209–210
lacrimal sac massage for, 206
nonsurgical management of, 206
probing for, 207, 207–208, 208*f*
surgical management of, 206–210, 208*f*, 209*f*
turbinate infracture for, 208–209
development of, 169
National Association of Parents of Children With Visual
Impairments, 417*t*
National Association for the Visually Handicapped,
417*t*
National Dissemination Center for Children with
Disabilities, 417*t*
National Down Syndrome Society, 418*t*
National Easter Seal Society, 418*t*
National Eye Institute, on nystagmus terminology,
317–318
National Fragile X Foundation, 418*t*
National Health Information Center, 418*t*
National Library Service for the Blind and Physically
Handicapped, 417*t*
National Organization for Albinism and
Hypopigmentation, 417*t*
Nausea and vomiting, after strabismus surgery, 161

NAVH. *See* National Association for the Visually Handicapped

Nd:YAG laser therapy, cycloablation/cyclophotocoagulation, for glaucoma, 241

NDP gene, in Norrie disease, 296

Near point of convergence, 81

Near reflex
accommodative convergence and, 37
assessment of, 81
spasm of, esotropia and, 97
voluntary application of, 37

Near visual acuity, testing, 74
nystagmus and, 319

Negative angle kappa, 77, 78*f*

NEI. *See* National Eye Institute

Neisseria
gonorrhoeae (gonococcus), conjunctivitis caused by
in children, 189
in neonates, 187, 187*f*
meningitidis (meningococcus), conjunctivitis caused by, 189

NEMO (NF-kB essential modulator) gene, in incontinentia pigmenti, 379

Neonatal hemangiomatosis, diffuse, 340

Neonates. *See also* Infants
conjunctivitis in, 186–188, 187*f*. *See also* Ophthalmia neonatorum
ocular infections in, 181–186. *See also specific type*
screening eye examinations in, 250–251

Neostigmine, for myasthenia gravis diagnosis, 138

Neovascularization, in retinopathy of prematurity, 280–287
screening for, 285, 286*t*

Nephritis, tubulointerstitial, uveitis and, 271–272

Nephroblastoma. *See* Wilms tumor

Neptazane. *See* Methazolamide

Nerve fibers, medullated (myelinated), 306, 306*f*

Nettleship-Falls albinism, 298, 300*t*, 301

Neural/neurogenic tumors, orbital, 333*t*, 343

Neurilemoma (neurinoma/schwannoma), of orbit, 343

Neuritis, optic. *See* Optic neuritis

Neuroblastoma, 336–337, 336*f*
Horner syndrome in, 230, 336, 336*f*
of orbit, 336–337, 336*f*

Neurocristopathy, 212–214, 213*f*. *See also* Anterior segment, dysgenesis of; Axenfeld-Rieger syndrome

Neurocutaneous syndromes (phakomatoses), 363–381, 364*t*. *See also specific type*

Neurofibromas
acoustic, 371
nodular cutaneous and subcutaneous, 366
plexiform, 343, 366–367, 367*f*
eyelid involvement and, 367, 367*f*
glaucoma and, 367, 370
of orbit, 343, 367

Neurofibromatosis (von Recklinghausen disease), 363–371
type 1, 363–365, 364*t*, 365–371
choroidal lesions in, 352, 366
diagnostic criteria for, 365

glaucoma and, 238, 367, 370
glial cell lesions in, 366–367, 367*f*, 368*f*
iris mamillations associated with, 226
Lisch nodules associated with, 225, 225*f*, 365–366, 366*f*, 370
melanocytic lesions in, 355–356, 366*f*
miscellaneous manifestations of, 369–371
nodular neurofibromas in, 366
optic pathway/optic nerve gliomas and, 343, 367–369, 368*f*
plexiform neurofibromas in, 343, 366–367, 367*f*
eyelid involvement and, 367, 367*f*
glaucoma and, 367, 370
orbital involvement and, 343, 367
type 2, 363, 371

Neurofibromin, 365

Neurofibrosarcoma, 367

Neuroglial lesions, in neurofibromatosis, 366–367, 367*f*, 368*f*

Neuroimaging
in cortical visual impairment, 416
in hyphema, 409
in optic nerve hypoplasia, 415
in orbital tumors, 334
hemangiomas, 340
in retinoblastoma, 356, 356*f*
in Sturge-Weber syndrome, 376, 376*f*
in tuberous sclerosis, 372, 373*f*

Neurologic disorders, optic nerve hypoplasia and, 308, 309

Neuroma, acoustic, in neurofibromatosis type 2, 371

Neurometabolic disorders, retinal findings in, 302–303

Neuromuscular abnormalities, constant exotropia and, 105

Neuronal ceroid-lipofuscinosis, 398, 401*t*

Neuroretinitis, 312, 313*f*

Neutral-density filter effect, 62

Neutral zone. *See also* Null point
in congenital motor nystagmus, 321

Nevus
of choroid, 352
conjunctival, 349, 349*f*
flammeus (port-wine stain), 342
of orbit, 342
in Sturge-Weber syndrome, 238, 342, 375, 376, 376*f*
in von Hippel–Lindau disease, 374
iris, 351
nevocellular, congenital, 349–350, 350*f*
of Ota (oculodermal melanocytosis), 350

New York Times Large-Print Weekly, 418*t*

Newborns. *See also* Infants
ocular infections in, 181–186. *See also specific type*
conjunctivitis, 186–188, 187*f*. *See also* Ophthalmia neonatorum
screening eye examinations in, 250–251

Newcastle Control Score, in intermittent exotropia, 100

NF. *See* Neurofibromatosis

NF-kB essential modulator *(NEMO)* gene, in incontinentia pigmenti, 379

NF1 gene, 363–365

NF2 gene, 365
NICHCY. *See* National Dissemination Center for Children with Disabilities
Niemann-Pick disease, 400*t*
Night blindness, congenital stationary, 291–292
NLD. *See* Nasolacrimal duct
NLS. *See* National Library Service for the Blind and Physically Handicapped
NOAH. *See* National Organization for Albinism and Hypopigmentation
Nodular episcleritis, 351
Nodular neurofibromas, cutaneous and subcutaneous, in neurofibromatosis, 366
Nonaccommodative acquired esotropia, 90*t*, 95–98
Nonalternating suppression, 50–51
Noncomitant deviations. *See* Incomitant (noncomitant) deviations
Nonoptic reflex systems, 37
Nonproliferative diabetic retinopathy (NPDR). *See* Diabetic retinopathy, nonproliferative
Nonrefractive accommodative esotropia (high accommodative convergence/accommodative esotropia), 94–95
    management of, 82, 94–95
Nonsteroidal anti-inflammatory drugs (NSAIDs)
    for ocular allergy, 198, 199*t*
    for uveitis, 277*t*
Normal retinal correspondence, 39
Norrie disease, 296
Norrin protein, in Norrie disease, 296
NRC. *See* Normal retinal correspondence
Nuclear cataracts, 247–248, 248*f*, 250*t*
Null point, 317
    in congenital motor nystagmus, 321
    in downbeat nystagmus, 325–326
    in latent nystagmus, 323
    nystagmus surgery and, 328, 328*f*, 329
Nystagmus, 288–289, 289*t*, 317–330, 319*t*
    acquired, 324–326
    in albinism, 298
    in aniridia, 223
    cataracts and, 252
    congenital, 288–289, 289*t*, 321–323, 321*t*, 323*f*, 324*f*
    convergence-retraction (induced convergence-retraction), 325
    in decreased vision, 414, 415
    differential diagnosis of, 326, 327*f*
    dissociated, 326
    downbeat, 325–326
    with esotropia, 90*t*, 92, 321
    evaluation of, 318–320, 319*t*, 320*t*
    funduscopic evaluation in, 320, 320*t*
    gaze positions affecting, 317, 318*f*
    in hereditary retinal disorders, 288–289, 289*t*
    history in, 318, 319*t*
    infantile, 288–289, 289*t*, 321–323, 321*t*, 323*f*, 324*f*
    in internuclear ophthalmoplegia, 141
    jerk, 317
    latent/manifest latent (fusion maldevelopment), 322–323, 323*f*, 324*f*
        dissociated vertical deviation and, 116, 117, 323

    monocular, 326
    motor (congenital), 321
    nomenclature associated with, 317–318
    ocular examination in, 318–320, 320*t*
    ocular motility testing in, 320
    opsoclonus and, 325
    in optic nerve hypoplasia, 308, 320, 415
    optokinetic (OKN), 319, 413
        assessment of, 319, 413
        in congenital motor nystagmus, 321
    pendular, 317
    periodic alternating, 322
    prisms for, 326–328
    pupil assessment in, 319–320, 320*t*
    see-saw (vision loss), 325
    sensory (congenital), 322, 414
    spasmus nutans, 324–325
    with strabismus, surgery for, 329
    surgery for, 328–329, 328*f*, 329*t*
    transient, 320
    treatment of, 326–330, 328*f*, 329*t*
    types of, 320–326
    visual acuity testing in, 73, 318–319
Nystagmus blockage syndrome, 321
    surgery for, 329

OA1 albinism, 300*t*, 301. *See also* Ocular albinism
OA1 gene, 300*t*, 301
OAV. *See* Oculoauriculovertebral (OAV) spectrum
Obligatory suppression, 51
Oblique muscles, 13, 14–15, 14*f*, 15*f*, 16*f*, 17*t*, 18*f*. *See also* Inferior oblique muscles; Superior oblique muscles
    action of, 14–15, 29, 29*t*
        gaze position and, 31–32, 33*f*, 34*f*
        3-step test in evaluation of, 83–86, 85*f*
    anatomy of, 14–15, 14*f*, 15*f*, 16*f*, 17*t*, 18*f*
        surgery and, 24
    field of action of, 29
    myokymia affecting, 142–143
    overaction of, 113–116, 114*f*, 115*f*
        A-pattern deviations associated with, 107, 109*f*
        apparent (pseudo-overaction), 116
        in infantile esotropia, 92
        V-pattern deviations associated with, 107, 108*f*
        vertical deviations caused by, 113–116, 114*f*, 115*f*
    paralysis of, 118–121, 119*f*
    pseudo-overaction of, 116
    pulley system of, 22, 22*f*, 23
        A- and V-pattern deviations and, 109–110, 110*f*
    strengthening procedures for, 152
    weakening procedures for, 147, 148*t*, 151–152
        for A- and V-pattern deviations, 110, 111, 112
        for infantile esotropia, 92
        for inferior oblique muscle paralysis, 122
        for superior oblique muscle paralysis, 120–121
        for vertical deviations, 114–115, 116
Oblique tenotomy
    for Brown syndrome, 131–132
    for third nerve (oculomotor) paralysis, 133

Obstetric history
    corneal opacities and, 217
    decreased vision and, 414
    nystagmus and, 318
    strabismus/amblyopia and, 71
OCA1 (albinism), 298
OCA1A (albinism), 298, 299*t*
OCA1B (albinism), 298, 299*t*
OCA2 (albinism), 299*t*, 301, 301*f*
OCA2 gene, in albinism, 299*t*, 301
OCA3 (albinism), 299*t*, 301
OCA4 (albinism), 299*t*, 301
Occipital (primary visual/calcarine/striate) cortex, 42
    development of, 44, 45*f*
        abnormal visual experience affecting, 46–49, 47*f*,
            48*f*
Occlusion amblyopia, 64, 67–68
    eye trauma and, 403
Occlusion therapy. *See also* Patching
    for amblyopia, 66–67
        cataract surgery and, 259
        compliance issues and, 66–67, 68
        complications of, 67–68
Ocular adnexa
    in craniosynostosis syndromes, 391–392
    development of, 169
    infections of, 194–197, 196*f*
Ocular albinism, 298, 300*t*, 301
    autosomal recessive, 301
    X-linked (Nettleship-Falls), 298, 300*t*, 301
Ocular alignment
    decreased vision and, 414
    tests of, 74–80
    unsatisfactory, after strabismus surgery, 155
Ocular allergy, 197–200. *See also* Allergic reactions/
        allergies
Ocular dominance columns, 43*f*, 44
    visual development and, 44, 45*f*
        abnormal visual experiences affecting, 46, 47, 47*f*
Ocular hypertelorism, 173, 384
Ocular melanocytosis (melanosis oculi), 350, 350*f*
Ocular motility, 32–37. *See also specific type of eye
        movement*
    assessment of, 81–83
        convergence and, 81–82
        fusional vergence and, 82–83
        motor tests in, 83
        ocular rotations and, 81
        prism adaptation test in, 86
        3-step test in, 83–86, 85*f*
    binocular eye movements and, 34–37
        conjugate (versions), 34, 35, 36*f*
        disconjugate (vergences), 34, 35–37. *See also*
            Vergences
            assessment of, 86–87
        in infants, 413
    cortical/supranuclear pathways in control of, 37
    disorders of
        in ataxia-telangiectasia, 378
        history/presenting complaint in, 71
        in inborn errors of metabolism, 400–401*t*

    nystagmus/spontaneous, 320. *See also* Nystagmus
    saccadic dysfunction and, ocular motor apraxia
        and, 141–142
    growth/development and, 170
    monocular eye movements (ductions) and, 33–34
    motor units and, 32–33
Ocular motor apraxia, congenital, 141–142
Ocular rotations
    assessing, 81
    in myasthenia gravis, 137
Ocular surface, inflammatory conditions affecting,
        350–351
Ocular (intraocular) surgery, for uveitis, 278
Ocular toxocariasis. *See Toxocara* (toxocariasis)
Ocular trauma. *See* Trauma
Oculoauriculovertebral (OAV) spectrum, 392–393
Oculocardiac reflex, 161
Oculocerebrorenal syndrome (Lowe syndrome), 302
    cataract and, 247*t*, 302
    glaucoma and, 239, 302
Oculocutaneous albinism, 298–301, 299*t*
Oculodermal melanocytosis (nevus of Ota), 350
Oculodigital reflex, 413
Oculoglandular syndrome, Parinaud, 189–190, 190*f*
Oculomotor nerve palsy. *See* Third nerve (oculomotor)
        paralysis
Oculorenal syndromes, familial, 302
Ocupress. *See* Carteolol
Ocusert Delivery System. *See also* Pilocarpine
    for glaucoma, 243
Oguchi disease, 292
Oil droplet appearance, in lenticonus and lentiglobus,
        249
Oligoarticular (pauciarticular)-onset juvenile idiopathic
        (chronic/rheumatoid) arthritis (oligoarthritis), 269,
        269*t*
    eye examination schedule for children with, 271*t*
    uveitis in, 269
One toy, one look rule, for pediatric examination, 3
ONH. *See* Optic nerve (cranial nerve II), hypoplasia of
Open-angle glaucoma. *See also* Glaucoma
    clinical manifestations and diagnosis of, 234–238,
        234*f*, 235*t*, 236*f*, 237*f*
    genetics of, 233
    juvenile, 234
    natural history of, 238
    pathophysiology of, 234
    primary
        congenital, 233–238, 234*f*, 235*t*, 236*f*, 237*f*
        juvenile, 234
    secondary, 238–240
    treatment of, 240–243, 240*f*, 242*f*
Ophthalmia neonatorum, 186–188, 187*f*
    chemical, 188
    chlamydial, 187–188
    gonococcal, 187, 187*f*
    herpes simplex causing, 188. *See also* Conjunctivitis,
        herpes simplex virus causing
    prophylaxis for, 186, 188
Ophthalmic artery, extraocular muscles supplied
        by, 16

Ophthalmopathy, thyroid (Graves). *See* Thyroid eye disease
Ophthalmoplegia
  chronic progressive external, 137, 139*t*
  internuclear, 141
Opsoclonus, 325
  neuroblastoma and, 336
Optic atrophy, 310–311, 311*t*, 415
  Behr, 311
  in craniosynostosis, 391
  dominant, 310–311
  in inborn errors of metabolism, 400–401*t*
  Leber hereditary optic neuropathy and, 311
Optic chiasm. *See* Chiasm
Optic disc (optic nerve head). *See also* Optic nerve
  aplasia of, 309
  atrophy of. *See* Optic atrophy
  coloboma of, 306, 306*f*, 415
  congenital/developmental abnormalities of, 305–310
  disorders of, 305–315
  drusen of, 314–315, 315*f*
    papilledema/pseudopapilledema and, 314–315, 315*f*
  edema of, 314*t*. *See also* Papilledema; Pseudopapilledema
    in craniosynostosis, 391
    in leukemia, 298, 298*f*, 354
    papilledema and, 312
    pseudopapilledema and, 313–315, 314*t*, 315*f*
  in glaucoma, evaluation of, 237, 237*f*
  hypoplasia of, 308–309, 308*f*, 320, 414–415
  in leukemia, 298, 298*f*, 354
  in megalopapilla, 307–308
  morning glory, 305, 305*f*, 415
  tilted (Fuchs coloboma), 307, 307*f*
Optic nerve (cranial nerve II). *See also* Optic disc
  aplasia of, 309
  atrophy of. *See* Optic atrophy
  coloboma of, 306, 306*f*, 415
  congenital abnormalities of, 305–310
  disorders of, 305–315
    in craniosynostosis, 391
  evaluation of
    in glaucoma, 237, 237*f*
    in nystagmus, 320
  hypoplasia of, 308–309, 308*f*, 320, 414–415
  in leukemia, 298, 298*f*
Optic nerve (optic pathway/chiasm) glioma (pilocytic astrocytoma), 343, 367–369, 368*f*
  in neurofibromatosis, 343, 367–369, 368*f*
  orbital involvement in, 343
Optic nerve pits, 310, 310*f*
Optic nerve sheath meningioma, optic glioma differentiated from, 368
Optic neuritis, 311–312
Optic neuropathy, Leber hereditary, 311
Optic tract, 43*f*, 44
Optical (optic) axis, 12
Optical degradation, for amblyopia, 67
OptiPranolol. *See* Metipranolol

Optokinetic nystagmus (OKN), 319, 413
  assessment of, 319, 413
  in congenital motor nystagmus, 321
Optotypes, evaluation of visual acuity and, 4, 73
  crowding bars and, 65, 65*f*, 73
Orbit
  congenital disorders of, 173–175, 174*f*, 175*f*
  cysts of, 332*t*, 343–344, 344*f*
    aneurysmal bone, 343
    dermoid, 343–344, 344*f*
    epidermoid, 343
    with microphthalmos (colobomatous cyst), 345, 346*f*
  development of, 169
  dysmorphic, 173–175, 174*f*, 175*f*
  fascial system of, 19–24, 20*f*
  floor of, fractures of, 124–126, 125*f*, 411
    vertical deviations and, 124–126, 125*f*
  fractures of, 124–126, 125*f*, 411, 411*f*
    vertical deviations and, 124–126, 125*f*
  infection/inflammation of, 194–197
  lateralization of (orbital hypertelorism), 173, 384
  measurement of, 173, 174*f*
  myositis affecting, 347
  roof of, fractures of, 411, 411*f*
  surgery of, for volume expansion in craniosynostosis, 392
  tumors of, 331–347, 332–333*t*. *See also specific type*
    benign, 338–343
    bony, 342–343
    connective tissue, 343
    cystic, 332*t*, 343–344, 344*f*
    differential diagnosis of, 331–334
    ectopic tissue masses, 343–346
    histiocytic, 332*t*, 337–338, 338*f*
    inflammatory disorders simulating, 332*t*, 346–347, 347*f*
    metastatic, 333*t*, 336–338, 336*f*, 338*f*
    primary malignant, 334–336, 335*f*
    vascular, 332*t*, 338–342, 339*f*, 341*f*
Orbital cellulitis, 195–197, 196*f*
  fungal (mucormycosis), 197, 197*f*
  after strabismus surgery, 156, 156*f*
Orbital hypertelorism, 173, 384
Orbital layer of extraocular muscle, 18
  pulley system and, 18, 21, 22, 22*f*, 23
Orbital pseudotumor, 272, 346–347, 347*f*
Orbital varices, 342
Orbital veins, 18
Orbitopathy, thyroid/thyroid-associated/Graves. *See* Thyroid eye disease
"Organic amblyopia," 64
Ornithine transcarbamylase deficiency, 398
Orthophoria/orthotropia, 9
Orthoptics
  for convergence insufficiency, 106
  fusional vergences and, 82
  for intermittent exotropia, 102
  for residual exotropia, 103
  for suppression, 52
Ossifying fibroma, of orbit, 343

Osteoma, choroidal, 353
Osteomyelitis, maxillary, 197
Osteosarcoma, of orbit, 336
Ota, nevus of (oculodermal melanocytosis), 350
Overcorrection, in exodeviation, value of, 103, 151
Overdepression in adduction, 115
Overelevation in adduction, 114
Ovoid bodies, in neurofibromatosis, 369
Ox eye (buphthalmos/megaloglobus)
    in glaucoma, 238
    in neurofibromatosis, 370
Oxycephaly, 383
Oxygen therapy, retinopathy of prematurity and, 281

P cells (parvocellular neurons/system), 43, 43f, 44
    development of, 43, 43f, 44
        abnormal visual experience affecting, 46, 48
P gene. See OCA2 gene
Pachymetry/pachymeter, 236
Palpebral fissures, 169
    congenital widening of (euryblepharon), 177
    slanting of, 178
        A- and V-pattern deviations and, 110, 110f
        in Treacher Collins syndrome, 178, 393–394, 394f
    surgery affecting, 24–25
    vertical height of, in ptosis, 179
Palpebral vernal keratoconjunctivitis, 198–199, 199f
PAN. See Periodic alternating nystagmus
Panum's area of single binocular vision, 40, 40f, 49
Panuveitis, 267, 268t, 274–275, 274f. See also Uveitis
    familial juvenile systemic granulomatosis (Blau
        syndrome) and, 274–275
    sarcoidosis and, 274, 274f
    Vogt-Koyanagi-Harada (VKH) syndrome and, 275
Papillae, Bergmeister, 307
Papilledema, 312
    in craniosynostosis, 391
    in leukemia, 298
    pseudopapilledema and, 313–315, 314t, 315f
    pseudotumor cerebri and, 312, 313
Papillomas, eyelid, 348
Paradoxical diplopia, 52, 53f
Paradoxical pupillary phenomena, 319, 319t, 414
Paralytic strabismus, Hering's law and, 35
Paranasal sinus infection
    orbital cellulitis caused by, 195, 196, 196f
    preseptal cellulitis caused by, 195
Parasol retinal ganglion cells, 42, 43f
Parinaud oculoglandular syndrome, 189–190, 190f
Pars planitis, 272, 273f. See also Uveitis
    diagnosis of, 268t
Partially accommodative esotropia, 95
Parvocellular neurons (P cells/system), 43, 43f, 44
    development of, 43, 43f, 44
        abnormal visual experience affecting, 46, 48
Patching
    acute esotropia caused by, 96
    for amblyopia, 66–67
        after cataract surgery, 259
        compliance issues and, 66–67, 68

for consecutive esotropia, 103
for corneal abrasion, 407
for dissociated vertical deviation, 117
for esotropia in sixth nerve paralysis, 98
for intermittent exotropia, 102
occlusion amblyopia caused by, 64, 67–68
for residual exotropia, 103
Pauciarticular (oligoarticular)-onset juvenile idiopathic
    (chronic/rheumatoid) arthritis (oligoarthritis), 269,
    269t
eye examination schedule for children with, 271t
uveitis in, 269
PAX6 gene
    in aniridia, 223–224, 233
    in foveal hypoplasia, 292
PCG. See Congenital glaucoma (primary congenital
    glaucoma)
Pediatric cataract. See Cataract
Pediatric corneal transplantation, 219
Pediatric glaucoma. See Glaucoma
Penalization
    for amblyopia, 67
    for dissociated vertical deviation, 117
Pendular nystagmus, 317
Penetrating injuries, 408–409, 408f
Penicillins, for syphilis, 186
Perennial allergic conjunctivitis, 198
Peribulbar anesthesia, for extraocular muscle surgery,
    160
Perimacular folds, in shaking injury, 405
Perimetry, Goldmann, in strabismus/amblyopia
    evaluation, 83
Perinatal ocular infection, 181–186. See also specific type
Periodic alternating nystagmus, 322
Periorbital ecchymosis
    in child abuse, 404
    in neuroblastoma, 336, 336f
Peripapillary staphyloma, 310, 415
Peripheral fusion, 41
    in monofixation syndrome, 60
Peripheral suppression, 50
Peritomy incision, for extraocular muscle surgery, 154
Periventricular leukomalacia, 309
Perkins tonometer, 236
Peroxisomal disorders, retinal degeneration in, 398
Persistent fetal vasculature (persistent hyperplastic
    primary vitreous), 250, 250t, 252f, 279–280, 279f, 307
    cataract and, 250, 250t, 252f, 279, 280
    glaucoma and, 250, 280
    lensectomy and, 256
    microcornea and, 212
Persistent pupillary membranes, 228, 229f
Peters anomaly, 215–216, 215f
    glaucoma and, 238
Pfeiffer syndrome, 388
PFV. See Persistent fetal vasculature
PHACE(S) syndrome, 339, 339f
Phakoma/phakomatoses (neurocutaneous syndromes),
    363–381, 364t. See also specific type
    retinal. See Retina, phakomas of

Pharmacologic penalization, for amblyopia, 67
Pharyngoconjunctival fever, 191
Phenylephrine, for fundus examination in premature
    infant, 285
Pheochromocytoma, in von Hippel–Lindau disease, 374
Philadelphia practical classification, for retinoblastoma,
    358
Phlyctenular keratoconjunctivitis, 351
-phoria (suffix), 10
Phorias. See Heterophorias
Phospholine. See Echothiophate
Photocoagulation
    for retinal angiomas, 375
    for retinopathy of prematurity, 286
Photophobia
    in achromatopsia, 291
    in primary congenital glaucoma, 234
Photoreceptors
    density/distribution of, 44–45
    development of, 44–45
PHPV (persistent hyperplastic primary vitreous). See
    Persistent fetal vasculature
Phthisis bulbi, retinoblastoma regression and, 356
Physiologic (simple/essential) anisocoria, 229
Physostigmine, for atropine intoxication, 88
Phytanic acid storage disease. See Refsum disease/
    syndrome
Pierre Robin sequence (anomaly/deformity), 171, 394
Pigment epithelium. See Iris pigment epithelium;
    Retinal pigment epithelium
Pilocarpine, for glaucoma, 243
Pilocytic astrocytoma, optic. See Optic nerve (optic
    pathway/chiasm) glioma
Pilopine/Pilopine gel. See Pilocarpine
Pits, optic nerve, 310, 310f
Pituitary gland disorders, optic nerve hypoplasia and,
    308–309, 415
PITX2/RIEG1 gene, in Axenfeld-Rieger syndrome, 214,
    233
Plagiocephaly, 383, 385f
    deformational, 386
    in Saethre-Chotzen syndrome, 388
Pleomorphic rhabdomyosarcoma, 335
Plexiform neurofibromas, 343, 366–367, 367f
    eyelid involvement and, 367, 367f
    glaucoma and, 367, 370
    of orbit, 343, 367
Plica semilunaris, incorporation of during strabismus
    surgery, 157, 157f
Plus disease, retinopathy of prematurity and, 282t, 283,
    284f
PMMA. See Polymethylmethacrylate
Poland syndrome, Möbius syndrome and, 140
Polar cataracts, 247, 247t, 248f, 250t
Polyarticular-onset juvenile idiopathic (chronic/
    rheumatoid) arthritis (polyarthritis), 269t
    eye examination schedule for children with, 271t
    rheumatoid factor (RF)-negative, 269, 269t
        uveitis in, 269
Polycoria, 230

Polydystrophy, pseudo–Hurler, 400t
Polymethylmethacrylate (PMMA) intraocular lenses,
    249
Polyposis, familial adenomatous (Gardner syndrome),
    retinal manifestations of, 352
Port-wine stain (nevus flammeus), 342
    of orbit, 342
    in Sturge-Weber syndrome, 238, 342, 375, 376, 376f
    in von Hippel–Lindau disease, 374
POS. See Parinaud oculoglandular syndrome
Positions of gaze. See Gaze, positions of
Positive angle kappa, 77, 78f
    in retinopathy of prematurity, 287, 287f
Posterior capsule, lensectomy with intraocular lens
    implantation and, 257
Posterior embryotoxon, 212, 212f
    in Axenfeld-Rieger syndrome, 212, 212f, 213
Posterior fixation suture (fadenoperation), 148t
    for dissociated vertical deviation, 153
Posterior keratoconus, central (posterior corneal
    depression), 215
Posterior lenticonus/lentiglobus, 249, 249f, 250t
Posterior polar cataract, 247t
Posterior segment, glaucoma associated with
    abnormalities of, 239
Posterior subcapsular cataract, 249, 250t
Posterior synechiae, 231
Posterior uveitis, 267, 272–274, 273f, 275. See also
    Uveitis
    differential diagnosis of, 268t
    laboratory tests for, 277t
    masquerade syndromes and, 276t
    toxocariasis and, 273–274, 273f
    toxoplasmosis and, 272
Postoperative care of ophthalmic surgery patient,
    cataract surgery and, 259–260
Postoperative endophthalmitis, after strabismus surgery,
    156
Povidone-iodine, for ophthalmia neonatorum
    prophylaxis, 188
Power (optical), intraocular lens, determination of, 258
pRB protein, retinoblastoma and, 356
Prednisolone, for hyphema, 410
Preferential looking, for visual acuity testing, 62, 63f,
    72t, 73, 170–171, 413
Pregeniculate visual loss, 414–415
Pregnancy
    alcohol use during (fetal alcohol syndrome),
        craniofacial malformations and, 394–395, 395f
    cytomegalovirus infection during, 184
    herpes simplex virus infection during, 185
    history of
        corneal opacities and, 217
        decreased vision and, 414
        nystagmus and, 318
        strabismus/amblyopia and, 71
    lymphocytic choriomeningitis virus infection during,
        186
    maternally transmitted eye infection and, 181–186
        ophthalmia neonatorum and, 186–188, 187f

rubella during, 183
syphilis during, 185, 221
toxoplasmosis during, 182
Prematurity, retinopathy of. *See* Retinopathy, of prematurity
Pre-plus disease, retinopathy of prematurity and, 283
Preseptal cellulitis, 194–195
after strabismus surgery, 156
Press-On prism
for consecutive esotropia, 103
for esotropia in sixth nerve paralysis, 98
for nystagmus, 326
Prethreshold disease, in retinopathy of prematurity, 285, 285*t*
oxygen therapy for, 281
treatment criteria and, 286
Prevent Blindness America, 417*t*
Primary deviation, 35
Primary glaucoma. *See* Glaucoma
Primary position of gaze, 13, 27, 80, 80*f*
extraocular muscle action and, 30, 30*f*
Primary vitreous, persistent hyperplasia of. *See* Persistent fetal vasculature
Prism adaptation test, 86
Prism and cover test
alternate (alternate cover test), 74–75, 76*f*
for intermittent exotropia evaluation, 100
simultaneous, 75–76
Prisms
for acute esotropia, 96
for basic (acquired) esotropia, 96
for consecutive esotropia, 103
for convergence insufficiency, 106
for convergence paralysis, 106
for induced tropia test, 72–73
for intermittent exotropia, 102
for monofixation syndrome evaluation, 57–58, 57*f*
for nystagmus, 326–328
for postoperative diplopia, 155
for residual exotropia, 103
for superior oblique muscle paralysis, 120
for thyroid eye disease, 135–136
Probing of lacrimal system
for congenital dacryocele, 205
for congenital nasolacrimal duct obstruction, 207, 207–208, 208*f*
Progressive (chronic progressive) external ophthalmoplegia, 137, 139*t*
Project-O-Chart, 87
Propine. *See* Dipivefrin
Propranolol, for hemangiomas, 340
Proptosis (exophthalmos/exorbitism), 173
in craniosynostosis, 388
in idiopathic orbital inflammatory disease, 346, 347*f*
in neuroblastoma, 336
in orbital cellulitis, 195, 196*f*
in orbital lymphangioma, 341
in rhabdomyosarcoma, 335
in teratoma, 344, 345*f*
in thyroid eye disease, 135, 136, 136*f*, 346, 347*f*

Prostaglandin analogues, for glaucoma, 242–243
Prostigmin. *See* Neostigmine
Proximal (instrument) convergence, 37
Proximal fusion, tenacious, in intermittent exotropia, 100–101
PSC. *See* Posterior subcapsular cataract
Pseudo-Brown syndrome, 130
Pseudocolobomas, in Treacher Collins syndrome, 394
Pseudoesotropia, 89, 90*t*
Pseudoexotropia, 99
in retinopathy of prematurity, 287, 287*f*
Pseudogliomas, in incontinentia pigmenti, 380
Pseudo-Hurler polydystrophy, 400*t*
Pseudohypopyon, in retinoblastoma, 354
Pseudo-overaction, oblique muscle, 116
Pseudopapilledema, 313–315, 314*t*, 315*f*
Pseudophakic glaucoma, 239
Pseudopolycoria, 230–231, 231*f*
Pseudoproptosis, 334
Pseudoptosis, 179*t*
in third nerve paralysis, 132
Pseudoretinitis pigmentosa
in congenital rubella, 183
in congenital syphilis, 185
Pseudostrabismus, in retinopathy of prematurity, 287, 287*f*
Pseudotumor
cerebri (idiopathic intracranial hypertension), 312–313
orbital, 272, 346–347, 347*f*
Psoriatic arthritis, 269*t*, 270–271
Pterygium, excision of, medial rectus muscle damage/strabismus and, 143
Ptosis (blepharoptosis), 178–179, 179*t*
acquired, 179*t*
in blepharophimosis syndrome, 178, 179*f*
botulinum toxin causing, 164
in chronic progressive external ophthalmoplegia, 137
congenital, 178, 179*t*
Marcus Gunn jaw-winking, 180
in monocular elevation deficiency (double elevator palsy), 123, 123*f*
in myasthenia gravis, 137, 138*f*, 139*t*
in orbital rhabdomyosarcoma, 335, 335*f*
plexiform neuroma of eyelid causing, 367, 367*f*
synkinesis in, 180
third nerve paralysis causing, 132, 133*f*
Pull-over (stay) sutures, 149
Pulley hindrance, 24
Pulley system, 21–24, 22*f*, 23*f*
A- and V-pattern deviations and, 109–110, 110*f*
orbital muscle layer and, 18, 21, 22, 22*f*, 23
pseudo-Brown syndrome and, 130
rectus muscles and, 21–22, 22*f*, 23, 23*f*
vertical deviations and, 114
Puncta, 203
atresia/stenosis of, 203
supernumerary, 204
Pupil-sparing third nerve (oculomotor) paralysis, 132
Pupillary axis, 12

Pupillary (central) cysts, 227
Pupillary defects, size/shape/location abnormalities, 228–231, 231*f*
Pupillary light reflex (pupillary response to light)
    decreased vision and, 413, 414
    in newborn, 170
    in nystagmus evaluation, 319, 320*t*
    paradoxical, 319, 319*t*, 414
Pupillary membrane, persistent, 228, 229*f*
Pupils, 169–170
    abnormalities of, 228–231, 231*f*
    Adie tonic, 229
    displacement of (corectopia), 230
    examination of
        decreased vision and, 414
        in nystagmus, 319–320, 320*t*
    shape of, abnormalities in (dyscoria), 223
    size of, abnormalities in, 170, 228–230. *See also* Anisocoria
    white. *See* Leukocoria
Pursuit eye movements/pursuit pathways/system, smooth, 37
    asymmetry of, 91
PVL. *See* Periventricular leukomalacia
Pyogenic granuloma, 351
Pyridoxine (vitamin B$_6$), for homocystinuria, 399

Racemose angioma (Wyburn-Mason syndrome), 342, 364*t*, 381, 381*f*
Radiation therapy
    increased sensitivity to, in ataxia-telangiectasia, 378
    for retinoblastoma, 358
Random-Dot E test, 87
Random-dot stereopsis tests, 87
Randot test, 87
RB1 (retinoblastoma) gene, 356
Reader's Digest Large Print, 418*t*
Recession (extraocular muscle), 23*f*, 24, 148*t*
    and anteriorization, 148*t*
Recession-resection procedures
    monocular, 150–151, 150*t*
    for nystagmus (Kestenbaum-Anderson procedure), 328–329, 329*t*
Recessive optic atrophy, 311
Reciprocal innervation, Sherrington's law of, 34
Reconstructive surgery, for craniofacial malformations, 392
Recording for the Blind and Dyslexic, 417*t*
Recruitment, 33
Rectus muscles, 13, 13–14, 14*f*, 16*f*, 17*t*, 18*f*
    action of, 13, 14, 17*t*, 28–29, 29*t*
        gaze position and, 30, 30*f*, 31, 31*f*, 32*f*
        3-step test in evaluation of, 83–86, 85*f*
    anatomy of, 13, 13–14, 14*f*, 16*f*, 17*t*, 18*f*
        growth/development and, 170
        surgery and, 24
    for comitant vertical deviations, 152
    fascial capsules of, 19–20
        surgery and, 24
    field of action of, 29

horizontal, 13, 14*f*. *See also* Lateral rectus muscles; Medial rectus muscles
    A-pattern deviations associated with dysfunction of, 107–108
    action of, 13, 28, 29*t*
        gaze position and, 30, 30*f*
    anatomy of, 13, 14*f*
    surgery of
        for A- and V-pattern deviations, 110, 111, 111*f*
        for nystagmus, 328, 329, 329*t*
    V-pattern deviations associated with dysfunction of, 107–108
insertion relationships of, 16, 18*f*
    growth/development and, 170
intermuscular septum of, 22
    surgery and, 24
pulley system for, 21–22, 22*f*, 23, 23*f*
    A- and V-pattern deviations and, 109–110, 110*f*
    pseudo-Brown syndrome and, 130
surgery of, 150, 150*t*, 152–154
    for A- and V-pattern deviations, 110, 111, 111*f*
    anatomy and, 24
    anterior segment ischemia and, 158–159, 158*f*
    for consecutive esotropia, 103
    for constant exotropia, 103
    for convergence insufficiency, 106
    for dissociated vertical deviation, 117, 153
    for Duane syndrome, 129
    eyelid position changes after, 159, 159*f*
    for hypo- and hypertropia, 152–153
    for infantile esotropia, 92
    for inferior oblique muscle paralysis, 122
    for intermittent exotropia, 102–103
    lost/slipped muscle and, 159–160, 160*f*
    for monocular elevation deficiency (double elevator palsy), 124
    for nystagmus, 154, 328, 329, 329*t*
    for orbital floor fracture, 126
    for sixth nerve paralysis, 135
    for superior oblique muscle paralysis, 120, 121
    for third nerve (oculomotor) paralysis, 133
    for thyroid eye disease, 136
    in thyroid eye disease, 135, 139*t*
vertical, 14, 14*f*. *See also* Inferior rectus muscles; Superior rectus muscles
    A-pattern deviations associated with dysfunction of, 109
    action of, 14, 28–29, 29*t*
        gaze position and, 31, 31*f*, 32*f*
    anatomy of, 14, 14*f*
    surgery of
        for A- and V-pattern deviations, 111
        for dissociated vertical deviation, 117, 153
        eyelid position changes after, 159, 159*f*
        for hypo- and hypertropia, 152–153
        for nystagmus, 329
    V-pattern deviations associated with dysfunction of, 109
Red eye, 188–193, 189*t*. *See also* Conjunctivitis

Red-glass test
    in ocular alignment assessment, 79
    in sensory adaptation testing, 53–55, 54*f*
Red-green test
    Lancaster, 80
    Worth 4-dot, 55, 55*f*, 87
        in binocular sensory cooperation evaluation, 87
        in sensory adaptation testing, 55, 55*f*
Red oculocutaneous albinism (OCA3), 299*t*, 301
Red reflex
    in cataract, 250–251
    in lenticonus and lentiglobus, 249
Reese-Ellsworth classification of retinoblastoma, 358, 359*t*
Refraction, clinical, cycloplegic, 87–88, 88*t*
Refractive accommodative esotropia, 93
Refractive errors, 169, 169*f*
    amblyopia caused by
        ametropic, 64
        anisometropic, 63
    changes in after strabismus surgery, 155
    correction/treatment of, in amblyopia treatment, 66
Refractive surgery, strabismus after, 143
Refsum disease/syndrome, infantile, 401*t*
Regional gigantism, 367
Renal cell carcinoma, in von Hippel–Lindau disease, 374
Renal disease, uveitis and, 271–272
Reoperation, surgical planning and, 147
Resection (extraocular muscle), 23*f*, 24, 147
Response accommodative convergence/accommodation ratio, 81. See also Accommodative convergence/accommodation ratio
Reticulum cell sarcoma, uveitis differentiated from, 276*t*
Retina. See also under Retinal
    development of, 44, 44–45
    disorders of. See specific type and Retinal disease; Retinopathy
    hamartomas of, 352
    in HIV infection/AIDS, 184, 304
    neovascularization of, disorders of in retinopathy of prematurity, 280–287
        screening for, 285, 286*t*
    phakomas of, in tuberous sclerosis, 372–374, 373*f*
    splitting of, in shaking injury, 405–406, 406*f*
    systemic disease affecting, 296–304
Retina International, 418*t*
Retinal angiomatosis (von Hippel–Lindau disease), 364*t*, 374–375, 375*f*
    retinoblastoma differentiated from, 358
Retinal correspondence, 39–40, 40*f*
    anomalous, 39, 51*f*, 52–53, 53*f*
        harmonious, 55
        testing in, 52, 53–59
        unharmonious, 55
    normal, 39
Retinal degenerations, in metabolic diseases, 398
Retinal detachment
    in child abuse, 404
    in retinopathy of prematurity, 287

surgery for
    in retinopathy of prematurity, 287
    strabismus and, 143
    uveitis and, differential diagnosis and, 276*t*
Retinal disease, 279–304
    in decreased vision, 415
    early-onset, 279–288
    hereditary, 288–292
        macular dystrophies, 292–294
        vitreoretinopathies, 294–296
    in metabolic disorders, 398
    systemic diseases and, 296–304
    vascular
        in incontinentia pigmenti, 380, 380*f*
        microaneurysms, in nonproliferative diabetic retinopathy, 297
        in retinopathy of prematurity, 280–287
            screening for, 285, 286*t*
        in Wyburn-Mason syndrome, 342, 381, 381*f*
Retinal folds, in shaking injury, 405
Retinal hemorrhages
    in leukemia, 297
    in shaking injury, 405, 405*f*
Retinal neovascularization, disorders of in retinopathy of prematurity, 280–287
    screening for, 285, 286*t*
Retinal nerve fibers, myelinated (medullated), 306, 306*f*
Retinal pigment epithelium (RPE)
    congenital hypertrophy of, 352, 353*f*
    hamartoma of, 352
    tumors of, 352–353, 353*f*
Retinal rivalry, 49, 50*f*
Retinitis
    cytomegalovirus
        congenital (cytomegalic inclusion disease), 184, 184*f*
        in HIV infection/AIDS, 184
    in toxoplasmosis, 181, 182, 182*f*
Retinitis pigmentosa, 398
    uveitis differentiated from, 276*t*
Retinoblastoma, 354–361
    chemotherapy of, 358–359, 360*f*
    classification of, 358, 359*t*
    clinical evaluation/diagnosis of, 356–358, 356*f*, 357*f*
    diffuse infiltrating, 355
    endophytic, 354, 355*f*
    enucleation for, 358
    exophytic, 355, 355*f*
    extraocular, 360, 361
    fleurettes in, 358
    genetics of, 356–357, 357*f*
        counseling and, 356–357, 357*f*
    leukocoria in, 354, 355*f*
        differential diagnosis and, 358, 359*t*
    monitoring patient with, 361
    nonocular, 360, 361
    rosettes in, 358
    secondary malignancies and, 359, 361
    spontaneous regression of, 356
    strabismus in, 354

treatment of, 358–360
trilateral, 360
uveitis differentiated from, 276*t*
vitreous seeding and, 354, 355*f*
Retinoblastoma *(RB1)* gene, 356
Retinoblastoma Support News (newsletter), 417*t*
Retinochoroiditis
in congenital herpes simplex, 185
in cytomegalic inclusion disease, 184, 184*f*
Retinocytoma, 356
Retinogeniculocortical pathway, 42, 42–44, 43*f*
development of, 42, 43, 43*f*, 44
abnormal visual experience affecting, 46–49, 47*f*,
48*f*
Retinopathy
in congenital rubella syndrome, 183, 183*f*
of incontinentia pigmenti, 380, 380*f*, 381
in leukemia, 297
of prematurity, 280–287
angle kappa and, 287, 287*f*
classification of, 282–285, 282*t*, 283*f*, 284*f*, 285*t*
diagnosis of, 285
management of, 285–286, 286*f*, 286*t*
screening examinations for, 285, 286*t*
sequelae and complications of, 286–287, 287*f*
Retinoschisis
foveal, 294
juvenile, 294–295, 295*f*
traumatic, in shaking injury, 405–406, 406*f*
Retinoscopy, in cataract, 251
Retrobulbar anesthesia
for extraocular muscle surgery, 160–161
strabismus after, 143
Retrogeniculate visual loss/cortical visual impairment,
415–416
Retrolental fibroplasia. *See* Retinopathy, of prematurity
RF-negative polyarthritis, 269, 269*t*
uveitis in, 269
Rhabdomyomas, in tuberous sclerosis, 372
Rhabdomyosarcoma, of orbit, 334–335, 335*f*
Rheumatoid arthritis, juvenile. *See* Juvenile idiopathic
(chronic/rheumatoid) arthritis
Rheumatoid factor, in juvenile idiopathic (chronic/
rheumatoid) arthritis, uveitis and, 269, 269*t*
Rieger anomaly/syndrome, 213. *See also* Axenfeld-
Rieger syndrome
Right gaze (dextroversion), 35
Riley-Day syndrome (familial dysautonomia), 221
Rivalry pattern, 49, 50*f*
RLF (retrolental fibroplasia). *See* Retinopathy, of
prematurity
Rod monochromatism, 291
ROP. *See* Retinopathy, of prematurity
Rosettes, in retinoblastoma, 358
Rotation, center of, 27, 27*f*
RP. *See* Retinitis pigmentosa
RPE65 gene/RPE65 protein, in Leber congenital
amaurosis, 290
Rubella, congenital, 183–184, 183*f*
Rufous oculocutaneous albinism (OCA3), 299*t*, 301

Saccades/saccadic system, 37
in ataxia-telangiectasia, 378
dysfunction of, ocular motor apraxia and, 141–142
inability to initiate, 141–142
testing velocity of, 83
Saccadic initiation failure (ocular motor apraxia),
141–142
Saethre-Chotzen syndrome, 389, 390*f*
Salmon patches, in syphilitic keratitis, 221
Salt-and-pepper fundus
rubella and, 183, 183*f*
syphilis and, 185
Sandhoff disease (GM$_2$ gangliosidosis type II), 303, 401*t*
Sanfilippo syndrome, 400*t*
Sarcoidosis, 274, 274*f*
uveitis in, 274, 274*f*
Sarcoma
Ewing, of orbit, 337
granulocytic (chloroma), 337
orbital, 334–336, 335*f*
reticulum cell, uveitis differentiated from, 276*t*
Satellite lesions, in toxoplasmosis, 182
Scaphocephaly, 383
Scheie syndrome, 400*t*
corneal opacities and, 217
Schwalbe line/ring, prominent (posterior embryotoxon),
212, 212*f*
in Axenfeld-Rieger syndrome, 212, 212*f*, 213
Schwannoma (neurilemoma/neurinoma), of orbit, 343
Sclera, perforation of
extraocular muscle/strabismus surgery and, 25,
155–156
traumatic, 408
Scleral buckle, for retinopathy of prematurity, 287
Sclerocornea, 216–217, 216*t*
glaucoma and, 238
Sclerosis, tuberous (Bourneville disease), 364*t*, 371–374,
372*f*, 373*f*
Scopolamine, for cycloplegia/cycloplegic refraction, 88,
88*t*
Scotomata
of monofixation syndrome, 59–60
Bagolini glasses in evaluation of, 57
4Δ base-out prism test in evaluation of, 57–58, 57*f*
Worth 4-dot test in evaluation of, 55
suppression, diplopia after strabismus surgery and, 155
Screening/diagnostic tests
for JIA-associated uveitis, 270, 271*t*
for neonates, 250–251
for retinopathy of prematurity, 285, 286*t*
Seasonal allergic conjunctivitis, 198, 198*t*, 199*t*
Secondary deviation, 35
Secondary glaucoma. *See* Glaucoma
Secondary positions of gaze, 27
See-saw (vision loss) nystagmus, 325
Seizures, in tuberous sclerosis, 372
Senior-Loken syndrome, 302
Sensory defects/deprivation
congenital nystagmus and, 322, 414
esodeviation and, 96–97

exotropia and, 104–105
visual development affected by, 46–47, 47f
Sensory fusion, 41
Sensory visual system, 39–60
abnormalities of binocular vision and, 49–50, 50f
adaptations in strabismus and, 50–60, 51f
testing, 53–59
assessment of binocular vision and, 86–87
neurophysiological aspects of, 42–49, 43f, 45f, 47f, 48f
physiology of normal binocular vision and, 39–42, 40f, 41t
Septo-optic dysplasia (de Morsier syndrome), 308
Sequence (congenital anomalies), 171
Seventh nerve (facial) palsy, Möbius syndrome/
sequence and, 140
Sexual abuse, gonococcal conjunctivitis and, 189
Shagreen patch, in tuberous sclerosis, 372
Shaking injury (shaken baby syndrome), 404–407, 405f, 406f
Sherrington's law of reciprocal innervation, 34
Shield ulcer, 200
Sialidoses, 400t
Sickle Cell Association, 418t
Sickle cell disease, traumatic hyphema and, 409
Sickle cell preparations ("preps"), 409
Silver nitrate, for ophthalmia neonatorum prophylaxis, 188
chemical conjunctivitis caused by, 188
Simulated divergence excess exotropia, 101
Simultaneous prism and cover test, 75–76
Single binocular vision
Panum's area of, 40, 40f, 49
testing field of, 83, 84f
Sinus surgery, endoscopic, medial rectus laceration/
strabismus and, 143
Sinusitis
Brown syndrome caused by, 130
orbital cellulitis caused by, 195, 196, 196f
preseptal cellulitis caused by, 195
Sixth nerve (abducens) paralysis, 98, 134–135, 134f
incomitant esodeviation caused by, 98
Möbius syndrome/sequence and, 140
surgery for, 153
Skew deviation
in infants, 413
inferior oblique muscle paralysis as form of, 121
Skin
congenital nevocellular nevi of, 349–350, 350f
disorders of
in incontinentia pigmenti, 379–380, 380f
in tuberous sclerosis, 372, 372f
Skull base, 383, 384f
suture fusion and, 386, 386f
Sleep test, for myasthenia gravis, 137
Slipped muscle, in extraocular muscle surgery, 24, 160, 160f
esodeviations and, 97–98
Slit-lamp examination
in cataract, 252–253
in glaucoma, 236–237
Sly syndrome, 400t

Smart System II PC Plus test, 87
SmartSight website, 330, 417
Smith-Lemli-Opitz syndrome, 398
Smoking, thyroid disease and, 135
Smooth pursuit eye movements/system, 37
asymmetry of, 91
Snellen acuity, 72t, 73
in strabismic amblyopia, 62
Snellen charts, 72t, 73
monofixation assessment and, 60
SO. See Superior oblique muscles
Spasm of near reflex, esotropia and, 97
Spasmus nutans/spasmus nutans syndrome, 324–325
Spectacle lenses (spectacles)
after cataract surgery, 258, 259
for consecutive esotropia, 103
for convergence insufficiency, 106
for high accommodative convergence/
accommodative esotropia, 94, 95
for intermittent exotropia, 102
for partially accommodative esotropia, 95
with prisms. See Prisms
for refractive accommodative esotropia, 93
Spherophakia, 260, 260f
Spielmeyer-Vogt disease, 401t
Spina Bifida (toll-free telephone), 418t
Spiral of Tillaux, 16, 18f
Spondylitis, juvenile ankylosing, 271
Spread of comitance, in superior oblique muscle
paralysis, 120
SR. See Superior rectus muscles
Staphylococcus/Staphylococcus aureus
conjunctivitis caused by, 189
orbital cellulitis caused by, 195
preseptal cellulitis caused by, 195
Staphylomas, peripapillary, 310, 415
Starfish cataract, 251f
Stargardt disease (juvenile macular degeneration/fundus
flavimaculatus), 292–293, 293f
Stationary night blindness, congenital, 291–292
Stay (pull-over) sutures, 149
Stereo Fly test, 87
Stereoacuity
development of, 170–171
testing, 87
in monofixation syndrome, 60
Stereopsis, 40–41, 40f, 41–42
depth perception differentiated from, 42
in intermittent exotropia, 101
in monofixation syndrome, 60
testing, 87
Stevens-Johnson syndrome (erythema multiforme
major), 200–201, 201f
Stickler syndrome, 295
Stimulus accommodative convergence/accommodation
ratio, 81. See also Accommodative convergence/
accommodation ratio
Stimulus deprivation amblyopia, 64
eye trauma and, 403
visual development affected by, 46–47, 47f, 61–62

STOP-ROP (Supplemental Therapeutic Oxygen for Prethreshold ROP) study, 281
Strabismic amblyopia, 62–63, 63*f*
  visual development and, 48–49, 48*f*, 61–62
Strabismus, 9–164. *See also* Deviations; Diplopia
  A-pattern, 107–112, 109*f. See also* A-pattern deviations
  acquired, 11
  age of onset and, 11, 71, 100
  amblyopia and, 62–63, 63*f. See also* Amblyopia
    visual development and, 48–49, 48*f*, 61–62
  anomalous retinal correspondence in, 51*f*, 52–53, 53*f*
    testing for, 52, 53–59
  botulinum toxin for, 163–164
  in Brown syndrome, 122*t*, 130–132, 131*f*
  in chronic progressive external ophthalmoplegia, 137, 139*t*
  in cataract, 252
  classification of, 10–11
  congenital, 11
  in congenital fibrosis syndrome, 138–140
  convergent, 9
  cover tests in, 74–76, 75*f*, 76*f*
  in craniosynostosis, 390–391, 391*f*
  cyclovertical, surgery planning and, 146
  definition of, 9
  diagnosis of, 71–88. *See also* Ocular motility, assessment of
  diagnostic positions of gaze and, 80, 80*f*
  dissimilar image tests in, 78–79, 79*f*
  dissimilar target tests in, 79–80
  divergent, 9
  in Duane syndrome, 127–130, 128*f*
  esodeviations, 89–98, 90*t*
  exodeviations, 99–106
  extorsional, 10
  extraocular muscle anatomy and, 13–25, 14*f*, 16*f*, 17*t*
  extraocular muscle field of action and, 29
  fixus, 139
  full-time patching for amblyopia and, 66
  high myopia and, 141
  history/presenting complaint in, 71
  infantile, 11
  infantile esotropia and, 90
  in inferior oblique muscle paralysis, 122*t*
  in internuclear ophthalmoplegia, 141
  intorsional, 10
  light reflex tests in, 76–78, 77*f*, 78*f*
  manifest, 9
  in Möbius syndrome, 140–141, 140*f*
  monofixation syndrome in, 59
  motor physiology and, 27–37
  motor tests in evaluation of, 83
  in myasthenia gravis, 137–138, 138*f*, 139*t*
  nystagmus surgery and, 329
  ocular alignment tests in, 74–80
  in ocular motor apraxia, 141–142
  in optic nerve hypoplasia, 308, 414–415
  paralytic, Hering's law and, 35

  in pregeniculate visual loss, 414
  prism adaptation test in, 86
  pulley system pathology and, 23, 109–110, 110*f*
    pseudo-Brown syndrome and, 130
  in retinoblastoma, 354
  secondary, botulinum toxin injections causing, 164
  sensory adaptations in, 50–60, 51*f*
    testing for, 53–59
  sensory physiology/pathology and, 39–60
  in sixth nerve (abducens) paralysis, 98, 134–135, 134*f*
  in superior oblique myokymia, 142–143
  suppression in, 50–52, 51*f*
    testing for, 51, 53–59
  terminology related to, 9–11
  in third nerve (oculomotor) paralysis, 132–134, 133*f*
  3-step test in, 83–86, 85*f*
  in thyroid eye disease, 135–136, 136*f*, 139*t*
  V-pattern, 107–112, 108*f. See also* V-pattern deviations
  vertical, 10. *See also* Vertical deviations
  visual acuity testing in, 71–74, 72*t*
  visual development affected by, 48–49, 48*f*
Strabismus surgery, 145–162. *See also specific type or disorder and* Extraocular muscle surgery
  acuity considerations and, 145–146
  adjustable sutures used in, 148–149
  anesthesia for, 160–162
  complications of, 154–160
  cyclovertical strabismus and, 146–147
  for dissociated vertical deviation, 117, 153
  for esodeviations and exodeviations, 150–151, 150*t*
  extraocular muscle anatomy and, 23*f*, 24–25
  guidelines for, 149–154, 150*t*
  for hypo- and hypertropia, 152–153
  incisions for, 154
  incomitance and, 146
  indications for, 145
  infections after, 156, 156*f*
  monocular recession-resection procedures, 150–151, 150*t*
  oblique muscle procedures and, 148*t*, 151–152
  planning, 145–147
  posterior fixation in, 148*t*, 149
  prior surgery and, 147
  pull-over (stay) sutures used in, 149
  rectus muscle procedures and, 152–154
  strengthening procedures in, 147–148, 152
  symmetric, 150, 150*t*
  techniques for, 147–149, 148*t*
  transposition procedures in, 149, 153
  weakening procedures in, 147, 148*t*, 151–152
Strawberry hemangioma. *See* Hemangiomas
Strengthening procedures (extraocular muscle), 147–148, 152
Streptococcus
  cellulitis caused by
    orbital, 195
    preseptal, 194, 195
  conjunctivitis caused by, 189

pneumoniae (pneumococcus)
   conjunctivitis caused by, 189
   orbital cellulitis caused by, 195
   preseptal cellulitis caused by, 195
pyogenes (group A β-hemolytic), orbital cellulitis caused by, 195
Striate cortex (Brodmann area 17), 42
   development of, 44, 45*f*
      abnormal visual experience affecting, 46–49, 47*f*, 48*f*
Stroma, iris, cysts of, 227
Stromal corneal dystrophies, congenital hereditary, 216*t*, 219
Sturge-Weber syndrome (encephalofacial/ encephalotrigeminal angiomatosis), 342, 364*t*, 375–378, 376*f*, 377*f*
   glaucoma associated with, 238, 377, 378
   port-wine stain in, 238, 342, 375, 376, 376*f*
Subarachnoid hemorrhage, in shaking injury, 405, 406
Subcapsular cataract, posterior, 249, 250*t*
Subconjunctival hemorrhage, in child abuse, 404
Subluxed/subluxated lens, 261, 262*f*. *See also* Ectopia lentis
Subperiosteal abscess, in orbital cellulitis, 195, 196, 196*f*
Succinylcholine, malignant hyperthermia caused by, 161
Sulfite oxidase deficiency, 264
Sulfur metabolism, in sulfite oxidase deficiency, 264
"Sunsetting," in infants, 413
Superior oblique muscles, 14–15, 14*f*, 15*f*, 16*f*, 17*t*, 18*f*
   action of, 15, 17*t*, 29, 29*t*
      gaze position and, 31–32, 33*f*
      3-step test in evaluation of, 83–86, 85*f*
   anatomy of, 14–15, 14*f*, 15*f*, 16*f*, 17*t*, 18*f*
      surgery and, 24
   field of action of, 29
   myokymia affecting, 142–143
   overaction of
      A-pattern deviations associated with, 107, 109*f*
      in inferior oblique muscle paralysis, 122*t*
      vertical deviations caused by, 113, 115–116, 115*f*
   paralysis (paresis/palsy) of, 118–121, 119*f*
      Hering's law and, 35, 36*f*
      after tenotomy for Brown syndrome, 131–132
   surgery of, 152
      for A- and V-pattern deviations, 110, 111
      for inferior oblique muscle paralysis, 122
      for superior oblique myokymia, 142–143
      for vertical deviation, 116
Superior oblique myokymia, 142–143
Superior oblique tendon, 14–15, 15*f*, 16*f*
   tucking procedure on, 120, 152
Superior oblique tenotomy
   for Brown syndrome, 131–132
   for superior oblique myokymia, 142–143
   for third nerve (oculomotor) paralysis, 133
Superior orbital vein, 18
Superior rectus muscles, 14, 14*f*, 16*f*, 17*t*, 18*f*
   action of, 14, 17*t*, 29*t*
      gaze position and, 31, 31*f*
      3-step test in evaluation of, 83–86, 85*f*

anatomy of, 14, 14*f*, 16*f*, 17*t*, 18*f*
   surgery and, 23*f*, 24–25
   surgery of
      for A-pattern deviation, 111
      for dissociated vertical deviation, 153
      eyelid position changes after, 159
      for inferior oblique muscle paralysis, 122
      for nystagmus, 329
      for orbital floor fracture, 126
      for superior oblique muscle paralysis, 120
Supernumerary puncta, 204
Supplemental Therapeutic Oxygen for Prethreshold ROP (STOP-ROP) study, 281
Suppression, 50–52, 51*f*
   testing in, 51, 53–59, 87
Suppression scotoma, diplopia after strabismus surgery and, 155
Supraduction. *See* Elevation of eye
Supranuclear (cortical) pathways, 37
Surgical (consecutive) esodeviation, 97–98
   management of, 103
Sursumduction/sursumversion. *See* Elevation of eye
Sutures (surgical)
   adjustable, for strabismus surgery, 148–149
   allergic reaction to, 156, 157*f*
   pull-over (stay), for strabismus surgery, 149
Sweep VEP, 171
SWS. *See* Sturge-Weber syndrome
Symblepharon, in Stevens-Johnson syndrome, 201
Symmetric surgery, 150, 150*t*
Syndactyly
   in Apert syndrome, 388, 389*f*
   in Fraser syndrome, 175
   in Saethre-Chotzen syndrome, 388, 390*f*
Syndrome (genetic), definition of, 171
Synechiae, posterior, 231
Synergist muscles, 34
Synkinesis, in Marcus Gunn jaw-winking syndrome, 180
Synkinetic near reflex. *See* Near reflex
Syphilis
   congenital/intrauterine, 185–186, 221
   interstitial keratitis caused by, 185, 186, 221

Tachyzoites, in toxoplasmosis transmission, 181
Tangent screen, in strabismus/amblyopia evaluation, 83
Tarsal kink, congenital, 176–177
Tarsorrhaphy, for craniosynostosis-induced corneal exposure, 389
Tay-Sachs disease (GM_2 gangliosidosis type I), 303, 398, 401*t*
TCOF1 gene, in Treacher Collins syndrome, 394
Tear film (tears), evaluation of, in ptosis, 179
Tearing/epiphora
   congenital, 203, 206
   in craniosynostosis, 391–392
   in nasolacrimal duct obstruction, 206, 208
   in primary congenital glaucoma, 203, 234, 235*t*
   in punctal disorders, 203
Tears (artificial), for Stevens-Johnson syndrome, 201

Telangiectasias
    in ataxia-telangiectasia (Louis-Bar syndrome),
        378–379, 379*f*
    conjunctival, 378, 379*f*
Telecanthus, 174, 386
    in blepharophimosis syndrome, 178, 179*f*
Teller acuity cards, 62, 63*f*, 73, 170
Tenacious proximal fusion, in intermittent exotropia,
    100–101
Tenectomy, 148*t*
Tenon capsule, 19, 20, 20*f*, 21*f*
    extraocular muscle surgery and, 25
        advancement of, 157
        excessive advancement and, 157
        scarring of (adherence syndrome), 158
Tenotomy, 148*t*
    superior oblique
        for Brown syndrome, 131–132
        for third nerve (oculomotor) paralysis, 133
Tensilon test, for myasthenia gravis diagnosis, 138, 138*f*,
    139*t*
Teratomas, orbital, 344–345, 345*f*
Tertiary positions of gaze, 28
Tetracyclines, for ophthalmia neonatorum prophylaxis,
    188
The Arc of the United States, 418*t*
Thermal injury (burns), 407
Third nerve (oculomotor) paralysis, 132–134, 133*f*
    inferior oblique muscle paralysis caused by, 121
    superior oblique muscle paralysis caused by, 118
    surgery for, 153
3-step test, 83–86, 85*f*
    in inferior oblique muscle paralysis, 121
    in superior oblique muscle paralysis, 118, 119
Threshold disease, in retinopathy of prematurity, 283,
    284*f*
    treatment criteria and, 285–286, 286*f*
Thyroid-associated ophthalmopathy/orbitopathy. *See*
    Thyroid eye disease
Thyroid eye disease, 135–136, 136*f*, 139*t*
    proptosis and, 135, 136, 136*f*, 346, 347*f*
TIGR/myocilin (TIGR/MYOC) gene, in glaucoma, 233
Tillaux, spiral of, 16, 18*f*
Tilted disc syndrome (Fuchs coloboma), 307, 307*f*
Timolol, for glaucoma, 242
Timoptic. *See* Timolol
TINU. *See* Tubulointerstitial nephritis uveitis
TNO test, 87
Tolmetin, for uveitis, 277
Tonic convergence, 36
Tonic pupil (Adie pupil), 229
Tono-Pen, for IOP measurement, 236
Tonometry (tonometer), 236
    in congenital/infantile glaucoma, 236
    Perkins, 236
Topamax. *See* Topiramate
Topical anesthesia
    for extraocular muscle surgery, 160
    for foreign-body removal, 5
Topical medications. *See* Eyedrops

Topiramate, glaucoma and, 239
TORCHES, 181
Torsion, 29
Torsional deviations, 11
Torsional fusional vergence, 82
Touton giant cells, in juvenile xanthogranuloma, 351
Toxocara (toxocariasis), 273–274
    canis, 273
    uveitis caused by, 273–274, 273*f*
Toxoplasma (toxoplasmosis), 181–183, 182*f*
    congenital, 182, 182*f*
    gondii, 181
Toys, for pediatric examination, 3, 4*f*
Trabeculectomy, 241
    uveitic glaucoma and, 278
Trabeculotomy, for glaucoma, 240–241
Trachoma, 190
Trachoma-inclusion conjunctivitis (TRIC) agent, 187
Tranexamic acid, for hyphema, 410
Transillumination, iris, 231
    in albinism, 231, 298, 301*f*
Transplantation, corneal, 219
Transposition procedures, extraocular muscle, 149, 153
Transscleral laser cycloablation, for glaucoma, 241
Trauma, 403–411
    abuse and, 404–407, 405*f*, 406*f*
    blunt injury and, 409–411, 410*f*, 411*f*
    cataract caused by, 251*f*
    chemical injuries and, 407
    hyphema and, 409–411, 410*f*
    management of, 403
    orbital fractures and, 124–126, 125*f*, 411, 411*f*
    penetrating injury and, 408–409, 408*f*
    shaking injury and, 404–407, 405*f*, 406*f*
    superficial injury and, 407–408
Traumatic hyphema, 409–411, 410*f*
    sickle cell disease and, 409
Traumatic retinoschisis, in shaking injury, 405–406, 406*f*
Travatan/Travatan Z. *See* Travoprost
Travoprost, for glaucoma, 242–243
Treacher Collins syndrome (mandibulofacial
    dysostosis), 393–394, 394*f*
    palpebral fissure slanting in, 178, 393–394, 394*f*
Treponema pallidum, 185
TRIC (trachoma-inclusion conjunctivitis) agent, 187
Trichotillomania, 177
Trochlea, 14–15, 16*f*
    in Brown syndrome, 130
Trochlear nerve palsy. *See* Fourth nerve (trochlear)
    palsy
-tropia (suffix), 10
Tropias, 10. *See also* Heterotropias/tropias
    induced, testing visual acuity and, 72–73
    intermittent, 10
        esotropia, 89
        exotropia, 99–103
Tropicamide, for cycloplegia/cycloplegic refraction, 88,
    88*t*
True divergence excess exotropia, 101
Trusopt. *See* Dorzolamide

TS. *See* Tuberous sclerosis
TSC1/TSC2 genes, in tuberous sclerosis, 371
Tuberous sclerosis (Bourneville disease), 364*t*, 371–374, 372*f*, 373*f*
Tubulointerstitial nephritis uveitis (TINU), 271–272
Tucking procedure, 120, 152
Tumor necrosis factor inhibitors, for uveitis, 278
Tumors, 331–361, 332–333*t*
   classification of, 332–333*t*
   eyelid/epibulbar, 333*t*, 347–351
   intraocular, 351–361
   orbital, 331–347, 332–333*t*
Turbinate, infracture of, for congenital nasolacrimal duct obstruction, 208–209
Turribrachycephaly, 387*f*, 389*f*
Turricephaly, 383
TWIST gene, 387
   in Saethre-Chotzen syndrome, 388
TYR gene mutations, in albinism, 298, 299*t*
Tyrosinase activity, in albinism, 298, 299*t*, 300
Tyrosinase gene mutations, in albinism, 298, 299*t*
TYRP1 gene, in OCA3 (albinism), 299*t*, 301

UC. *See* Uncentral fixation/acuity
Ultrasonography/ultrasound
   in orbital evaluation, hemangioma diagnosis and, 340
   in retinoblastoma, 356
UM. *See* Unmaintained fixation/acuity
Uncentral fixation/acuity, 72
Uncrossed diplopia, 54, 54*t*
Unharmonious anomalous retinal correspondence, 55
United Cerebral Palsy Association, 418*t*
Unmaintained fixation/acuity, 72
Unsteady fixation/acuity, 72
Upgaze. *See* Elevation of eye
US. *See* Unsteady fixation/acuity
Uvea (uveal tract)
   melanoma of, uveitis differentiated from, 276*t*
   in neurofibromatosis, melanocytic tumors and, 365–366, 366*f*
Uveitis, 267–278
   anterior, 267, 267–272, 270*f*, 271*t*
   cataracts and, surgery in patients with, 278
   classification of, 267, 268*t*
   in cytomegalic inclusion disease, 184
   diagnosis/differential diagnosis of, 268*t*, 275, 277*t*
   familial juvenile systemic granulomatosis (Blau syndrome) and, 274–275
   intermediate/pars planitis, 267, 268*t*, 272, 273*f*
   in juvenile idiopathic (chronic/rheumatoid) arthritis, 268–271, 270*f*, 271*t*
   in Kawasaki disease, 202
   laboratory tests for, 275, 277*t*
   masquerade syndromes and, 275, 276*t*
   panuveitis, 267, 268*t*, 274–275, 274*f*
   posterior, 267, 272–274, 273*f*
      differential diagnosis of, 268*t*
   in psoriatic arthritis, 270–271
   sarcoidosis and, 274, 274*f*
   in toxocariasis, 273–274, 273*f*
   treatment of, 275–278
   tubulointerstitial nephritis and, 271–272
   Vogt-Koyanagi-Harada (VKH) syndrome and, 275

V1 to V6 areas of brain. *See* Visual (calcarine/occipital) cortex
V-pattern deviations, 107–112, 108*f*
   in Brown syndrome, 122*t*, 131
   in craniosynostosis, 391, 391*f*
   definition of, 107
   esotropia, 107–112, 108*f*
      treatment of, 112
   exotropia, 107–112, 108*f*
      treatment of, 112
   pulley system pathology and, 23, 109–110, 110*f*
   in superior oblique muscle paralysis, 119
   surgical treatment of, 110–111, 111*f*, 112
Varicella-zoster virus/varicella (chickenpox), conjunctivitis in, 192–193, 193*f*
Varices, orbital, 342
Vascular endothelial growth factor (VEGF), retinopathy of prematurity and, 281
Vascular malformations, orbital, 341–342, 341*f*
Vascular system, of extraocular muscles, 16–18
   surgery and, 25
Vascular tumors, of orbit, 332*t*, 338–342, 339*f*, 341*f*
Vasoconstrictors, for allergic conjunctivitis, 198, 199*t*
Vectograph slide test, 87
VEGF. *See* Vascular endothelial growth factor
Veins, extraocular muscles supplied by, 18
Velocardiofacial syndrome, posterior embryotoxon in, 212
Velocity, saccadic system evaluation and, 83
Venous malformations (varices), orbital, 342
Venous system, of extraocular muscles, 18
   surgery and, 25
VEP/VER. *See* Visually evoked cortical potentials (visual evoked response)
Vergences/vergence system (eye movements), 34, 35–37
   assessment of, 86–87
   fusional, 41, 41*t*, 82–83
      assessment of, 82
   in infants, 413
   supranuclear control and, 37
Vernal keratoconjunctivitis, 198–200, 199*f*
Versions, 34, 35, 36*f*
   assessment of, 81
Vertical deviations, 10, 11, 113–126
   botulinum toxin causing, 164
   comitant, 113
      surgery for, 152
   dissociated, 116–118, 117*f*
      surgery for, 117, 153
   incomitant (noncomitant), 113
      strabismus surgery planning and, 146
   inferior oblique muscle overaction and, 113, 113–115, 114*f*
   orbital floor (blowout) fractures and, 124–126, 125*f*
   superior oblique muscle overaction and, 113, 115–116, 115*f*

Vertical fusional vergence, 41*t*, 82
Vertical incomitance, 113
    strabismus surgery planning and, 146
Vertical rectus muscles, 14, 14*f*. *See also* Inferior rectus
    muscles; Superior rectus muscles
    A-pattern deviations associated with dysfunction of,
        109
    action of, 14, 28–29, 29*t*
        gaze position and, 31, 31*f*, 32*f*
    anatomy of, 14, 14*f*
    surgery of
        for A- and V-pattern deviations, 111
        for dissociated vertical deviation, 117, 153
        eyelid position changes after, 159, 159*f*
        for hypo- and hypertropia, 152–153
        for nystagmus, 329
        for superior oblique muscle paralysis, 120
    V-pattern deviations associated with dysfunction of,
        109
Vertical retraction syndrome, 140
Vertical vergence, 36
Vestibular nystagmus, central instability (periodic
    alternating nystagmus), 322
VHL. *See* von Hippel–Lindau disease
Vieth-Müller circle, 39, 40*f*
Vincristine, for hemangiomas, 340
Virchow's law, 383, 385*f*
Viruses
    conjunctivitis caused by
        in children, 190–193
        in neonates, 188
    optic neuritis caused by, 311–312
Visceral larva migrans, 273
Vision
    binocular. *See* Binocular vision
    development of, 44–46, 45*f*, 413
        abnormal visual experience affecting, 46–49, 47*f*, 48*f*
        delayed, 416
    neurophysiology of, 42–49, 43*f*, 45*f*, 47*f*, 48*f*
    physiology of, 39–42, 40*f*, 41*t*
Vision loss (see-saw) nystagmus, 325
Vision rehabilitation, 416–417
    for nystagmus, 330
Visual acuity
    in albinism, 298
    in amblyopia, 62, 65, 71–74, 72*t*
    after cataract surgery, 260
    in congenital glaucoma, 233, 243
    development of, 170–171
    fusional vergences and, 82
    in Leber congenital amaurosis, 289
    in optic nerve hypoplasia, 308
    in Stargardt disease, 293
    in strabismic amblyopia, 62
    after strabismus surgery, 155
    strabismus surgery planning and, 145–146
    testing, 71–74, 72*t*
        in amblyopia, 65, 71–74, 72*t*
        in nystagmus, 73, 318–319
        in strabismus, 71–74, 72*t*

Visual axis, 12, 14*f*, 39
    accommodative convergence and, 37
    muscle action/gaze position and, 30
Visual confusion, 49, 50*f*
Visual (calcarine/occipital) cortex, 42
    development of, 44, 45*f*
        abnormal visual experience affecting, 46–49, 47*f*, 48*f*
Visual field defects, in optic nerve hypoplasia, 308
Visual field testing, Goldmann perimetry, 83
Visual loss/impairment. *See also* Low vision
    in albinism, 298
    amblyopia causing, 61–69
    in cataract, 252
    craniosynostosis and, 390
    in glaucoma, 233, 243
    in hereditary retinal disease, 289
    in leukemia, 297
    in nystagmus, 318–319
    in retinopathy of prematurity, 286–287, 287*f*
Visual pathways. *See also* Retinogeniculocortical
        pathway
    development of, 45–46
Visually evoked cortical potentials (visual evoked
        response), 72*t*, 171, 413
Visuscope, for strabismic amblyopia testing, 63
Vitamin B$_6$ (pyridoxine), for homocystinuria, 399
Vitamin B$_{12}$, for homocystinuria, 399
Vitelliform macular dystrophy, juvenile-onset. *See* Best
        disease
Vitelliform macular dystrophy gene *(VMD2)*, 294
Vitrectomy
    with capsulectomy, for cataract
        lensectomy with intraocular lens implantation and,
            258
        lensectomy without intraocular lens implantation
            and, 256, 257*f*
    for retinal detachment, in retinopathy of prematurity,
        287
Vitrectorhexis, 255
Vitreoretinal dystrophies, Goldmann-Favre, 296
Vitreoretinal traction, in retinopathy of prematurity, 281
Vitreoretinopathies
    familial exudative, 296
    hereditary, 294–296
Vitreous
    disorders of, 279–304. *See also specific type*
    primary, persistent hyperplasia of. *See* Persistent fetal
        vasculature
Vitreous hemorrhage, shaking injury and, 405, 407
Vitreous seeds, in retinoblastoma, 354, 355*f*
Vitritis, in cytomegalovirus retinitis, 184
VKC. *See* Vernal keratoconjunctivitis
VLM. *See* Visceral larva migrans
VMD2 (vitelliform macular dystrophy) gene, 294
Vogt-Koyanagi-Harada (VKH) syndrome, 275
Vogt triad, in tuberous sclerosis, 371
Volkmann type cataract, 247*t*
Voluntary convergence, 37
von Hippel–Lindau disease, 364*t*, 374–375, 375*f*
    retinoblastoma differentiated from, 358

von Recklinghausen disease. *See* Neurofibromatosis
Vortex veins, 18
    extraocular muscle surgery and, 25

Waardenburg syndrome, dystopia canthorum in, 175,
    175*f*
WAGR syndrome, 224
Weakening procedures (extraocular muscle), 147, 148*t*,
    151–152
    inferior oblique muscle, 151–152
        for superior oblique muscle paralysis, 120
        for V-pattern deviations, 110, 112
        for vertical deviations, 114–115
    superior oblique muscle, 152
        for A-pattern deviations, 110, 111, 112
        for vertical deviation, 116
Weill-Marchesani syndrome, 264
White-eyed blowout fracture, 125
White pupil. *See* Leukocoria
"White spot" (hypopigmented macule/ash-leaf spot), in
    tuberous sclerosis, 372, 372*f*
Wildervanck syndrome, Duane syndrome and, 127
Wilms tumor, aniridia and, 224
Wilms tumor *(WT1)* gene, aniridia and, 224
Wilson disease (hepatolenticular degeneration),
    220–221, 398
    cataracts associated with, 247*t*
Wofflin nodules, 227
Wolfram (DIDMOAD) syndrome, 297
Worth 4-dot test, 55, 55*f*, 87
    in binocular sensory cooperation evaluation, 87
    in sensory adaptation testing, 55, 55*f*
WT1 (Wilms tumor) gene, aniridia and, 224

Wyburn-Mason syndrome (racemose angioma), 342,
    364*t*, 381, 381*f*

x-axis of Fick, 27, 27*f*
X-linked disorders
    Aicardi syndrome, 292, 292*f*
    albinism (Nettleship-Falls), 298, 300*t*, 301
    Alport syndrome, 302
    blue-cone monochromacy, 291
    congenital stationary night blindness, 291
    familial exudative vitreoretinopathy, 296
    incontinentia pigmenti (Bloch-Sulzberger syndrome),
        379
    Lowe syndrome, 302
    Norrie disease, 296
    retinoschisis, 294–295, 295*f*
        electroretinogram patterns in, 295
X-pattern exotropia, 23
Xalatan. *See* Latanoprost
Xanthogranuloma, juvenile, 226, 351, 352*f*
    glaucoma associated with, 351
    of iris, 226, 351, 352*f*
    uveitis differentiated from, 276*t*

y-axis of Fick, 27, 27*f*
Yoke muscles, 35
    cardinal positions of gaze and, 28*f*, 35, 80
    Hering's law of motor correspondence and, 35

z-axis of Fick, 27, 27*f*
Zellweger syndrome, 398
Zonular (lamellar) cataracts, 247*f*, 247*t*, 248, 248*f*, 250*t*
    pulverulent, 247*t*